From Molecules to Materials, Devices and Processes: The Chemical Basis of Novel Technologies

From Molecules to Materials, Devices and Processes: The Chemical Basis of Novel Technologies

Guest Editors

Giuseppina Raffaini
Fabio Ganazzoli

MDPI

Basel • Beijing • Wuhan • Barcelona • Belgrade • Novi Sad • Cluj • Manchester

Guest Editors

Giuseppina Raffaini
Department of Chemistry,
Materials, and Chemical
Engineering "Giulio Natta"
Politecnico di Milano
Milano
Italy

Fabio Ganazzoli
Department of Chemistry,
Materials, and Chemical
Engineering "Giulio Natta"
Politecnico di Milano
Milano
Italy

Editorial Office
MDPI AG
Grosspeteranlage 5
4052 Basel, Switzerland

This is a reprint of the Special Issue, published open access by the journal *Molecules* (ISSN 1420-3049), freely accessible at: www.mdpi.com/journal/molecules/special_issues/O8G0TVX1RU.

For citation purposes, cite each article independently as indicated on the article page online and using the guide below:

Lastname, A.A.; Lastname, B.B. Article Title. *Journal Name* **Year**, *Volume Number*, Page Range.

ISBN 978-3-7258-3250-7 (Hbk)
ISBN 978-3-7258-3249-1 (PDF)
https://doi.org/10.3390/books978-3-7258-3249-1

Contents

About the Editors . . . . **vii**

Giuseppina Raffaini and Fabio Ganazzoli
From Molecules to Materials, Devices and Processes: The Chemical Basis of Novel Technologies
Reprinted from: *Molecules* **2025**, *30*, 357, https://doi.org/10.3390/molecules30020357 . . . . . . **1**

Simone Naddeo, Davide Gentile, Fatima Margani, Gea Prioglio, Federica Magaletti and Maurizio Galimberti et al.
Pyrrole Compounds from the Two-Step One-Pot Conversion of 2,5-Dimethylfuran for Elastomer Composites with Low Dissipation of Energy
Reprinted from: *Molecules* **2024**, *29*, 861, https://doi.org/10.3390/molecules29040861 . . . . . . **7**

Francesco Moriggi, Vincenzina Barbera, Maurizio Galimberti and Giuseppina Raffaini
Adsorption Affinities of Small Volatile Organic Molecules on Graphene Surfaces for Novel Nanofiller Design: A DFT Study
Reprinted from: *Molecules* **2023**, *28*, 7633, https://doi.org/10.3390/molecules28227633 . . . . . . **26**

Chiara Ruini, Erika Ferrari, Caterina Durante, Giulia Lanciotti, Paolo Neri and Anna Maria Ferrari et al.
Integrated Approach of Life Cycle Assessment and Experimental Design in the Study of a Model Organic Reaction: New Perspectives in Renewable Vanillin-Derived Chemicals
Reprinted from: *Molecules* **2024**, *29*, 2132, https://doi.org/10.3390/molecules29092132 . . . . . . **43**

Arianna Rossetti, Alessandro Sacchetti, Fiorella Meneghetti, Greta Colombo Dugoni, Matteo Mori and Carlo Castellano
Synthesis and Characterization of New Triazole-Bispidinone Scaffolds and Their Metal Complexes for Catalytic Applications
Reprinted from: *Molecules* **2023**, *28*, 6351, https://doi.org/10.3390/molecules28176351 . . . . . . **59**

Nicola Melis, Danilo Loche, Swapneel V. Thakkar, Maria Giorgia Cutrufello, Maria Franca Sini and Gianmarco Sedda et al.
Magnetic Aerogels for Room-Temperature Catalytic Production of Bis(indolyl)methane Derivatives
Reprinted from: *Molecules* **2024**, *29*, 2223, https://doi.org/10.3390/molecules29102223 . . . . . . **80**

Elisa I. García-López, Narimene Aoun and Giuseppe Marcì
An Overview of the Sustainable Depolymerization/Degradation of Polypropylene Microplastics by Advanced Oxidation Technologies
Reprinted from: *Molecules* **2024**, *29*, 2816, https://doi.org/10.3390/molecules29122816 . . . . . . **95**

Pierfrancesco Atanasio, Rubia Y. S. Zampiva, Luca Buccini, Corrado Di Conzo, Anacleto Proietti and Francesco Mura et al.
Graphene Quantum Dots from Agricultural Wastes: Green Synthesis and Advanced Applications for Energy Storage
Reprinted from: *Molecules* **2024**, *29*, 5666, https://doi.org/10.3390/molecules29235666 . . . . . . **115**

Yongsheng Zhou, Siyun Zhou, Cuiwen Lu, Yihao Zhang and Haiyan Zhao
Enrichment of Trypsin Inhibitor from Soybean Whey Wastewater Using Different Precipitating Agents and Analysis of Their Properties
Reprinted from: *Molecules* **2024**, *29*, 2613, https://doi.org/10.3390/molecules29112613 . . . . . . **134**

Saad Javaid, Alessandra Zanoletti, Angela Serpe, Elza Bontempi, Ivano Alessandri and Irene Vassalini
Glassy Powder Derived from Waste Printed Circuit Boards for Methylene Blue Adsorption
Reprinted from: *Molecules* **2024**, *29*, 400, https://doi.org/10.3390/molecules29020400 . . . . . . **149**

Anela Kovačević, José Alejandro Ricardo García, Marilena Tolazzi, Andrea Melchior and Martina Sanadar
Selective Co(II) and Ni(II) Separation Using the Trihexyl(tetradecyl)phosphonium Decanoate Ionic Liquid
Reprinted from: *Molecules* **2024**, *29*, 4545, https://doi.org/10.3390/molecules29194545 . . . . . . **161**

Biagia Musio, Rosa Ragone, Stefano Todisco, Antonino Rizzuti, Egidio Iorio and Mattea Chirico et al.
Non-Targeted Nuclear Magnetic Resonance Analysis for Food Authenticity: A Comparative Study on Tomato Samples
Reprinted from: *Molecules* **2024**, *29*, 4441, https://doi.org/10.3390/molecules29184441 . . . . . . **180**

Francesca Baldassarre, Daniele Schiavi, Veronica Di Lorenzo, Francesca Biondo, Viviana Vergaro and Gianpiero Colangelo et al.
Cellulose Nanocrystal-Based Emulsion of Thyme Essential Oil: Preparation and Characterisation as Sustainable Crop Protection Tool
Reprinted from: *Molecules* **2023**, *28*, 7884, https://doi.org/10.3390/molecules28237884 . . . . . . **193**

Muhamad Tahriri Rozaini, Denys I. Grekov, Mohamad Azmi Bustam and Pascaline Pré
Low-Hydrophilic HKUST–1/Polymer Extrudates for the PSA Separation of CO_2/CH_4
Reprinted from: *Molecules* **2024**, *29*, 2069, https://doi.org/10.3390/molecules29092069 . . . . . . **216**

Selene Varliero, Samira Jamali Alamooti, Francesco Pietro Campo, Giovanni Cappello, Stefano Cappello and Stefano Caserini et al.
Assessing the Limit of CO_2 Storage in Seawater as Bicarbonate-Enriched Solutions
Reprinted from: *Molecules* **2024**, *29*, 4069, https://doi.org/10.3390/molecules29174069 . . . . . . **238**

Vincenzo Villani
Viscosity Flow Curves of Agar and the *Bounded Ripening Growth* Model of the Gelation Onset
Reprinted from: *Molecules* **2024**, *29*, 1293, https://doi.org/10.3390/molecules29061293 . . . . . . **257**

About the Editors

Giuseppina Raffaini

Giuseppina Raffaini is an Associate Professor at the Politecnico di Milano in the Department of Chemistry, Materials, and Chemical Engineering "Giulio Natta". After classical studies, Giuseppina Raffaini obtained her Ms Sc. in Chemistry at the Università degli Studi di Milano under the supervision of Prof. Mario Raimondi, then a post-graduate diploma at the "Advanced School in Polymer Science Giulio Natta" at the Politecnico di Milano under the supervision of Prof. Fabio Ganazzoli and an inter-university master's in Biomaterials under the supervision of Prof. Matteo Santin. In 2005, she obtained her PhD cum laude in Materials Engineering at the Politecnico di Milano. In 2008, she became an Assistant Professor and in 2014, an Associate Professor at the Politecnico di Milano. In October 2018, she obtained the Abilitazione Scientifica Nazionale as a Full Professor (03/CHEM-06). After her initial studies in quantum chemistry and in coarse-grained models for branched polymers and dendrimers, her expertise expanded to molecular mechanics and molecular dynamics simulations at the atomistic level of molecules, biological macromolecules, and polymeric, ceramic, and metallic materials. Her main research interests include protein and drug adsorption on biomaterial surfaces and 3D nanocrystals, organic inhibitors to prevent corrosion in reinforced concrete, cyclodextrins, their inclusion complexes,and nanoaggregates in drug delivery systems for cancer therapy, and the adsorption of chiral molecules and oligopeptides on DNA for gene delivery purposes. She is the co-author of about 80 original peer-reviewed ISI papers. She is a member of ACS, AICIng, DCT-SCI, SIB (Italian Association for Biomaterials), and CD-TEC (Italian Association of Chemistry and Technology for Cyclodextrins) and is a full member of Sigma Xi (The Scientific Research Honor Society).

Fabio Ganazzoli

Fabio Ganazzoli obtained his degree in Chemistry (5 years) at the Università di Milano and then his post-graduate diploma at the School in Polymer Science "G. Natta" at the Politecnico di Milano. In 1983, he became a research assistant; in 1992, an associate professor; and since 2003, he has been a full professor of Chemistry at the Politecnico di Milano. His research interests are 1) computer simulations of protein adsorption on biomaterials and of surface phenomena; 2) computer simulations of biological and synthetic macromolecules, biomaterials, and supramolecular complexes; and 3) equilibrium and dynamical properties of polymers and dendrimers studied with statistical mechanical methods. He has published about 150 scientific papers, with an h index of 33 and more than 3100 citations (Scopus, January 2025). He is a member of the Editorial Board of *Molecules* (since 2019) and he was Guest Editor with Giuseppina Raffaini of the Special Issue "Topology Effects on Polymer Properties" of *Polymers* (2019-2020). He has been on the Executive Board of the Italian Association of Chemistry for Engineering, AICIng (2019–2023), and he is on the Executive Board of the Division of Chemistry for the Technologies of the Italian Chemical Society (since 2020).

molecules

MDPI

Editorial

From Molecules to Materials, Devices and Processes: The Chemical Basis of Novel Technologies

Giuseppina Raffaini [1,2,*] and Fabio Ganazzoli [1,2,*]

1 Department of Chemistry, Materials and Chemical Engineering "G. Natta", Politecnico di Milano, Via Luigi Mancinelli 7, 20131 Milan, Italy
2 INSTM, National Consortium of Materials Science and Technology, Local Unit Politecnico di Milano, 20131 Milano, Italy
* Correspondence: giuseppina.raffaini@polimi.it (G.R.); fabio.ganazzoli@polimi.it (F.G.)

1. Introduction

This Special Issue was launched in connection with the joint XIII National Congress of AICIng (the Italian Association of Chemistry for Engineering) and the II National Congress of the Division of Chemistry for the Technologies of the Italian Chemical Society, held at the Politecnico di Milano (Italy) from 25 to 28 June 2023. The aim of the Congress was to present and discuss recent advances in fundamental and applied chemistry in the fields of new or improved technologies, comprising compounds, materials or processes.

2. Scope of the Special Issue

On the Special Issue's web page (https://www.mdpi.com/journal/molecules/special_issues/O8G0TVX1RU last accessed on 16 January 2025), we pointed out that chemistry provides a molecular-level tool, allowing for significant advances in current and novel technologies in a wide range of fields. In this Special Issue, we collected selected relevant examples of the chemical foundations of the technologies that produced the new, scientific, and technologically innovative results obtained in Italy and elsewhere, in which various methodologies and approaches were used to design new products, materials, or processes in a wide range of fields.

It must be noted that there is a common thread to the papers collected in the present Special Issue, which is the sustainability of the products, materials and processes, as seen from a chemical viewpoint, and their novel technological applications. Sustainability is considered here in different ways, ranging from green chemistry (in a strict sense) to the circular economy (especially the waste-to-product processes), as well as the performance of the modified materials, including composites such as tires in the automotive sector or the eco-sustainable synthesis of nanomaterials for energy. Other sustainability issues encountered in agriculture include the food traceability of crops, including the detection of possible fraud or industrial processing and the preparation of biocompatible and biodegradable natural pesticides to allow for sustainable crop production with a minimal or negligible environmental impact. In addition, new materials with improved performances, processes, or materials related to renewable energy or to energy storage are presented, and the increasingly important topic of environmental remediation is discussed.

3. Overview of the Papers in the Special Issue

Green chemistry [1–3] is a major consideration in the design of products, materials, or processes that aim to minimize or eliminate unwanted or possibly hazardous byproducts,

Received: 31 December 2024
Accepted: 14 January 2025
Published: 17 January 2025

Citation: Raffaini, G.; Ganazzoli, F. From Molecules to Materials, Devices and Processes: The Chemical Basis of Novel Technologies. *Molecules* **2025**, *30*, 357. https://doi.org/10.3390/molecules30020357

improving their atom economy as much as possible. In this way, both the environmental impact and the use of non-renewable resources are minimized or completely avoided [4]. A fitting example of this approach is provided by Naddeo et al. (Contribution 1), who carried out a one-pot synthesis of 2,5-hexanedione (HD) via a ring-opening reaction of 2,5-dimethylfuran (DF), obtaining a very high yield. The HD was then used for the synthesis of pyrrole derivatives with various amines, again obtaining a very high yield, with water as the only byproduct. This process had a very high carbon efficiency and a very small E-factor, shown as the ratio of the waste mass to the product mass, which is a remarkable result. It should be added that, in the same paper, one of the pyrrole derivatives was used to functionalize the carbon black used as a filler in an elastomeric composite; this functionalized carbon black showed enhanced mechanical properties, which could improve the sustainability of tires in the automotive sectors [5,6], and, as such, is presently undergoing industrial-scale development. A somewhat related paper (Contribution 2) carried out a theoretical study of the adsorption of linear and cyclic molecules, both saturated and unsaturated, on a pristine graphene surface using DFT methods after a first study based on the molecular mechanics and molecular dynamics of the adsorption process [7]. The adsorption energies and the charge difference density were used to understand the intermolecular interactions at play. The adsorption energy was found to be dependent on the number of π electrons, with the most favorable results being provided by pyrrole-oxidized derivatives, providing a quantitative measure of the stability of the surface modifications offered by the physisorption of small molecules. This procedure allows for the production of novel fillers that could improve the mechanical properties of polymer composites [8] such as those used in tires.

Quantitative assessments of the environmental impact of a model organic synthesis, such as that carried out by Ruini et al. (Contribution 3), are strongly related to the green chemistry philosophy. This study achieved process optimization through a multivariate experimental design, aiming to maximize the yield of the desired product and, at the same time, to minimize the environmental impact, as quantified using the life cycle assessment (LCA) methodology [9,10]. The selected reaction was a nucleophilic substitution of a phenolic compound, namely vanillin, which was obtained from a renewable source, lignin. The approach presented in this paper, using a combination of an experimental design and a life cycle assessment, appears to be a step forward in measuring and improving the sustainability of organic synthesis processes.

Another type of organic synthesis was investigated in Contribution 4, in which different bispidine derivatives were prepared. Bispidine is a bicyclic diamine that may act as a ligand towards metal cations, particularly when additional nitrogen atoms are introduced via derivatization, with potential applications in many fields. In this paper, triazole derivatives of bispidine were prepared using the click reaction, which provided a high yield, particularly when performed under microwave irradiation. Note that this procedure appears to be in line with the principles of atomic efficiency, which is a common issue in green chemistry. Furthermore, the zinc(II) and copper(II) complexes of some of the obtained bispidine were also shown to be efficient catalysts for the Henry reaction, which is an established C-C bond-formation reaction. Once again, excellent yields were obtained under microwave irradiation, which appears to be a useful tool in many reactions to enhance the product yield.

A different methodology was employed to study the organic synthesis of bis(indolyl) methanes (Contribution 5), which are natural bis-heterocyclic compounds that are important organic intermediates in the pharmaceutical and chemical industries. The unique approach adopted in this paper is the proposed use of magnetic aerogels as catalysts, exploiting their high and open porosity and tunability and their ability to stabilize active metal-based nanocrystals. The investigated catalysts were highly porous $NiFe_2O_4/SiO_2$ aerogel nanocomposites containing ferrite nanocrystals with a size of about 10 nm. These aerogels were acidic catalysts that provided an excellent yield of bis(indolyl)methane when starting from stoichiometric amounts of indole and 4-nitro-benzaldehyde.

A different aspect of the sustainability of products or processes is the circular economy [11], which focuses on the means of recycling or reusing existing materials and products as much as possible, thus positively affecting environmental use and waste management. Several papers in this Special Issue provide examples of the circular economy. One review paper (Contribution 6) provided an overview of the current state of the art in the field of depolymerization or the degradation of polypropylene. For this polymer, the relevant technologies focus on advanced oxidation. In fact, the thermal recycling of this thermoplastic polymer was carried out for only a fraction of the discarded material, with the best choice being the back-transformation of polypropylene in the starting monomer, which can be purified and then repolymerized. However, these technologies are also of great importance in the removal of microplastics from water and wastewater [12–14], where they are found as pollutants originating from domestic and personal care products, with a direct environmental impact.

Among the other papers that deal with the circular economy, the study carried out by Atanasio et al. (Contribution 7) investigated the one-pot synthesis of graphene quantum dots from carbon aerogels obtained from rice husk, an abundant form of agricultural waste. Interestingly, the cellulose derived from the rice husk after gelification and carbonization was shown to produce quantum dots without the use of any solvent via ball-milling, obtaining the goals of the green chemistry approach. In turn, the quantum dots were then used as electrode materials for supercapacitors and Li-ion batteries, showing their usefulness as nanomaterials in advanced systems of energy storage [15–17].

Another paper (Contribution 8) studied a different waste of agricultural origin, namely soybean whey wastewater, in order to enrich soybean trypsin inhibitors. This procedure may have the twofold effect of reducing the environmental pollution of soybean whey and of recovering trypsin inhibitors, which have important physiological functions in the health food and pharmaceutical fields.

Concerning different types of waste, another paper (Contribution 9) considered the possibility of recycling a fast-growing type of e-waste (i.e., electronic waste) consisting of waste printed circuit boards. The glassy substrate of the non-metal fraction of the electronic boards was treated with acidic leaching with the help of microwave heating and was shown to be an excellent adsorbent against methylene blue, matching the performance of activated carbon. In view of the ever-increasing production of e-waste, this work offers the interesting possibility of recycling the printed boards after removing the metals, such as copper, for instance, and noble metals such as gold. Another contribution (Contribution 10) addressed the issue of the separation of Co(II) from Ni(II) in extractive metallurgy, as well as from spent Li-ion batteries, where these metals are present in the cathode; hence, this paper may also be relevant to the circular economy. The proposed method explores the use of a room-temperature ionic liquid via liquid–liquid extraction in a strongly acidic medium and through the polymer inclusion membranes formed of PVC and the same ionic liquid. The latter procedure was found to be the best one, since it used a lower amount of ionic liquid and allowed for the efficient separation of the metal cations in a single stage [18].

Other approaches investigated the issue of food control and the traceability of foodstuffs, particularly tomato samples (Contribution 11). In this case, using NMR spectra obtained in different laboratories via spectroscopic fingerprint data, one could assess the geographical origin of the tomatoes, as well as possible fraud, production, and industrial processing with high reliability using a metabolomic analysis conducted via a statistical multivariate data analysis. Another paper (Contribution 12) dealt with the issue of sustainability in agriculture through the preparation of pesticides based on essential oils stabilized in an appropriate oil-in-water emulsion. The essential oils were obtained through supercritical CO_2 extraction (in keeping with the requirements of green chemistry) and were encapsulated in stabilizing cellulose nanocrystals crosslinked with calcium chloride into an optimized ratio. These sustainable eco-friendly systems were active biopesticides in both in vitro and in vivo tests on olive seedlings, with the additional advantage of the use of a biocompatible and biodegradable nanocellulose stabilizer.

Finally, we should mention one approach to sustainability from a somewhat different perspective, namely the topic of renewable energy and environmental remediation. The separation of CO_2 from the biogas obtained from the anaerobic digestion of various organic wastes is important to obtain biomethane, which is useful in gas grids. One paper in this Special Issue (Contribution 13) tackled this problem by using a commercial metal–organic framework (MOF) extruded with a polymer in order to increase its stability, finding that hydrophobic polymers such as polyurethane were the best choice in view of the water sensitivity of the MOF. As a result, the CO_2 separation was also more complete than that obtained with the isolated MOF. In a different context, the removal and sequestration of CO_2 from the atmosphere due to industrial exhausts were investigated in another paper (Contribution 14). Here, the disposal of CO_2 in a geological formation was not considered; instead, the contribution focused on the possibility of storing it in seawater in the form of bicarbonate ions, avoiding the formation of calcium carbonate, which would release one half of the previously disposed CO_2. The limits of CO_2 storage in seawater at its natural pH and salinity (using the Mediterranean Sea as an example) were thus investigated both in the laboratory and in a pilot plant.

Finally, a more fundamental study (Contribution 15) addressed the problem of sol–gel transition, particularly the onset of gelation in polymer solutions, comparing a new theoretical model with the onset of gelation in agar probed via viscosimetric experiments. This is a technologically relevant problem in the preparation of hydrogels, for instance, which are important in the food sector and in the cosmetic and pharmaceutical industries, among others, as well as in the preparation of 3D scaffolds such as those used in tissue engineering [19].

4. Conclusions

In conclusion, we believe that the papers collected in this Special Issue provide an interesting overview of the current chemical approaches to novel technologies in terms of compounds, materials, and processes that are being carried out in Italy and elsewhere. The common thread is sustainability, which is considered from different viewpoints across a wide spectrum of problems and methodologies.

Acknowledgments: Giuseppina Raffaini and Fabio Ganazzoli gratefully acknowledge all the authors' contributions. We gratefully thank the Editorial Staff for their help in the management of the Special Issue, and all those involved in its preparation.

Conflicts of Interest: The authors declare no conflicts of interest.

List of Contributions

1. Naddeo, S.; Gentile, D.; Margani, F.; Prioglio, G.; Magaletti, F.; Galimberti, M.; Barbera, V. Pyrrole compounds from the two-step one-pot conversion of 2,5-dimethylfuran for elastomer composites with low dissipation of energy. *Molecules* **2024**, *29*, 861. https://doi.org/10.3390/molecules29040861.

2. Moriggi, F.; Barbera, V.; Galimberti, M.; Raffaini, G. Adsorption affinities of small volatile organic molecules on graphene surfaces for novel nanofiller design: a DFT study. *Molecules* **2023**, *28*, 7633. https://doi.org/10.3390/molecules28227633.
3. Ruini, C.; Ferrari, E.; Durante, C.; Lanciotti, G.; Neri, P.; Ferrari, A.M.; Rosa, R. Integrated approach of life cycle assessment and experimental design in the study of a model organic reaction: new perspectives in renewable vanillin-derived chemicals. *Molecules* **2024**, *29*, 2132. https://doi.org/10.3390/molecules29092132.
4. Rossetti, A.; Sacchetti, A.; Meneghetti, F.; Colombo Dugoni, G.; Mori, M.; Castellano, C. Synthesis and characterization of new triazole-bispidinone scaffolds and their metal complexes for catalytic applications. *Molecules* **2023**, *28*, 6351. https://doi.org/10.3390/molecules28176351.
5. Melis, N.; Loche, D.; Thakkar, S.V.; Cutrufello, M.G.; Sini, M.F.; Sedda, G.; Pilia, L.; Frongia, A.; Casula, M.F. Magnetic aerogels for room-temperature catalytic production of bis(indolyl)methane derivatives. *Molecules* **2024**, *29*, 2223. https://doi.org/10.3390/molecules29102223.
6. García-López, E.I.; Aoun, N.; Marcì, G. An overview of the sustainable depolymerization/degradation of polypropylene microplastics by advanced oxidation technologies. *Molecules* **2024**, *29*, 2816. https://doi.org/10.3390/molecules29122816.
7. Atanasio, P.; Zampiva, R.Y.S.; Buccini, L.; Di Conzo, C.; Proietti, A.; Mura, F.; Aurora, A.; Marrani, A.G.; Passeri, D.; Rossi, M.; Pasquali, M.; Scaramuzzo, F.A. Graphene quantum dots from agricultural wastes: Green synthesis and advanced ap-plications for energy storage. *Molecules* **2024**, *29*, 5666. https://doi.org/10.3390/molecules29235666.
8. Zhou, Y.; Zhou, S.; Lu, C.; Zhang, Y.; Zhao, H. Enrichment of Trypsin Inhibitor from Soybean whey wastewater using dif-ferent precipitating agents and analysis of their properties. *Molecules* **2024**, *29*, 2613. https://doi.org/10.3390/molecules29112613.
9. Javaid, S.; Zanoletti, A.; Serpe, A.; Bontempi, E.; Alessandri, I.; Vassalini, I. Glassy powder derived from waste printed circuit boards for methylene blue adsorption. *Molecules* **2024**, *29*, 400. https://doi.org/10.3390/molecules29020400.
10. Kovačević, A.; Ricardo García, J.A.; Tolazzi, M.; Melchior, A.; Sanadar, M. Selective Co(II) and Ni(II) separation using the trihexyl(tetradecyl)phosphonium decanoate ionic liquid. *Molecules* **2024**, *29*, 4545. https://doi.org/10.3390/molecules29194545.
11. Musio, B.; Ragone, R.; Todisco, S.; Rizzuti, A.; Iorio, E.; Chirico, M.; Pisanu, M.E.; Meloni, N.; Mastrorilli, P.; Gallo, V. Non-targeted nuclear magnetic resonance analysis for food authenticity: a comparative study on tomato samples. *Molecules* **2024**, *29*, 4441. https://doi.org/10.3390/molecules29184441.
12. Baldassarre, F.; Schiavi, D.; Di Lorenzo, V.; Biondo, F.; Vergaro, V.; Colangelo, G.; Balestra, G.M.; Ciccarella, G. Cellulose nanocrystal-based emulsion of thyme essential oil: preparation and characterisation as sustainable crop protection tool. *Molecules* **2023**, *28*, 7884. https://doi.org/10.3390/molecules28237884.
13. Rozaini, M.T.; Grekov, D.I.; Bustam, M.A.; Pré, P. Low-Hydrophilic HKUST−1/Polymer Extrudates for the PSA Separation of CO_2/CH_4. *Molecules* **2024**, *29*, 2069. https://doi.org/10.3390/molecules29092069.
14. Varliero, S.; Jamali Alamooti, S.; Campo, F.P.; Cappello, G.; Cappello, S.; Caserini, S.; Comazzi, F.; Macchi, P.; Raos, G. As-sessing the limit of CO_2 storage in seawater as bicarbonate-enriched solutions. *Molecules* **2024**, *29*, 4069. https://doi.org/10.3390/molecules29174069.
15. Villani, V. Viscosity flow curves of agar and the bounded ripening growth model of the gelation onset. *Molecules* **2024**, *29*, 1293. https://doi.org/10.3390/molecules29061293.

References

1. Sheldon, R.A.; Brady, D. Green Chemistry, Biocatalysis, and the Chemical Industry of the Future. *ChemSusChem* **2022**, *15*, e202102628. [CrossRef] [PubMed]
2. Tobiszewski, M.; Marc, M.; Galuszka, A.; Namiesnik, J. Green Chemistry Metrics with Special Reference to Green Analytical Chemistry. *Molecules* **2015**, *20*, 10928–10946. [CrossRef]
3. Sheldon, R.A.; Arends, I.W.C.E.; Hanefeld, U. *Green Chemistry and Catalysis*; Wiley-VCH: Hoboken, NJ, USA, 2007. [CrossRef]

4. Lozano, F.J.; Lozano, R.; Freire, P.; Jiménez-Gonzalez, C.; Sakao, T.; Ortiz, M.G.; Trianni, A.; Carpenter, A.; Viveros, T. New perspectives for green and sustainable chemistry and engineering: Approaches from sustainable resource and energy use, management, and transformation. *J. Clean. Prod.* **2018**, *172*, 227–232. [CrossRef]
5. Deng, S.; Chen, R.; Duan, S.; Jia, Q.; Hao, X.; Zhang, L. Research progress on sustainability of key tire materials. *SusMat* **2023**, *3*, 581–608. [CrossRef]
6. Hassan, M.R.; Rodrigue, D. Application of Waste Tire in Construction: A Road towards Sustainability and Circular Economy. *Sustainability* **2024**, *16*, 3852. [CrossRef]
7. Raffaini, G.; Ganazzoli, F. Classical atomistic simulations of protein adsorption on carbon nanomaterials. *Curr. Opin. Colloid Interface Sci.* **2019**, *41*, 11–26. [CrossRef]
8. Shah, A.U.H.A.; Ullah, S.; Bilal, S.; Rahman, G.; Seema, H. Reduced Graphene Oxide/Poly(Pyrrole-co-Thiophene) Hybrid Composite Materials: Synthesis, Characterization, and Supercapacitive Properties. *Polymers* **2020**, *12*, 1110. [CrossRef] [PubMed]
9. Kirchai, R.E., Jr.; Gregory, J.R.; Olivetti, E.A. Environmental life-cycle assessment. *Nat. Mater.* **2017**, *16*, 693–697. [CrossRef] [PubMed]
10. Kralisch, D.; Ott, D.; Gericke, D. Rules and benefits of Life Cycle Assessment in green chemical process and synthesis design: A tutorial review. *Green Chem.* **2015**, *17*, 123–145. [CrossRef]
11. Stahel, W. The circular economy. *Nature* **2016**, *531*, 435. [CrossRef] [PubMed]
12. Jani, V.; Wu, S.; Venkiteshwaran, K. Advancements and Regulatory Situation in Microplastics Removal from Wastewater and Drinking Water: A Comprehensive Review. *Microplastics* **2024**, *3*, 98–123. [CrossRef]
13. Adegoke, K.A.; Adu, F.A.; Oyebamiji, A.K.; Bamisaye, A.; Adigun, R.A.; Olasoji, S.O.; Ogunjinmi, O.E. Microplastics toxicity, detection, and removal from water/wastewater. *Mar. Pollut. Bull.* **2023**, *187*, 114546. [CrossRef] [PubMed]
14. Cheng, Y.L.; Kim, J.-G.; Kim, H.-B.; Choi, J.H.; Tsang, Y.F.; Baek, K. Occurrence and removal of microplastics in wastewater treatment plants and drinking water purification facilities: A review. *J. Chem. Eng.* **2021**, *410*, 128381. [CrossRef]
15. Liu, W.; Li, M.; Jiang, G.; Li, G.; Zhu, J.; Xiao, M.; Zhu, Y.; Gao, R.; Yu, A.; Feng, M.; et al. Graphene Quantum Dots-Based Advanced Electrode Materials: Design, Synthesis and Their Applications in Electrochemical Energy Storage and Electrocatalysis. *Adv. Energy Mater.* **2020**, *10*, 2001275. [CrossRef]
16. Hoang, V.C.; Dave, K.; Gomes, V.G. Carbon quantum dot-based composites for energy storage and electrocatalysis: Mechanism, applications and future prospects. *Nano Energy* **2019**, *66*, 104093. [CrossRef]
17. Suganya, G.; Arivanandhan, M.; Kalpana, G. Giant energy storage capacity of graphene quantum dots prepared by facile method. *Diam. Relat. Mater.* **2024**, *151*, 111798. [CrossRef]
18. Tan, S.; Zhang, D.; Chen, Y.; Helfrecht, B.A.; Baxter, E.T.; Cao, W.J.; Wang, X.B.; Nguyen, M.-T.; Johnson, G.E.; Prabhakaran, V. Complexation of heavy metal cations with imidazolium ionic liquids lowers their reduction energy: Implications for electrochemical separations. *Green Chem.* **2024**, *26*, 1566–1576. [CrossRef]
19. Yu, H.; Jiang, X.; Ji, W.; Song, W.; Cao, Y.; Yan, F.; Luo, C.; Yuan, B. The new low viscosity and high-temperature resistant composite hydrogel. *Chem. Pap.* **2023**, *77*, 3561–3570. [CrossRef]

molecules

MDPI

Article

Pyrrole Compounds from the Two-Step One-Pot Conversion of 2,5-Dimethylfuran for Elastomer Composites with Low Dissipation of Energy

Simone Naddeo, Davide Gentile, Fatima Margani, Gea Prioglio, Federica Magaletti, Maurizio Galimberti * and Vincenzina Barbera *

Department of Chemistry, Materials and Chemical Engineering "G. Natta", Politecnico di Milano, Via Mancinelli 7, 20131 Milano, Italy; simone.naddeo@polimi.it (S.N.); davide.gentile@polimi.it (D.G.); fatima.margani@polimi.it (F.M.); gea.prioglio@polimi.it (G.P.); federica.magaletti@polimi.it (F.M.)
* Correspondence: maurizio.galimberti@polimi.it (M.G.); vincenzina.barbera@polimi.it (V.B.)

Abstract: A one-pot, two-step process was developed for the preparation of pyrrole compounds from 2,5-dimethylfuran. The first step was the acid-catalyzed ring-opening reaction of 2,5-dimethylfuran (DF), leading to the formation of 2,5-hexanedione (HD). A stoichiometric amount of water and a sub-stoichiometric amount of sulfuric acid were used by heating at 50 °C for 24 h. Chemically pure HD was isolated, with a quantitative yield (up to 95%), as revealed by ^{1}H-NMR, ^{13}C-NMR, and GC-MS analyses. In the second step, HD was used as the starting material for the synthesis of pyrrole compounds via the Paal–Knorr reaction. Various primary amines were used in stoichiometric amounts. ^{1}H-NMR, ^{13}C-NMR, ESI-Mass, and GC-Mass analyses confirmed that pyrrole compounds were prepared with very good/excellent yields (80–95%), with water as the only co-product. A further purification step was not necessary. The process was characterized by a very high carbon efficiency, up to 80%, and an E-factor down to 0.128, whereas the typical E-factor for fine chemicals is between 5 and 50. Water, a co-product of the second step, can trigger the first step and therefore make the whole process circular. Thus, this synthetic pathway appears to be in line with the requirements of a sustainable chemical process. A pyrrole compound bearing an SH group (SHP) was used for the functionalization of a furnace carbon black (CB). The functionalized CB (CB/SHP) was utilized in place of silica, resulting in a 15% mass reduction of reinforcing filler, in an elastomeric composite based on poly(styrene-co-butadiene) from solution anionic polymerization and poly(1,4-cis-isoprene) from *Hevea Brasiliensis*. Compared to the silica-based composite, a reduction in the Payne effect of about 25% and an increase in the dynamic rigidity (E′ at 70 °C) of about 25% were obtained with CB/SHP.

Keywords: green chemistry; circular; almost null E-factor; 2,5-dimethylfuran; pyrrole compounds

Citation: Naddeo, S.; Gentile, D.; Margani, F.; Prioglio, G.; Magaletti, F.; Galimberti, M.; Barbera, V. Pyrrole Compounds from the Two-Step One-Pot Conversion of 2,5-Dimethylfuran for Elastomer Composites with Low Dissipation of Energy. *Molecules* **2024**, *29*, 861. https://doi.org/10.3390/molecules29040861

Academic Editor: Mathias O. Senge

Received: 16 January 2024
Revised: 5 February 2024
Accepted: 6 February 2024
Published: 15 February 2024

1. Introduction

Responsible consumption and production and climate action are among the sustainable development goals of the United Nations [1]. To achieve these goals, the replacement of fossil resources with renewable biomass for the production of chemicals has emerged as a major research topic [2–7]. Lignocellulosic biomass has an estimated annual production of 180 billion metric tons [4]; hence, it is an almost endless reservoir.

Among the chemicals derived from lignocellulosic sources, a strategic role is played by furanic compounds [8–19]. In particular, furfural and 5-hydroxymethylfurfural are versatile chemical platforms [16,19] and give rise to a great variety of downstream substances, such as 2,5-dimethylfuran (DF). DF is indeed prepared through the hydrogenolysis of 5-hydroxymethylfurfural [20], apart from direct synthesis from fructose by means of tandem dehydration/hydrogenolysis [21–23].

DF has been prevailingly investigated for conversion to p-xylene [24,25]. Few other reactions have been reported, including conversion to hydrodeoxygenated products [26], to chiral oxyndoles [27], and to 2,5-hexanedione (HD), which is an intermediate for a wide range of synthetic processes and is largely used in the chemical industry with great commercial value.

The use of bio-sources in place of oil to produce HD is of growing interest. HD has been prepared through the Pd/C-catalyzed hydrogenation of 5-hydroxymethylfurfural (HMF) in water and under CO_2 atmosphere at high pressure (30–40 bar) and high temperature (150 °C) [28]. Analogously, the hydrogenation of 5-hydroxymethylfurfural (HMF) in ethanol at 140 °C by using an iridium complex as a catalyst led to 1-hydroxyhexan-2,5-dione [29]. Scientific papers were published on the acid-catalyzed ring opening of DF for the synthesis of HD. The reactions were performed in pure D_2O at 250 °C for 30 min [30] in the presence of a cationic resin and an excess of H_2O (H_2O:DF = 3:1) at room temperature for 72 h [31]; in the presence of 10% sulfuric acid in H_2O and glacial acetic acid at 85 °C [32]; and in the presence of 10% by mole of a strong acid in H_2O and 1/1 mixtures of H_2O and an organic solvent at T = 60–80 °C [33]. Moreover, the ring-opening reaction of DF is achieved by using sulfuric acid and ruthenium catalysts in 2-propanol at 80–90 °C [34]. The use of the acid is thus mandatory for the ring-opening reaction of DF. However, it was reported that prolonged contact of HD with the acidic media led to the formation of oligomeric products [35]. Hence, the methods reported in the literature for the preparation of HD from DF present some drawbacks, such as the use of organic solvents and/or an excess of water; high temperatures; and, in particular, in view of scaling up on an industrial scale, the formation of by-products.

The synthesis of a pyrrole compound (PyC) via the Paal–Knorr reaction of primary amine and 1,4-dicarbonyl compounds was performed in neat conditions by using different synthetic approaches, such as microwaves [36] or mechanochemistry in the presence of organic acids [37]. Pyrrole derivatives were also obtained by using flow chemistry methods [38], from microscale to production scale. With the aim of scaling up the process, some of the authors developed the neat Paal–Knorr reaction by simply mixing and heating primary amines and HD in the absence of solvent(s) and catalysts, achieving high atom efficiency [39–41]. The PyCs were used for the neat functionalization of sp^2 carbon allotropes [41,42] and inorganic oxy-hydroxides such as silica [43].

The research on PyCs was focused on two families of compounds, *Janus* molecules [44,45] bearing either hydroxy- or sulfur-based functional groups. Both families of PyCs had a twofold reactivity, based on the pyrrole ring and on the substituent of the nitrogen atom. The pyrrole ring promoted the functionalization of the sp^2 carbon allotropes through a domino reaction (shown in Figure S1 in the Supplementary Materials) with the carbocatalytic oxidation of PyC in the benzylic position, followed by the cycloaddition reaction of PyC with the graphitic substrate [45]. This functionalization reaction was characterized by the absence of co- and by-products, by yields ranging from 60% to 90% in the case of graphene layers [39,40], and, thus, by high carbon efficiency. The most studied PyC, with hydroxy functional groups in the substituent of the nitrogen atom, was 2-(2,5-dimethyl-1*H*-pyrrol-1-yl)-1,3-propanediol (serinol pyrrole, SP), whose chemical structure is reported below in the text [39,41]. The hydroxy groups promote the condensation reaction of SP with silica with excellent/quantitative yield without the need for solvents or catalysts [42]. The most investigated PyCs with sulfur-based functional groups were 2-(2,5-dimethyl-1*H*-pyrrol-1-yl)ethane-1-thiol (SHP) and 1,2-bis(2-(2,5-dimethyl-1*H*-pyrrol-1-yl)ethyl)disulfide (SSP). Their chemical structure is reported below in the text. The -SH and -SS- functional groups were reported to react with the unsaturated elastomers [46]. The functionalization of silica and of sp^2 carbon allotropes, mainly carbon black, with the two mentioned families of PyCs improved the properties of elastomeric composites for a large-scale application such as that in tire compounds [46,47]. The development on an industrial scale was announced by a major player in the tire field [48].

The objectives of the research here reported were to develop a sustainable synthesis of PyCs, with a view of large-scale production, and to demonstrate that a pyrrole compound obtained from such a synthesis makes a significant contribution to the sustainability of a large-scale product such as a tire. Therefore, one of the objectives of the research was to carry out a one-pot synthesis in which HD was synthesized from DF. The obtained HD was then used as the starting material in reactions with different primary amines, achieving excellent/quantitative yield and no waste, thus aiming at very high carbon efficiency and very low E-factor [49–51]. In particular, experimental conditions for the ring-opening reaction of DF had to be suitable to allow the efficient reaction of HD with the primary amine, avoiding the formation of by-products. It is worth noting that the synthesis of a PyC leads to water as the co-product. The use of an excess of water for the preparation of HD from DF, as documented in the above-mentioned literature, would be detrimental to this equilibrium reaction. Moreover, an excess of acid could lead to the formation of oligomeric products, based not only on HD but also on the pyrrole compound, as reported in the literature [35].

In this work, the synthesis of pyrrole compounds was performed in two steps: (i) ring-opening reaction of DF to HD, and (ii) ring closure of HD to form the pyrrole rings, through the reaction with a primary amine. Several primary amines were investigated.

Water is the nucleophile that allows the ring opening of the furan ring and it is also the co-product of the Paal–Knorr reaction. These characteristics make the process circular. The scheme in Figure 1 shows that the cyclic process promoted by water leads to the formation of PyC having 100% carbon economy. In the synthesis here reported, solvents were not used, in line with the basic rules of green chemistry [49–51]. Hence, a quantitative yield is the only necessary condition to have high carbon efficiency and low E-factor [51].

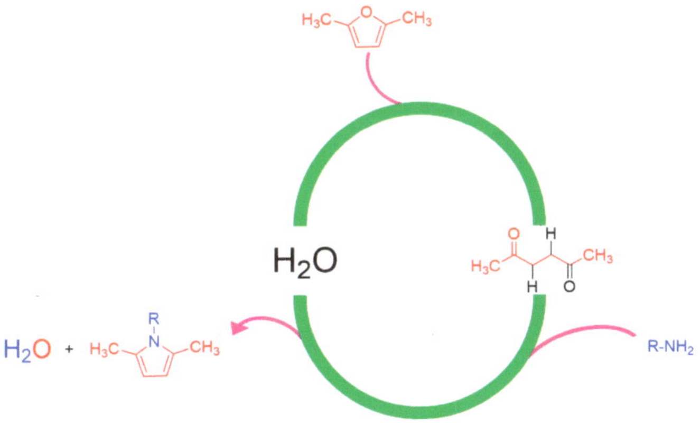

Figure 1. The water cycle for the synthesis of pyrrole compounds in a two-step, one-pot process. The valorization of all the atoms involved is also underlined.

A further objective of this work was to use a pyrrole compound prepared through the one-pot two-step process in an elastomeric composite characterized by low dissipation of energy and also suitable for large-scale tire application. As mentioned above, SP was used as a coupling agent for silica in composites suitable for tire compounds [42]. It is well-known that silica is the filler of choice [52–55] for the preparation of low-dissipation-energy tires because silica elastomer composites are characterized by low hysteresis. However, silica-based composites have several technical drawbacks. Firstly, the silanols of the silica surface lead to high compound viscosity, short storage time, difficult processability, corrosion, abrasion of metal surfaces and need of special mixing equipment [56]. On the other hand, silica silanols are abl to establish a chemical bond with the elastomer chains, through the use of coupling agent. Generally, a sulphur-based silane such as bis(triethoxysilylpropyl)tetrasulfide (TESPT) is used for this aim. However, TESPT increases the adhesiveness of the composites to the metal parts of the equipment, which require special treatments. Moreover, the condensation reaction of TESPT with the silanols of silica releases ethanol. The combustion of ethanol produces CO_2. Serinol Pyrrole (SP) was used in place of TESPT. As a matter of fact, the use of SP would allow us to avoid the release of about 8.0×10^7 Kg of CO_2 on a worldwide basis [43]. Furthermore, it would be highly desirable to reproduce the properties of a silica-based elastomer composite, without using silica as the filler and without using a coupling agent for the filler.

Hence, the objective of the research here reported was to replace silica by using a functionalized furnace carbon black (CB in the following phrases) with a pyrrole compound. The pyrrole compound selected for the functionalization of CB was SHP, obtained from cysteamine as the primary amine. The procedure used for the functionalization of CBN234 was already reported [46]. The aim was to reproduce the dynamic mechanical properties of the silica-based composite. The elastomers were a solution-polymerized poly(styrene-co-butadiene) (S-SBR) and poly(1,4-cis-isoprene) from *Hevea brasiliensis* (natural rubber, NR), typically used in a tire tread. The hypothesis behind the use of CB/SHP was to exploit the chemical reactivity of the thiol group with the unsaturations of the elastomer chains. The ultrafast thiol-ene reaction based on cysteine has been reported [57,58] and the reaction of thiol groups with internal double bonds has been documented [59]. In a recent paper [46], some of the authors showed the ability of SHP to react with squalene, used as a model compound of the unsaturated elastomer. The increase in the dynamic rigidity of the elastomer composite, by using CB/SHP in place of CB [46], was attributed to the chemical bond between CB and the elastomer chains. In this work, for the first time, CB/SHP was used in place of silica with the aim to prepare an elastomer composite for low dissipation of energy. The composites were prepared by means of melt blending in an internal mixer and were cured with a sulfur-based system. The cross-linking reaction was studied, and the dynamic mechanical properties in the shear and in the axial mode were determined.

2. Results and Discussion

2.1. Synthesis of Pyrrole Compounds

A one-pot two-step process was performed for the synthesis of pyrrole compounds starting from DF. The first step was the conversion of DF (**1**) into HD (**2**) and the second step was the ring closure to the pyrrole compound (**3**), via the Paal–Knorr reaction of HD with a primary amine.

As shown in Figures 1 and 2, the ring-opening reaction of DF to HD and the ring-closing reaction to pyrrole are both water-dependent processes.

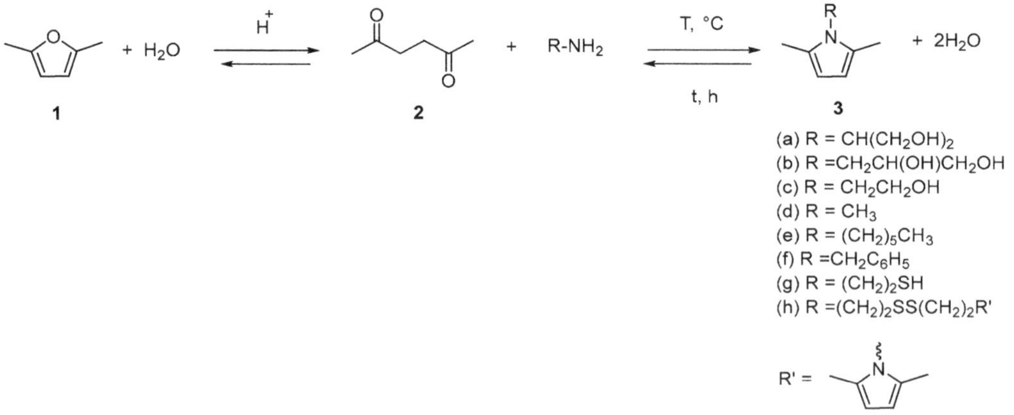

Figure 2. The one-pot, two-step synthetic process that yields variously substituted pyrroles (**3a–h**) with almost null E-factor.

Step 1. Ring-opening reaction of DF to HD.

The ring-opening reaction of DF to HD is a reaction without co-products, hence with 100% atom economy. It is an acid-catalyzed equilibrium reaction that requires at least a stoichiometric amount of water to ensure the formation of HD. As the conversion of DF to HD is a neat reaction, two considerations can be made. (i) The reaction is triggered by water and acid, with the proton transfer from the protonated water to the furan ring. It takes place at room temperature, with the heterocycle insoluble in water. (ii) As the furan is converted to HD, water is consumed. Therefore, there is no water in the reaction mixture, at the end of the first step. Investigation of (a) the amount of water and (b) the amount and the type of acid was carried out to assess their effect on the yield of the reaction. Data are given in Table 1 and details are in the experimental section.

Table 1. Step 1 of the process. Synthesis of HD from DF and H_2O in the presence of an acid.

Entry	Ingredient: Type and Amount				Yield (%)
	DF (mmol)	H_2O (mmol)	Acid Catalyst		
			Type	mol % [a]	
1	47	141	H_2SO_4 [b]	15	95
2	47	94	H_2SO_4 [b]	15	97
3	47	70	H_2SO_4 [b]	15	99
4	47	47	H_2SO_4 [b]	15	98
5	47	47	H_2SO_4 [b]	4	95
6	47	47	H_2SO_4 [b]	1.7	17
7	47	47	H_2SO_4 [b]	0.1	13
8	47	47	HCl [c]	4	97
9	47	47	HBr [d]	4	97
10	47	47	HNO_3 [e]	4	<5
11	47	47	CH_3COOH [f]	4	0

[a] with respect to DF; [b] 97% w; [c] 37% w; [d] 48% w; [e] 69.5% w; [f] glacial.

(a) Effect of the amount of water. Firstly, the effect of water was investigated by using 15 mol% of H_2SO_4 (pKa = −3) with respect to DF. This amount of acid was to be considered the limit value to avoid the formation of by-products, in particular of the HD oligomers, documented in the literature with 16 mol % of H_2SO_4 [35].

Entry 1 was carried out with an excess of water (H_2O/DF = 3/1). Entries 2–4 were carried out with a decreasing amount of water (about 30% less for each entry), reaching an equimolar amount of H_2O and DF in Entry 4, without observing a decrease in the yield to HD, which was quantitative. It was observed that a slightly lower yield was achieved with the largest amount of water. Without going too far into inferences not supported by experimental results, it could be said that an excess of water favors the reverse reaction, since water acts as a proton transfer agent that could hinder the direct reaction. The ^{1}H-NMR spectra of Entries 1, 2, 3, and 4 are shown in Figures S2–S7 respectively, in the Supplementary Material. Residual water was detected in the spectra of the reaction mixtures, when an amount of water larger than the stoichiometric one was used. The quantitative yield of HD obtained with a DF/H_2O molar ratio = 1 is a relevant result for the one-pot process, since water is the co-product of the Paal–Knorr reaction, and its presence should be avoided at the beginning of the reaction.

(b) Amount and type of acid. Moving from the experimental conditions of Entry 4, the amount of sulfuric acid was reduced from 4 to 1.7 and to 0.1 (mol% with respect to DF) (Table 1, Entries 5, 6, and 7, respectively). The yield was almost quantitative by also using 4% of H_2SO_4, whereas it dropped to low values when the amount of mineral acid was further

reduced, at 17% and 13%, respectively. ^{1}H-NMR spectra of the final reaction mixtures of Entries 6 and 7 are reported in Figures S8 and S9, respectively, in the Supplementary Material. To account for these results, the interaction between the H_3O^+ from the acids and the basic centers in DF and H_2O could be considered. In 2,5-dimethylfuran, one of the two sp^2 lone pair electrons is available for reacting with protons, while the other one is involved in the heterocyclic aromatic system. When mineral acid is added to the reaction mixture, it reacts with the lone pair of the oxygen atom in the water molecule, which is more basic. In the reaction mixtures of Entries 6 and 7, with the low amount of H_3O^+, water was preferentially protonated and the ring opening of DF occurred only to a very minor extent. Acids with different pK_a values, higher and lower than the pKa of H_2SO_4, were examined, keeping constant their amount equal to 4 mol% with respect to DF. The following acids were tested: HBr (pKa = −9), HCl (pKa = −8.08), HNO_3 (pKa = −1.3), and CH_3COOH (pKa = 4.88). Data are in Entries 8–11 in Table 1. Reactions performed with strong mineral acid, like hydrochloric and hydrobromic acid, allowed us to convert DF to HD with quantitative yield (Entries 8–9 of Table 1). Reaction performed in the presence of nitric acid (Entry 10 in Table 1) led to the formation of a number of by-products, whose chemical nature was not assessed. HD was not obtained with acetic acid (Entry 11 in Table 1). These findings suggest the usage of a strong mineral acid for the protonation of the DF ring, which leads, consequently, to the ring opening and then to the conversion to HD. Highly oxidizing acid should be avoided. All the ^{1}H-NMR spectra of Entries 8, 9, 10, and 11 are reported in Figures S10–S12, respectively, in the Supplementary Material.

Based on these experimental findings, HD for the reaction with a primary amine (Step 2 of the process) was prepared with the following experimental conditions: molar ratio DF/H_2O = 1/1 (47.0 mmol each), 4 mol% of H_2SO_4, 50 °C, 24 h. The kinetics of the ring-opening reaction, in these conditions, was studied by means of ^{1}H-NMR spectroscopies of the reaction mixture, analyzing samples at increasing times: 2, 3, 3.5, 5, 8, and 24 h. The NMR spectra are in Figure S2 in the Supplementary Material. Most of the reaction occurred after 8 h, as shown by the substantial decrease in the intensity of the methyl group in the NMR spectrum in Figure S2 and by the curves in the graph in Figure S3. Nonetheless, 24 h was adopted as the reaction time and co- or by-products were not observed.

Step 2. Paal–Knorr reaction of primary amines with HD derived from DF.

The reaction scheme for the synthesis of the pyrrole compounds is in Figure 2.

The following primary amines were used: 2-amino-1,3-propandiol (serinol), 1-amino-2,3-propandiol (isoserinol), ethanolamine, methylamine, hexanamine, benzylamine, cysteamine, and cystamine. HD and the acid catalyst were present in the reaction mixture at the end of the first step. The amine was then added to the mixture without any further purification. This approach mimics the settings of a traditional Paal–Knorr reaction, apart from the absence of solvent. The reactions are characterized by very good atom economy (from 75% to 90%), the only co-product being water, which is, however, the reagent of the first step of the process. The detailed procedures are reported in the experimental section. In brief, neat reactions were carried out in temperatures ranging from 25 °C to 155 °C for 2–2.5 h. Data are in Table 2. The yield of all the reactions performed with the primary amines was at least very good ($\geq$80%), and in some cases was excellent (>90%). The atom efficiency was from 61% (Entry 1) to 77% (Entry 5) and the carbon efficiency of the whole two-step process was from 74% (Entry 8) to 94% (Entry 4). Low values of E-factor were obtained, from 0.8 to 0.13. Complete characterization of pyrroles **3a–3h** is available in the Supplementary Material. ^{1}H-NMR spectra and GC-Mass chromatograms are from Figures S13–S37 (for the detailed list, see the Supplementary Material).

Table 2. Step 2 of the process: synthesis of pyrrole compounds from primary amines and HD from Step 1.

Entry	Primary Amine [a]	T (°C)	Time (h)	Pyrrole Compound Yield	Carbon Efficiency [b]	E-Factor [d]
1 [a]	Serinol	150	2.5	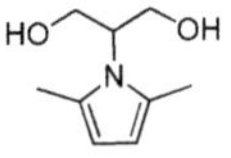 80%	80% [c]	0.097
2	Isoserinol	50	2	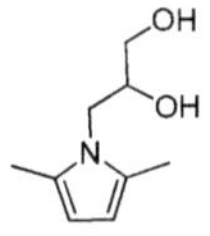 92%	92%	0.084
3	Ethanolamine	155	2	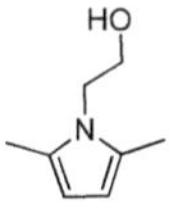 93%	93%	0.101
4	Methylamine	room temperature	2	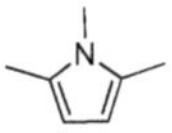 94% 94%	94%	0.128
5	Hexylamine	60	2	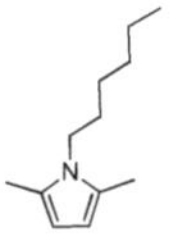 85%	85%	0.086
6	Benzylamine	100	2	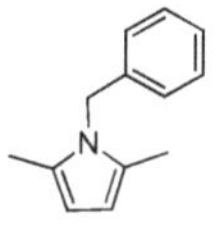 80%	80%	0.088
7	Cysteamine	Room temperature	4	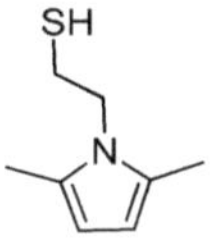 79%	79%	0.076
8	Cystamine	80	2	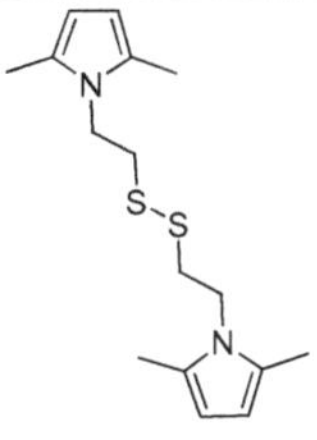 74%	74%	0.080

[a] 47 mmol of primary amine was added to the solution of 2,5-hexanedione obtained from DF. No purification was needed. [b] The carbon efficiency was calculated considering the whole process. [c] The 80% yield obtained with serinol was also probably due to the presence of water in the serinol sample used for the reaction. [d] The E-factor was calculated considered the total amount of waste produced in both steps.

Primary amines are also available as hydrochlorides. To check the possibility of using the hydrochlorides in the one-pot two-step process, the synthesis of SHP and SSP was also performed from cysteamine hydrochloride and cystamine dihydrochloride. Sodium acetate was added to release the free amino group of cysteamine and cystamine from the hydrochloride salt. Good yields were obtained, from 73% to 78%, according to the principles of Green Metrics [49–51]. The lower atom economy and reaction mass efficiency are due to the use of sodium acetate. Hence, the process based on the hydrochloride salts, though feasible, is not advisable to pursue sustainability. The synthesis and characterization of SHP and SSP from hydrochloride salts are reported in the Supplementary Materials.

In previous works by some of the authors, pyrrole compounds were prepared by using oil-derived HD. The yields were worse in the case of 1-hexyl-2,5-dimethyl-*1H*-pyrrole (73%) [40] and 1,2,5-Trimethylpyrrole (86.9%) [42] and better in the case of 2-(2,5-dimethyl-1*H*-pyrrol-1-yl)propane-1,3-diol (96%) [40] (the water in the serinol sample used in the present work affected the yield). Hence, the process here reported at least does not make the reaction yield worse.

2.2. *Elastomer Composites with CB/SHP as the Reinforcing Filler*

As reported in the introduction, the CB/SHP adduct was used in place of silica in an elastomer composite suitable for tire tread. Silica is the preferred filler in tire tread elastomer composites with low dissipation of energy, thanks to its reactivity with the elastomer chains, mediated by the sulfur-based silane. The objective of this study was to replace silica with a functionalized carbon black, CB/SHP, in an elastomer matrix based on S-SBR, whose vinyl groups were reported to react with CB/SHP. The preparation and characterization of the CB/SHP adduct used in this work has been recently reported [46]. Silica was used as the reinforcing filler in the reference composite. The composites based on either silica or CB/SHP contained the same volume amount of filler (silica and CB). The use of CB allowed us to save 15% by mass of the reinforcing filler. Reference composites were prepared as well with pristine CB and the same vulcanization system of the silica-based composite ("CB" composite) and with the same amount of sulfur atoms present in the CB/SHP composite ("CB + S" composite). The composites were prepared via melt blending in an internal mixer, by using the same traditional mixing procedure as reported in the experimental section.

Crosslinking

The crosslinking was performed with a sulfur-based system. Details are in the experimental section. The rheometric curves are in Figure 3 and data of M_L, M_H, $(M_H - M_L)$, t_{s1}, t_{90}, and curing rate are in Table S1, in the Supplementary Material.

The replacement of silica with CB led to a reduction in the composite viscosity, as indicated by the M_L values, to a lower extent with CB/SHP. The M_H and $(M_H - M_L)$ values, which can be correlated with both the crosslinking and the filler networks [46], were remarkably higher in the presence of silica and appear to depend on the amount of sulfur atoms for the composites containing CB; in fact, they are higher for the (CB/SHP) and (CB+ S) composites. The induction time of vulcanization (t_{s1}) was lower for the (silica) composite, whereas the optimum time (t_{90}) was lower for the CB-based composites, and the highest curing rate was for the composite with CB/SHP.

The lower viscosity of the CB-based composite was expected, in consideration of the lower surface activity of CB, and is in line with the objectives of this work. The higher M_L value obtained with CB/SHP suggests that CB/SHP could react with the vinyl groups of S-SBR during the processing. The higher M_H and $(M_H - M_L)$ values of the (silica) composite can be explained, at least in part, by the formation of the filler network. The higher curing efficiency of the CB-based composites is due to the replacement of silica with the carbonaceous filler and the higher curing rate observed with CB/SHP can be explained by the reactivity of the thiol group with the elastomer chains.

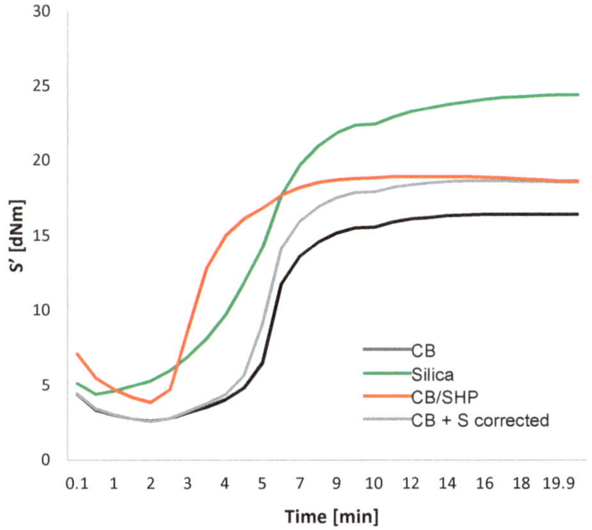

Figure 3. Curing curves of the elastomer composites. The recipes are reported in the experimental section.

2.3. Dynamic Mechanical Properties in the Shear Mode

Dynamic mechanical properties were determined, for the crosslinked samples, in the shear mode by means of strain sweep experiments, by using a strain amplitude in the range from 0.1% to 25% at a frequency of 1 Hz and a temperature of 50 °C. Details are in the experimental section. The storage G′ and the loss G″ moduli were measured. The graphs showing the dependence on the strain amplitude of G′ and of Tan delta (G″/G′ ratio) are in Figure 4a,b, respectively, and data of $G'\gamma_{min}$, $G'\gamma_{max}$, $\Delta G'$, $\Delta G'/G'\gamma_{min}$, G''_{max}, and Tan δ_{max} are in Table S2 in the Supplementary Material. G′ at minimum strain is an index of the presence of the filler network. The $\Delta G'$ and $\Delta G'/G'\gamma_{min}$ values were taken as the indexes of the non-linearity of the modulus, which is known as the Payne effect [60–63].

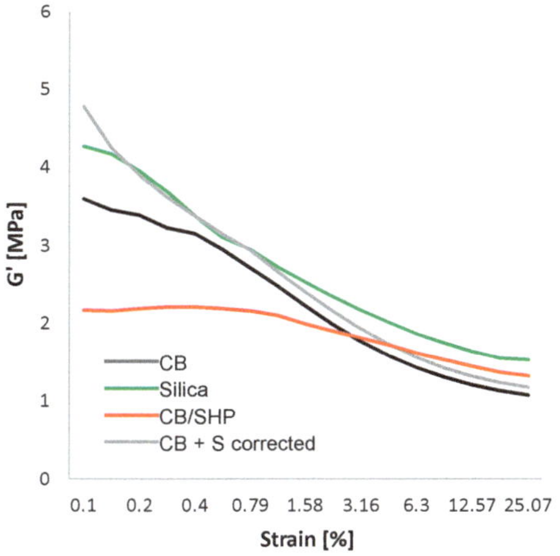

(a)

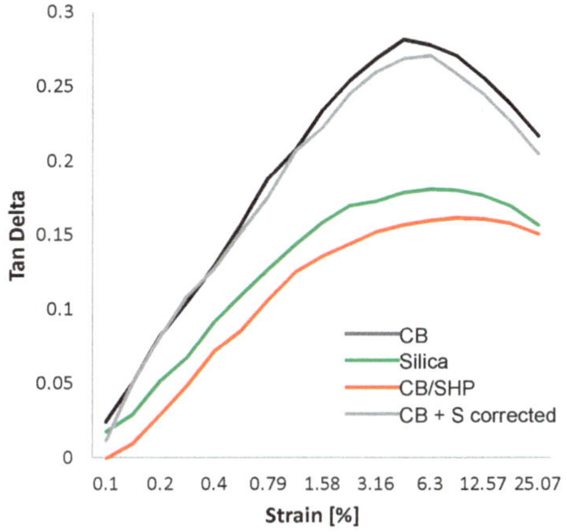

(b)

Figure 4. G′ vs. strain amplitude (**a**) and Tan Delta versus strain amplitude (**b**) for composites of Table 1.

With CB/SHP, remarkably lower values of $G'\gamma_{min}$, $\Delta G'/G'\gamma_{min}$, G''_{max}, and Tan δ_{max} were obtained. The reduction, compared to the (silica) composite and to the (CB + S) composite, is indeed appreciable. In particular, the reduction in $\Delta G'/G'\gamma_{min}$ was about 25% and 33%, respectively. It is worth observing in Figure 5a the crossover of the curves of the (CB) and (CB/SHP) composites; the curve due to the (CB/SHP) composite is well below the other curves at minimum strain and is above them at high strain. These findings indicate that the difference between the (silica) composite and the (CB/SHP) and (CB + S) composites is not due to the amount of sulfur in the composites. It can be thus commented that CB/SHP reacts with the elastomer chains, and this brings about the reduction in the filler network.

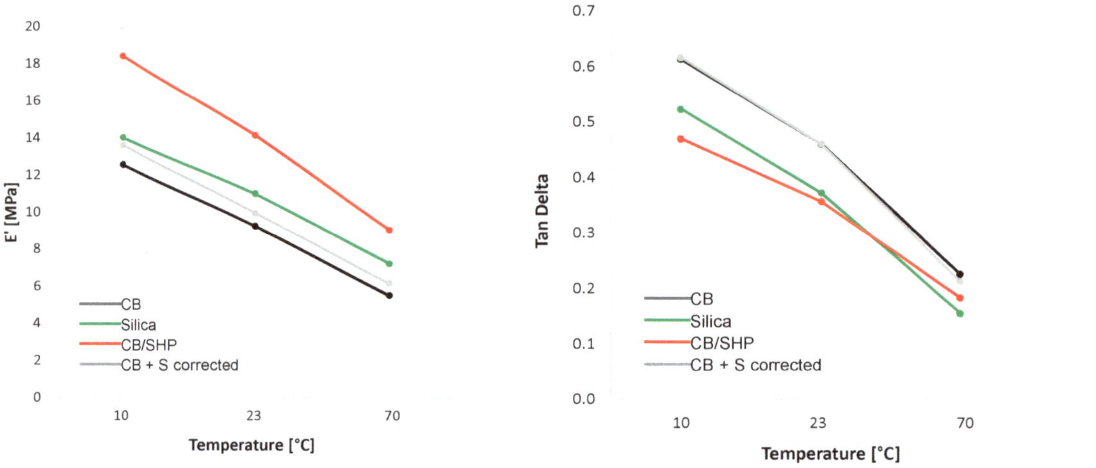

(**a**) (**b**)

Figure 5. (**a**) E′ vs. temperature curves and (**b**) Tan Delta vs. temperature curves for the composites whose ricepise is reported in Table 4 in the experimental Part.

2.4. Dynamic Mechanical Properties in the Axial Mode

Axial dynamic mechanical analyses in compression were carried out by first applying a pre-strain of 25%, then a dynamic sinusoidal strain of 3.5% at a frequency of 100 Hz. Storage modulus (E′) and loss modulus (E″) were measured at 10 °C, 23 °C, and 70 °C. Data are reported in Table 3 and the dependence of E′ and Tan Delta on the temperature is shown in Figure 5a,b, respectively.

CB/SHP led to higher dynamic rigidity with respect to all the other composites, at all the temperatures. E′ at 70 °C of the (CB/SHP) composite was higher than E′ of the (silica) and the (CB + S) composites of about 25% and 46%, respectively. It is worth observing that the ($E'_{70\,°C} - E'_{10\,°C}$) difference is similar for the (silica) and the (CB/SHP) composite. This is a very meaningful finding, as the reduction in the dynamic rigidity with temperature is a very important feature for a tire tread compound. The tan delta values of the CB/SHP composite are lower at 10 °C and 23 °C and similar at 70 °C, compared to the values of the (silica) composite. The values of E′ are lower and the values of Tan delta are higher for the (CB + S) composite. Hence, the content of sulfur in the CB-based composites is not the parameter which steers the dynamic mechanical properties of the composites. These results can be reasonably justified by the reaction of CB/SHP with the elastomer chains. It is indeed worth adding that a higher dynamic rigidity gives the opportunity to reduce the filler content, thus reducing the hysteresis of the composite. In a recent work [46], it was shown that CB-SHP is more efficient than CB-SSP in promoting the dynamic-mechanical reinforcement of the elastomer composite. For example, it was shown that the dynamic rigidity increased more than 20% and the hysteresis decreased by about 10%, at 70 °C, by using CB/SHP and CB/SSP in place of 33% and 66% of CB, respectively. It was hypothesized that only one of the two pyrrole rings of CB-SSP could react with the carbon substrate.

Table 3. E′, E″, and Tan delta values at 10 °C, 23 °C, and 70 °C for composites of Table 1.

		Composite Based on			
Property	**Temperature (°C)**	**Silica**	**CB/SHP**	**CB + S**	**CB**
E′ (MPa)	10	14.02	18.42	13.62	12.56
	23	11.00	14.15	9.95	9.27
	70	7.23	9.05	6.18	5.52
E″ (MPa)	10	7.34	8.67	8.41	7.72
	23	4.11	5.07	4.59	4.27
	70	1.13	1.67	1.32	1.25
Tan Delta	10	0.52	0.47	0.62	0.61
	23	0.37	0.36	0.46	0.46
	70	0.16	0.18	0.21	0.23
$\Delta E'$ ($E'_{70°C} - E'_{10°C}$) (MPa)		6.79	7.44	9.37	7.04

The recipes of the elastomer composites are reported in Table 4 in the experimental section.

The results obtained with CB/SHP demonstrate the key role of CB functionalization and are very important for improving the sustainability of elastomer composites. In fact, carbon black can rightly be considered not an example of sustainability, but new carbon fillers are appearing on the scene, such as char from tires [64] and biochar [65]. The low surface area and the lack of structure make these carbon materials unsuitable as tire compounds, and only the reactivity brought by functionalization can enable their use.

3. Experimental Section

3.1. Materials

3.1.1. For the Preparation of Pyrrole Compounds

Reagents and solvents, commercially available, were purchased and used without further purification.

Sulfuric acid 95–97% purity, acetic acid solution, hexylamine, methylamine solution (40% in weight), ethanolamine, benzylamine, cysteamine, and cystamine were purchased from Sigma Aldrich. Hydrochloric acid solution (37% w) and nitric acid solution (69.5% w) were purchased from Carlo Erba. Bromidic acid solution (48% w) was purchased from Fluka. 2-Amino-1,3-propanediol (serinol) and 1-amino-2,3-propandiol (isoserinol) were kindly provided by Bracco.

3.1.2. For the Preparation of CB/SHP Adduct

CBN234 with a carbon content not lower than 98 wt%, a surface area of 113 m^2/g, an average elemental particle size of 27 nm, and an average aggregate size of 152 nm was from Cabot Corporation, Ravenna, Italy.

3.1.3. For the Preparation of Rubber Composites

Solution styrene-butadiene rubber (S-SBR) was poly (styrene-co-butadiene) from anionic polymerization promoted by an organo-lithium initiator: SPRINTAN SLR-4630 (TRINSEO), with 25% styrene, 37.5 parts of TDAE oil, typical glass transition temperature = −28 °C, Mooney viscosity (ML(1 + 4)100 °C) = 55 MU.

Natural rubber was poly(1,4-cis-isoprene) from Hevea brasiliensis: STR20 (Eatern GR Thailand – Chonburi).

Silica ZEOSIL 1165MP (Solvay). The product was in the form of white micropearls. The specific surface area was 140–180 m^2/g, loss on drying (2 h @ 105 °C) $\leq$ 8.0%, soluble salts (as Na_2SO_4) $\leq$ 2.0%.

CBN234 was of the same commercial grade reported above.

Stearic acid was provided by Sogis (Sospiro, Italy), ZnO was provided by Zincol Ossidi (Ferrania, Italy), N′-phenyl-p-phenylenediamine (6PPD) was provided by Crompton (Mumbai, India), sulfur was provided by Solfotecnica (Ravenna, Italy), and N-ter-butyl-2-benzothiazyl sulfenamide (TBBS) was provide by Flexsys (St. Louis, MO, USA).

3.1.4. Synthesis of Pyrrole Derivatives

It was performed in one pot and two steps.

Step 1. General procedure for the synthesis of 2,5-hexanedione (2) (STEP 1)

The procedure adopted for Entry 1 of Table 1 is reported as follows. The same procedure was followed for the other entries, except that the amount of water and/or the amount of acid were changed. The water in the reaction partially came from the acid solution.

In a round-bottomed flask, equipped with a condenser, distilled water (47.0 mmol, 0.85 mL), sulfuric acid (4 mol%, 1.88 mmol), and 2,5-dimethylfuran (47.0 mmol, 5.0 mL) were put in sequence. Then, the oil bath was set at 50 °C and the reaction was stirred for 24 h. The final mixture was analyzed by ^{1}H-NMR spectroscopy. 2,5-hexanedione (HD) (**2**) was obtained as a dark brown liquid with a yield of 95% and used without any further purification in STEP 2. Water was detected in negligible traces. The relative yield of 2,5-hexanedione and the amount of the unreacted 2,5-dimethylfuran were determined by ^{1}H-NMR spectroscopy, considering the ratio of the signals of DF and HD, respectively.

Step 2. General procedure for the synthesis of pyrrole compounds

Reaction of 2,5-HD with primary amines

The selected primary amine, either serinol (38.0 mmol), isoserinol (47.0 mmol), ethanolamine (47.0 mmol), methylamine solution (40% in weight water solution) (47.0 mmol), hexylamine (47.0 mmol), benzylamine (47.0 mmol), cysteamine (47.0 mmol), or cystamine (23.5 mmol), was introduced in a 50 mL round-bottomed flask, containing the 2,5-hexanedione (**2**), obtained in Step 1, in equimolar ratio. The mixtures were stirred for 2 h at different temperatures (indicated below). The chemical purity of the products was determined by means of ^{1}H-NMR, ^{13}C-NMR, and GC-Mass spectroscopies. The reaction yield was calculated considering the final amount (mmol) of the pyrrole compound compared to the starting amount of 2,5-dimethylfuran (mmol).

The coupling constants and chemical shift values from ^{1}H-NMR and ^{13}C-NMR analyses of the PyC prepared in this work have been compared with literature values. The data are in Tables S1 and S2, respectively, in the Supplementary Material. The values are very similar when the analyses are performed in the same solvent. The use of different solvents led to different values.

2-(2,5-dimethyl-1H-pyrrol-1-yl)propane-1,3-diol (Serinol pyrrole) (**3a**)

Reaction temperature: 150 °C. Dark viscous red liquid was obtained: 6.73 g, 80% yield.

Atom Economy ($A.E_c$) = 82%; Atom efficiency ($A.E_f$) = 65%, Reaction Mass Efficiency(RME) = 72%, E-Factor = 0.097.

^{1}H-NMR (d_6-DMSO), δ, (ppm): 5.55 (s, 2H), 4.78 (t, J = 5.5 Hz, 2H), 4.09 (m, J = 6.7 Hz, 1H), 3.76 (dt, J_1 = 11.5 Hz, J_2 = 6.0 Hz, 2H), 3.64 (dt, J_1 = 11.1 Hz, J_2 = 7.1 Hz, J_3 = 5.5 Hz, 2H), 2.15 (s, 6H). ^{13}C-NMR (CDCl3), δ, (ppm): 128.97, 107.09, 62.61, 60.30, 14.15

GC-Mass: retention time = 17.309 min; molecular peak = 169 m/z.

ESI-Mass: $[M - H]^-$: Calculated exact mass = 168.11 m/z; found exact mass = 168.0 m/z.

3-(2,5-dimethyl-1H-pyrrol-1-yl)propane-1,2-diol (iso-Serinol pyrrole) (**3b**)

Reaction temperature: 50 °C. Viscous red liquid was obtained: 8.60 g, 92% yield.

$A.E_c$ = 82%; $A.E_f$ = 75%, RME = 89%, E-Factor = 0.084.

^{1}H-NMR (d_6-DMSO), δ, (ppm): 5.57 (s, 2H), 4.82 (s, 1H), 4.69 (s, 1H), 3.85 (dd, J_1 = 18.0 Hz, J_2 = 7.30 Hz 1H), 3.58 (dd, 2H), 3.31 (dd, 2H), 2.14 (s, 6H). ^{13}C-NMR ($CDCl_3$), δ, (ppm): 128.44, 105.74, 71.71, 64.12, 46.21, 12.82.

GC-Mass: retention time = 17.064 min; molecular peak = 169 m/z.

ESI-Mass: $[M + H]^+$: Calculated exact mass = 170.11 m/z; found exact mass = 170.2 m/z,

2-(2,5-dimethyl-1H-pyrrol-1-yl)ethanol (ethanol pyrrole, EP) (**3c**)

Reaction temperature: 155 °C. Dark brown viscous liquid was obtained: 6.27 g, 93% yield.

$A.E_c$ = 79%; $A.E_f$ = 73%, RME = 76%, E-Factor = 0.101.

^{1}H-NMR (d_6-DMSO), δ, (ppm): 5.58 (s, 2H, CH-pyr), 4.83 (s, J = 5.3 Hz, 1H, OH), 3.77. (t, J = 6.5 Hz, 2H, CH_2), 3.49 (m, J = 6.1 Hz, 2H, CH_2), 2.14 (s, 6H, CH_3).

^{13}C-NMR (CDCl3), δ, (ppm): 128.17, 105.57, 62.24, 45.67, 12.72.

GC-Mass: retention time = 13.973 min; molecular peak = 139 m/z.

ESI-Mass: $[M + Na]^+$: Calculated exact mass = 162.31 m/z; found exact mass = 162.3 m/z.

1,2,5-trimethyl-1H-pyrrole (trimethyl pyrrole, TMP) (**3d**)

Reaction temperature: 25 °C. Dark brown liquid was obtained: 4.97 g, 94% yield.

$A.E_c$ = 75%; $A.E_f$ = 70%, RME = 72%. E-Factor = 0.128.

^{1}H-NMR ($CDCl_3$), δ, (ppm): 5.78, s, 2H; 3.39, s, 3H; 2.22, s, 6H.

^{13}C-NMR ($CDCl_3$), δ, (ppm): 127.83, 104.70, 30.00, 12.55.

GC-Mass: retention time = 9.286 min; molecular peak = 109 m/z.

ESI-Mass: $[2M + H]^+$: Calculated exact mass = 219.31 m/z; found exact mass $[2M + H]^+$ = 219.2 m/z.

1-hexyl-2,5-dimethyl-1H-pyrrole (hexyl pyrrole, HP) (**3e**)

Reaction temperature: 60 °C. Dark brown liquid was obtained: 7.67 g, 85% yield.

$A.E_c$ = 90%; $A.E_f$ = 76%, RME = 75.9%, E-Factor = 0.086.

^{1}H-NMR (DMSO-d_6), δ, (ppm): 5.58 (s, 2H), 3.68 (t, J = 15.6 Hz, 2H), 3.13 (s, 6H), 1.49 (m, 14.4 Hz, 2H), 1.31–1.25 (m, J = 14.0 Hz, 6H), 0.86 (t, J = 6.7 Hz, 3H). ^{13}C-NMR ($CDCl_3$), δ, (ppm): 127.41, 105.06, 43.81, 31.66, 31.14, 26.79, 22.71, 14.12, 12.60.

GC-Mass: retention time = 15.754 min; molecular peak = 179 m/z.

ESI-Mass: $[2M + H]^+$: Calculated exact mass = 359.16 m/z; found exact mass = [2M + H] = 359.5 m/z.

1-benzyl-2,5-dimethyl-1H-pyrrole (benzyl pyrrole, BP) (**3f**)

Reaction temperature: 100 °C. Dark brown viscous liquid was obtained: 6.93 g, 80% yield.

$A.E_c$ = 83.7%; $A.E_f$ = 66%, RME = 75.9%, E-Factor = 0.088.

^{1}H-NMR (DMSO-d_6), δ, (ppm): 7.30 (m, J = 7.4 Hz, 2H, Ar benz), 7.22 (t, J = 7.3 Hz, 1H; Ar benz), 6.85 (d, J= 8.2 Hz, 2H; Ar benz), 5.71 (s, 2H, Ar pyr), 5.03 (s, 2H, CH_2), 2,06 (s, 6H, CH_3).

^{13}C-NMR ($CDCl_3$), δ, (ppm): 138.69, 128.82, 128.11, 127.11, 127.03, 125.78, 105.55, 46.85, 12.56.

GC-Mass: retention time = 17.291 min; molecular peak = 185 m/z.

ESI-Mass: $[M + H]^+$: Calculated exact mass = 186.26 m/z; found exact mass = 186.3.

2-(2,5-Dimethyl-1H-pyrrol-1-yl)ethane-1-thiol (SHP) (**3g**)

Dark brown liquid was obtained: 5.31g. yield of 79%.

$A.E_c$ = 81%; $A.E_f$ = 64%, RME = 65%, E-Factor = 0.076.

^{1}H-NMR ($CDCl_3$), δ (ppm): 5.78, (s, 2H, Ar), 3.93 (m, J = 7.75 Hz, 2H, -CH_2), 2.75–2.66 (m, J_1 = 7.7 Hz, J_2 = 15.8 Hz, 2H, -CH_2), 2.24 (s, 6H, -CH_3), 1.36 (t, J = 8.5 Hz, 1H, -SH).

^{13}C-NMR (d_6-DMSO), δ (ppm): 126.81, 104.74, 46.16, 24.09, 12.18.

GC-Mass analysis retention time = 14.50 min, molecular peak = 155 m/z.

1,2-Bis(2-(2,5-dimethyl-1H-pyrrol-1-yl)ethyl)disulfide (SSP) (**3h**)

A dark orange solid was obtained: 5.39 g, 74% yield.

$A.E_c$ = 65%; $A.E_f$ = 48%, RME = 58%, E-Factor = 0.080.

^{1}H-NMR ($CDCl_3$), δ (ppm): 5.78 (s, 4H, Ar), 4.12–4.02 (m, J = 7.9 Hz 4H, CH_2), 2.87–2.83 (m, J = 7.9 Hz 4H, CH_2), 2.25 (s, 12H, CH_3).

^{13}C-NMR ($CDCl_3$), δ (ppm): 127.43, 105.90, 43.22, 37.94, 12.64.

GC-Mass: retention time = 25.76 min; molecular peak = 308 m/z.

ESI-Mass: $[M + Na]^+$: Calculated exact mass = 331.13 m/z; found exact mass = 331.2 m/z.

3.1.5. Preparation and Characterization of the CB/PyC Adduct

The preparation and characterization of the CB/SHP adduct have been reported elsewhere [46]. In brief, CB and SHP were mixed with the help of acetone and sonication. Upon removing the solvent at reduced pressure, the physical mixture was heated at 150 °C for 2 h. The organic solvent and sonication were used at the lab scale to allow the preparation of a homogeneous mixture but were avoided at the pre-industrial scale, where a spray-dry can be used. TGA was carried out on the adduct, and the weight loss between 150 °C and 900 °C allowed us to estimate an amount of the modifier in the adduct equal to 7 parts per 100 parts of CB.

3.2. *Preparation of Elastomeric Composites*

3.2.1. Recipes

The recipes of the elastomer composites are reported in Table 4. The amount of the ingredients is expressed in parts per hundred rubber (phr). In the text below, the composites are indicated with reference to the reinforcing filler, indicated in brackets. For example, the composite with CB/SHP is indicated as the (CB/SHP) composite.

Table 4. S-SBR/NR-based composites with silica, CB, CB/SHP adduct as reinforcing fillers [a].

	Composite Based on			
Ingredient	**Silica**	**CB/SHP**	**CB + S**	**CB**
S-SBR 4630	70	70	70	70
NR	30	30	30	30
Silica	65	0	0	0
Silane TESPT	5.2	0	0	0
CB N234	0	0	55	55
CB N234-SHP	0	58.70	0	0
Sulphur S_8	1.80	1.80	2.57	1.80
Sulphur atoms [b]	3.04	2.57	2.57	1.80

[a] Other ingredients used for each composite: ZnO 2.5 phr, stearic acid 2 phr, wax 1 phr, 6PPD 2 phr, TBBS 1.8 phr, PVI 0.5 phr. [b] Total sulfur content, including the silane TESPT and SHP.

3.2.2. Mixing Procedure

The composites were prepared via melt blending by using a Brabender® internal mixer whose volume was 55 cc (Brabender® PL-2000 Plasti-Corder Torque Rheometer, Brabender GmbH & Co. KG, Duisburg, Germany). The procedure is shown in the infographic in Figure 6.

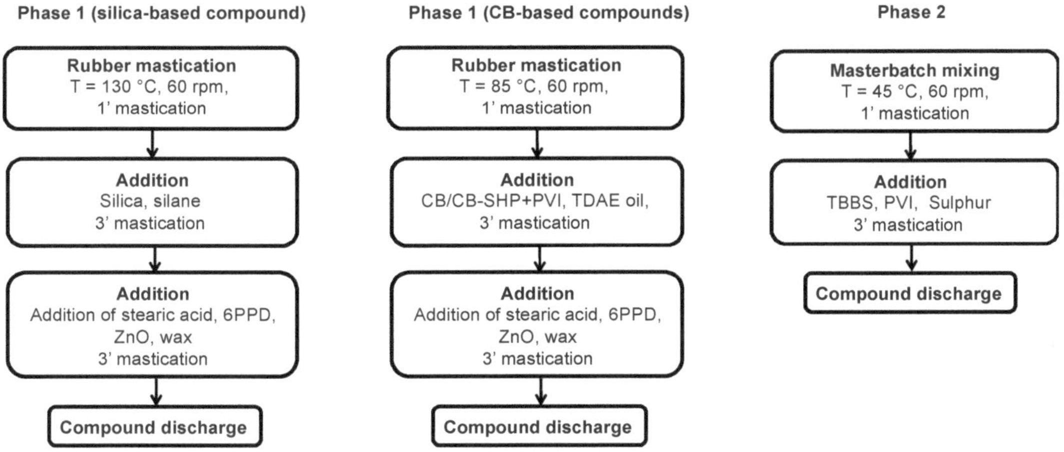

Figure 6. Block diagram of elastomeric composites reported in Table 1.

3.3. Characterization Methods

3.3.1. Characterization of Pyrrole Compounds

NMR spectra were recorded on a Bruker 400 MHz instrument (100 MHz) at 298 K. Chemical shifts were reported in ppm with the solvent residual peak as the internal standard (DMSO-d_6: δH = 2.50 ppm; $CDCl_3$: δH = 7.26 ppm).

Mass spectra were recorded by using electrospray ionization (ESI) with a Bruker Esquire 3000 plus ion-trap mass spectrometer instrument equipped with an ESI Ion Trap LC/MSn System.

The instrument for GC-MS analysis was an Agilent 5973 (Agilient technologies, Santa Clara, CA, USA) network mass selective detector with a 6890 Series GC system mass spectrometer. The column used for all analyses was a J&W GC Column HP-5MS [(5%-phenyl)-methylpolysiloxane] 30 m, with 0.25 mm internal diameter and 0.25 μm film thickness.

3.3.2. Characterization of CB/SHP Adduct

CB/SPH adduct was characterized as reported in reference [46].

3.3.3. Characterization of Elastomer Composites

Crosslinking

A rubber process analyzer (RPA, Alpha Technologies, Hudson, OH, USA) was used for performing the crosslinking reaction of each rubber composite. A total of 0 g of elastomeric composites was placed in the rheometer. A first thermal ramp was performed on the sample in order to cancel the thermomechanical history. A strain sweep from 0.1−25% of strain amplitude at 50 °C was applied to non-crosslinked samples. Then, the sample was kept at 50 °C for 10 min, and another strain sweep at 50 °C was applied. Then, the temperature was increased from 50 °C to 170 °C, and the crosslinking reaction occurred. The crosslinking reaction was performed at 170 °C for 20 min. The oscillation angle adopted was 6.28° at a frequency of 1.7 Hz. The minimum torque (M_L), the maximum torque (M_H), the time needed to have a torque equal to ML + 1 dNm (t_{S1}), and the time needed to reach 90% of the maximum torque (t_{90}) were measured at the end of the analysis.

3.3.4. Dynamic Mechanical Analyses in Shear Strain Sweep Tests

Shear dynamic mechanical properties were evaluated by using a rubber process analyzer (RPA).

A strain sweep at low deformations (0.1–25% strain) was applied to the crude sample.

The temperature then was kept at 50 °C for ten minutes and subjected to another strain sweep at 50 °C before being vulcanized. After 20 min at 50 °C, the crude elastomeric composites were subjected to a strain sweep of 0.1–25%. The frequency of the oscillation was 1 Hz. The measured properties were shear storage, G′, and loss moduli G″.

3.3.5. Dynamic Mechanical Characterization in the Axial Mode

An instron dynamic device was used for the determination of the dynamic mechanical properties in the traction compression mode according to the following methods. A test piece of the crosslinked elastomeric composition was preloaded up to 25%. The dimensions of the cylinder were as follows: length = 25 mm; diameter = 12 mm. The obtained cylinders were kept at the prefixed temperature (10, 23, and 70 °C) for the whole duration of the test. Longitudinal deformation with respect to the initial length was applied, and then the sample was submitted to a dynamic sinusoidal strain having an amplitude of ±3.5% with respect to the length under pre-load. The experimental data were measured at a frequency of 100 Hz. The dynamic mechanical properties are expressed in terms of dynamic storage modulus (E′) and loss factor (Tan Delta) values. The Tan Delta value is calculated as a ratio between loss (E″) and storage modulus (E′).

4. Conclusions

This work demonstrates that pyrrole compounds can be prepared via a one-pot, two-step synthesis, through the acid-catalyzed ring-opening reaction of a cellulosic derivative such as DF to HD, followed by the Paal–Knorr reaction of HD with a primary amine. In the process, the key role is played by water, the reagent in the ring opening of DF, and the co-product of the pyrrole synthesis. Water could thus create a circular process. The amount of water and acid in the first step was tuned to have a high yield in the second step and to avoid the formation of by-products. Excellent yield to HD was achieved with mild reaction conditions (50 °C and 8 h as the time needed to achieve most of the yield) by using a stoichiometric amount of water and a sub-stoichiometric amount of sulfuric acid. The formation of HD oligomers was prevented. HD was used without any purification for the Paal–Knorr reaction in the presence of different primary amines. Pyrrole compounds were obtained with good, very good, and excellent yields, without by-products. The chemical purity of the products of the first and second steps was confirmed by ^{1}H-NMR, ^{13}C-NMR, and GC-Mass spectroscopies. Pyrrole compounds can thus be prepared with excellent carbon efficiency and with an almost null E-factor.

Adduct of CB with SHP, the pyrrole compound prepared from cysteamine, was used in place of silica in elastomer composites, saving 15% by mass of reinforcing filler and obtaining a reduction in the Payne effect of about 25% and an increase in dynamic rigidity (E′ at 70 °C) of about 25%. The higher dynamic rigidity paves the way for the reduction in filler content, thus reducing hysteresis.

As mentioned in the introduction, a primary company in the tire field announced the use of pyrrole compounds as coupling agents for reinforcing fillers, both silica and carbon black. The global market for tires is forecast to reach 2.7 billion units by 2025. By estimating 10 kg as the total weight of the compounds in a tire, 30 as the weight% of the reinforcing filler, and 5% as the average amount of the coupling agent, 40×10^7 kg of pyrrole compounds could be needed for the whole tire market, a remarkable amount that would indeed require a sustainable synthesis. By considering a more reasonable market penetration (the company that promotes this technology has a market share of about 5%), a tonnage of about 2×10^4 tons could be estimated. This tonnage is in the typical range of fine chemicals, whose production is characterized by an E-factor of 5 (kg waste/kg product), as reported in the well-known table of E-factors. It is thus worth observing that the E-factor for the preparation of the pyrrole compounds here presented is much lower. The process reported in this manuscript appears to be in line with the teaching of green chemistry: "*what needed was not end-of-pipe remediation of waste but waste prevention at source by developing clear processes*". The lower E-factor for the preparation of chemicals, the lower weight, the Payne effect, and the hysteresis of elastomeric composites for tire compounds can indeed make a remarkable contribution to the sustainability of a large-scale product such as a tire. Moreover, to implement the sustainability of the synthetic protocols, sources of energy, such as microwave or ultrasound irradiation, could be used.

Supplementary Materials: The following supporting information can be downloaded at: https://www.mdpi.com/article/10.3390/molecules29040861/s1, S1. Reaction mechanism for the functionalization of sp2 carbon allotropes with pyrrole compound; S2. Kinetic studies; S2. Screening of the amount of water; S3. Screening of the amount of acid; S4. Screening of the type of acids, S5. Characterization of bio-pyrroles; S6. Synthesis of SHP and SSP starting from hydrochloride salt; S7. Green metrics calculation for bio-pyrroles [66,67]; S8. Rheometric data.

Author Contributions: Conceptualization, S.N., M.G. and V.B.; Methodology, S.N. and V.B.; Validation, S.N., D.G. and V.B.; Formal analysis, S.N., F.M. (Fatima Margani), G.P. and F.M. (Federica Magaletti); Investigation, S.N., M.G. and V.B.; Resources, M.G. and V.B.; Data curation, D.G.; Writing—original draft, S.N., M.G. and V.B.; Writing—review & editing, S.N., D.G., G.P., M.G. and V.B.; Supervision, M.G. and V.B.; Project administration, V.B.; Funding acquisition, M.G. and V.B. All authors have read and agreed to the published version of the manuscript.

Funding: This research was funded by Made in Italy–Circular and Sustainable (MICS) Extended Partnership funded by the European Union Next-Generation EU (Piano Nazionale di Ripresa e Resilienza (PNRR)–Missione 4, Componente 2, Investimento 1.3–D.D. 1551.11-10-2022, PE00000004) for financial support.

Institutional Review Board Statement: Not applicable.

Informed Consent Statement: Not applicable.

Data Availability Statement: Data will be made available on request.

Acknowledgments: Activities of Simone Naddeo, Fatima Margani, Gea Prioglio, and Federica Magaletti were financially supported by Pirelli Tyre.

Conflicts of Interest: The authors declare that they have no conflicts of interest.

References

1. The 17 Goals for the Sustainable Development, United Nations, Department of Economic and Social Affairs. Available online: https://sdgs.un.org/goals (accessed on 27 January 2022).
2. Ragauskas, A.J.; Williams, C.K.; Davison, B.H.; Britovsek, G.; Cairney, J.; Eckert, C.A.; Frederick, W.J.; Hallet, J.P.; Leak, D.J.; Liotta, C.L.; et al. The path forward for biofuels and biomaterials. *Science* **2006**, *311*, 484–489. [CrossRef] [PubMed]
3. Huang, K.; Peng Xong, L.; Wu, W.; Chen, Y.; Maravelias, C.T. Greenhouse gas emission mitigation potential of chemicals produced from biomass. *ACS Sustain. Chem. Eng.* **2021**, *9*, 14480–14487. [CrossRef]
4. Bozell, J.J.; Petersen, G.R. Technology development for the production of biobased products from biorefinery carbohydrates—The US Department of Energy's "Top 10" revisited. *Green Chem.* **2010**, *12*, 539. [CrossRef]
5. Varma, R.S. Biomass-derived renewable carbonaceous materials for sustainable chemical and environmental applications. *ACS Sustain. Chem. Eng.* **2019**, *7*, 6458–6470. [CrossRef]
6. Cho, E.J.; Trinh, L.T.P.; Song, Y.; Lee, Y.G.; Bae, H.J. Bioconversion of biomass waste into high value chemicals. *Bioresour. Technol.* **2020**, *298*, 122386. [CrossRef] [PubMed]
7. Wu, X.; Luo, N.; Xie, S.; Zhang, H.; Zhang, Q.; Wang, F.; Wang, Y. Photocatalytic transformations of lignocellulosic biomass into chemicals. *Chem. Soc. Rev.* **2020**, *49*, 6198–6223. [CrossRef] [PubMed]
8. Newth, F.H. The formation of furan compounds from hexoses. *Adv. Carbohydr. Chem.* **1951**, *6*, 83.
9. Feather, M.S.; Harris, J.F. Dehydration reactions of carbohydrates. *Adv. Carbohydr. Chem.* **1973**, *28*, 161.
10. Kuster, B.F.M. 5-Hydroxymethylfurfural (HMF). A review focussing on its manufacture. *Starch/Staerke* **1990**, *42*, 314. [CrossRef]
11. Moreau, C.; Belgacem, M.N.; Gandini, A. Recent catalytic advances in the chemistry of substituted furans from carbohydrates and in the ensuing polymers. *Top. Catal.* **2004**, *27*, 11–30. [CrossRef]
12. Tong, X.; Ma, Y.; Li, Y. Biomass into chemicals: Conversion of sugars to furan derivatives by catalytic processes. *Appl. Catal. A Gen.* **2010**, *385*, 1–13. [CrossRef]
13. Ståhlberg, T.; Fu, W.; Woodley, J.M.; Riisager, A. Synthesis of 5-(Hydroxymethyl) furfural in ionic liquids: Paving the way to renewable chemicals. *ChemSusChem.* **2011**, *4*, 451–458. [CrossRef]
14. Lima, S.; Antunes, M.M.; Pillinger, M.; Valente, A.A. Ionic liquids as tools for the acid-catalyzed hydrolysis/dehydration of saccharides to furanic aldehydes. *ChemCatChem* **2011**, *3*, 1686–1706. [CrossRef]

15. Román-Leshkov, Y.; Chheda, J.N.; Dumesic, J.A. Phase modifiers promote efficient production of hydroxymethylfurfural from fructose. *Science* **2006**, *312*, 1933–1937. [CrossRef]
16. van Putten, R.J.; Van Der Waal, J.C.; De Jong, E.D.; Rasrendra, C.B.; Heeres, H.J.; de Vries, J.G. Hydroxymethylfurfural, a versatile platform chemical made from renewable resources. *Chem. Rev.* **2013**, *113*, 1499–1597. [CrossRef] [PubMed]
17. Kashparova, V.P.; Chernysheva, D.V.; Klushin, V.A.; Andreeva, V.E.; Kravchenko, O.A.; Smirnova, N.V. Furan monomers and polymers from renewable plant biomass. *Russ. Chem. Rev.* **2021**, *90*, 750. [CrossRef]
18. Dedes, G.; Karnaouri, A.; Topakas, E. Novel routes in transformation of lignocellulosic biomass to furan platform chemicals: From pretreatment to enzyme catalysis. *Catalysts* **2020**, *7*, 743. [CrossRef]
19. Li, J.; Muller, E.; Pera-Titus, M.; Jérôme, F.; Vigier, K.D.O. Synthesis of functionalized tetrahydrofuran derivatives from 2, 5-dimethylfuran through cascade reactions. *Green Chem.* **2019**, *21*, 2601–2609. [CrossRef]
20. Hu, L.; Lin, L.; Liu, S. Chemoselective hydrogenation of biomass-derived 5-hydroxymethylfurfural into the liquid biofuel 2, 5-dimethylfuran. *Ind. Eng. Chem. Res.* **2014**, *53*, 9969–9978. [CrossRef]
21. Román-Leshkov, Y.; Barrett, C.J.; Liu, Z.Y.; Dumesic, J.A. Production of dimethylfuran for liquid fuels from biomass-derived carbohydrates. *Nature* **2007**, *447*, 982–985. [CrossRef] [PubMed]
22. Thananatthanachon, T.; Rauchfuss, T.B. Efficient production of the liquid fuel 2, 5-dimethylfuran from fructose using formic acid as a reagent. *Angew. Chem.* **2010**, *122*, 6766–6768. [CrossRef]
23. Dutta De, S.; Saha, B. One-pot conversions of lignocellulosic and algal biomass into liquid fuels. *ChemSusChem.* **2012**, *5*, 1826–1833. [PubMed]
24. Yin, J.; Shen, C.; Feng, X.; Ji, K.; Du, L. Highly selective production of p-xylene from 2,5-dimethylfuran over hierarchical NbO x-based catalyst. *ACS Sustain. Chem. Eng.* **2018**, *6*, 1891–1899. [CrossRef]
25. Chang, C.C.; Cho, H.J.; Yu, J.; Gorte, R.J.; Gulbinski, J.; Dauenhauer, P.; Fan, W. Lewis acid zeolites for tandem Diels–Alder cycloaddition and dehydration of biomass-derived dimethylfuran and ethylene to renewable p-xylene. *Green Chem.* **2016**, *18*, 1368. [CrossRef]
26. Sullivan, R.J.; Latifi, E.; Chung, B.K.M.; Soldatov, D.V.; Schlaf, M. Hydrodeoxygenation of 2,5-hexanedione and 2,5-dimethylfuran by water-air and acid-stable homogeneous ruthenium and iridium catalysts. *ACS Catal.* **2014**, *4*, 4116–4128. [CrossRef]
27. Xu, L.; Chen, H.; Liu, J.; Zhou, L.; Liu, Q.; Lan, Y.; Xiao, J. Chiral phosphoric acid-catalyzed asymmetric C(sp^3)–H functionalization of biomass-derived 2,5-dimethylfuran via two sequential Cope-type rearrangements. *Org. Chem. Front.* **2019**, *6*, 1162–1167. [CrossRef]
28. Liu, F.; Audemar, M.; De Oliveira Vigier, K.; Clacens, J.M.; De Campo, F.; Jérôme, F. Palladium/carbon dioxide cooperative catalysis for the production of diketone derivatives from carbohydrates. *ChemSusChem.* **2014**, *7*, 2089–2095. [CrossRef]
29. Li, H.; Guo, H.; Fang, Z.; Aida, T.M.; Smith, R.L. Cycloamination strategies for renewable N-heterocycles. *Green Chem.* **2020**, *22*, 582–611. [CrossRef]
30. Kaneda, K.; Ueno, S.; Imanaka, T.; Shimotsuma, E.; Nishiyama, Y.; Ishii, Y. Baeyer-Villiger oxidation of ketones using molecular oxygen and benzaldehyde in the absence of metal catalysts. *Org. Chem.* **1994**, *59*, 2915–2917. [CrossRef]
31. Iovel, I.; Goldberg, Y.; Shymanska, M. Hydroxymethylation of furan and its derivatives in the presence of cation-exchange resins. *J. Mol. Catal.* **1989**, *57*, 91–103. [CrossRef]
32. Zhang, J.; Zhang, S.; Peng, C.; Chen, Y.; Tang, Z.; Wu, Q. Continuous synthesis of 2,5-hexanedione through direct C–C coupling of acetone in a Hilbert fractal photo microreactor. *Adv. Mater. Res.* **2012**, *518*, 3947–3950. [CrossRef]
33. Waidmann, C.R.; Pierpont, A.W.; Batista, E.R.; Gordon, J.C.; Martin, R.L.; West, R.M.; Wu, R. Functional group dependence of the acid catalyzed ring opening of biomass derived furan rings: An experimental and theoretical study. *Catal. Sci. Technol.* **2013**, *3*, 106–115. [CrossRef]
34. Gilkey, M.J.; Vlachos, D.G.; Xu, B. Poisoning of Ru/C by homogeneous Brønsted acids in hydrodeoxygenation of 2,5-dimethylfuran via catalytic transfer hydrogenation. *Appl. Catal. A Gen.* **2017**, *542*, 327–335. [CrossRef]
35. Li, Y.; Lv, G.; Wang, Y.; Deng, T.; Wang, Y.; Hou, X.; Yang, Y. Synthesis of 2,5-Hexanedione from Biomass Resources Using a Highly Efficient Biphasic System. *Chem. Select* **2016**, *6*, 1252–1255. [CrossRef]
36. Vidal, T.; Petit, A.; Loupy, A.; Gedye, R.N. Re-examination of microwave-induced synthesis of phthalimides. *Tethraedon Lett.* **1990**, *40*, 3957–3960. [CrossRef]
37. Balme, G.; Bossharth, E.; Monteiro, N. Pd-assisted multicomponent synthesis of heterocycles. *Eur. J. Org. Chem.* **2003**, *21*, 4101–4111. [CrossRef]
38. Nieuwland, P.J.; Segers, R.; Koch, K.; van Hest, J.C.; Rutjes, F.P. Fast scale-up using microreactors: Pyrrole synthesis from micro to production scale. *Org. Process Res. Dev.* **2011**, *15*, 783–787. [CrossRef]
39. Galimberti, M.; Barbera, V.; Guerra, S.; Conzatti, L.; Castiglioni, C.; Brambilla, L.; Serafini, A. Biobased Janus molecule for the facile preparation of water solutions of few layer graphene sheets. *RSC Adv.* **2015**, *5*, 81142–81152. [CrossRef]
40. Barbera, V.; Bernardi, A.; Palazzolo, A.; Rosengart, A.; Brambilla, L.; Galimberti, M. Facile and sustainable functionalization of graphene layers with pyrrole compounds. *Pure Appl. Chem.* **2018**, *90*, 253–270. [CrossRef]
41. Locatelli, D.; Barbera, V.; Brambilla, L.; Castiglioni, C.; Sironi, A.; Galimberti, M. Tuning the solubility parameters of carbon nanotubes by means of their adducts with Janus pyrrole compounds. *Nanomaterials* **2020**, *10*, 1176. [CrossRef]

42. Locatelli, D.; Bernardi, A.; Rubino, L.; Gallo, S.; Vitale, A.; Bongiovanni, R.; Barbera, V.; Galimberti, M. Biosourced Janus Molecules as Silica Coupling Agents in Elastomer Composites for Tires with Lower Environmental Impact. *ACS Sustain. Chem. Eng.* **2023**, *11*, 2713–2726. [CrossRef]
43. De Gennes, P.-G. Soft matter (nobel lecture). *Angew. Chem. Int. Ed.* **1992**, *31*, 842–845. [CrossRef]
44. Casagrande, C.; Fabre, P.; Raphaël, E.; Veyssié, M. Janus beads: Realization and behaviour at water/oil interfaces. *Europhys. Lett.* **1989**, *9*, 251–255. [CrossRef]
45. Barbera, V.; Brambilla, L.; Milani, A.; Palazzolo, A.; Castiglioni, C.; Vitale, A.; Galimberti, M. Domino reaction for the sustainable functionalization of few-layer graphene. *Nanomaterials* **2018**, *9*, 44. [CrossRef]
46. Prioglio, G.; Naddeo, S.; Giese, U.; Barbera, V.; Galimberti, M. Bio-Based Pyrrole Compounds Containing Sulfur Atoms as Coupling Agents of Carbon Black with Unsaturated Elastomers. *Nanomaterials* **2023**, *13*, 2761. [CrossRef]
47. Magaletti, F.; Margani, F.; Monti, A.; Dezyani, R.; Prioglio, G.; Giese, U.; Barbera, V.; Galimberti, M. Adducts of Carbon Black with a Biosourced Janus Molecule for Elastomeric Composites with Lower Dissipation of Energy. *Polymers* **2023**, *15*, 3120. [CrossRef] [PubMed]
48. Pirelli Tyre; Annual Report: The Human Dimension. 2020, 106. Available online: https://corporate.pirelli.com/var/files2020/EN/PDF/PIRELLI_ANNUAL_REPORT_2020_ENG.pdf (accessed on 4 October 2022).
49. Curzons, A.D.; Constable, D.J.; Mortimer, D.N.; Cunningham, V.L. So you think your process is green, how do you know?—Using principles of sustainability to determine what is green—A corporate perspective. *Green Chem.* **2001**, *3*, 1–6. [CrossRef]
50. Sheldon, R.A. The E factor 25 years on: The rise of green chemistry and sustainability. *Green Chem.* **2017**, *19*, 18–43. [CrossRef]
51. Sheldon, R.A. Metrics of green chemistry and sustainability: Past, present, and future. *ACS Sustain. Chem. Eng.* **2018**, *6*, 32–48. [CrossRef]
52. Chevalier, Y.; Morawski, J.C. Precipitated Silica with Morphological Properties, Process for Producing It and Its Application, Especially as a Filler. Legrand. EP0157703 B1, 6 April 1984.
53. Leblanc, J.L. Rubber-filler interactions and rheological properties in filled compounds. *Progr. Polym. Sci.* **2002**, *27*, 627–687. [CrossRef]
54. Legrand, A.P. On the silica edge. In *The Surface Properties of Silicas*; Legrand, A.P., Ed.; Wiley and Sons: New York, NY, USA, 1998; pp. 1–20.
55. Donnet, J.B.; Custodero, E. Reinforcement of Elastomers by Particulate Fillers. In *The Science and Technology of Rubber*, 3rd ed.; Mark, J.E., Erman, B., Eirich, F.R., Eds.; Elsevier: Amsterdam, The Netherlands, 2005; pp. 367–400.
56. Fröhlich, J.; Niedermeier, W.; Luginsland, H.D. The effect of filler-filler and filler-elastomer interaction on rubber reinforcement. *Compos. Part A* **2005**, *36*, 449–460. [CrossRef]
57. Hoyle, C.E.; Bowman, C.N. Thiol–ene click chemistry. *Angew. Chem. Int. Ed.* **2010**, *49*, 1540–1573. [CrossRef]
58. Wang, X.; Liang, H.; Jiang, J.; Wang, Q.; Luo, Y.; Feng, P.; Zhang, C.A. Cysteine derivative-enabled ultrafast thiol–ene reaction for scalable synthesis of a fully bio-based internal emulsifier for high-toughness waterborne polyurethanes. *Green Chem.* **2020**, *22*, 5722–5729. [CrossRef]
59. Sato, M.; Mihara, S.; Amino, N.; Dierkes, W.K.; Blume, A. Reactivity study of mercapto–silane and sulfide–silane with polymer. *Rubber Chem. Technol.* **2020**, *93*, 319–345. [CrossRef]
60. Dillon, J.H.; Prettyman, I.B.; Hall, G.L. Hysteretic and elastic properties of rubberlike materials under dynamic shear stresses. *J. Appl. Phys.* **1944**, *15*, 309. [CrossRef]
61. Fletcher, W.P.; Gent, A.N. Nonlinearity in the dynamic properties of vulcanized rubber compounds. *Trans. Inst. Rubber Ind.* **1953**, *29*, 266. [CrossRef]
62. Payne, A.R. The dynamic properties of carbon black-loaded natural rubber vulcanizates. Part I. *J. Appl. Polym. Sci.* **1962**, *6*, 57. [CrossRef]
63. Warasitthinon, N.; Genix, A.C.; Sztucki, M.; Oberdisse, J.; Robertson, C.G. The Payne effect: Primarily polymer-related or filler-related phenomenon? *Rubber Chem. Technol.* **2019**, *92*, 599–611. [CrossRef]
64. Zhang, Y.; Zhang, Z.; Wemyss, A.M.; Wan, C.; Liu, Y.; Song, P.; Wang, S. Effective thermal-oxidative reclamation of waste tire rubbers for producing high-performance rubber composites. *ACS Sustain. Chem. Eng.* **2020**, *8*, 9079–9087. [CrossRef]
65. Jiang, C.; Bo, J.; Xiao, X.; Zhang, S.; Wang, Z.; Yan, G.; Wu, Y.; Wong, C.; He, H. Converting waste lignin into nano-biochar as a renewable substitute of carbon black for reinforcing styrene-butadiene rubber. *Waste Manag.* **2020**, *102*, 732–742. [CrossRef]
66. Vogel, A.I.; Tatchell, A.R.; Furnis, B.S.; Hannaford, A.J.; Smith, P.W.G. (Eds.) *Vogel's Textbook of Practical Organic Chemistry 1996*; Prentice Hall: Hoboken, NJ, USA, 1996; ISBN 978-0-582-46236-6.
67. Anastas, P.; Eghbali, N. Green chemistry: Principles and practice. *Chem. Soc. Rev.* **2010**, *39*, 301–312. [CrossRef] [PubMed]

molecules

MDPI

Article

Adsorption Affinities of Small Volatile Organic Molecules on Graphene Surfaces for Novel Nanofiller Design: A DFT Study

Francesco Moriggi, Vincenzina Barbera, Maurizio Galimberti * and Giuseppina Raffaini *

Department of Chemistry, Materials, and Chemical Engineering "Giulio Natta", Politecnico di Milano, Via Luigi Mancinelli 7, 20131 Milano, Italy; francesco.moriggi@polimi.it (F.M.); vincenzina.barbera@polimi.it (V.B.)

* Correspondence: maurizio.galimberti@polimi.it (M.G.); giuseppina.raffaini@polimi.it (G.R.)

Abstract: The adsorption of organic molecules on graphene surfaces is a crucial process in many different research areas. Nano-sized carbon allotropes, such as graphene and carbon nanotubes, have shown promise as fillers due to their exceptional properties, including their large surface area, thermal and electrical conductivity, and potential for weight reduction. Surface modification methods, such as the "pyrrole methodology", have been explored to tailor the properties of carbon allotropes. In this theoretical work, an ab initio study based on Density Functional Theory is performed to investigate the adsorption process of small volatile organic molecules (such as pyrrole derivatives) on graphene surface. The effects of substituents, and different molecular species are examined to determine the influence of the aromatic ring or the substituent of pyrrole's aromatic ring on the adsorption energy. The number of atoms and presence of π electrons significantly influence the corresponding adsorption energy. Interestingly, pyrroles and cyclopentadienes are 10 kJ mol^{-1} more stable than the corresponding unsaturated ones. Pyrrole oxidized derivatives display more favorable supramolecular interactions with graphene surface. Intermolecular interactions affect the first step of the adsorption process and are important to better understand possible surface modifications for carbon allotropes and to design novel nanofillers in polymer composites.

Keywords: adsorption; surface modification; DFT; nano-sized carbon allotropes; graphene; carbon nanotubes; supramolecular interactions; pyrrole methodology

Citation: Moriggi, F.; Barbera, V.; Galimberti, M.; Raffaini, G. Adsorption Affinities of Small Volatile Organic Molecules on Graphene Surfaces for Novel Nanofiller Design: A DFT Study. *Molecules* **2023**, *28*, 7633. https://doi.org/10.3390/molecules28227633

Academic Editor: Erich A. Müller

Received: 7 October 2023
Revised: 6 November 2023
Accepted: 10 November 2023
Published: 16 November 2023

1. Introduction

The adsorption process on solid surfaces plays a critical role in numerous scientific disciplines, ranging from chemistry and physics to materials science and nanotechnology [1–8]. Many phenomena can occur when molecules adsorb on solid surface. The ability to understand and manipulate the interactions between molecules and surfaces opens up avenues for designing novel materials with tailored surface properties and optimizing the performance of existing systems [9–15]. While experimental techniques provide valuable information about surface adsorption, a deeper understanding at the atomic level requires the use of numerical simulations that can help us study the possible mechanisms and dynamics driving these processes [16–22].

Density Functional Theory (DFT) calculations together with molecular mechanics (MM) and molecular dynamics (MD) methods can provide information that strongly complements experimental studies [23–38]. MM and MD simulations are interesting tools to describe both the bulk and surface properties of materials at the atomistic level [39–47]. The adsorption process of proteins, peptides, and small molecules can be investigated on the external surfaces of graphite and carbon allotropes in general. The comparisons between theoretical results and experimental data are interesting, such as those concerning favorable van der Waals interactions between graphene allotropes and proteins, an important aspect for biomaterials in contact with the blood [43]. The same favorable interactions explain the possible solubilization of carbon nanotubes synthesized in an amorphous phase due to protein adsorption on the external surface. Their solubilization is an important technology aspect to prepare aligned fibers in polymeric matrices of composite materials [47–49].

Considering the adsorption of a single molecule on a solid surface, Density Functional Theory has emerged as an interesting tool for studying the ground-state properties of condensed matter systems, particularly with regard to how surface interactions influence the electronic distribution in the molecular orbitals of the volatile organic molecules near a solid surface [50–53]. DFT offers a rigorous framework based on quantum mechanics, enabling accurate predictions of adsorption sites, binding energies, and electronic properties that closely align with experimental observations, allowing researchers to gain insights into the structural, electronic, and energetic aspects of adsorption, thus helping to clarify the fundamental principles that govern these phenomena [23,50–54].

In recent years, there has been a growing interest in surface modification techniques aiming to improve the properties of fillers used in advanced technological applications [55]. One prominent area where surface modification has shown significant potential is in the development of polymer composites for the tire industry [56–58]. By modifying the surfaces of fillers, scientists can achieve substantial improvements in mechanical strength, thermal stability, electrical conductivity, and other desired characteristics, thereby pushing the boundaries of material performance [59–62]. In this context, nano-sized carbon allotropes, such as graphene and carbon nanotubes, have emerged as promising candidates due to their exceptional properties [63,64]. Carbon allotropes display a remarkable combination of attributes that make them highly attractive as fillers in polymer composites [65–71]. Their large surface area provides an extended contact interface with the surrounding polymer matrix, enabling efficient load transfer and reinforcing the mechanical properties of the composite [66–68]. Additionally, carbon allotropes exhibit exceptional thermal and electrical conductivity, facilitating heat dissipation and electrical conduction pathways within the material. Furthermore, their incorporation into composites allows for a reduction in the volume ratio of fillers compared to traditional alternatives, which can lead to lighter and more cost-effective materials [53]. Given these advantages, tailoring the properties of carbon allotropes has become a topic of considerable scientific interest, driving the exploration of various surface modification methods [69–74].

Among the diverse approaches investigated, one particularly efficient and reliable procedure is known as the "pyrrole methodology", which involves the covalent modification of carbon allotrope surfaces using *N*-substituted pyrrole molecules [75,76], a method that enables the introduction of desirable functionalities onto the carbon allotrope surface. The grafting process begins with the initial adsorption of *N*-substituted pyrrole molecules onto the sp^2 carbon surface, which then undergoes oxidation and subsequent Diels–Alder cycloaddition, forming covalent bonds with the edges of the carbon allotrope plane. The adsorption and grafting mechanisms of the pyrrole methodology are governed by a complex interplay of supramolecular interactions, which dictate the stability, structure, and properties of the modified surface [77]. This approach has been employed to produce novel fillers in order to improve the mechanical properties of polymer nanocomposites [78,79].

Motivated by the potential of the pyrrole methodology and the need for a detailed understanding of the adsorption process, our study employed ab initio simulations based on DFT to gain deeper insights into the initial steps of the pyrrole methodology and investigate the adsorption behaviors of various compounds on carbon allotropes. Our objectives encompassed not only determining the optimal computational parameters for the simulations but also exploring the interactions between pyrrole molecules and graphene surfaces. Furthermore, we sought to examine the effects of substituents and oxidation on the adsorption process, allowing us to understand how different modifications influence the stability and reactivity of this system.

To broaden the scope of our investigation, we expanded our calculations to include other compounds, including alkanes, cyclopentanes, pyrrolidines, and cyclopentadiene derivatives. By exploring a broad range of molecular species, we aimed to uncover the underlying factors governing adsorption and shed light on the role of dispersion and π-π interactions in stabilizing these systems on graphene surfaces, an approach that has already been verified in the recent literature [80–83]. The structures of the systems were studied by calculating their adsorption energies and generating charge difference density plots. These detailed analyses allowed us to obtain a comprehensive understanding of the supramolecular interactions at play and their influence on the adsorption phenomena occurring on carbon allotrope surfaces. Table 1 shows a list of the compounds adsorbed on the pristine graphene samples studied. The pyrrole compounds used to develop the "pyrrole methodology" were obtained from the Paal Knorr reaction [84,85] of a primary amine with 2,5-hexanedione (HD). This synthetic pathway gave the chance to start from a biobased chemical. Indeed, HD was prepared through the ring opening reaction of 2,5-dimethylfuran, also by using a two-step one pot process [86,87]. The use of HD led to pyrrole molecules with two methyl groups in the alpha positions of the ring. In Section 2.4, theoretical results about 1,2,5-trimethylpyrrole and its oxidized derivatives on a pristine graphene surface will be discussed. The use as reinforcing fillers of sp^2 carbon allotropes, mainly carbon black, functionalized by means of the "pyrrole methodology" with pyrrole compounds as the ones studied in the research here reported, improved the properties of elastomeric composites for a large-scale application such as the one in tyre compounds [87,88]. The development on an industrial scale was announced by a major player in the tyre field [89]. This study is aimed at giving a contribution to the development of the "pyrrole methodology", elucidating its first step.

Table 1. A list of the studied compounds adsorbed on pristine graphene.

Compound	Structure Type	Structure
Alkane	Linear	**H–R**
Cyclopentane	Saturated cyclic	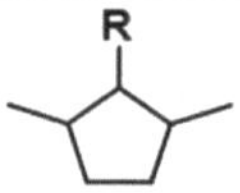
Pyrrolidine		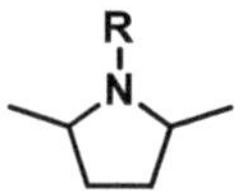
Cyclopentadiene	Unsaturated cyclic	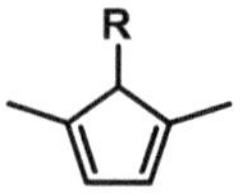
Pyrrole		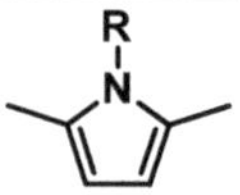

2. Results and Discussion

In this section, the results about the adsorption of the different aliphatic and aromatic compounds reported in Table 1 on the pristine graphite surface are reported and discussed.

2.1. Adsorption of Linear Alkanes on the Pristine Graphene Surface

As described in the Materials and Methods section, linear alkane compounds such as methane, ethane, propane, and butane were considered close to the pristine surface of graphene. The optimized structures are shown to the left of all four panels in Figure 1, while the adsorption distances and adsorption energies are listed in Table 2. As seen in the latter, the adsorption distances ranged from 3.46 Å (methane) to 3.65 Å (ethane), and the adsorption energies increased with increasing carbon atoms in the alkyl chain, indicating increased supramolecular interactions due to the forces of dispersion between the molecule and the graphene surface.

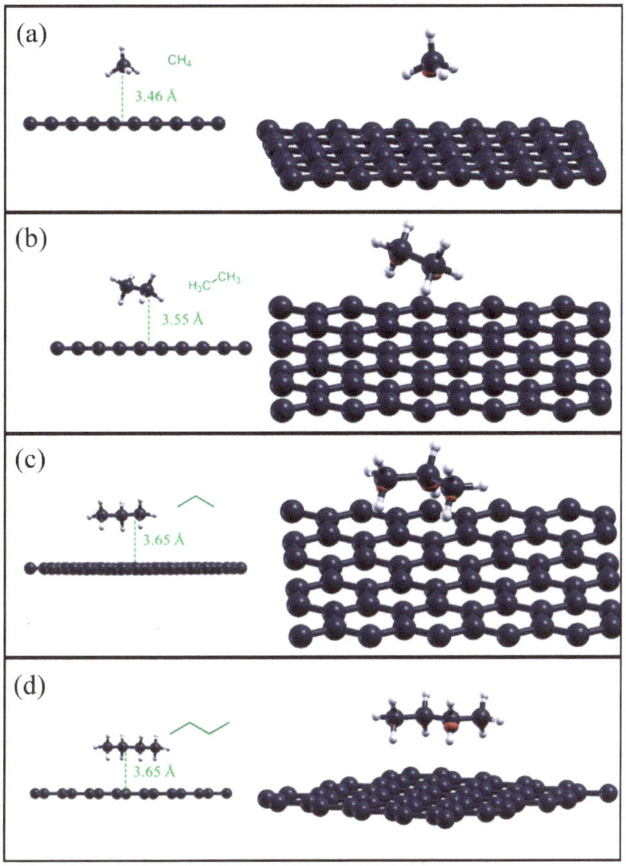

Figure 1. Optimized structures for the studied alkanes adsorbed on the pristine graphene surface (on the left), and their charge density difference plots (iso-surface value: 0.0003) on the surface (on the right). Methane adsorbed on graphene is reported in panel (**a**), ethane in panel (**b**), propane in panel (**c**), butane in panel (**d**), respectively.

Table 2. Adsorption distances and energies for alkane compounds adsorbed on the pristine graphene surface.

Compound	Distance, *d* (Å)	E_{ads} (kJ mol^{-1})
Methane	3.46	−13.2
Ethane	3.55	−18.7
Propane	3.65	−25.6
Butane	3.65	−32.7

The charge density difference iso-surfaces (value = 0.0003) shown to the right of all four panels in Figure 1 indicate the regions where there is charge transfer, and this information is useful for representing the nature of bonding between the elements present in the simulation. The small red clouds present for all adsorbents indicate a slight increase in charge density (charge per unit volume) pointing toward the graphene surface in the direction of the C–H bond. The red clouds are more evident for propane and butane in Figure 1c,d, respectively.

Regarding the ground-state geometries studied, upon considering the plane defined by all carbon atoms in the propane and butane chains, it can be gleaned that this plane is parallel to the graphene plane. As regards the interaction energy, we can observe that as the number of carbon atoms in the chain increases, the interactions with the solid surface increase proportionally, indicating a stabilizing effect due, as mentioned previously, to the favorable dispersion interactions between the C–H bonds and the graphene surface.

2.2. *Adsorption of Saturated Cyclic Compounds on the Pristine Graphene Surface*

The results relating to the saturated cyclic systems reported in Table 1 are presented and discussed in this section, considering both cyclopentane and pyrrolidine compounds.

2.2.1. Adsorption of Cyclopentane Compounds on the Pristine Graphene Surface

As described in the Materials and Methods section, cyclopentane compounds were considered adsorbed on the pristine graphene surface. The ground-state structures are shown on the left in Figure 2, while the adsorption distances and the adsorption energies are reported in Table 3.

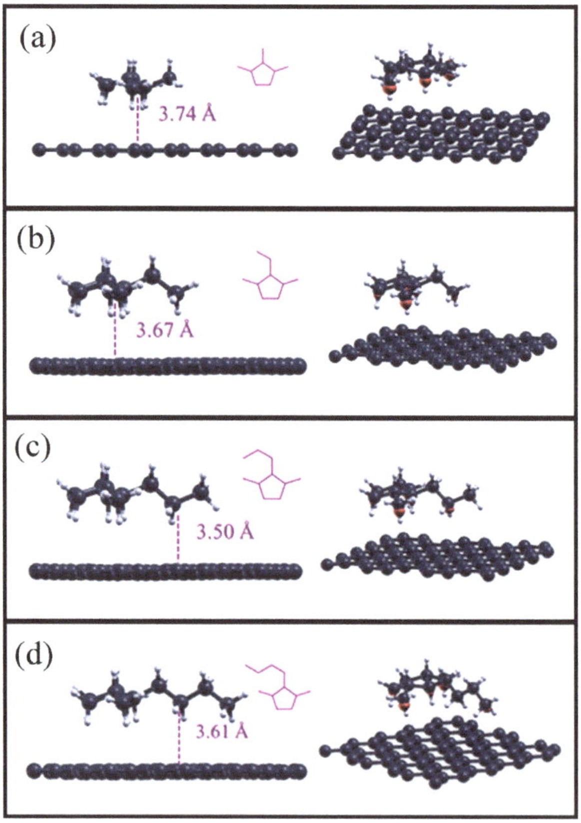

Figure 2. Optimized structures for the cyclopentane compounds adsorbed on the pristine graphene surface (on the left), and the charge density difference plots (iso-surface value: 0.0003) of the alkane compounds on the surface (on the right). 1,2,3-trimethylcyclopentane adsorbed on graphene is reported in panel (**a**), 2-ethyl-1,3-dimethylcyclopentane in panel (**b**), 2-propyl-1,3-dimethylcyclopentane in panel (**c**), 2-butyl-1,3-dimethylcyclopentane in panel (**d**), respectively.

Table 3. Adsorption distances and energies for cyclopentane compounds adsorbed on the pristine graphene surface.

Compound	Distance, *d* (Å)	E_{ads} (kJ mol^{-1})
1,2,3-trimethylcyclopentane	3.74	−48.1
2-ethyl-1,3-dimethylcyclopentane	3.67	−53.2
2-propyl-1,3-dimethylcyclopentane	3.50	−58.5
2-butyl-1,3-dimethylcyclopentane	3.61	−64.1

Compared to the previous results, considering the structures in the ground-state ranging from 1,2,3-trimethylcyclopentane to 2-butyl-1,3-dimethylcyclopentane, we observed a different arrangement of the structure of the alkyl residue -R with respect to the graphene plane: in fact, if we also consider for these structures the plane defined only by the carbon atoms linked to carbon 2 of the cyclopentane, this plane is now arranged perpendicular to the graphene surface, as reported in the panels on the left of Figure 2. The distances of carbon atoms closer to the graphene surface varied from 3.74 Å in 1,2,3-trimethylcyclopentane to 3.50 Å in 2-propyl-1,3-dimethylcyclopentane.

Concerning the strength of the interactions, the adsorption energies were higher when increasing the carbon atoms in linear chain, indicating, as with the alkane compounds, increased supramolecular interactions due to dispersion forces between these cyclopentane derivatives and the graphene surface.

Regarding the charge difference density plots (iso-surface value: 0.0003) shown on the right in all panels in Figure 2, and regarding the linear alkanes, the red clouds present for all the adsorbates indicate an increase in charge density that points toward the graphene surface.

As mentioned previously, regarding the geometry of the interactions in the calculated ground state, the alkyl chains that start from the cyclopentane are perpendicular to the graphene surface, and the adsorbate atoms that are close to the latter seem to contribute more to the overall supramolecular interactions. Moreover, because cyclopentanes are sp^3-hybridized, there are no planar geometry constraints; thus, the molecules, after adsorption, adjust themselves to maximize the interaction forces due to C–H bonds and the graphene surface.

2.2.2. Adsorption of Pyrrolidine Compounds on the Pristine Graphene Surface

As described in the Materials and Methods section, pyrrolidine derivatives adsorbed on the pristine graphene surface were studied. The lowest total energy structures are reported in the panels on the left in Figure 3, while the adsorption distances and their adsorption energies are listed in Table 4. Compared to the previous results, the calculated distances of pyrrolidine compounds in the calculated ground state were, on average, smaller, ranging from 3.46 Å to 3.58 Å for 1-propyl-2,5-dimethylpyrrolidine and 1-ethyl-2,5-dimethylpyrrolidine, respectively. Using the same methodologies for the analysis of the theoretical results, the adsorption energies were calculated, and their values were found to be lower, and therefore more stable in the system, for molecules with a greater number of carbon atoms, which were comparable in size to compounds of cyclopentane.

Considering the graphs of the charge density differences for the pyrrolidines (see the right side in all panels in Figure 3), one can see, as in the previous case, the positive (red) contribution to the charge transfer between the carbon atoms and the surface of graphene. Compared to saturated homoatomic systems (e.g., alkanes and cyclopentanes), however, the nitrogen atom appeared to deplete the graphene surface, as can be gleaned from the blue cloud under the pyrrolidine ring. This could be explained by the fact that nitrogen possesses a lone pair of electrons, which, in addition to the dispersion forces between the C–H bonds and the graphene surface, can interact with the graphene surface via a π-type bond.

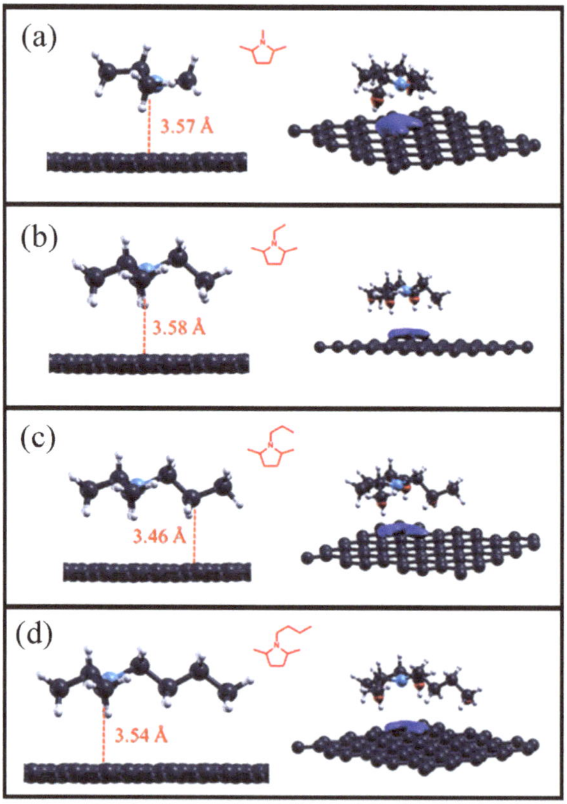

Figure 3. Optimized structures for pyrrolidine compounds adsorbed on the pristine graphene surface (on the left), and the charge density difference plots (iso-surface value: 0.0003) of alkane compounds on the surface (on the right). 1,2,5-trimethylpyrrolidine adsorbed on graphene is reported in panel (**a**), 1-ethyl-2,5-dimethylpyrrolidine in panel (**b**), 1-propyl-2,5-dimethylpyrrolidine in panel (**c**), 1-butyl-2,5-dimethylpyrrolidine in panel (**d**), respectively.

Table 4. Adsorption distances and energies for pyrrolidine compounds adsorbed on the pristine graphene surface.

Compound	Distance, d (Å)	E_{ads} (kJ mol^{-1})
1,2,5-trimethylpyrrolidine	3.57	−46.2
1-ethyl-2,5-dimethylpyrrolidine	3.58	−51.3
1-propyl-2,5-dimethylpyrrolidine	3.46	−56.5
1-butyl-2,5-dimethylpyrrolidine	3.54	−62.1

2.3. *Adsorption of Unsaturated Cyclic Compounds on the Pristine Graphene Surface*

The results regarding the unsaturated cyclic systems reported in Table 1 are presented and discussed in this section, considering both cyclopentadiene and pyrrole compounds.

2.3.1. Adsorption of Cyclopentadiene Compounds on Pristine Graphene Surface

As described in the Materials and Methods section, cyclopentadiene derivatives were adsorbed on the pristine graphene surface. The optimized structures are reported on the left in all panels in Figure 4, while the adsorption distances and calculated adsorption energies are shown in Table 5.

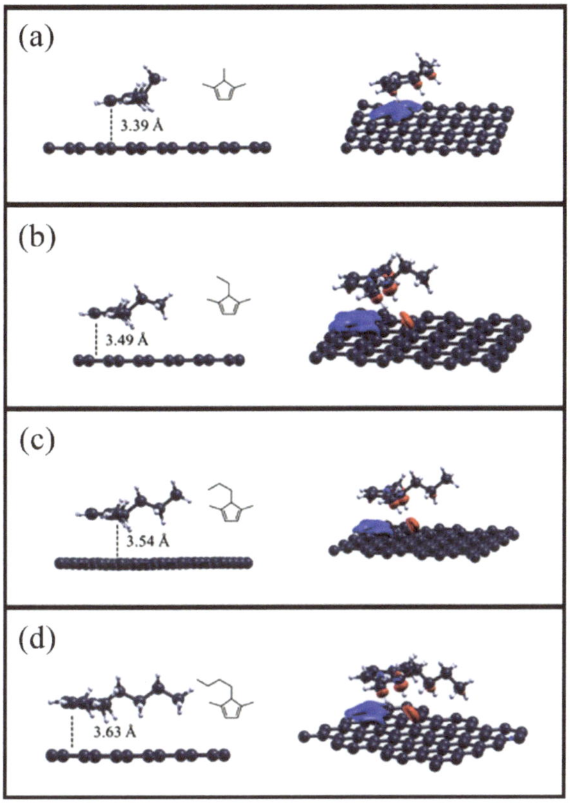

Figure 4. Optimized structures for cyclopentadiene compounds adsorbed on the pristine graphene surface (on the left), and the charge density difference plots (iso-surface value: 0.0003) of alkane compounds on the surface (on the right). 1,4,5-trimethylcyclopenta-1,3-diene adsorbed on graphene is reported in panel (**a**), 5-ethyl-1,4-dimethylcyclopenta-1,3-diene in panel (**b**), 5-propyl-1,4-dimethylcyclopenta-1,3-diene in panel (**c**), 5-butyl-1,4-dimethylcyclopenta-1,3-diene in panel (**d**), respectively.

Table 5. Adsorption distances and energies for cyclopentadiene compounds adsorbed on the pristine graphene surface.

Compound	Distance, *d* (Å)	E_{ads} (kJ mol^{-1})
1,4,5-trimethylcyclopenta-1,3-diene	3.57	−46.2
5-ethyl -1,4-dimethylcyclopenta-1,3-diene	3.58	−51.3
5-propyl -1,4-dimethylcyclopenta-1,3-diene	3.46	−56.5
5-butyl-1,4-dimethylcyclopenta-1,3-diene	3.54	−62.1

We can observe that the studied cyclopentadiene compounds, due to sp^2 hybridization, have a planar ring that is positioned parallel to the graphene surface to maximize the interaction area, with the distance d increasing as the number of atoms adsorbed increases.

Compared to the results for the previously reported saturated compounds, the calculated adsorption energies are higher but still follow the same trend, ranging from

−51.5 kJ mol^{-1} to −67.7 kJ mol^{-1} for 1,4,5-trimethylcyclopenta-1,3-diene and 5-butyl-1,4-dimethylcyclopenta-1,3-diene, respectively.

In the charge density difference plots shown in all panels on the right in Figure 4, we can observe that there are two contributions to the adsorption of cyclopentadiene derivatives on the graphene surface. Initially, dispersion interactions are significant, such as in alkane compounds, as indicated by the increase in charge density (red cloud) in the direction of the C–H bonds toward the graphene surface. Furthermore, the contribution of π interactions between the molecular π orbitals of the cyclopentadiene rings and the delocalized π orbitals of the graphene surface is important, highlighted in this case by the charge depletion (blue cloud) on the graphene surface.

2.3.2. Adsorption of Pyrrole Compounds on the Pristine Graphene Surface

As described in the Materials and Methods section, the theoretical results regarding the pyrrole derivatives adsorbed on the pristine graphene surface are shown and discussed in this section. The optimized structures can be seen in Figure 5, while the adsorption distances and calculated adsorption energies are listed in Table 6.

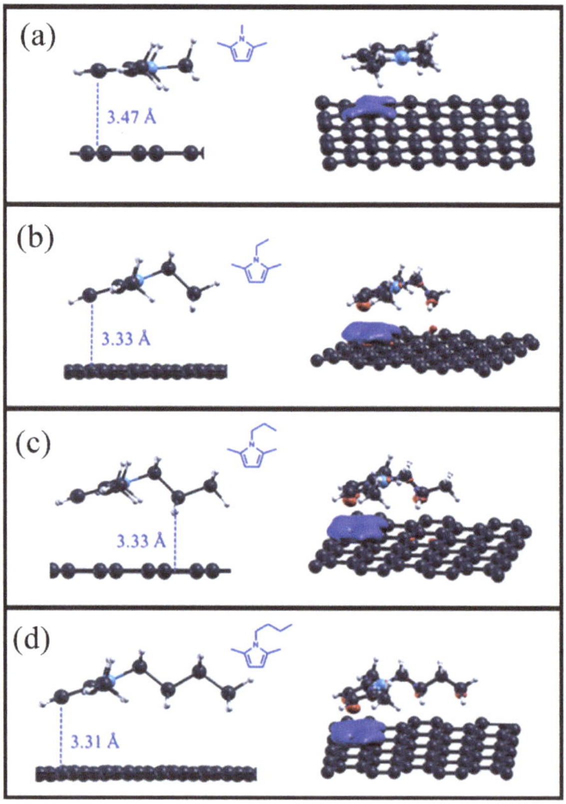

Figure 5. Optimized structures for pyrrole derivatives adsorbed on the pristine graphene surface (on the left), and the charge density difference plots (iso-surface value: 0.0003) of alkane compounds on the surface (on the right). 1,2,5-trimethylpyrrole adsorbed on graphene is reported in panel (**a**), 1-ethyl-2,5-dimethylpyrrole in panel (**b**), 1-propyl-2,5-dimethylpyrrole in panel (**c**), 1-butyl-2,5-dimethylpyrrole in panel (**d**), respectively.

Table 6. Adsorption distances and energies for pyrrole compounds adsorbed on the pristine graphene surface.

Compound	Distance, *d* (Å)	E_{ads} (kJ mol^{-1})
1,2,5-trimethylpyrrole	3.47	−55.3
1-ethyl-2,5-dimethylpyrrole	3.33	−54.9
1-propyl-2,5-dimethylpyrrole	3.33	−61.0
1-butyl-2,5-dimethylpyrrole	3.31	−66.3

Unlike unsaturated cyclopentadiene compounds, pyrroles are aromatic compounds, so the delocalized molecular orbitals in the ring constraint fix the carbon attached to the nitrogen in the same plane. This causes molecules that have a longer chain than that of 1,2,5-trimethylpyrrole to be slightly inclined and not perfectly parallel to the graphene surface, thus resulting in shorter adsorption distances between the molecule and the latter.

Even for these systems, the adsorption energy (E_{ads}) increases as the number of atoms in the molecule increases, specifically in the substituent of the linear alkyl chain, with values ranging from −55.4 kJ mol^{-1} to −66.3 kJ mol^{-1} for 1,2,5-trimethylpyrrole and 1-butyl-2,5-dimethylpyrrole, respectively.

In the graphs of the charge density differences reported on the right-hand panels in Figure 5 (iso-surface values: 0.0003), specifically regarding the cyclopentadiene derivatives, we can observe that two different contributions to the adsorption strength are important: the first contribution increases the density of charge between carbon atoms facing the direction of the C-H bond due to dispersion interactions, and the second contribution induces a charge depletion on the graphene surface due to π–π interactions.

In Figure 6, the adsorption energy on the pristine graphene surface has been plotted as a function of the number of atoms in the studied molecule. As expected, a linear correlation was found when increasing the number of carbon atoms present (see Table 7). Since there are no covalent or ionic bonds present between the molecule and the carbon substrate, the only forces exerted between these two systems are, as previously mentioned, due partly to dispersion and partly, if present in the case of adsorbates with free electron bonds in p-type orbitals, to π–π interactions. Further theoretical studies based on molecular mechanics and dynamics method on the role of the van der Waals contributions using a simulation previously proposed protocol [90] are an ongoing work.

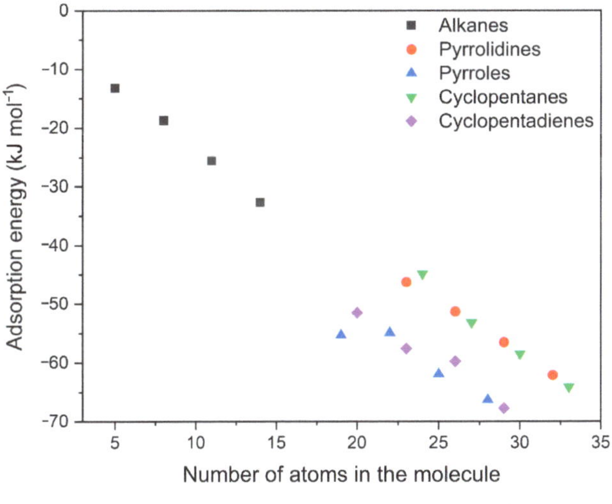

Figure 6. Adsorption energies of compounds adsorbed on the pristine graphene surface as a function of the number of atoms in the specific organic molecule.

Table 7. Information on the best linear fit with intercept equal to zero passing through the data related to the adsorption energy as a function of the number of atoms in the single molecules studied reported in Figure 6.

Compound	Slope	Standard Error	R^2
Alkanes	−2.3522	0.0426	0.9990
Pyrrolidines	−1.9616	0.0142	0.9998
Pyrroles	−2.5122	0.1050	0.9948
Cyclopentanes	−1.9371	0.0194	0.9997
Cyclopentadienes	−2.4005	0.0624	0.9980

For alkane and cyclopentane compounds, which lack these mechanisms, a possible adsorption mode is through the dispersion bond, while pyrrolidines, cyclopentadienes, and pyrroles, which have π electrons, can interact with the surface through π–π interactions. At the same number of atoms, cyclopentadiene and pyrrole compounds showed better stability and a gain of about 10 kJ mol^{-1} compared to their saturated counterparts, cyclopentanes and pyrrolidines, respectively. Interestingly, the pyrrole compounds, which interact better with the graphene surface, show a negative and greater slope in the best linear fit as reported in Table 7.

2.4. Adsorption of 1,2,5-Trimethylpyrrole and Its Oxidized Derivatives on Pristine Graphene Surface

To study the effect of oxidation, which, as described in the introduction, is a key step for the cycloaddition of pyrrole molecules onto carbon allotropes [77,91], 1,2,5-trimethylpyrrole and its oxidized derivatives were adsorbed on the pristine graphene surfaces and their adsorption energies calculated. In Figure 7, ground-state energy structures for TMP, TMP-CHO, and TMP-2CHO can be seen. For all the compounds, the value of the adsorption distance was found to be 3.46 Å. Figure 8 shows the adsorption energies as a function of the number of carbon atoms in the organic adsorbates. As can be seen from the E_{ads} values, the presence of an aldehyde group favors the adsorption process, with a decrease of about 3 kJ mol^{-1} per aldehyde. This means that the oxidation of pyrrole compounds enhances the supramolecular interactions between the latter and the graphene surface, as the oxygen increases the number of π interactions with the conjugated graphene system. Regarding the effect of oxidation, we can conclude that the presence of aldehyde groups improved the adsorption energy for 1,2,5-trimethylpyrrole on the pristine graphene surface.

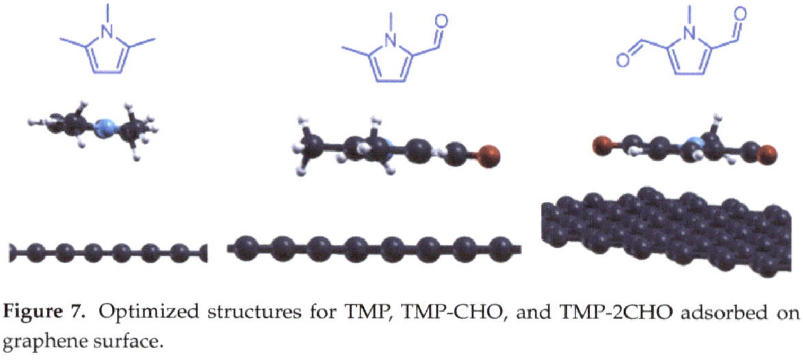

Figure 7. Optimized structures for TMP, TMP-CHO, and TMP-2CHO adsorbed on the pristine graphene surface.

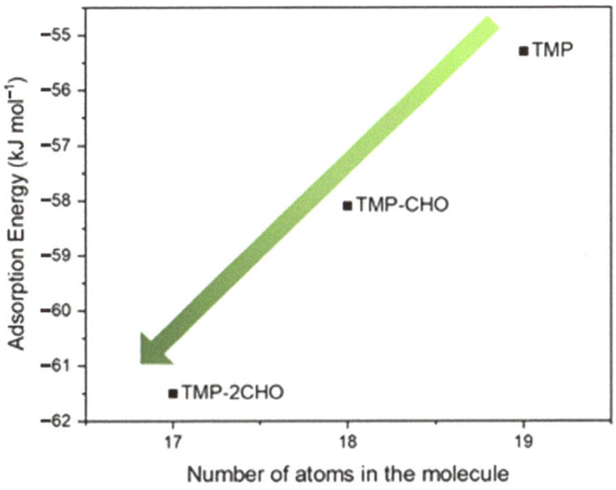

Figure 8. Adsorption energies for TMP, TMP-CHO, and TMP-2CHO on the pristine graphene surface versus the number of atoms in the molecule.

3. Materials and Methods

The specific initial geometries of volatile organic compounds near graphene layer were obtained after molecular mechanics and molecular dynamics simulations using a simulation protocol adopted in previous work [90] about the adsorption process on graphite, graphene surface. These data will be published in a future paper related to the adsorption of single volatile compounds on graphene surface and at larger concentration.

Optimal adsorption configurations were derived using pw.x software, part of the Quantum ESPRESSO suite of codes [92]. This package is widely used to simulate the behavior of materials and molecules, and pw.x software [93] specifically performs Density Functional theory (DFT) calculations related to the electronic structures of materials. A non-empirical generalized gradient approximation functional, namely, Perdew–Burke–Ernzerhof (PBE), was used [94], and standard solid-state ultrasoft pseudopotentials were employed to process the electron–ion interactions for all the atoms [95]. The kinetic energy cutoff of the plane wave basis set was fixed at 60 Ryd. For pristine graphene systems, a $3 \times 3 \times 1$ Monkhorst–Pack set was used to sample the Brillouin zones, while the other simulations were performed at the Γ point. To account for dispersion (Van der Waals) interactions, which, as mentioned in the introduction, are important in describing physisorption on graphene-based systems, the "DFT-D of Grimme" algorithm was used [96].

To model the pristine graphene sheet, a periodic unit cell with dimensions of $6 \times 5 \times 1$ was built. The unit cell contained 60 carbon atoms, and the lattice parameters were set to 12.30 Å, 12.78 Å, and 20.33 Å in the a, b, and c directions, respectively. To prevent any interaction that could introduce errors in the analysis, the c parameter (the height of the box in which the calculation was carried out) was adjusted to 20 Å, ensuring a sufficient separation between the graphene layers.

Regarding the different types of small organic molecules adsorbed on the surface of graphene, the analyzed compounds and their chemical structures are listed in Table 1. For the R group, linear alkyl chains were investigated by increasing the number of carbon atoms from methane to butane; the other molecules were cyclic saturated with cyclopentane, pyrrolidine, unsaturated cyclic cyclopentadiene, and pyrrole.

With regard to adsorption energy, it is important to highlight that to quantify the interaction force between the adsorbate and the investigated surface, adsorption energy (E_{ads}) was calculated as follows:

$$E_{ads} = E_{(S+A)} - E_A - E_S$$

Above, $E_{(S+A)}$ is the total energy of the adsorbate/surface system, E_A is the total energy of the molecule calculated with the same cell and electronic parameters of the whole system, and E_S is the total energy of the investigated surface. As a quantity strictly connected to the thermodynamics of adsorption, the more negative the value, the more favorable the process.

Charge density difference plots were used to visualize the charge transfer and charge disequilibria between atoms from the adsorbate, and surface charge density difference (CDD) maps were calculated using the pp.x software contained in the Quantum ESPRESSO Suite. $\Delta\rho$ was calculated using the following formula:

$$\Delta\rho = \rho_{(S+A)} - \rho_A - \rho_S$$

Above, $\rho_{(S+A)}$ is the charge density of the adsorbate/surface system, ρ_A is the charge density of the molecule (calculated with the same cell and electronic parameters of the whole system), and ρ_S is the charge density of the investigated surface. Following this methodology, $\Delta\rho$ (or, more specifically, its iso-surface) shows the variations in the charge density of the graphene–adsorbate system. In the figures, a difference in charge density is shown in red on an iso-surface on which the accumulation of charge is represented, while blue indicates depletion [97,98].

4. Conclusions

The DFT study of pyrroles and pyrrole derivatives adsorbed on graphene surface revealed that adsorption process is predominantly governed by dispersion forces and π–π bonding interactions. The number of atoms in the molecules considered and the presence of π electrons significantly influence the corresponding adsorption energy. A linear dependence of the adsorption energy is found as a function of the number of atoms in the adsorbed molecules. The pyrrole compounds display more favorable supramolecular interactions with graphene surface. In particular, at the same number of atoms in contact with the graphene surface pyrroles and cyclopentadienes are 10 kJ mol^{-1} more stable than the corresponding unsaturated ones. Furthermore, the presence of aldehydic groups in pyrrole derivatives improves the adsorption energy which is therefore more negative. This study provides valuable insights into supramolecular interactions and their influence on the first step of the adsorption process, contributing to the fundamental understanding of surface modifications for carbon allotropes and their applications in polymer composites.

Overall, the findings of this study offer valuable insights into the complex mechanisms governing adsorption on carbon allotrope surfaces. By elucidating the significant roles of dispersion forces and π–π bonding interactions, this research study contributes to a comprehensive understanding of surface modifications for carbon allotropes and their potential applications in the field of polymer composites. Further study on the adsorption process of these molecules on the graphene surface as single molecules and at higher concentrations will be performed using molecular mechanics and molecular dynamics methods to better understand the contribution of van der Waals interactions in the adsorption process in a more complex supramolecular structure as in previous work [90].

Author Contributions: Conceptualization, M.G. and G.R.; methodology, F.M. and G.R.; software, F.M. and G.R.; validation, F.M., V.B., M.G. and G.R.; formal analysis, F.M. and G.R.; investigation, F.M. and G.R.; resources, F.M., V.B., M.G. and G.R.; data curation, F.M. and G.R.; writing—original draft preparation, F.M. and G.R.; writing—review and editing, F.M., V.B., M.G. and G.R.; visualization, G.R.; supervision, M.G. and G.R.; project administration, M.G. and G.R.; funding acquisition, M.G. and G.R. All authors have read and agreed to the published version of the manuscript.

Funding: This research was funded by Made in Italy–Circular and Sustainable (MICS) Extended Partnership funded by the European Union Next-Generation EU (Piano Nazionale di Ripresa e Resilienza (PNRR)–Missione 4, Componente 2, Investimento 1.3–D.D. 1551.11-10-2022, PE00000004) for financial support. This research was also funded by ICSC—Centro Nazionale di Ricerca in High Performance Computing, Big Data, and Quantum Computing funded by European Union—NextGenerationEU. F.M., V.B. and M.G. gratefully acknowledge BIRLA Carbon for funding the research.

Data Availability Statement: Data are contained within the article.

Acknowledgments: The authors acknowledge CINECA HPC clusters (grant HP10CKOQOB) for the computational resources.

Conflicts of Interest: The authors declare no conflict of interest.

References

1. Magne, T.M.; Vieira, T.D.; Alencar, L.M.R.; Maia, F.F.M.; Gemini-Piperni, S.; Carneiro, S.V.; Fechine, L.M.U.D.; Freire, R.M.; Golokhvast, K.; Metrangolo, P.; et al. Graphene and its derivatives: Understanding the main chemical and medicinal chemistry roles for biomedical applications. *J. Nanostructure Chem.* **2022**, *12*, 693–727. [CrossRef]
2. Criado, A.; Melchionna, M.; Marchesan, S.; Prato, M. The Covalent Functionalization of Graphene on Substrates. *Angew. Chem. Int. Ed.* **2015**, *54*, 10734–10750. [CrossRef] [PubMed]
3. Park, W.; Shin, H.; Choi, B.; Rhim, W.K.; Na, K.; Keun Han, D. Advanced hybrid nanomaterials for biomedical applications. *Prog. Mater. Sci.* **2020**, *114*, 1–110.
4. Liu, S. Cooperative adsorption on solid surfaces. *J. Colloid Interface Sci.* **2015**, *450*, 224. [CrossRef]
5. Freund, H.J. Adsorption of gases on complex: Solid surfaces. *Angew. Chem. Int. Ed.* **1997**, *36*, 452. [CrossRef]
6. Carr, A.J.; Carr, A.; Lee, S.E.; Uysal, A. Ion and water adsorption to graphene and graphene oxide surfaces. *Nanoscale* **2023**, *15*, 14319. [CrossRef]
7. Krishna, R.H.; Chandraprabha, M.N.; Samrat, K.; Murthy, T.P.K.; Manjunatha, C.; Kumar, S.G. Carbon nanotubes and graphene-based materials for adsorptive removal of metal ions—A review on surface functionalization and related adsorption mechanism. *Appl. Surf. Sci. Adv.* **2023**, *16*, 100431.
8. Yang, G.; Li, L.; Lee, W.B.; Ng, M.C. Structure of Graphene and Its Disorders: A Review. *Sci. Technol. Adv. Mater.* **2018**, *19*, 613–648. [CrossRef]
9. Liu, Y.; Ge, Z.; Li, Z.; Chen, Y. High-power instant-synthesis technology of carbon nanomaterials and nanocomposites. *Nano Energy* **2021**, *80*, 1–61.
10. Ali, I.; Pakharukov, Y.; Shabiev, F.K.; Galunin, E.; Safargaliev, R.F.; Vasiljev, S.A.; Ezdin, B.S.; Burakov, A.E.; Alothman, Z.A.; Sillanpaa, M. Preparation of graphene based nanofluids: Rheology determination and theoretical analysis of the molecular interactions of graphene nanoparticles. *J. Mol. Liq.* **2023**, *390*, 122954. [CrossRef]
11. Old 6 Bahiraei, M.; Heshmatian, S. Graphene family nanofluids: A critical review and future research directions. *Energy Convers. Manag.* **2019**, *196*, 1222–1256. [CrossRef]
12. Kumar, K.V.; Gadipelli, S.; Wood, B.; Ramisetty, K.A.; Stewart, A.A.; Howard, C.A.; Brett, D.J.L.; Rodriguez-Reinoso, F. Characterization of the adsorption site energies and heterogeneous surfaces of porous materials. *J. Mater. Chem. A* **2019**, *7*, 10104. [CrossRef]
13. Lin, L.C.; Thirumavalavan, M.; Wang, Y.T.; Lee, J.F. Surface area and pore size tailoring of mesoporous silica materials by different hydrothermal treatments and adsorption of heavy metal ions. *Colloids Surf. A Physicochem. Eng. Asp.* **2010**, *319*, 223. [CrossRef]
14. Dong, D.M.; Hua, X.Y.; Li, Y.; Li, Z.H. Lead adsorption to metal oxides and organic material of freshwater surface coatings determined using a novel selective extraction method. *Environ. Pollut.* **2002**, *119*, 317. [CrossRef]
15. Zhang, W.; Wu, C.M.; Li, Y.R. Determination of the surface properties and adsorption states of nanoporous materials using the zeta adsorption isotherm. *Phys. Chem. Chem. Phys.* **2023**, *25*, 22669. [CrossRef]
16. Mao, K.; Gao, L.S.; Lv, X.C.; Gao, D.D.; Lv, J.Z.; Bai, M.L. Numerical simulation of forced convection heat transfer mechanism and comprehensive performance on hydrophobic structure surface. *Int. J. Therm. Sci.* **2023**, *184*, 107895. [CrossRef]
17. Kubota, T.; Watanabe, N.; Ohtsuka, S.; Iwasaki, T.; Ono, K.; Iriye, Y.; Samukawa, S. Numerical simulation on neutral beam generation mechanism by collision of positive and negative chlorine ions with graphite surface. *J. Phys. D Appl. Phys.* **2011**, *44*, 125203. [CrossRef]
18. Zhao, D.; Liu, X.Q. Study on the microscopic mechanism of adsorption and diffusion of hydrocarbon oil drops on coal surface using molecular dynamics simulations. *Int. J. Quantum. Chem.* **2023**, *123*, e27229. [CrossRef]
19. Zhao, L.F.; Liu, W.L.; Shen, Y.Z.; Xu, Y.J.S.; Jiang, B.; Tao, J. Ice adhesion mechanism on the patterned surface of aluminum matrix and array graphene based on molecular dynamics simulations. *Appl. Phys. Lett.* **2023**, *123*, 061602. [CrossRef]
20. James, J.N.; Sholl, D.S. Theoretical studies of chiral adsorption on solid surfaces. *J. Colloid Interface Sci.* **2008**, *13*, 60. [CrossRef]
21. Amrhar, O.; Lee, H.S.; Lgaz, H.; Berisha, A.; Ebenso, E.E.; Cho, Y.J. Computational insights into the adsorption mechanisms of anionic dyes on the rutile TiO_2 (110) surface: Combining SCC-DFT tight binding with quantum chemical and molecular dynamics simulations. *J. Mol. Liq.* **2023**, *377*, 121554. [CrossRef]
22. Dehmani, Y.; Lgaz, H.; Alrashdi, A.A.; Lamhasni, T.; Abouarnadasse, S.; Chung, I.M. Phenol adsorption mechanism on the zinc oxide surface: Experimental, cluster DFT calculations, and molecular dynamics simulations. *J. Mol. Liq.* **2021**, *324*, 114993. [CrossRef]
23. Yi, P.; Zuo, X.Z.; Lang, D.; Wu, M.; Dong, W.; Chen, Q.; Zhang, L.J. Competitive adsorption of methanol co-solvent and dioctyl phthalate on functionalized graphene sheet: Integrated investigation by molecular dynamics simulations and quantum chemical calculations. *J. Colloid Interface Sci.* **2021**, *605*, 354. [CrossRef] [PubMed]

24. Tang, H.; Zhang, S.Y.; Huang, T.L.; Cui, F.Y.; Xing, B.S. pH-Dependent adsorption of aromatic compounds on graphene oxide: An experimental, molecular dynamics simulation and density functional theory investigation. *J. Hazard. Mater.* **2020**, *395*, 122680. [CrossRef] [PubMed]
25. Sun, C.Z.; Liu, M.; Bai, B.F. Molecular simulations on graphene-based membranes. *Carbon* **2019**, *153*, 481–494. [CrossRef]
26. Qiu, Z.Y.; Li, P.; Li, Z.Y.; Yang, J.L. Atomistic Simulations of Graphene Growth: From Kinetics to Mechanism. *Acc. Chem. Res.* **2018**, *51*, 728–735. [CrossRef]
27. Ganazzoli, F.; Raffaini, G. Classical atomistic simulations of protein adsorption on carbon nanomaterials. *Curr. Opin. Colloid Interface Sci.* **2019**, *41*, 11–26. [CrossRef]
28. Yang, J.; Yang, X.N.; Li, Y.P. Molecular simulation perspective of liquid-phase exfoliation, dispersion, and stabilization for graphene. *Curr. Opin. Colloid Interface Sci.* **2015**, *20*, 339–345. [CrossRef]
29. Thapa, R.; Ugwumadu, C.; Nepal, K.; Trembly, J.; Drabold, D.A. Ab Initio Simulation of Amorphous Graphite. *Phys. Rev. Lett.* **2022**, *128*, 236402. [CrossRef]
30. Cutini, M.; Civalleri, B.; Corno, M.; Orlando, R.; Brandenburg, J.G.; Maschio, L.; Ugliengo, P. Assessment of Different Quantum Mechanical Methods for the Prediction of Structure and Cohesive Energy of Molecular Crystals. *J. Chem. Theory Comput.* **2016**, *12*, 3340. [CrossRef]
31. Brann, M.R.; Ma, X.Y.; Sibener, S.J. Isotopic Enrichment Resulting from Differential Condensation of Methane Isotopologues Involving Non-equilibrium Gas-Surface Collisions Modeled with Molecular Dynamics Simulations. *J. Phys. Chem. C* **2023**, *127*, 13286–13294. [CrossRef]
32. Jiang, M.M.; Zhang, C.; Liao, N.B.; Zhao, T.C.; Ge, J.Q. Self-cantilever phenomenon of graphite/graphenes micro/nano structure: Experiment and DFT simulation analysis. *Appl. Surf. Sci.* **2021**, *545*, 149009. [CrossRef]
33. Raffaini, G.; Catauro, M. Surface Interactions between Ketoprofen and Silica-Based Biomaterials as Drug Delivery System Synthesized. Sol-Gel: A Molecular Dynamics Study. *Materials* **2022**, *15*, 2759. [CrossRef]
34. Catauro, M.; Barrino, F.; Dal Poggetto, G.; Milazzo, M.; Blanco, I.; Ciprioti, S.V. Structure, drug absorption, bioactive and antibacterial properties of sol-gel SiO_2/ZrO_2 materials. *Ceram. Int.* **2020**, *46*, 29459. [CrossRef]
35. Johnson, R.P.; Jeong, Y.I.; Choi, E.; Chung, C.W.; Kang, D.H.; Oh, S.O.; Suh, H.; Kim, I. Biocompatible Poly(2-hydroxyethyl methacrylate)-b-poly(L-histidine) Hybrid Materials for pH-Sensitive Intracellular Anticancer Drug Delivery. *Adv. Funct. Mater.* **2012**, *22*, 1058. [CrossRef]
36. Xie, Y.H.; Kong, Y.; Gao, H.J.; Soh, A.K. Molecular dynamics simulation of polarizable carbon nanotubes. *Comput. Mater. Sci.* **2007**, *40*, 460–465. [CrossRef]
37. Li, J.; Liu, Q.H.; Flores, R.A.; Lemmon, J.; Bligaard, T. DFT simulation of the X-ray diffraction pattern of aluminum-ion-intercalated graphite used as the cathode material of the aluminum-ion battery. *Phys. Chem. Chem. Phys.* **2020**, *22*, 5969–5975. [CrossRef]
38. Pal, G.; Kumar, S. Modeling of carbon nanotubes and carbon nanotube-polymer composites. *Prog. Aerosp. Sci.* **2016**, *80*, 33–58. [CrossRef]
39. Raffaini, G.; Elli, S.; Ganazzoli, F. Computer simulation of bulk mechanical properties and surface hydration of biomaterials. *J. Biomed. Mater. Res. A* **2006**, *77A*, 618–626. [CrossRef]
40. Guo, W.M.; Bai, Q.S.; Dou, Y.H.; Wang, H.F.; Chen, S.D. Molecular Dynamics Study on the Effects of Substrate Grain Boundaries on the Adsorption State of Graphene: Implications for Nanoscale Lubrication. *ACS Appl. Nano Mater.* **2023**, *6*, 8093. [CrossRef]
41. Li, Q.L.; Zhu, S.M.; Hao, G.Z.; Hu, Y.B.; Wu, F.; Jiang, W. Fabrication of thermoresponsive metal-organic nanotube sponge and its application on the adsorption of endocrine-disrupting compounds and pharmaceuticals/personal care products: Experiment and molecular simulation study. *Environ. Pollut.* **2021**, *273*, 116466. [CrossRef]
42. Salehi, A.; Rash-Ahmadi, S. Effect of adsorption, hardener, and temperature on mechanical properties of epoxy nanocomposites with functionalized graphene: A molecular dynamics study. *J. Mol. Graph. Model.* **2022**, *117*, 108311. [CrossRef]
43. Mantero, S.; Piuri, D.; Montevecchi, F.M.; Vesentini, S.; Ganazzoli, F.; Raffaini, G. Albumin adsorption onto pyrolytic carbon: A molecular mechanics approach. *J. Biomed. Mater. Res.* **2002**, *59*, 329–339. [CrossRef]
44. Li, B.; Mi, C.W. Atomistic insights on the adsorption of long-chain undecane molecules on carbon nanotubes: Roles of chirality and surface hydroxylation. *Diam. Relat. Mater.* **2023**, *133*, 109706. [CrossRef]
45. Taheri, Z.; Pour, A.N. Studying of the adsorption and diffusion behaviors of methane on graphene oxide by molecular dynamics simulation. *J. Mol. Model.* **2021**, *27*, 59. [CrossRef] [PubMed]
46. Comer, J.; Chen, R.; Poblete, H.; Vergara-Jaque, A.; Riviere, J.E. Predicting Adsorption Affinities of Small Molecules on Carbon Nanotubes Using Molecular Dynamics Simulation. *ACS Nano* **2015**, *9*, 11761–11774. [CrossRef] [PubMed]
47. Raffaini, G.; Ganazzoli, F. Separation of chiral nanotubes with an opposite handedness by chiral oligopeptide adsorption: A molecular dynamics study. *J. Chromatogr. A* **2016**, *1425*, 221–230. [CrossRef] [PubMed]
48. Barinov, N.A.; Prokhorov, V.V.; Dubrovin, E.V.; Klinov, D.V. AFM visualization at a single-molecule level of denaturated states of proteins on graphite. *Colloids Surf. B-Biointerfaces* **2016**, *146*, 777–784. [CrossRef]
49. Karajanagi, S.S.; Yang, H.C.; Asuri, P.; Sellitto, E.; Dordick, J.S.; Kane, R.S. Protein-assisted solubilization of single-walled carbon nanotubes. *Langmuir* **2006**, *22*, 1392–1395. [CrossRef]
50. Hasnip, P.J.; Refson, K.; Probert MI, J.; Yates, J.R.; Clark, S.J.; Pickard, C.J. Density Functional Theory in the Solid State. *Philos. Trans. R. Soc. A Math. Phys. Eng. Sci.* **2014**, *372*. [CrossRef]

51. Ostovari, F.; Hasanpoori, M.; Abbasnejad, M.; Saleh, M.A. DFT calculations of graphene monolayer in presence of Fe dopant and vacancy. *Phys. B Condens. Matter.* **2018**, *541*, 6–13. [CrossRef]
52. Gecim, G.; Ozekmekci, M. A density functional theory study of molecular H_2S adsorption on (4,0) SWCNT doped with Ge, Ga and B. *Surf. Sci.* **2021**, *711*, 121876. [CrossRef]
53. Kamedulski, P.; Kaczmarek-Kedziera, A.; Lukaszewicz, J. Influence of intermolecular interactions on the properties of carbon nanotubes. *Bull. Mater. Sci* **2018**, *41*, 76. [CrossRef]
54. Lejaeghere, K.; Bihlmayer, G.; Björkman, T.; Blaha, P.; Blügel, S.; Blum, V.; Caliste, D.; Castelli, I.E.; Clark, S.J.; Dal Corso, A.; et al. Reproducibility in Density Functional Theory Calculations of Solids. *Science* **2016**, *351*, aad3000. [CrossRef]
55. Mittal, G.; Dhand, V.; Rhee, K.Y.; Park, S.J.; Lee, W.R. A Review on Carbon Nanotubes and Graphene as Fillers in Reinforced Polymer Nanocomposites. *J. Ind. Eng. Chem.* **2015**, *21*, 11–25. [CrossRef]
56. Al-Hartomy, O.A.; Al-Ghamdi, A.A.; Al-Salamy, F.; Dishovsky, N.; Slavcheva, D.; El-Tantawy, F. Properties of Natural Rubber-Based Composites Containing Fullerene. *Int. J. Polym. Sci.* **2012**, *2012*, 967276. [CrossRef]
57. Khuntawee, W.; Sutthibutpong, T.; Phongphanphanee, S.; Karttunen, M.; Wong-ekkabut, J. Molecular dynamics study of natural rubber-fullerene composites: Connecting microscopic properties to macroscopic behavior. *Phys. Chem. Chem. Phys.* **2019**, *21*, 19403–19413. [CrossRef] [PubMed]
58. Kitjanon, J.; Khuntawee, W.; Phongphanphanee, S.; Sutthibutpong, T.; Chattham, N.; Karttunen, M.; Wong-ekkabut, J. Nanocomposite of Fullerenes and Natural Rubbers: MARTINI Force Field Molecular Dynamics Simulations. *Polymers* **2021**, *13*, 4044. [CrossRef]
59. Rong, M.Z.; Zhang, M.Q.; Ruan, W.H. Surface Modification of Nanoscale Fillers for Improving Properties of Polymer Nanocomposites: A Review. *Mater. Sci. Technol.* **2006**, *22*, 787–796. [CrossRef]
60. Shen, X.; Wang, Z.; Wu, Y.; Liu, X.; Kim, J.K. Effect of Functionalization on Thermal Conductivities of Graphene/Epoxy Composites. *Carbon N. Y.* **2016**, *108*, 412–422. [CrossRef]
61. Patti, A.; Russo, P.; Acierno, D.; Acierno, S. The Effect of Filler Functionalization on Dispersion and Thermal Conductivity of Polypropylene/Multi Wall Carbon Nanotubes Composites. *Compos. Part B Eng.* **2016**, *94*, 350–359. [CrossRef]
62. Shen, C.; Oyadiji, S.O. The Processing and Analysis of Graphene and the Strength Enhancement Effect of Graphene-Based Filler Materials: A Review. *Mater. Today Phys.* **2020**, *15*, 100257. [CrossRef]
63. Tang, B.; Hu, G.; Gao, H.; Hai, L. Application of Graphene as Filler to Improve Thermal Transport Property of Epoxy Resin for Thermal Interface Materials. *Int. J. Heat Mass Transf.* **2015**, *85*, 420–429. [CrossRef]
64. Zhou, Z.; Wang, S.; Zhang, Y.; Zhang, Y. Effect of Different Carbon Fillers on the Properties of PP Composites: Comparison of Carbon Black with Multiwalled Carbon Nanotubes. *J. Appl. Polym. Sci.* **2006**, *102*, 4823–4830. [CrossRef]
65. Kwon, Y.J.; Park, J.B.; Jeon, Y.P.; Hong, J.Y.; Park, H.S.; Lee, J.U. A Review of Polymer Composites Based on Carbon Fillers for Thermal Management Applications: Design, Preparation, and Properties. *Polymers* **2021**, *13*, 1312. [CrossRef]
66. Kim, H.; Abdala, A.A.; MacOsko, C.W. Graphene/Polymer Nanocomposites. *Macromolecules* **2010**, *43*, 6515–6530. [CrossRef]
67. Dai, J.-F.; Wang, G.-J.; Ma, L.; Wu, C.-K.; Wang, G.-J.; Dai, J.-F.; Wang, G.-J.; Ma, L.; Wu, C.-K. Surface Porperties of Graphene: Relationship to Graphene-Polymer composites. *Rev. Adv. Mater. Sci.* **2015**, *40*, 60–71.
68. Cadek, M.; Coleman, J.N.; Ryan, K.P.; Nicolosi, V.; Bister, G.; Fonseca, A.; Nagy, J.B.; Szostak, K.; Béguin, F.; Blau, W.J. Reinforcement of Polymers with Carbon Nanotubes: The Role of Nanotube Surface Area. *Nano Lett.* **2004**, *4*, 353–356. [CrossRef]
69. Kim, S.W.; Kim, T.; Kim, Y.S.; Choi, H.S.; Lim, H.J.; Yang, S.J.; Park, C.R. Surface modifications for the effective dispersion of carbon nanotubes in solvents and polymers. *Carbon* **2012**, *50*, 3–33. [CrossRef]
70. Eitan, A.; Jiang, K.Y.; Dukes, D.; Andrews, R.; Schadler, L.S. Surface modification of multiwalled carbon nanotubes: Toward the tailoring of the interface in polymer composites. *Chem. Mater.* **2003**, *15*, 3198–3201. [CrossRef]
71. Zhao, W.; Song, C.H.; Pehrsson, P.E. Water-soluble and optically pH-sensitive single-walled carbon nanotubes from surface modification. *J. Am. Chem. Soc.* **2002**, *124*, 12418–12419. [CrossRef] [PubMed]
72. Sun, J.T.; Hong, C.Y.; Pan, C.Y. Surface modification of carbon nanotubes with dendrimers or hyperbranched polymers. *Polym. Chem.* **2011**, *2*, 998. [CrossRef]
73. Verma, B.; Balomajumder, C. Surface modification of one-dimensional Carbon Nanotubes: A review for the management of heavy metals in wastewater. *Environ. Technol. Innov.* **2020**, *17*, 100596. [CrossRef]
74. Atif, M.; Afzaal, I.; Naseer, H.; Abrar, M.; Bongiovanni, R. Review-Surface Modification of Carbon Nanotubes: A Tool to Control Electrochemical Performance. *ECS J. Solid State Sci. Technol.* **2020**, *9*, 041009. [CrossRef]
75. Barbera, V.; Bernardi, A.; Palazzolo, A.; Rosengart, A.; Brambilla, L.; Galimberti, M. Facile and Sustainable Functionalization of Graphene Layers with Pyrrole Compounds. *Pure Appl. Chem.* **2018**, *90*, 253–270. [CrossRef]
76. Galimberti, M.; Barbera, V.; Guerra, S.; Conzatti, L.; Castiglioni, C.; Brambilla, L.; Serafini, A. Biobased Janus Molecule for the Facile Preparation of Water Solutions of Few Layer Graphene Sheets. *RSC Adv.* **2015**, *5*, 81142–81152. [CrossRef]
77. Barbera, V.; Brambilla, L.; Milani, A.; Palazzolo, A.; Castiglioni, C.; Vitale, A.; Bongiovanni, R.; Galimberti, M. Domino Reaction for the Sustainable Functionalization of Few-Layer Graphene. *Nanomaterials* **2019**, *9*, 44. [CrossRef]
78. Galimberti, M.; Barbera, V.; Citterio, A.; Sebastiano, R.; Truscello, A.; Valerio, A.M.; Conzatti, L.; Mendichi, R. Supramolecular Interactions of Carbon Nanotubes with Biosourced Polyurethanes from 2-(2,5-Dimethyl-1H-Pyrrol-1-Yl)-1,3-Propanediol. *Polymer* **2015**, *63*, 62–70. [CrossRef]

79. Prioglio, G.; Agnelli, S.; Conzatti, L.; Balasooriya, W.; Schrittesser, B.; Galimberti, M. Graphene Layers Functionalized with a Janus Pyrrole-Based Compound in Natural Rubber Nanocomposites with Improved Ultimate and Fracture Properties. *Polymers* **2020**, *12*, 944. [CrossRef]
80. Dindorkar, S.S.; Sinha, N.; Yadav, A. Comparative Study on Adsorption of Volatile Organic Compounds on Graphene, Boron Nitride and Boron Carbon Nitride Nanosheets. *Solid State Commun.* **2023**, *359*, 115021. [CrossRef]
81. Lazar, P.; Karlický, F.; Jurecka, P.; Kocman, M.; Otyepková, E.; Šafářová, K.; Otyepka, M. Adsorption of Small Organic Molecules on Graphene. *J. Am. Chem. Soc.* **2013**, *135*, 6372–6377. [CrossRef] [PubMed]
82. Lee, J.; Min, K.A.; Hong, S.; Kim, G. Ab Initio Study of Adsorption Properties of Hazardous Organic Molecules on Graphene: Phenol, Phenyl Azide, and Phenylnitrene. *Chem. Phys. Lett.* **2015**, *618*, 57–62. [CrossRef]
83. Xu, H.; Guan, D.; Ma, L. The bio-inspired heterogeneous single-cluster catalyst Ni100–Fe_4S_4 for enhanced electrochemical CO_2 reduction to CH_4. *Nanoscale* **2023**, *15*, 2756. [CrossRef] [PubMed]
84. Knorr, L. Einwirkung des Diacetbernsteinsäureesters auf Ammoniak und primäre Aminbasen. *Chem. Ber.* **1885**, *18*, 299. [CrossRef]
85. Paal, C. Synthese von Thiophen-und Pyrrolderivaten. *Chem. Ber.* **1885**, *18*, 367. [CrossRef]
86. Barbera, V.; Galimberti, M.; Giannini, L.; Naddeo, S. Process for the Preparation of Diketones and Pyrrole Derivatives. Patent Application n. PCT/IB2022/062453, 19 December 2022.
87. Prioglio, G.; Naddeo, S.; Giese, U.; Barbera, V.; Galimberti, M. Bio-Based Pyrrole Compounds Containing Sulfur Atoms as Coupling Agents of Carbon Black with Unsaturated Elastomers. *Nanomaterials* **2023**, *13*, 2761. [CrossRef]
88. Magaletti, F.; Margani, F.; Monti, A.; Dezyani, R.; Prioglio, G.; Giese, U.; Barbera, V.; Galimberti, M.S. Adducts of Carbon Black with a Biosourced Janus Molecule for Elastomeric Composites with Lower Dissipation of Energy. *Polymers* **2023**, *15*, 3120. [CrossRef]
89. Pirelli Tyre; Annual Report: The Human Dimension. 2020, 106. Available online: https://corporate.pirelli.com/var/files2020/EN/PDF/PIRELLI_ANNUAL_REPORT_2020_ENG.pdf (accessed on 4 October 2022).
90. Raffaini, G.; Ganazzoli, F. Surface topography effects in protein adsorption on nanostructured carbon allotropes. *Langmuir.* **2013**, *29*, 4883. [CrossRef]
91. Barbera, V.; Brambilla, L.; Porta, A.; Bongiovanni, R.; Vitale, A.; Torrisi, G.; Galimberti, M. Selective Edge Functionalization of Graphene Layers with Oxygenated Groups by Means of Reimer-Tiemann and Domino Reimer-Tiemann/Cannizzaro Reactions. *J. Mater. Chem. A* **2018**, *6*, 7749–7761. [CrossRef]
92. Giannozzi, P.; Baroni, S.; Bonini, N.; Calandra, M.; Car, R.; Cavazzoni, C.; Ceresoli, D.; Chiarotti, G.L.; Cococcioni, M.; Dabo, I.; et al. QUANTUM ESPRESSO: A Modular and Open-Source Software Project for Quantum Simulations of Materials. *J. Phys. Condens. Matter* **2009**, *21*, 395502. [CrossRef]
93. QuantumEspresso PWscf User's Guide (v.7.2). Available online: https://www.quantum-espresso.org/Doc/pw_user_guide/ (accessed on 4 October 2022).
94. Perdew, J.P.; Burke, K.; Ernzerhof, M. Generalized Gradient Approximation Made Simple. *Phys. Rev. Lett.* **1996**, *77*, 3865–3868. [CrossRef] [PubMed]
95. Prandini, G.; Marrazzo, A.; Castelli, I.E.; Mounet, N.; Marzari, N. Precision and Efficiency in Solid-State Pseudopotential Calculations. *NPJ Comput. Mater.* **2018**, *4*, 72. [CrossRef]
96. Grimme, S.; Antony, J.; Ehrlich, S.; Krieg, H. A Consistent and Accurate Ab Initio Parametrization of Density Functional Dispersion Correction (DFT-D) for the 94 Elements H-Pu. *J. Chem. Phys.* **2010**, *132*. [CrossRef] [PubMed]
97. Zhuoran, L.; Xu, H.; Xu, W.; Peng, B.; Zhao, C.; Xie, M.; Lv, X.; Gao, Y.; Hu, K.; Fang, Y.; et al. Quasi-Topological Intercalation Mechanism of $Bi_{0.67}NbS_2$ Enabling 100 C Fast-Charging for Sodium-Ion Batteries. *Adv. Energy Mater.* **2023**, *13*, 202300790.
98. Xiao, W.; Kiran, G.K.; Yoo, K.; Kim, J.H.; Xu, H. The Dual-Site Adsorption and High Redox Activity Enabled by Hybrid Organic-Inorganic Vanadyl Ethylene Glycolate for High-Rate and Long-Durability Lithium–Sulfur Batteries. *Small* **2023**, *19*, 202206750. [CrossRef]

molecules

MDPI

Article

Integrated Approach of Life Cycle Assessment and Experimental Design in the Study of a Model Organic Reaction: New Perspectives in Renewable Vanillin-Derived Chemicals

Chiara Ruini [1,*], Erika Ferrari [2], Caterina Durante [2], Giulia Lanciotti [2], Paolo Neri [1], Anna Maria Ferrari [1,3] and Roberto Rosa [1,3,4]

1 Department of Sciences and Methods for Engineering, University of Modena and Reggio Emilia, v. Amendola 2, 42122 Reggio Emilia, Italy; paolo.neri@unimore.it (P.N.); annamaria.ferrari@unimore.it (A.M.F.); roberto.rosa@unimore.it (R.R.)
2 Department of Chemical and Geological Sciences, University of Modena and Reggio Emilia, v. Campi 103, 41125 Modena, Italy; erika.ferrari@unimore.it (E.F.); caterina.durante@unimore.it (C.D.)
3 Interdepartmental Center En&Tech, University of Modena and Reggio Emilia, Tecnopolo di Reggio Emilia, Piazzale Europa 1, 42123 Reggio Emilia, Italy
4 Department of Economics, Science, Engineering and Design, University of San Marino Republic, v. Consiglio dei Sessanta 99, 47891 Dogana, San Marino
* Correspondence: chiara.ruini@unimore.it

Abstract: This work is focused on performing a quantitative assessment of the environmental impacts associated with an organic synthesis reaction, optimized using an experimental design approach. A nucleophilic substitution reaction was selected, employing vanillin as the substrate, a phenolic compound widely used in the food industry and of pharmaceutical interest, considering its antioxidant and antitumoral potential. To carry out the reaction, three different solvents have been chosen, namely acetonitrile (ACN), acetone (Ace), and dimethylformamide (DMF). The syntheses were planned with the aid of a multivariate experimental design to estimate the best reaction conditions, which simultaneously allow a high product yield and a reduced environmental impact as computed by Life Cycle Assessment (LCA) methodology. The experimental results highlighted that the reactions carried out in DMF resulted in higher yields with respect to ACN and Ace; these reactions were also the ones with lower environmental impacts. The multilinear regression models allowed us to identify the optimal experimental conditions able to guarantee the highest reaction yields and lowest environmental impacts for the studied reaction. The identified optimal experimental conditions were also validated by experimentally conducting the reaction in those conditions, which indeed led to the highest yield (i.e., 93%) and the lowest environmental impacts among the performed experiments. This work proposes, for the first time, an integrated approach of DoE and LCA applied to an organic reaction with the aim of considering both conventional metrics, such as reaction yield, and unconventional ones, such as environmental impacts, during its lab-scale optimization.

Keywords: organic synthesis; LCA; DoE; ReCiPe2016; vanillin

Citation: Ruini, C.; Ferrari, E.; Durante, C.; Lanciotti, G.; Neri, P.; Ferrari, A.M.; Rosa, R. Integrated Approach of Life Cycle Assessment and Experimental Design in the Study of a Model Organic Reaction: New Perspectives in Renewable Vanillin- Derived Chemicals. *Molecules* **2024**, *29*, 2132. https://doi.org/10.3390/molecules29092132

Academic Editors: Fabio Ganazzoli and Giuseppina Raffaini

Received: 29 March 2024
Revised: 26 April 2024
Accepted: 29 April 2024
Published: 3 May 2024

1. Introduction

Vanillin (4-hydroxy-3-methoxybenzaldehyde) is a flavor used worldwide in food manufacturing and a precious fragrance agent in cosmetics [1]. Vanillin can be chemically synthesized starting from eugenol, ferulic acid (from rice), coniferyl alcohol (from spruce tree lignin), and guaiacol. Although these approaches can have economic advantages, chemical synthesis is typically characterized by high environmental impacts. A more sustainable approach is provided by biotechnology-based manufacturing [2] or direct extraction from plants rich in its content in their essential oils, mainly *Vanilla plantifolia* L., *Vanilla tahitensis* L., and *Vanilla pompona* L. [3]. Currently, in view of the circular economy, recycling, and exploitation of natural wastes, direct extraction has received reduced interest in favor of more sustainable bio-production from lignin [4]. Indeed, among all the lignin-derived fine chemicals, vanillin represents the only commercialized mono-aromatic compound obtained on a large scale [5]. Nowadays, more than 20% of the overall production of vanillin starts from lignin compounds [6], representing an alternative option for biomass feedstock exploitation [7]. Vanillin derived from lignin has the advantage of being a renewable compound that does not compete with food sources, thus not leading to food security issues, the latter being recognized as a top priority worldwide [7].

Vanillin stands out for a plethora of properties and applications. Firstly, it is a safe compound with well-established therapeutic activities, such as antitumor [8,9], antimutagenic [10], antidiabetic [11], antioxidant [12], and antimicrobial [13] properties.

From a chemical point of view, vanillin can be classified as a bifunctional aromatic compound since it bears two reactive groups, namely the aldehyde and the phenol groups, that can be used for the synthesis of several second-generation vanillin-derived chemicals. Additionally, these compounds can be exploited as building-block monomers for preparing polymeric materials with tuned properties for tailored applications, including coatings, adhesives, elastomers, and optoelectronic materials [14]. For these reasons, vanillin has the potential to be a renewable building block in the cutting-edge chemical industry. Among the chemical reactions that may involve the phenolic group in polymer synthesis, alkylation is particularly interesting in order to add new reactive groups, such as epoxides and vinyl, or simply to bridge vanillin units by an aliphatic/aromatic linkage. The alkylation of the phenolic oxygen is mostly performed through a nucleophilic substitution reaction carried out under basic conditions in the presence of an alkylating agent with a good leaving group, typically a bromide. In order to enhance the conversion, a large excess of the alkylating agent can be used, as well as a long reaction time and a high temperature [15], the latter few all being conditions that affect both the economic burden and the environmental impact of the overall process. As these aspects are of utmost importance, new approaches exploiting Design of Experiment (DoE) and Life Cycle Assessment (LCA) methodologies can be applied to improve the process, both in terms of high reaction yields and low environmental impacts. Indeed, DoE represents an extremely efficient tool to comprehensively understand the effect of selected factors (e.g., solvent, substrate, reactants/reagents, temperature, time, etc.) on the outcome of a given chemical reaction, typically quantified by the sole yield parameter, without any considerations related to the associated environmental impacts. In this latter regard, LCA represents a prominent methodology to quantify, in a trustworthy manner, the potential environmental impacts associated with the whole life cycle of a given product or process [16], and its use has also been recognized as being of paramount importance in the early design stages of a lab-scale procedure [17]. The as-calculated environmental impacts can therefore be implemented among the responses to be analyzed by DoE.

However, some examples can be found in the literature combining the use of LCA and Experimental Design to better evaluate a process by also accounting for its environmental performances. Their fields of application mainly fall within materials science and nanomaterials [18,19], or within the optimization of industrial processes not directly related to synthetic organic chemistry [20,21]. On the other hand, the present study aims to investigate a model organic synthesis process by concurrently employing DoE and LCA methodologies.

Different approaches can be employed in the design of experiments; however, when the explored factors are characterized by distinct natures (quantitative and qualitative), a conventional experimental design [22] is not able to simultaneously examine them, hence a D-optimal response-surface design emerges as the most appropriate option as it enables the consideration of irregular experimental domains and various types of variables [23].

Concerning the assessment of the environmental impacts, LCA methodology can be used to reliably optimize the environmental performances of chemical reactions by comparing the same synthesis conducted with slightly different variations (e.g., different solvents, different reagent amounts, or different reaction times). This approach can help to highlight the synthetic conditions with lower environmental impacts.

In this work, the integrated LCA/DoE approach was applied to a model alkylation reaction (Figure 1) performed on vanillin in order to both improve the conversion and reduce the impacts associated to environmental issues, i.e., wastes, energy consumption, and use of renewable resources. Midpoint (i.e., problem-oriented) results obtained from LCA were exploratorily analyzed by means of Principal Component Analysis (PCA) [24] to gain initial insights and an overarching understanding of the variables under investigation. Subsequently, LCA endpoint (i.e., damage-oriented) results, alongside reaction yield, served as response variables in the Design of Experiments. The obtained dataset was inspected using multilinear regression analysis to obtain the best reaction conditions able to maximize the reaction yield while minimizing the associated environmental impacts.

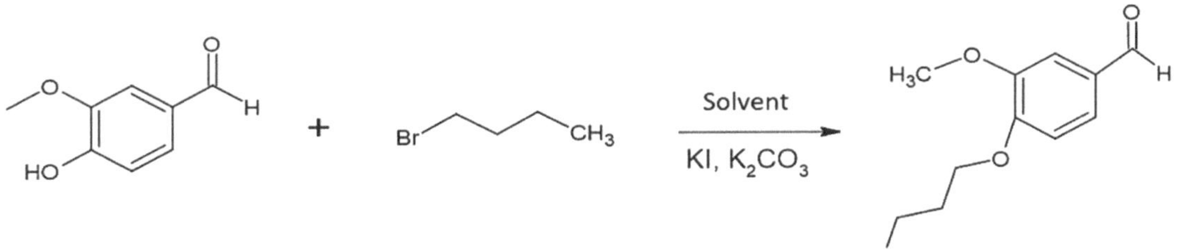

Figure 1. Scheme of the investigated reaction: O-alkylation of vanillin with 1-bromobutane.

The aim of this work is therefore to propose, for the first time, an integrated approach of DoE and LCA applied to an organic synthesis. In this way, it should be possible to best optimize a chemical reaction, an organic one in the case of this work, obtaining the optimal reaction conditions to concurrently maximize the reaction yield and minimize the environmental impacts associated with that synthesis by significantly reducing the number of experiments needed.

2. Results and Discussion

2.1. *Synthesis*

The model reaction selected for the investigation is a nucleophilic substitution performed in a basic environment (K_2CO_3) in three different solvents: acetonitrile (ACN), dimethylformamide (DMF), and acetone (Ace). The presence of KI allows the substitution of bromide, providing a better leaving group (iodine). According to the experimental plan, the reaction was performed in different conditions, as reported in Table 1, and the yields of the final product for each run are summarized in Figure 2 and Table S1 in the Supplementary Information.

Table 1. DoE Experimental Plan (* replicates of the center points).

Experiment	Solvent	Time (h)	KI	K_2CO_3	BrBu
R1	DMF	8	2	1	1
R2	ACN	24	2	1	2
R3	Ace	24	2	1	1
R4 *	DMF	16	1	1.5	1.5
R5 *	DMF	16	1	1.5	1.5
R6	Ace	8	0	1	2
R7 *	Ace	16	1	1.5	1.5
R8 *	Ace	16	1	1.5	1.5

Table 1. *Cont.*

Experiment	Solvent	Time (h)	KI	K_2CO_3	BrBu
R9	DMF	24	0	2	2
R10	Ace	8	0	2	1
R11	ACN	8	2	2	1
R12	Ace	24	2	2	1
R13	ACN	24	0	2	2
R14 *	ACN	16	1	1.5	1.5
R15	DMF	24	0	1	1
R16 *	ACN	16	1	1.5	1.5
R17	Ace	8	2	1	2
R18	ACN	8	0	1	1
R19	DMF	8	2	2	2

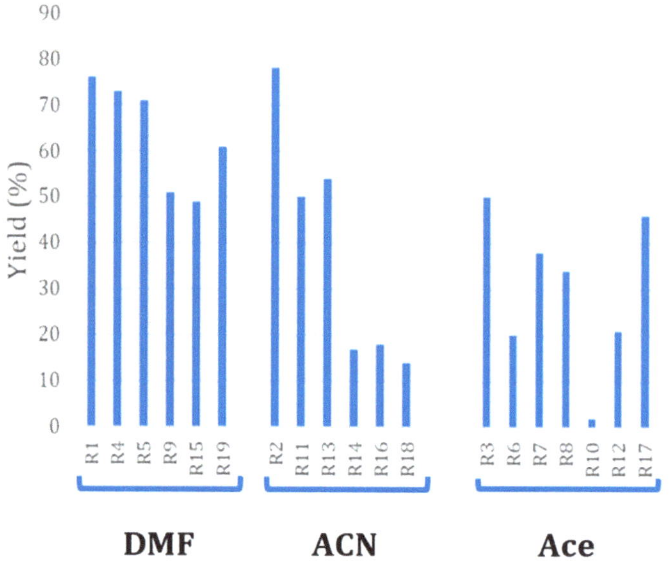

Figure 2. Bar diagram plot representing the yield of pure product (3-methoxy-4butoxy-benzaldehyde) in each experiment. Results are grouped according to the used solvent.

A total of 26% of all experiments (5/19) provided a yield > 60%, and among them, four out of five runs were carried out in DMF and only one in ACN. None of the synthesis performed in acetone allowed a yield > 60%. A total of 47% of the experiments permitted a yield above 50%. Among them, 59% were carried out in DMF, 33% in ACN, and only 11% in Acetone. All the other experiments (10 out of 19) gave low yields (<50%) and were mostly carried out in Acetone (six out of ten).

Although it is not possible to directly compare the experiments, since they were performed in different conditions according to the experimental plan, it is possible to derive some interesting outcomes. Firstly, all the experiments carried out in DMF resulted in a higher averaged yield with respect to ACN and acetone (67.5% vs. 38.5% and 27.5% for ACN and acetone, respectively). The higher yield levels reached using DMF could be attributed to a higher solubility of reactants and products in the reaction medium as well as the higher temperature at which the reaction was carried out. The higher solubility of carbonate and iodide in ACN rather than in Ace, providing a more basic environment and higher availability of the good leaving group, may account for the greater yields observed in this solvent. Secondly, none of the experiments performed without KI reached a yield greater than 60%, suggesting that the presence of this salt is an important factor in triggering the reaction.

2.2. Green Chemistry Metrics

To preliminarily better understand the environmental acceptability of this reaction, some green chemistry metrics were determined. The ones considered are mass intensity (MI), atom economy (AE), atom efficiency (AEf), carbon efficiency (CE), reaction mass efficiency (RME), EcoScale, and environmental factor (E-Factor), calculated according to [25–28]. The results are reported in Table 2 and their graphical representation is reported in Figures S1–S4 in the Supplementary Information. The results of these green chemistry metrics are coherent with the yields obtained for the nineteen performed reactions. In particular, the MI is higher for reactions with lower yields (such as R10, the reaction with the lowest yield and the highest MI value) and lower for reactions with higher yields (as in the case of R1, R2, and R4). The same trend is also exhibited in the AEf and E-Factor results. For the CE parameter, the results are higher for reactions with higher yields, meaning that there is a much better conversion of reagents into the final product. The values obtained for the EcoScale parameter range from 19% to 57%, even in cases following the yield trend (higher yields for higher EcoScale results). Altogether, these results confirm that reactions with higher yields result in better parameters, i.e., reactions that are greener than the others. However, since the as-calculated metrics are focused on the sole synthesis phase, thus neglecting several contributions related to the production and transport of reagents, solvents, and the electricity mix employed, as well as equipment, emissions, and waste treatments, their environmental performances need to be assessed in a more reliable way by applying a more holistic methodology such as LCA.

Table 2. Green Chemistry metrics results for the nineteen performed reactions.

Experiment	Mass Intensity (MI) g/g	Atom Economy (AE) %	Atomy Efficiency (Aef) %	Carbon Efficiency (CE) %	Reaction Mass Efficiency (RME) %	EcoScale %	E-Factor (g/g)
R1	54.90	71.97	54.69	72.90	51.60	56.00	0.94
R2	76.72	71.97	56.13	58.31	37.93	57.00	1.64
R3	117.79	71.97	35.98	50.13	36.08	43.00	1.77
R4	63.24	71.97	52.53	58.04	39.49	54.50	1.53
R5	61.28	71.97	51.10	59.44	40.37	53.50	1.48
R6	284.15	71.97	14.39	15.16	9.85	28.00	9.15
R7	159.95	71.97	27.35	31.16	21.07	37.00	3.75
R8	174.93	71.97	24.47	28.47	19.30	35.00	4.18
R9	86.53	71.97	36.70	36.18	23.55	43.50	3.25
R10	2648.43	71.97	1.44	2.12	1.52	19.00	64.87
R11	123.89	71.97	35.98	48.37	34.81	43.00	1.87
R12	299.04	71.97	15.11	19.41	13.81	28.50	6.24
R13	108.03	71.97	38.86	39.84	25.98	45.00	2.85
R14	366.46	71.97	12.23	13.55	9.24	26.50	9.82
R15	86.79	71.97	35.26	47.60	34.24	42.50	1.92
R16	341.12	71.97	12.95	14.72	9.97	27.00	9.03

Table 2. *Cont.*

Experiment	Mass Intensity (MI) g/g	Atom Economy (AE) %	Atomy Efficiency (Aef) %	Carbon Efficiency (CE) %	Reaction Mass Efficiency (RME) %	EcoScale %	E-Factor (g/g)
R17	130.50	71.97	33.10	33.30	21.60	41.00	3.63
R18	470.05	71.97	10.08	12.10	8.67	25.00	10.53
R19	70.68	71.97	43.90	45.49	29.72	48.50	2.36

2.3. *Life Cycle Assessment*

The potential environmental impacts associated with the organic synthesis of 4-butoxy-3-methoxybenzaldehyde at midpoint level (i.e., problem-oriented) are depicted in Figure 3 as a heat map showing the relative percentage impacts among the nineteen syntheses assessed for each of the eighteen impact categories.

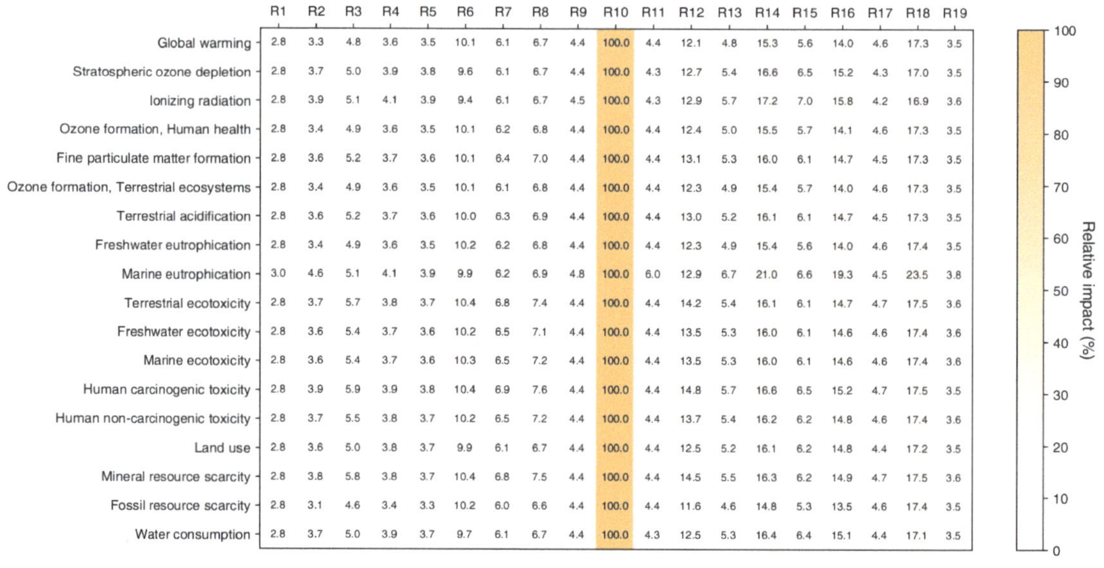

Figure 3. Relative percentage environmental impacts at midpoint level (ReCipe, 2016; H) associated with the production of 1 g of 4-butoxy-3-methoxybenzaldehyde for each of the nineteen reactions, referring to the eighteen impact categories considered.

The quantitative results are instead detailed in Table S2 in the Supplementary Information. These results have been calculated for the synthesis of 1 g of product for each of the nineteen reactions. As can be seen, for every impact category considered by the ReCiPe 2016 midpoint method, the reaction with the highest relative impact is reaction R10, conducted in Acetone with a reaction time of 8 h and without using KI as a reagent. This reaction is the one with the lowest yield (2%) and, as a direct consequence of that, it is also the synthesis with the highest environmental impact. Indeed, with respect to the other reactions, the obtainment of 1 g of the final product would require higher amounts of reagents and higher energy consumption, thus necessarily leading to higher environmental impacts.

By grouping the results of the eighteen impact categories into the opportune damage categories (i.e., Human health, Ecosystems, and Resources) and referring to them at the point at which the environmental effects potentially occur, the endpoint results are obtained. The endpoint Single Score results (thus obtained after normalization and weighting operations performed by the impact assessment method selected) associated with the preparation of 1 g of 4-butoxy-3-methoxybenzaldehyde for each of the nineteen reactions are reported in Table 3. The environmental impacts are expressed in terms of eco-indicator points, Pt (the smaller its value is, the lower the potential environmental impact of that product or process results).

Table 3. Endpoint Single Score results (ReCiPe, 2016; H) for the synthesis of 1 g or the production of 1 g of 4-butoxy-3-methoxybenzaldehyde for each of the nineteen reactions.

Reaction	Yield (%)	Human Health (Pt)	Ecosystems (Pt)	Resources (Pt)
R1	76	5.99×10^{-1}	2.11×10^{-2}	2.01×10^{-2}
R2	78	7.51×10^{-1}	2.55×10^{-2}	2.18×10^{-2}
R3	50	1.10×10^{0}	3.69×10^{-2}	3.24×10^{-2}
R4	73	7.88×10^{-1}	2.72×10^{-2}	2.42×10^{-2}
R5	71	7.64×10^{-1}	2.64×10^{-2}	2.35×10^{-2}
R6	20	2.17×10^{0}	7.63×10^{-2}	7.36×10^{-2}
R7	38	1.35×10^{0}	4.62×10^{-2}	4.24×10^{-2}
R8	34	1.48×10^{0}	5.09×10^{-2}	4.67×10^{-2}
R9	51	9.46×10^{-1}	3.33×10^{-2}	3.16×10^{-2}
R10	2	2.14×10^{0}	7.55×10^{-1}	7.19×10^{-1}
R11	50	9.38×10^{-1}	3.30×10^{-2}	3.16×10^{-2}
R12	21	2.75×10^{0}	9.26×10^{-2}	8.12×10^{-2}
R13	54	1.09×10^{0}	3.72×10^{-2}	3.20×10^{-2}
R14	17	3.38×10^{0}	1.17×10^{-1}	1.05×10^{-1}
R15	49	1.26×10^{0}	4.30×10^{-2}	3.63×10^{-2}
R16	18	3.08×10^{0}	1.07×10^{-1}	9.51×10^{-2}
R17	46	9.80×10^{-1}	3.44×10^{-2}	3.33×10^{-2}
R18	14	3.71×10^{0}	1.31×10^{-1}	1.25×10^{-1}
R19	61	7.58×10^{-1}	2.67×10^{-2}	2.54×10^{-2}

From Table 3, it can immediately be seen that the most affected damage category is Human Health, independently from the reaction considered, followed by Ecosystems and then Resources. Even in this case, as for the midpoint results, it is reaction R10 that had the highest environmental impact. Instead, the reactions with the highest yields (i.e., R1, R2, R4, and R5, with a yield > 70%) are the ones with the lowest environmental impact; again, a high yield can be translated into a lower consumption of reagents, together with reduced energy demand, to obtain 1 g of the final product.

2.4. Midpoint PCA Analysis

To comprehensively understand the impact of selected factors, namely the solvent, substrate, reactants/agent, and reaction time, on both the yield of a nucleophilic substitution reaction on vanillin and its environmental implications, a D-optimal response-surface design was employed [23]. The dataset was inspected using multilinear regression analysis to obtain the best reaction conditions able to maximize yield while minimizing environmental impact. LCA midpoint results (Table S2) were subjected to principal component analysis (PCA) to gain insights into the relationships between different experiments and to identify the factors that most influence environmental impact. Data were autoscaled to ensure equal weighting of all midpoint variables and the PCA model was developed using two principal components (PCs), which explained a cumulative variance of 99%. From a synergistic evaluation of the scores and loadings plots, reported in Figures 4a and 4b, respectively, it is possible to note that the first principal component (PC1) clearly distinguished experiment R10 (conducted in acetone) from the other experiments (Figure 4a).

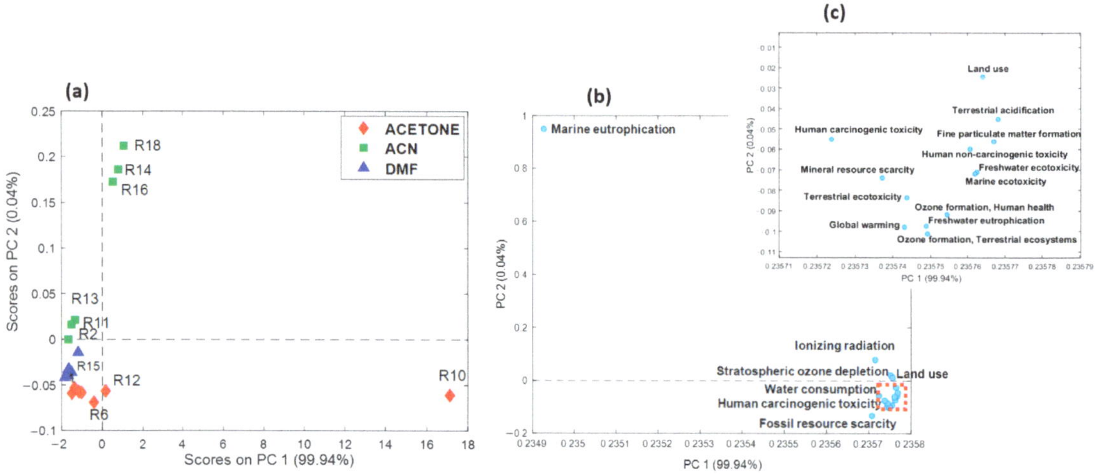

Figure 4. Score (**a**) and loading (**b**) plots of PCA applied on the LCA midpoint dataset. (**c**) Zoom-in of the loadings present within the red dashed area of (**b**).

This experiment, with the highest PC1 scores, presented a higher environmental impact across all midpoint categories (positive PC1 loadings, Figure 4b,c). The second principal component (PC2) distinguished the products of experiments R14, R16, and R18 (conducted in acetonitrile) from the others. These experiments had higher PC2 scores, associated with a higher impact on marine eutrophication (highest positive PC2 score, Figure 4b). A decreasing trend in PC2 scores was observed from products in acetonitrile to those in DMF and finally to those in acetone, with the exception of experiment R10 in acetone. The Marine Eutrophication impact category had higher PC2 loadings for products obtained in acetonitrile, with a decrease in products obtained with acetone (except for experiment R10). Therefore, PCA identified experiment R10 as having the overall highest environmental impact, and marine eutrophication was identified as an impact category particularly sensitive to the type of solvent used.

2.5. D-Optimal Design Results

In Figure 5, the LCA Single Score endpoint results obtained for each reaction conducted according to the DoE experimental plan were reported. In the previous Table 3, the yields and Single Score endpoint results are reported together.

In order to get a deep overview of the influence of all the investigated factors, four different regression models were developed separately for the four responses: yield (y1), human health (y2), ecosystems (y3), and resources (y4). The explained variance for each model and the significant coefficients are reported in Table 4.

Regarding the yield, a positive significant coefficient indicates that higher values of the corresponding factor led to higher yields. Conversely, a negative coefficient indicates that the lowest value of the factor results in the maximum yield. This is the opposite of the other LCA impact data responses, as their optimal values should be as low as possible.

For yield, both the DMF and KI terms are positive and significant, suggesting that the highest yield is achieved when using DMF as a solvent and a high KI content. The other three LCA responses (human health, ecosystems, and resources) exhibit similar trends. Considering the significant coefficients, time, Br, and KI, K_2CO_3 content and the interaction between KI and K_2CO_3 play key roles in predicting LCA responses. Although the solvent exerts a profound impact on the yield of the reactions, from the MLR results, it appears to be insignificant based on LCA data compared to the other terms. To achieve the lowest possible LCA data values, it seems crucial to use longer reaction times and higher Br quantities. Determining the optimal values for KI and K_2CO_3 requires considering their interaction term, as significant interactions impact the optimum. In multivariate models with significant interactions, surface plots are crucial for understanding the effect of factors. The optimum may depend on the interaction between factors, not just on their individual effects. Therefore, surface plots illustrating the effects of KI and K_2CO_3 on the three LCA data responses are presented in Figure 6a–c. Across all cases, the best compromise to achieve optimal results (lowest values) seems to be with the highest value for KI and the lowest value for K_2CO_3.

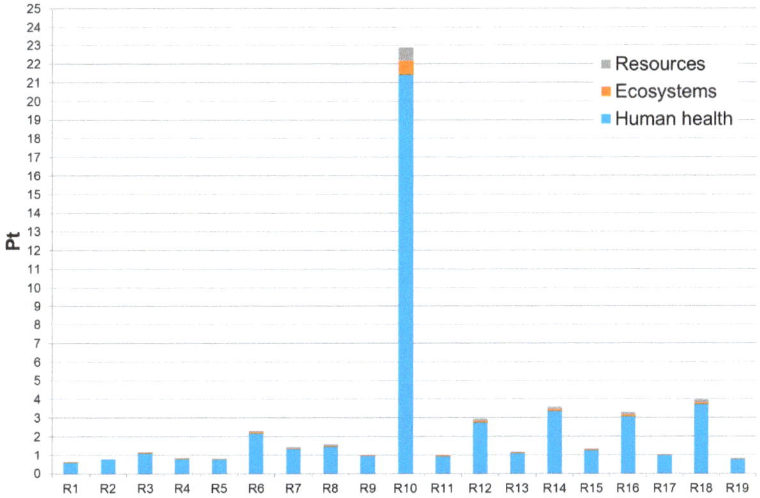

Figure 5. Endpoint single score results (ReCiPe, 2016; H, A) for the synthesis of 1 g of 4-butoxy-3-methoxybenzaldehyde for each of the nineteen reactions (R1–R19).

Table 4. MLR regression coefficients.

		y1: Yield (R^2: 87%)	y2: Human Health (R^2: 94%)	y3: Ecosystem (R^2: 94%)	y4: Resources (R^2: 94%)
b_1	solvent	DMF	n.s	n.s	n.s
b_2	time	n.s.	(−)	(−)	(−)
b_3	Br	n.s.	(−)	(−)	(−)
b_4	KI	(+)	(−)	(−)	(−)
b_5	K_2CO_3	n.s.	(+)	(+)	(+)
b_4b_5	KI*K_2CO_3	n.s.	(−)	(−)	(−)

n.s.: not-significant term; (−): lower level; (+): higher level.

Therefore, in this preliminary phase of the study, it is hypothesized that to obtain the optimal results in terms of highest yield and lowest LCA data, the following conditions should be applied: DMF for the conduction reaction, a high molar ratio of potassium iodide to vanillin, a high molar ratio of Br to vanillin, a long reaction time, and a low molar ratio of K_2CO_3 to vanillin. Considering these optimal conditions, the theoretical yield predicted using the MLR model is 95.8% ± 8.7%. In order to validate the MLR model, an additional run was carried out following the conditions reported in Table 5. As reported in Table 5, the experimentally obtained yield for the additional synthesis performed was 93%, which is in the predicted variability range.

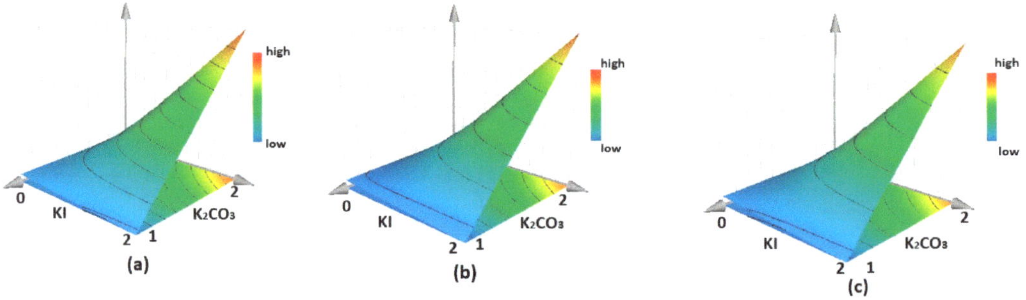

Figure 6. Surface plots showing the effects of KI and K_2CO_3 on human health (**a**), ecosystems (**b**), and resources (**c**) responses.

Table 5. Environmental impact assessment results at Endpoint level (Single Score, ReCiPe 2016; H) obtained considering the optimal conditions predicted by the MLR model, and the yield experimentally determined on the synthesis performed in the optimal conditions predicted.

Reaction	**Solvent**	**Time (h)**	**Br**	**KI**	**K_2CO_3**	**Yield (%)**	**Human Health (Pt)**	**Ecosystems (Pt)**	**Resources (Pt)**
Optimal Reaction	DMF	24	2	2	1	93	3.84×10^{-1}	1.38×10^{-2}	1.48×10^{-2}

Using these optimal conditions and considering the experimental yield of 93%, the environmental impacts, at endpoint level, were calculated and reported in Table 5.

With respect to the endpoint results associated with the nineteen reactions, previously reported in Table 3, the values characterizing the optimal reaction are indeed the lowest ones, independently by the damage category considered (i.e., Human Health, Ecosystems, and Resources). In particular, the experimentally obtained increase in the reaction yield (up to 93%) led to a reduction in the overall potential environmental impacts ranging from 35.5% (with respect to R1) up to 98.2% (with respect to R10).

3. Materials and Methods

All the chemicals and solvents were purchased from Merck (Merck KGaA, Darmstadt, Germany) in the highest purity grade available and used without further purification unless otherwise specified. Nuclear Magnetic Resonance (NMR) spectra were recorded on a Bruker Biospin FT-NMR AVANCE III HD (600 MHz) spectrometer equipped with a CryoProbe BBO H&F 5 mm in inverse detection (Bruker corporation 40 Manning Road Billerica, MA, USA). The nominal frequencies were 150.90 MHz for ^{13}C and 600.13 MHz for ^{1}H, respectively.

3.1. General Synthesis of 4-Butoxy-3-methoxybenzaldehyde

KI and K_2CO_3 were suspended in the selected solvent using a two-neck round-bottom flask (50 mL) and kept under magnetic stirring for 5 min. The mixture was then warmed up at the temperature specified in Table S1 and 1-bromobutane was added, followed by vanillin (van). The reaction was maintained at the same temperature under continuous stirring for the planned reaction time. The final reaction mixture was filtered off to get rid of the salts, and the solvent was removed under reduced pressure by a rotary evaporator. The crude was a light-yellow sticky oil. Yield was estimated by weighing the product and performing NMR analysis using $CDCl_3$ as a solvent (20 mg of crude were used). A representative example of the ^{1}H NMR spectrum of the product is shown in Figure S5 in the Supplementary Information.

All the specific reaction details for each run are reported in the Experimental plan in Tables 1 and S1.

3.2. Experimental Design Procedure

The optimization of the studied nucleophilic substitution reaction was systematically approached using DoE techniques, aimed at assessing the impact of selected parameters on reaction yield while simultaneously minimizing the environmental footprint. Three solvents (i.e., *N,N*-dimethylformamide (DMF), acetone (Ace), and acetonitrile (ACN)) were specifically chosen for conducting the reaction, each associated with distinct reaction temperatures tailored to their respective boiling points.

In addition to solvent variation, the DoE also investigated the following factors: (1) reaction duration (hours), (2) molar ratio of potassium iodide to vanillin, (3) molar ratio of potassium carbonate to vanillin, and (4) molar ratio of bromobutane to vanillin.

The experimental settings were planned following a D-Optimal Design approach [23], with a center point replicated twice for each solvent. Experiments were randomized and yield and LCA endpoint results were used as responses to be modelled. A linear model was fitted, and the G-efficiency criterion [29] was utilized to determine the optimal experimental layout. This criterion evaluates the performance of D-optimal designs across varying numbers of design runs, with each design being computed based on D-optimality principles, aiming to maximize the determinant of the information matrix related to the candidate set. In particular, G-efficiency is computed as detailed in Equation (1), where p is the number of terms in the model, n is the number of runs in the design, and $d_{\max}$ is the maximum relative prediction variance across the candidate set according to Equation (2), where x is a row in the candidate set and X is the selected design.

$$\text{G-effinciency: } 100 \times p/n \times d_{\max} \quad (1)$$

$$d = \mathrm{x}(\mathrm{X}'\mathrm{X})^{-1}\mathrm{x}' \quad (2)$$

The factors under investigation, along with their corresponding levels (range of variability), are reported in Table 6.

Table 6. Factors investigated by D-Optimal Design.

Factors	Abbreviation	Type	Actual Value
Solvent (x_1)	Ace	Qualitative	Acetone
	ACN		Acetonitrile
	DMF		*N,N*-dimethylformamide
Reaction time (x_2)	t	Quantitative	8–16–24 h
KI/van molar ratio (x_3)	KI	Quantitative	0–1–2
K_2CO_3/van molar ratio (x_4)	K_2CO_3	Quantitative	1–1.5–2
BrBu/van molar ratio (x_5)	BrBu	Quantitative	1–1.5–2

In summary, a total of 19 experiments, reported in Table 1, were carried out and a multilinear regression model (MLR) was built to develop a predictive model for the chosen response. The applied experimental design allowed the estimation of the coefficients of the mathematical model reported in the following Equation (3), where y represents the response variable (reaction yield or endpoint LCA results refer to human health, ecosystems, or resources areas of protection, AoP), b_i are the linear coefficients, and b_{ij} are the coefficients of the interactions. The significance of each term was computed at a significance level of 5%.

Modde 13.0.2 software was utilized to plan the D-Optimal design and to compute the response surface models.

$$y = b_0 + b_1x_1 + b_2x_2 + b_3x_3 + b_4x_4 + b_5x_5 + b_{23}x_2x_3 + b_{24}x_2x_4 + b_{25}x_2x_5 + b_{34}x_3x_4 + b_{35}x_3x_5 + b_{45}x_4x_5 \quad (3)$$

3.3. *Life Cycle Assessment (LCA)*

LCA was applied according to the ISO14040-14044 [30,31], as detailed hereafter.

Goal and scope definition

Goal definition

The goal of this study was to quantify the potential environmental impacts associated with the organic lab-scale synthesis of 4-butoxy-3-methoxybenzaldehyde, from "cradle to gate", thus from raw materials extraction up to the isolation of the desired product.

System, functional unit, and function of the system

The system object of this study is the chemical synthesis of the viscous oil 4-butoxy-3-methoxybenzaldehyde in order to use its environmental impact data as responses for the experimental design approach. The functional unit selected for this study is 1 g of the product obtained after the synthesis and the workup procedures. The system boundaries consider the chemical synthesis of 4-butoxy-3-methoxybenzaldehyde, followed by the workup and purification phase to obtain the final product. The flowchart summarizing the system boundaries is reported in Figure 7.

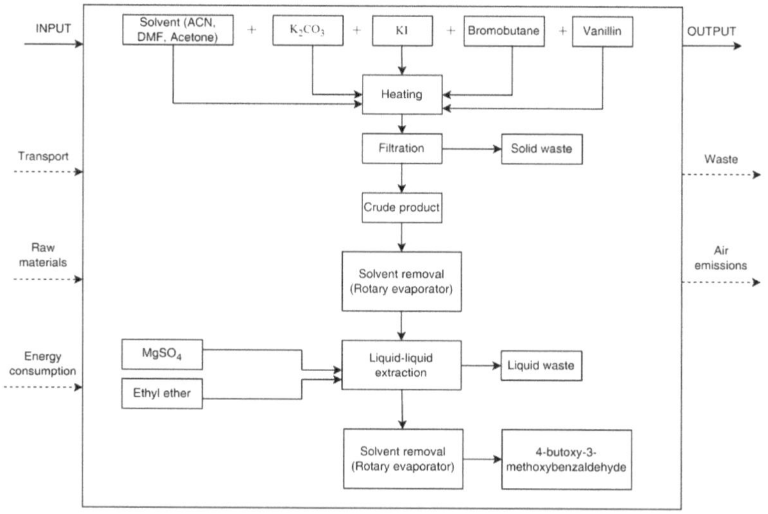

Figure 7. Flowchart summarizing the system boundaries considered in the LCA analysis.

3.4. *Life Cycle Inventory and Life Cycle Impact Assessment (LCIA)*

The data for the LCI were mostly primary data, collected from the experimental activity performed by some of the authors on a laboratory scale. The modelling of the processes was done employing datasets from the Ecoinvent database (EID, version 3.9.1). In particular, an attributional approach was followed, employing the "Allocation at the point of substitution" (i.e., APOS) system model.

The chemicals not present in the Ecoinvent database, such as Vanillin and Bromobutane, were modelled, respectively, according to the synthesis proposed by Taber et al. [32] and Williamson et al. [33]. Regarding transportation, 100 km was considered for the transport contributions. In particular, road freight transport by diesel EURO 6 lorries was assumed with two different lorry capacities of 3.5–7.5 and 16–32 t, respectively, for transportation of reagents and small laboratory equipment and large laboratory equipment. The potential emissions that could have happened during the chemical synthesis were considered, especially the working losses, Lw [34], which were considered and calculated as detailed in Equation (4).

$$L_W = \frac{V}{V_m}\left(\frac{273.15}{T}\right)\left(\frac{P_i^{sat}}{760}\right)(MW)K_N K_P \quad (4)$$

The equation is described as follows: V is the volume of the chemical (l), Vm is the molar volume (l) of ideal gas at 0 °C and 1 atm, T is the average temperature (K), Pisat is the vapor pressure of the liquid (mmHg), MW is the molecular weight of the chemical (g/mol), K_N is the turnover factor (dimensionless and equal to 1 in the present study), and K_P is the working loss product factor (dimensionless), equal to 1 for organic liquids.

A total of 99% of each emitted substance was considered to be retained by an aspiration system associated with an activated carbon filter. The inventory of the plants and laboratory equipment necessary for the synthesis process is detailed in Tables S3–S18. The inventory for the synthesis of vanillin is detailed in Tables S19–S20. The inventory for the synthesis of Bromobutane is detailed in Tables S21–S23. The complete inventories, for each of the 19 runs that were experimentally performed regarding the chemical synthesis of the product 4-butoxy-3-methoxybenzaldehyde, are detailed in Tables S24–S42. The inventories were modelled in SimaPro 9.5.0.1 [35]. The Life Cycle Impact Assessment (LCIA) phase was conducted by using the global scale-oriented method ReCiPe2016, both at midpoint and endpoint levels, with a hierarchist (H) perspective and average weighting set (A) [36]. This method is one of the most widely accepted and applied global methods, comprising a high number of impact categories [37].

4. Conclusions

A nucleophilic substitution reaction was performed in a basic environment (K_2CO_3) in three different solvents (i.e., *N,N*-dimethylformamide (DMF), acetone (Ace), and acetonitrile (ACN)), employing vanillin as a substrate and bromobutane as an alkylating agent. The reaction was conducted in the presence of KI to allow the substitution of bromide, providing a better leaving group (i.e., iodine). Nineteen reactions were experimentally carried out according to the experimental plan obtained by using DoE techniques, aimed at assessing the impact of selected parameters on maximizing reaction yield while simultaneously minimizing environmental footprint. The parameters considered were the type of solvent used, reaction duration (hours), molar ratio of potassium iodide to vanillin, molar ratio of potassium carbonate to vanillin, and molar ratio of bromobutane to vanillin. Based on primary data obtained from the laboratory experiments, an LCA study was conducted on all nineteen reactions. The environmental impacts were obtained, both at midpoint and endpoint levels, and they were used as a further response for a D-optimal design study, together with the experimentally determined yields. Looking at the experimental results, all the reactions carried out in DMF resulted in a higher average yield with respect to ACN and Ace. Moreover, none of the experiments performed without KI reached a yield greater than 60%, suggesting that the presence of this salt is an important factor in triggering the reaction. This was confirmed by analyzing the LCA results. Indeed, both midpoint and endpoint results highlighted that the reaction with the lower yield (i.e., R10) is the one conducted without the KI salt and using acetone as a solvent. This also resulted in the highest environmental impact for R10. The results from the LCA analysis were then used as a response, along with the reaction yield, for a D-optimal study. The results obtained confirmed that the highest yield is achieved when DMF is used as the solvent, employing a high KI content. The other three LCA responses (human health, ecosystems, and resources) exhibit similar trends. Considering these results, some optimal experimental conditions were predicted by the multilinear regression model developed: DMF as a solvent, a high molar ratio of potassium iodide to vanillin, a high molar ratio of Br to vanillin, a long reaction time, and a low molar ratio of K_2CO_3 to vanillin. The theoretical yield predicted considering these conditions is 95.8% ± 8.7%. To confirm the predicted optimal conditions, an additional run was carried out following the conditions reported in Table 5. The obtained yield was 93%.

A validating LCA analysis confirmed that the optimal experimental conditions, together with the experimentally obtained yield of 93%, allow us to obtain the lowest potential environmental impacts, with significant reductions up to −98.2%, as calculated at the endpoint level as a single score. This outcome confirms the validity of the experimental design and its ability to predict optimal conditions by performing a reduced number of experiments.

This work proposes, for the first time, an integrated approach of DoE and LCA applied to a model organic reaction by concurrently considering conventional metrics, such as reaction yield, and metrics that are typically neglected during lab-scale optimization, i.e., associated environmental impacts.

Supplementary Materials: The following supporting information can be downloaded at: https://www.mdpi.com/article/10.3390/molecules29092132/s1, Figures S1–S4: green chemistry metrics; Figure S5: NMR spectra; Table S1: experimental details; Table S2: LCA midpoint results; Tables S3–S42: LCI inventory tables. References [32,33,38] are cited in the supplementary materials.

Author Contributions: Conceptualization, E.F. and R.R.; methodology, E.F., C.D., R.R. and C.R.; software, C.D., C.R., G.L. and P.N.; validation, C.D. and C.R.; formal analysis, G.L. and C.R.; investigation, G.L. and E.F.; resources, E.F., C.D., A.M.F. and R.R.; data curation, E.F., C.D. and C.R.; writing—original draft preparation, C.R., E.F. and C.D.; writing—review and editing, E.F., C.D., C.R. and R.R.; visualization, E.F., C.D. and R.R.; supervision, E.F., A.M.F. and R.R. All authors have read and agreed to the published version of the manuscript.

Funding: This research received no external funding.

Institutional Review Board Statement: Not applicable.

Informed Consent Statement: Not applicable.

Data Availability Statement: The raw data supporting the conclusions of this article will be made available by the authors on request.

Conflicts of Interest: The authors declare no conflicts of interest.

References

1. Sinha, A.K.; Sharma, U.K.; Sharma, N. A comprehensive review on vanilla flavor: Extraction, isolation and quantification of vanillin and other constituents. *Int. J. Food Sci. Nutr.* **2008**, *59*, 299–326. [CrossRef] [PubMed]
2. van den Heuvel, R.H.H.; Fraaije, M.W.; Laane, C.; van Berkel, W.J.H.; Heuvel, R.H.H.V.D.; Berkel, W.J.H.V. Enzymatic synthesis of vanillin. *J. Agric. Food Chem.* **2001**, *49*, 2954–2958. [CrossRef] [PubMed]
3. Priefert, H.; Rabenhorst, J.; Steinbüchel, A. Biotechnological production of vanillin. *Appl. Microbiol. Biotechnol.* **2001**, *56*, 296–314. [CrossRef] [PubMed]
4. Silpa, V.; Athira, V.A.; Nandulal, A.M. Industrial crops and props. *Ind. Crops Props* **2023**, *200 Pt B*, 116839. [CrossRef]
5. Holladay, J.; Bozell, J.; White, J.; Johnson, D. Top Value-Added Chemicals from Biomass. *ACS Sustain. Chem. Eng.* **2016**, *4*, 35–46. [CrossRef]
6. Li, H.; Chen, X.; Xiong, L.; Zhang, L.; Chen, X.; Wang, C.; Huang, C.; Chen, X. Production, separation, and characterization of high purity xylobiose from enzymatic hydrolysis of alkaline oxidation pretreated sugarcane bagasse. *Bioresour. Technol.* **2020**, *299*, 122625. [CrossRef] [PubMed]
7. Harvey, B.G.; Sahagun, C.M.; Guenthner, A.J.; Groshens, T.J.; Cambrea, L.R.; Reams, J.T.; Mabry, J.M. A High-Performance Renewable Thermosetting Resin Derived from Eugenol. *ChemSusChem* **2014**, *7*, 1964–1969. [CrossRef] [PubMed]
8. Rakoczy, K.; Szlasa, W.; Saczko, J.; Kulbacka, J. Therapeutic role of vanillin receptors in cancer. *Adv. Clin. Exp. Med.* **2021**, *30*, 1293–1301. [CrossRef] [PubMed]

9. Naz, H.; Tarique, M.; Khan, P.; Luqman, S.; Ahamad, S.; Islam, A.; Ahmad, F.; Hassan, M.I. Evidence of vanillin binding to CAMKIV explains the anti-cancer mechanism in human hepatic carcinoma and neuroblastoma cells. *Mol. Cell Biochem.* **2018**, *438*, 35–45. [CrossRef]
10. King, A.A.; Shaughnessy, D.T.; Mure, K.; Leszczynska, J.; Ward, W.O.; Umbach, D.M.; Xu, Z.; Ducharme, D.; Taylor, J.A.; Demarini, D.M.; et al. Antimutagenicity of cinnamaldehyde and vanillin in human cells: Global gene expression and possible role of DNA damage and repair. *Mutat. Res.* **2007**, *616*, 60–69. [CrossRef]
11. Salau, V.F.; Erukainure, O.L.; Olofinsan, K.O.; Msomi, N.Z.; Ijomone, O.M.; Islam, M.S. Vanillin improves glucose homeostasis and modulates metabolic activities linked to type 2 diabetes in fructose-streptozotocin induced diabetic rats. *Arch. Physiol. Biochem.* **2024**, *130*, 169–182. [CrossRef] [PubMed]
12. Karathanos, T.V.; Mourtzinos, I.; Yannakopoulou, K.; Andrikopoulos, N.K. Study of the solubility, antioxidant activity and structure of inclusion complex of vanillin with β-cyclodextrin. *Food Chem.* **2007**, *101*, 652–658. [CrossRef]
13. Fitzgerald, D.J.; Stratford, M.; Gasson, M.J.; Ueckert, J.; Bos, A.; Narbad, A. Mode of antimicrobial action of vanillin against Escherichia coli, Lactobacillus plantarum and Listeria innocua. *J. Appl. Microbiol.* **2004**, *97*, 104–113. [CrossRef] [PubMed]
14. Qiang, H.; Wang, J.; Liu, H.; Zhu, Y. From vanillin to biobased aromatic polymer. *Polym. Chem.* **2023**, *14*, 4255–4274. [CrossRef]
15. Foyer, G.; Chanfi, B.H.; Boutevin, B.; Caillol, S.; David, G. New Method for the Synthesis of Formaldehyde-Free Phenolic Resins from Lignin-Based Aldehyde Precursors. *Eur. Polym. J.* **2016**, *74*, 296–309. [CrossRef]
16. Kirchai, R.E., Jr.; Gregory, J.R.; Olivetti, E.A. Environmental life-cycle assessment. *Nat. Mater.* **2017**, *16*, 693–697. [CrossRef]
17. Pini, M.; Rosa, R.; Neri, P.; Ferrari, A.M. LCA Application to Chemical Synthesis at Laboratory Scale. In *Life Cycle Assessment in the Chemical Product Chain: Challenges, Methodological Approaches and Applications*; Maranghi, S., Brondi, C., Eds.; Springer: Cham, Switzerland, 2020; pp. 101–123.
18. Rivera, J.L.; Sutherland, J.W. A design of experiments (DOE) approach to data uncertainty in LCA: Application to nanotechnology evaluation. *Clean. Techn Environ. Policy* **2015**, *17*, 1585–1595. [CrossRef]
19. Pinto, A.H.; Cho, D.R.; Oliynyk, A.O.; Silverman, J.R. Green Chemistry Applied to Transition Metal Chalcogenides through Synthesis, Design of Experiments, Life Cycle Assessment, and Machine Learning [Internet]. In *Green Chemistry—New Perspectives*; IntechOpen: London, UK, 2022. [CrossRef]
20. Antonacci, A.; Matheis, R.; Del Pero, F.; Thirunavukkarasu, D.; Delogu, M. Design of experiments framework for performance and environmental assessment in automotive context. *Proc. Inst. Mech. Eng. Part D J. Automob. Eng.* **2023**. [CrossRef]
21. Silva, A.L.D.; Filleti, R.A.P.; Christoforo, A.L.; Silva, J.E.; Ometto, R.A. Application of Life Cycle Assessment (LCA) and Design of Experiments (DOE) to the Monitoring and Control of a Grinding Process. *Procedia CIRP* **2015**, *29*, 508–513. [CrossRef]
22. Benedetti, B.; Tronconi, A.; Turrini, F. Determination of polycyclic aromatic hydrocarbons in bud-derived supplements by magnetic molecular imprinted microparticles and GC-MS: D-optimal design for a fast method optimization. *Sci. Rep.* **2023**, *13*, 17544. [CrossRef]
23. Leardi, R.D. Optimal designs. *Encycl. Anal. Chem.* **2018**, *1*, 11. [CrossRef]
24. Li Vigni, M.; Durante, C.; Cocchi, M. Chapter 3—Exploratory Data Analysis. In *Data Handling in Science and Technology*; Marini, F., Ed.; Elsevier: Amsterdam, The Netherlands, 2013; pp. 55–126. [CrossRef]
25. Milovanović, V.M.; Petrović, Z.D.; Novaković, S.; Bogdanović, G.A.; Petrović, V.P.; Simijonović, D. Green synthesis of benzamide-dioxoisoindoline derivatives and assessment of their radical scavenging activity—Experimental and theoretical approach. *Tetrahedron* **2020**, *76*, 131456. [CrossRef]
26. McElroy, C.R.; Constantinou, A.; Jones, L.C.; Summerton, L.; Clark, J.H. Towards a holistic approach to metrics for the 21st century pharmaceutical industry. *Green Chem.* **2015**, *17*, 3111–3121. [CrossRef]
27. Constable, D.J.C.; Curzons, A.D.; Cunningham, V.L. Metrics to "green" chemistry—Which are the best? *Green Chem.* **2002**, *4*, 521–527. [CrossRef]
28. Brahmachari, G.; Karmakar, I.; Nurjamal, K. Ultrasound-assisted expedient and green synthesis of a new series of diversely functionalized 7-aryl/heteroarylchromeno [4,3-d]Pyrido [1,2-a]Pyrimidin-6(7H)-Ones via one-pot multicomponent reaction under sulfamic acid catalysis at ambient conditions. *ACS Sustain. Chem. Eng.* **2018**, *6*, 1101811028. [CrossRef]
29. Eriksson, L.; Johansson, E.; Kettaneh-Wold, N.; Wikstrom, C.; Wold, S. *Design of Experiments: Principles and Applications*; Third Revised and Enlarged Edition; Umetrics Academy: Umeaa, Sweden, 2008; ISBN 978-91-973730-4-3.
30. *ISO 14040:2006*; Environmental Management—Life Cycle Assessment—Principles and Framework. ISO: Geneva, Switzerland, 2006.
31. *ISO 14044:2006*; Environmental Management—Life Cycle Assessment—Requirements and Guidelines. ISO: Geneva, Switzerland, 2006.
32. Taber, D.F.; Patel, S.; Hambleton, M.T.; Winkel, E.E. Vanillin Synthesis from 4-Hydroxybenzaldehyde. *J. Chem. Educ.* **2007**, *84*, 1158. [CrossRef]
33. Williamson, K.L.; Minard, R.D.; Masters, K.M. *Macroscale and Microscale Organic Experiments*, 5th ed.; Houghton Mifflin Company: Boston, MA, USA, 2007.
34. Smith, R.L.; Ruiz-Mercado, G.J.; Meyer, D.E.; Gonzalez, M.A.; Abraham, J.P.; Barrett, W.M.; Randall, P.M. Coupling computer-aided process simulation and estimations of emissions and land use for rapid life cycle inventory modeling. *ACS Sustain. Chem. Eng.* **2017**, *5*, 3786–3794. [CrossRef]

35. Pr'e Sustainability. Stationsplein 121, 3818 LE Amersfoort, The Netherlands. Available online: https://simapro.com/contact/ (accessed on 11 January 2024).
36. Huijbregts, M.A.J.; Steinmann, Z.J.N.; Elshout, P.M.F.; Stam, G.; Verones, F.; Vieira, M.; Zijp, M.; Hollander, A.; van Zelm, R. ReCiPe2016: A harmonized life cycle impact assessment method at midpoint and endpoint level. *Int. J. Life Cycle Assess.* **2017**, *22*, 138–147. [CrossRef]
37. Rosa, R.; Pini, M.; Cappucci, G.M.; Ferrari, A.M. Principles and indicators for assessing the environmental dimension of sustainability within green and sustainable chemistry. *Curr. Opin. Green Sustain. Chem.* **2022**, *37*, 100654. [CrossRef]
38. Yoffe, D.; Frim, R.; Ukeles, S.D.; Dagani, M.J.; Barda, H.J.; Benya, T.J.; Sanders, D.C. Bromine Compounds. In *Ullmann's Encyclopedia of Industrial Chemistry*, 7th ed.; John Wiley & Sons: Weinheim, Germany, 2013; pp. 1–31. [CrossRef]

molecules

MDPI

Article

Synthesis and Characterization of New Triazole-Bispidinone Scaffolds and Their Metal Complexes for Catalytic Applications

Arianna Rossetti [1,2,*], Alessandro Sacchetti [1,2], Fiorella Meneghetti [3,*], Greta Colombo Dugoni [1], Matteo Mori [3] and Carlo Castellano [4]

1 Department of Chemistry, Materials and Chemical Engineering "G. Natta", Politecnico di Milano, Via Mancinelli 7, 20131 Milano, Italy; alessandro.sacchetti@polimi.it (A.S.); greta.colombodugoni@polimi.it (G.C.D.)
2 INSTM—Local Unit c/o Politecnico di Milano, Via Mancinelli 7, 20131 Milano, Italy
3 Department of Pharmaceutical Sciences, University of Milan, Via L. Mangiagalli 25, 20133 Milano, Italy; matteo.mori@unimi.it
4 Department of Chemistry, University of Milan, Via C. Golgi 19, 20133 Milano, Italy; carlo.castellano@unimi.it
* Correspondence: arianna.rossetti@polimi.it (A.R.); fiorella.meneghetti@unimi.it (F.M.)

Abstract: Bispidines are a family of ligands that plays a pivotal role in various areas of coordination chemistry, with applications in medicinal chemistry, molecular catalysis, coordination polymers synthesis, and molecular magnetism. In the present work, triazole moieties were introduced using the CuAAC click-reaction, with the aim of expanding the number of coordination sites on the bispidine core. The 1,2,3-triazole rings were thus synthesized on propargyl-derived bispidines after reaction with different alkyl azides. The new class of triazole-bispidines was characterized, and their chelation capabilities were evaluated with different metals through NMR titration, ESI-MS spectrometry, and single-crystal X-ray diffraction (SC-XRD). Finally, the suitability of these molecules as metal ligands for the catalytic Henry reaction was demonstrated with copper and zinc.

Keywords: bispidine; click chemistry; metal coordination; NMR titration; crystal structure; triazoles; catalysis; Henry reaction

Citation: Rossetti, A.; Sacchetti, A.; Meneghetti, F.; Colombo Dugoni, G.; Mori, M.; Castellano, C. Synthesis and Characterization of New Triazole-Bispidinone Scaffolds and Their Metal Complexes for Catalytic Applications. *Molecules* **2023**, *28*, 6351. https://doi.org/10.3390/molecules28176351

Academic Editor: Andrea Bencini

Received: 14 July 2023
Revised: 7 August 2023
Accepted: 12 August 2023
Published: 30 August 2023

1. Introduction

Bispidines are a family of ligands that have been extensively applied in the last two decades in various areas of coordination chemistry due to their interesting properties. They are based on the 3,7-diazabicyclo[3.3.1]nonane scaffold and are found in the structure of some natural products, such as sparteine and cytisine [1]. The diazabicyclo[3.3.1]nonane core is a bi-dentate ligand, relying on the coordination activity of the two nitrogen atoms. It can be conveniently prepared by a classical multi-Mannich reaction approach, allowing for the obtainment of many differently decorated structures capable of efficiently coordinating metals in a highly preorganized way. By the introduction of specific substituents, many tetra-, penta-, hexa-, hepta-, and octadentate ligands have been reported in the literature [1–8]. Most of their applications are related to the rigidity of the bispidine backbone, which confers unique structural and electronic properties to the ligand, namely a relatively large cavity allowing for efficient metal ion encapsulation. In this respect, bispidines are expected to lead to very stable complexes with a pronounced selectivity for the size (and electronic requirements) of the metal ion. Hence, these ligands have been successfully applied in many fields, including medicinal chemistry [5,9], molecular catalysis [6,10], coordination polymers synthesis [7,11], and molecular magnetism [12].

To expand the number of coordination sites on the bispidine core, a classical approach is to introduce additional sp^2 nitrogen atoms, usually by adding one or more pyridine rings in different positions of the diazabicyclo scaffold [2,13]. For the same purpose, pyrazole rings, macrocyclic amides, and oxygen-containing substituents such as alcohols or carboxylate groups have also been proposed [2,13]. Recently, the introduction of the picoline residue by Comba allowed coordination numbers higher than eight to be achieved [5]. Additionally, the use of different coordinating atoms can be useful in tuning the interaction with the cation towards an increased selectivity of the ligands for the metals.

In our ongoing studies on the properties and applications of bispidines [2,6,11], we decided to introduce the 1,2,3-triazole ring on the bispidine core to expand the coordination capabilities of this ligand. The 1,2,3-triazole has gained great interest in the last decades due to the success of the Cu alkyne-azide cycloaddition, the so-called CuAAC click-reaction [14]. These functional-group-tolerant and easily synthesizable heterocycles have gradually become important building blocks in organic synthesis, not only as linkers between chemical or biological components, but also as efficient coordinating agents for metal ions [15–17]. The importance of 1,2,3-triazole-based ligands in catalyzed chemical transformations has recently been reported in the literature [18]. Moreover, the presence of three consecutive sp^2 nitrogen atoms has been shown to confer to the 1,2,3-triazole ring particular electron-donating capabilities [19].

In the present work, we synthesized the 1,2,3-triazole ring on a propargyl-derived bispidine core through a copper-catalyzed azide-alkyne Huisgen 1,3-dipolar cycloaddition (CuAAC, click reaction) with different alkyl azides. Hence, a small library of symmetrical tetradentate bispidines was prepared with an efficient reaction protocol involving the use of the microwaves, in order to reduce the reaction time while improving the yields. The chelating properties of the triazole-based bispidines thus synthesized were deeply investigated by means of SC-XRD and NMR. Finally, the efficacy of these molecules as metal ligands for the catalytic Henry reaction was demonstrated with two different metals: copper and zinc.

2. Results and Discussion

2.1. Synthesis of the Bispidine-Triazole Ligands

The key intermediate for the preparation of the new bispidine ligands was the bis-propargyl derivative **1** (Scheme 1). In a first attempt, we tried to obtain this compound by reacting 1,3-diphenylacetone with two equivalents of propargylamine and an excess of formaldehyde by a classical Mannich reaction. However, the very low yields prompted us to try a different approach, starting from the preparation of the dibenzyl analogue **2**, which was easily synthesized in high yields according to a procedure inspired by Black and co-workers [3]. The removal of the benzyl group through a palladium-catalyzed hydrogenation afforded the bispidine **3**, together with a lower amount of mono-benzylated derivative **4**, which were separated through column chromatography. The further reaction of **3** with propargyl bromide and sodium carbonate as an inorganic base afforded the desired intermediate **1**. Product **4**, obtained by the partial hydrogenation of **2**, was also employed in basic conditions with propargyl bromide to prepare the unsymmetrical bispidine **5**.

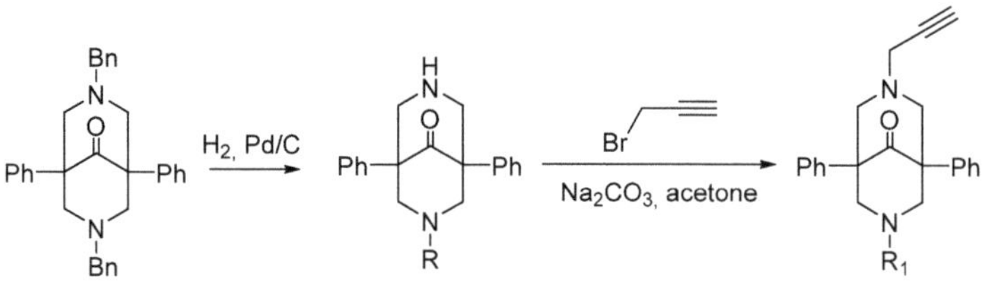

2

3 R = H
4 R = Bn

1 R_1 = $-CH_2C{\equiv}CH$
5 R_1 = Bn

Scheme 1. Synthesis of propargyl precursors **1** and **5**.

Once intermediates **1** and **5** were achieved, we studied the CuAAC 1,3-dipolar cycloaddition on our scaffolds. As a reference reaction for establishing the best set-up conditions, we employed **1** and the benzyl azide **6a**. Firstly, the CuAAC reaction was performed with

2 eq. of the azide in a 1:1 acetone/water mixture, using $CuSO_4$ and sodium ascorbate at 50 °C. After 24 h, the reaction of **1** with the benzyl azide **6a** afforded the desired product with a poor yield (23%). When the reaction was performed under microwave (MW) irradiation at 50 °C, the product was obtained after 1 h in 95% yield (Scheme 2).

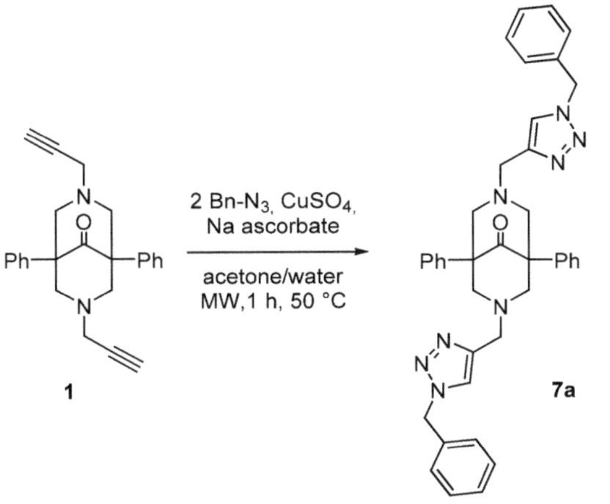

Scheme 2. Click reaction of **1** with azide **6a**.

The removal of the copper catalyst from the crude was quite troublesome, because, as expected, the newly formed bispidine ligand **7a** bound to the Cu cation very efficiently; therefore, a simple aqueous wash as work-up was not sufficient. Several attempts were made to remove the metal by ligand exchange, washing the organic layer with aqueous solutions of various amines, such as ammonia, trimethylamine, and ethylenediamine at different concentrations. In every instance, the desired bispidines were extracted in low yields, probably due to the degradation of the product in the basic conditions of the work-up. Finally, we managed to cleanly isolate the product by washing the organic phase with a 1 M aqueous solution of ethylenediaminetetraacetic acid (EDTA). With this protocol, the desired compound was isolated in high yields and without the need for further purifications.

Once established the optimum for the reaction set-up, a library of aryl- and alkyl-azides was selected (**6a–j**, Scheme 3) to be reacted with **1** or **5** to evaluate the potential chelation capabilities of the resulting derivatives.

All the azido-derivatives **6a–j** were efficiently prepared by reaction of sodium azide with the corresponding alkyl or benzyl bromide in *N*,*N*-dimethylformamide (DMF) under MW irradiation at 100 °C for 15 min. The synthesized azides were selected to tune both the coordination properties and the solubility of the bispidine derivatives, thus allowing the design of efficient ligands for their final applications. For instance, two pyridine-based azides were prepared: the 2-(azidomethyl)pyridine **6d** and 4-(azidomethyl)pyridine **6e**; the presence of these aromatic rings was designed in an attempt to further expand the coordination capabilities of the final bispidine ligands. The aliphatic 1-azidooctane **6f** and 1-azidoundecane **6g** were considered to increase the lipophilicity of the final products and promote their solubility in poorly polar organic solvents. With the same purpose, in addition to the benzyl azide **6a**, the aromatic 1-(azidomethyl)-4-chlorobenzene **6b**, and 1-(azidomethyl)-4-nitrobenzene **6c** were also prepared. On the contrary, 3-azidopropan-1-ol **6h** was prepared to improve the solubility of the target ligand in protic polar solvents, such as alcohols and water. Finally, the bis-azido derivatives 1,2-bis(azidomethyl)benzene **6i** and 1,3-diazidohexane **6j** were investigated to evaluate the feasibility of obtaining macrocyclic ligands.

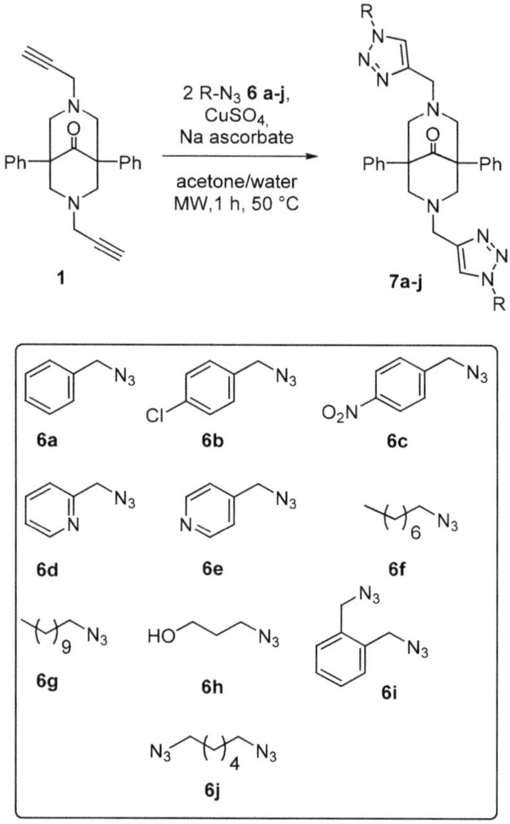

Scheme 3. Click reaction of **1** with azides **6a–j**.

Following the optimized procedure for the CuAAC reaction, a family of triazole-bispidine derivatives (**7a–j**) was thus prepared by coupling **1** with the corresponding azides (**6a–j**).

As shown in Table 1, most of the bis-triazole bispidines were obtained in good/excellent yields with both aromatic and aliphatic compounds (**7a–h**). On the contrary, the use of diazide linkers to produce macrocycles was unsuccessful, and products 7**i–j** were detected in traces.

Table 1. Library of the synthesized bis-triazole bispidines.

Compound	R	Yield (%)
7a	benzyl	95
7b	*p*-Cl-benzyl	75
7c	*p*-NO_2-benzyl	78
7d	2-(azidomethyl)pyridine	84
7e	4-(azidomethyl)pyridine	83
7f	*n*-octyl	86
7g	*n*-undecyl	73
7h	3-hydroxypropyl	85
7i	-CH_2PhCH_2-	traces
7j	-$CH_2(CH_2)_4CH_2$-	traces

The unsymmetrical propargyl-bispidine **5** was employed as a substrate for the CuAAC cycloaddition in the same reaction conditions (Scheme 4). Azides **6a** and **6g** were used as reference compounds, and the subsequent products **8a** and **8b** were isolated in high yields.

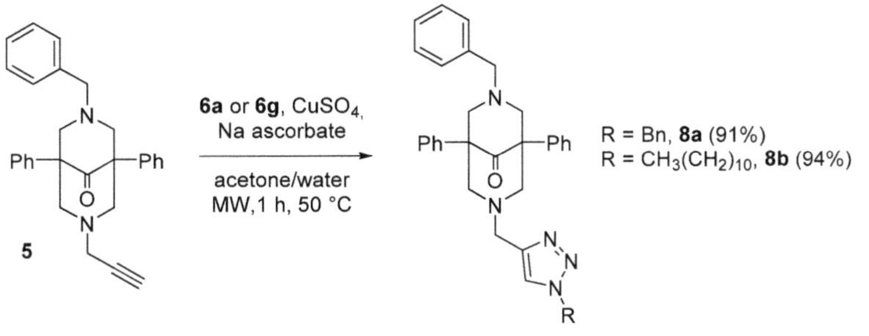

Scheme 4. Click reaction of **5** with azides **6a** or **6g**.

2.2. NMR Studies on the Coordination Chemistry

An extensive investigation of the coordination chemistry was conducted by performing ^{1}H-NMR titrations of the synthesized bispidines with various metals (such as Zn, La, and Pd). The objective was to analyze how the chelation number changed based on the different substituents incorporated into the frameworks. The chelation number, which represents the atoms directly coordinating to the central metal ion in a chelate complex, is evidently influenced by the geometry and electron configuration of the metal ion, as well as the coordinating sites of the ligand.

As a start, we studied the formation of the complexes of compounds **7b** and **7d** with Zn(II), and of **7a,d,h** with La(III) (Figure 1). These cations were selected as representative of bi- and trivalent metals.

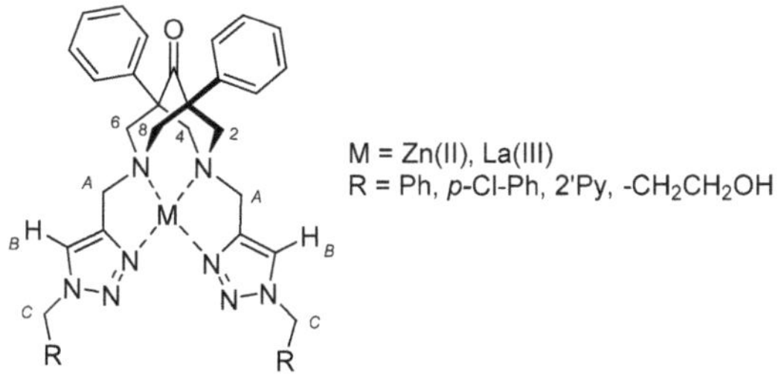

Figure 1. Coordination geometry of ligands **7a,b,d,h** and their metal complexes.

To investigate the coordination chemistry, ^{1}H-NMR titration studies were performed in CD_3CN as the deuterated solvent. Spectra were recorded after the addition of precise aliquots of the metal into the ligand solution. Upon addition of the salt, a progressive minor broadening of some signals was observed, with the concomitant appearance of new peaks (Figure 2). In all the tested samples, the addition of an equivalent of metal resulted in the formation of a single new species, which was attributed to the ligand-metal complex in a 1:1 ratio; further addition of the metal did not cause any significant change in the spectrum. This behavior is typical of very tight complexes (i.e., showing a very low dissociation constant) in a slow exchange regime between the complex and the free-ligand species.

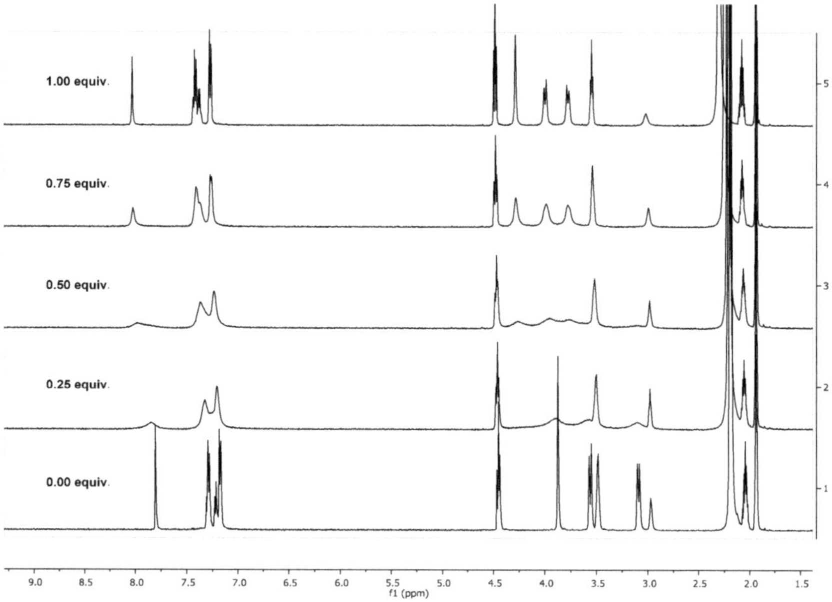

Figure 2. ^{1}H-NMR titration of compound **7h** with $La(NO_3)_3$.

Once established the stoichiometry of the complexes via NMR titration, the products were also prepared by stirring a solution of the ligand in acetonitrile with a stoichiometric amount of $Zn(NO_3)_2$ or $La(NO_3)_3$ for 24 h. The resulting precipitate was filtered and analyzed by ^{1}H-NMR in CD_3CN. In Table 2, the comparison of the chemical shifts of the free ligands and their complexes is reported.

Table 2. Comparison of the free ligands **7a**,**b**,**d**,**h** and their metal complexes: list of the Δδ in the ^{1}H-NMR spectra.

Entry	Compound	Δδ for $H_{2,4,6,8}$ eq (ppm)	Δδ for $H_{2,4,6,8}$ ax (ppm)	Δδ for H_A (ppm)	Δδ for H_B (ppm)	Δδ for H_C (ppm)
1	**7b·Zn(II)**	0.46	0.44	0.18	0.50	0.15
2	**7d·Zn(II)**	0.50	0.61	0.27	0.24	0.15
3	**7d·La(III)**	0.45	0.70	0.43	0.23	0.03
4	**7a·La(III)**	0.46	0.71	0.42	0.24	0.04
5	**7h·La(III)**	0.45	0.70	0.40	0.40	0.05

Concerning compound **7b** and its Zn(II)-complex **7b·Zn(II)**, the most evident shifts were detected for the methylene hydrogens of the bispidine core ($H_{2,4,6,8}$), with values of $\Delta\delta = 0.44$ ppm and $\Delta\delta = 0.46$ ppm towards low fields for axial and equatorial hydrogens, respectively (Table 2, entry 1). Similarly, the triazole hydrogen H_B was deshielded by $\Delta\delta = 0.50$ ppm. The benzylic methylene group's H_C also showed a $\Delta\delta = 0.15$ ppm shift. These data suggest a coordination with the metal cation involving both the sp^3 nitrogen of the bispidine core and one of the sp^2 nitrogen atoms of the 1,2,3-triazole system. The result is a tetracoordinated metal center, formed by the four nitrogen atoms of the bispidine and triazole rings (Figure 1).

Similarly, the metal coordination of ligand **7d** was also investigated with Zn(II). In this case, it was interesting to evaluate whether the pyridine ring could be involved in the coordination of the zinc ion. In Table 2 (entry 2), the comparison of the free ligand **7d** and its 1:1 Zn(II)-complex **7d·Zn(II)** is displayed. The most evident shifts were for the methylene hydrogens of the bispidine core, with values of $\Delta\delta$ = 0.50 ppm and $\Delta\delta$ = 0.61 ppm towards low fields for equatorial and axial hydrogens, respectively. Similarly, the triazole hydrogen H_B was deshielded by $\Delta\delta$ = 0.24 ppm. The methylene group's H_C also showed a $\Delta\delta$ = 0.15 ppm shift. The pyridine hydrogens showed no significant shift; a deshielding of $\Delta\delta$ = 0.05–0.10 ppm was observed, the same value measured for all the aromatic protons. This result indicated that the pyridine nitrogen was not involved in the coordination of the metal ion, since no important deshielding effects could be observed on the neighboring hydrogens. Again, the coordination resulted in a tetracoordinated metal center, formed by the four nitrogen atoms of the bispidine and triazole rings (Figure 1).

A ^{1}H-NMR titration experiment was also performed for compound **7h** in CD_3CN by adding aliquots of $La(NO_3)_3$ into the ligand solution. After the first additions, a strong broadening of the signals was observed in the whole spectrum, with the exception of the 3-hydroxypropyl portion, thus indicating that no coordination occurred at this part of the molecule. After the addition of 1 equivalent of metal, a single species formed, and the resolution of the spectrum improved (Figures 2 and 3). The pattern of the titration suggests that with less than 1 equivalent of metal, more species are present, indicating that in these conditions, the coordination is not complete, but a rapid exchange regime between complexed and free ligand is established.

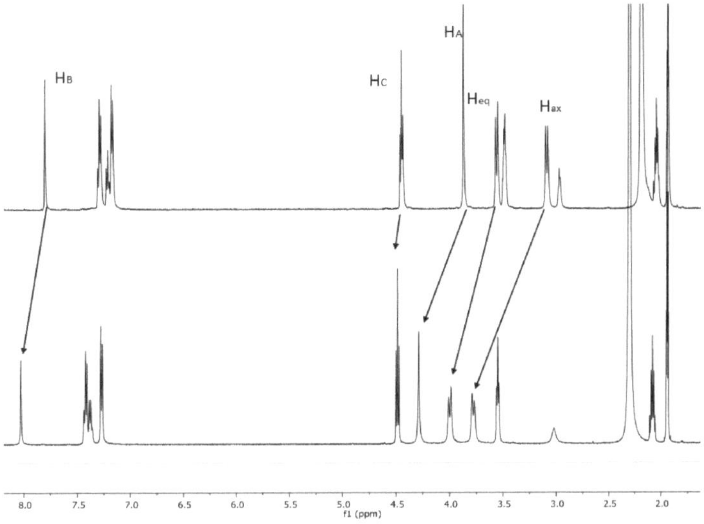

Figure 3. ^{1}H-NMR spectrum of compound **7h** and its La(III)-complex **7h·La(III)**.

To summarize, very similar effects were observed for the complexation of La(III) with ligands **7a,d,h**. Compared to the Zn(II) complexes, the methylene protons H_A showed a higher value of $\Delta\delta$, whereas a smaller value was observed for H_C.

Among the analyzed products, complexes **7d,h-La(III)** have an extra coordinating atom, namely the pyridine nitrogen in **7d**, and the hydroxy group of the 3-hydroxypropyl chain in **7h**. As for the complex **7d·Zn(II)**, these atoms did not seem to be involved in the coordination of the metal, considering that no significative shifts were observed for the adjacent hydrogen atoms.

Concerning the mono-substituted triazole-bispidines, the complexation of bispidine **8a** with $PdCl_2$ was investigated (Figure 4, Table 3). In this case, we were interested in exploring the possibility of obtaining a so-called 'Pincer-like' complex through the formation of a C–Pd bond with the aromatic ring of the benzyl residue. This kind of complexes have been previously reported by Bulygina et al. [20]. Worth notice is that the palladacycles are stable compounds, characterizable by NMR, and are efficient catalysts in C–C bond-forming reactions. The complexation reaction of **8a** with $PdCl_2$ was performed in acetonitrile at room temperature for 48 h. The obtained solid **8a·Pd(II)** was characterized by ^{1}H-NMR in CD_3CN, similar to the previous ones (Figure 5). As observed for the other ligands, all the signals of the hydrogen atoms adjacent to the chelating centers were shifted upfield as a consequence of the formation of the complex (Table 3). The hydrogens neighboring the bispidine nitrogen atoms showed the highest shifts ($\Delta\delta$ = 0.66–0.84 ppm). The presence of the newly formed C–Pd bond was confirmed by the fact that in the spectrum of the complex, a doublet appeared at 7.91 ppm (J = 7.5 Hz, 1H). As indicated by the COSY spectrum (Figure 6), this signal correlates with a group of peaks at 7.00–7.12 ppm (a doublet and two triplets, J = 7.0–7.5 Hz), typical of an ortho-disubstituted aromatic spin system. These data suggest the formation of a C–Pd bond in the ortho position of the benzyl substituent, with the proton in ortho to the palladium center shifted downfield to 7.91 ppm as a doublet; conversely, the other three hydrogen atoms of the phenyl ring are shifted upfield. These observations are in agreement with what previously reported in the literature for similar benzyl bispidine–palladium complexes [21].

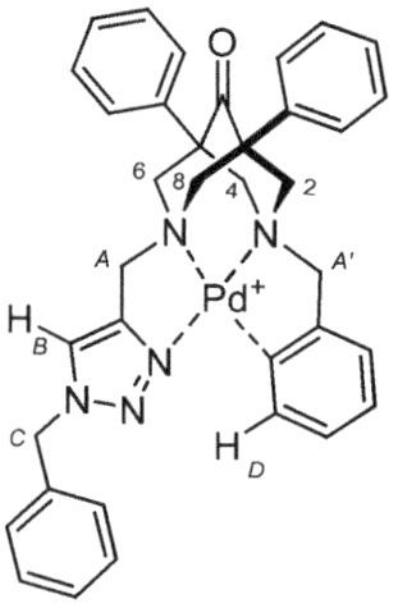

Figure 4. Coordination geometry of ligand **8a** complexed with Pd(II).

Table 3. List of the $\Delta\delta$ in the ^{1}H-NMR spectrum for complex **8a·Pd(II)**.

$\Delta\delta$ for $H_{2,4,6,8}$ eq (ppm)	$\Delta\delta$ for $H_{2,4,6,8}$ ax (ppm)	$\Delta\delta$ for $H_{A\text{-}A}$ (ppm)	$\Delta\delta$ for H_B (ppm)	$\Delta\delta$ for H_C (ppm)	$\Delta\delta$ for H_D (ppm)
0.82–0.84	0.80	0.66	0.28	0.18	0.68

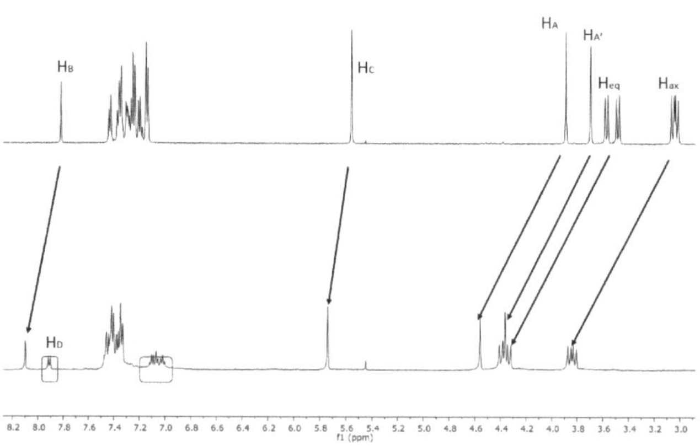

Figure 5. ^{1}H-NMR spectrum of compound **8a** and its Pd(II) complex **8a·Pd(II)**. The benzyl aromatic portion of the complex is highlighted in squares.

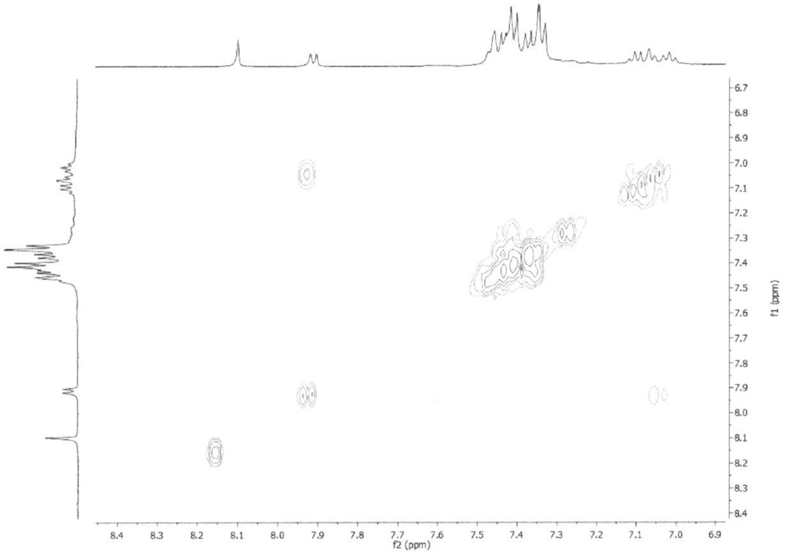

Figure 6. Aromatic portion of the ^{1}H-^{1}H COSY of compound **8a·Pd(II)**.

2.3. ESI-MS Studies on the Coordination Chemistry

With regard to the zinc-based complexes, further items of information were collected from electrospray ionization mass spectrometry (ESI-MS) analyses. The spectrum of compound **7b·Zn(II)** (Figure 7, left) showed the presence of one main signal as a complex pattern composed of many peaks, with the base peak at *m*/*z* 830.4, which is consistent with the elemental composition $[C_{39}H_{36}Cl_2N_9O_4Zn]^+$, assignable to the complex $\mathbf{[7b{\cdot}Zn(II){\cdot}NO_3]^+}$. This observation was confirmed by the comparison of the experimental pattern with the simulated isotopic pattern (Figure 7, right). Other much less intense peaks were observed due to anion exchange during the electro nebulization process. For example, a pattern with the base peak at *m*/*z* 803.4, consistent with $[C_{39}H_{36}Cl_3N_8OZn]^+$, was ascribed to the formation of the $\mathbf{[7b{\cdot}Zn(II){\cdot}Cl]^+}$ cation (Figure 8).

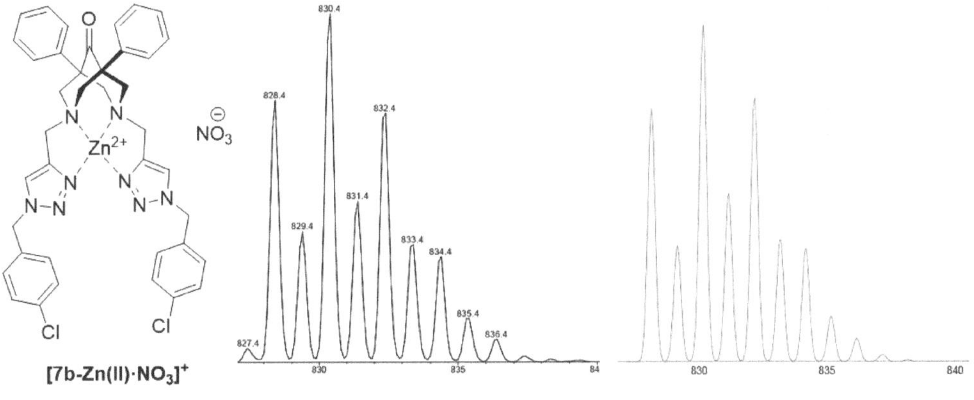

Figure 7. Comparison of the experimental ESI-MS spectrum of compound $\mathbf{[7b{\cdot}Zn(II){\cdot}NO_3]^+}$ (**left**) and the simulation of the isotopic pattern for the elemental composition $[C_{39}H_{36}Cl_2N_9O_4Zn]^+$ (**right**).

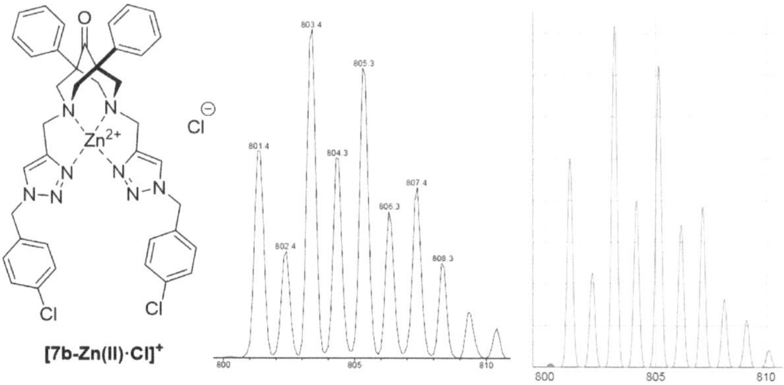

Figure 8. Comparison of the experimental ESI-MS spectrum of compound **[7b·Zn(II)·Cl]**$^+$ (**left**) and the simulation of the isotopic pattern for the elemental composition $[C_{39}H_{36}Cl_3N_8OZn]^+$ (**right**).

Similar patterns were observed for the complexes **[7d·Zn(II)·NO$_3$]**$^+$, $[C_{37}H_{36}N_{11}O_4Zn]^+$, base peak at m/z 762.22., and **[7d·Zn(II)·Cl]**$^+$, $[C_{37}H_{36}ClN_{10}OZn]^+$, base peak at m/z 735.21. The spectra and the simulation of the isotopic patterns, consistent with the elemental compositions reported above, are shown in Figures S30 and S31, respectively.

The ESI-MS analysis was also crucial to confirm the formation of the Pincer-like complex for **8a·Pd(II)**. In this case, the base peak was found at m/z 658.5. The observed value was consistent with the elemental composition $[C_{36}H_{34}N_5OPd]^+$, corresponding to the monocationic complex. Again, a very good agreement between the experimental and the predicted peak pattern was observed (Figure S32).

2.4. *Single-Crystal X-ray Characterization of the Free Ligand* **8a**

Among the synthesized products, we analyzed ligand **8a** by means of SC-XRD to provide an unambiguous description of its structure and derive useful information on the spatial arrangement of the N-benzyl triazole moiety with respect to the bispidine core. This feature influences the chiral space around the metal, determining the chelating capabilities of the ligand. These data helped us to rationalize the behavior of the compounds, also considering that the stereochemistry of these molecules is a major determinant of their chelating properties.

Compound **8a** crystallized in the monoclinic space group Cc, with four crystallographically independent molecules (**I**, **A**, **B**, and **C**) related by pseudosymmetry in the asymmetric unit ($Z' = 4$); conformer **I** is represented in Figure 9. Low-temperature (150 K) data were found to be pseudo-merohedrally twinned via twin law $-1\ 0\ 0, 0\ -1\ 0, 1\ 0\ 1$, detected by the TwinRotMat routine in PLATON [22].

In the crystal, the conformation of the bispidine core was the same in all four independent molecules, whereas the benzyl substituent of the triazole ring was differently oriented. The similarity between the four molecules was calculated by using the "Molecule Overlay" routine in Mercury [23]: the RMSD for the non-hydrogen atoms of molecules **I** and **B** was 0.1589 Å, whereas for molecules **A** and **C**, a smaller value of 0.1454 Å was observed. The bispidine was in boat–chair conformation, with the portion bearing the triazole moiety in boat conformation, the two phenyl groups arranged in anti-geometry, and the benzyl ring in endo position. This finding was in agreement with our previous results [6], which indicated that the introduction of large substituents on the nitrogen promotes a boat conformation of the piperidine. The puckering parameters of the ring in chair conformation were: $Q_T = 0.629(3)$ Å, $\varphi = -151(3)°$, and $\vartheta = 174(3)°$. Conversely, the piperidine in boat conformation showed the following puckering parameters: $Q_T = 2.442(3)$ Å, $\varphi = -34.6(2)°$, and $\vartheta = 156(1)°$ [24]. The crystal packing was consolidated by van der Waals contacts and weak Cπ-H···O-type interactions. Notably, the intermolecular contacts did not influence the conformation of the bicycle because the aromatic moieties were not involved in stacking interactions.

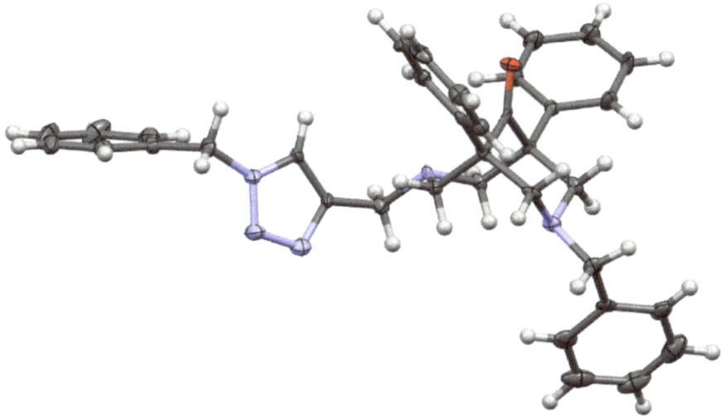

Figure 9. Thermal ellipsoid representation (40% probability) of one of the symmetrically independent molecules (**I**) in the crystal cell of **8a**. Color code: C = grey; H = white; N = blue; O = red.

2.5. Molecular Modeling

To collect more information on the structure of both the ligands and the complexes, a computational study was performed. Firstly, the role of the triazole rings on the conformational behavior of the bispidine was considered. To this end, the model molecules **9** and **10** (Figure 10) were used to shorten the computational times, with the approximation that the residues on the triazole ring would not significantly affect the conformation of the fused piperidine rings of the bispidine core. Three possible arrangements of this core can exist, namely the chair–chair (cc), the boat–chair (bc), and the boat–boat (bb) conformations. A conformational analysis (Monte Carlo search with Molecular Mechanics energy minimization) was performed; the most favorable conformers were then optimized at the DFT-B3LYP/6-311G(d) level in vacuo.

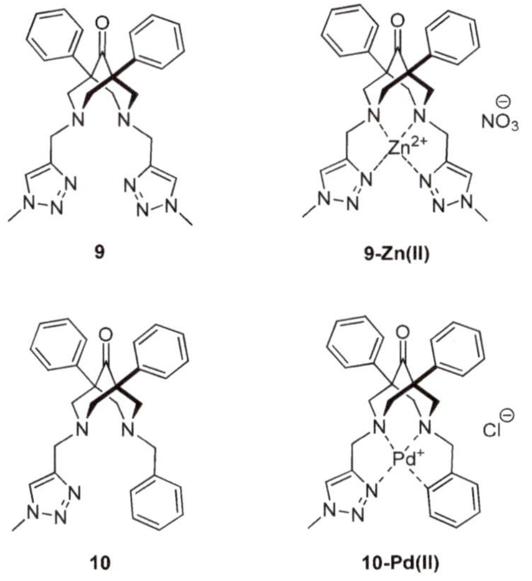

Figure 10. Model molecules **9** and **10** designed for conformational studies in silico.

To obtain more information on the coordination capability of the ligands, the complexes **9·Zn(II)** and **10·Pd(II)** were also submitted to energy optimization at the DFT-

B3LYP/LANL2DZ level. In both cases, the presence of the anion (nitrate and chloride anion, respectively) in the first coordination sphere was also considered.

In compound **9·Zn(II)**, the four coordinating nitrogen atoms lay on the same plane, forming a square of about 3 Å, with the Zn-N bond lengths in the range 2.1–2.3 Å (Figure 11). The metal ion occupies the apex of the resulting square-based pyramid, and the angles of inclination of this pyramid are in the range of 17–21°. The nitrate anion is 2.1 Å far from the metal. Similarly, for **10·Pd(II)** a square-based pyramid was found (Figure 11), even if in this case the angle of inclination was only 8.2°, very close to a square planar geometry. The chloride anion is at 3.0 Å from the palladium ion, and the C–Pd bond length is 2.0 Å. The Pd-N bond lengths vary from 2.1 to 2.3 Å. In both structures, the bispidine skeleton is bent towards the opposite side of the apex of the pyramid.

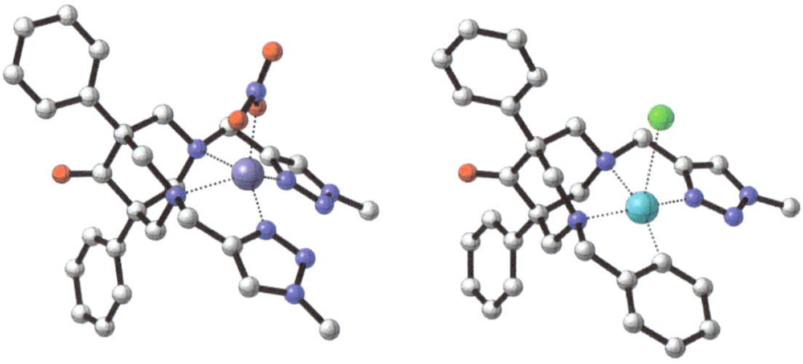

Figure 11. Optimized structures of **9·Zn(II)** and **10·Pd(II)** complexes. Color code: C = grey; O = red; N = blue; Cl = green; Zn = violet; Pd = light blue.

These results are in agreement with the experimental data gathered by NMR, MS, and SC-XRD. Most notably, the modeled conformation of the complexes supported the chelation number definitions resulting from the NMR investigations.

2.6. Catalysis Applications of the Complexes

Considering the extraordinary chelation capability of our library of triazole bispidines, tests were performed to investigate their possible use as catalysts. In detail, we focused on the Henry reaction for the copper- and zinc-based compounds. The Henry reaction is a very useful C–C bond-forming reaction, consisting in the nucleophilic addition of a nitronate (the carbanion of a nitroalkane) to an electrophilic aldehyde or ketone [25]. The main product is a β-nitro alcohol (Scheme 5), which can be further transformed into amino-alcohols, useful for the synthesis of many drugs and natural products [26,27].

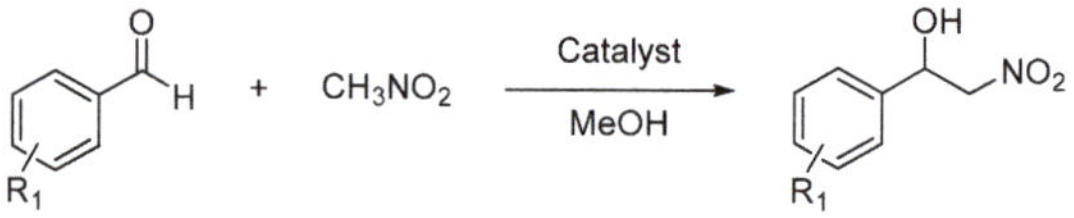

Scheme 5. Scheme of a general Henry reaction.

The reaction occurs under basic conditions, or with the assistance of an organometallic catalyst. One of the most commonly used metals is copper, combined with different amino ligands [28]. More recently, the use of zinc in combination with nitrogen-based ligands has been demonstrated to be a valid alternative, with the great advantage of the much lower toxicity of this metal [29].

Ligand **7a** was thus selected as the reference compound for testing the reaction conditions, in combination with both zinc and copper as metals. The reactions were initially performed in ethanol at room temperature for 24 h with 5 equivalents of nitromethane with respect to the aldehyde. Different loadings of catalyst were thus screened, as well as the influence of the addition of triethylamine in the reaction mixture (Table 4, entries 1–4). Notably, the zinc complex with the bispidine proved to be active at only 2% mol loading of the catalyst, with a 79% conversion for p-nitrobenzaldehyde (Table 4, entry 2). The complete conversion was achieved with 15% mol of catalyst. The addition of triethylamine caused a reduction of the yield (Table 4, entry 4). This effect was probably due to triethylamine coordinating the catalyst, thus inhibiting its activity. It is important to underline that the copper-based complex proved to be less efficient in the same conditions, with only a 22% conversion for p-nitrobenzaldehyde, when the catalyst was used at 2% mol, and a 56% conversion instead of completeness when employed at 15% mol (Table 4, entries 5 and 6, respectively).

Table 4. Screening of the Henry reaction using **7a·Zn** triazole bispidine as catalysts. Conditions: aldehyde (1 eq), nitromethane (5 eq), methanol (0.2 M), 1 h, 80 °C under microwave irradiation.

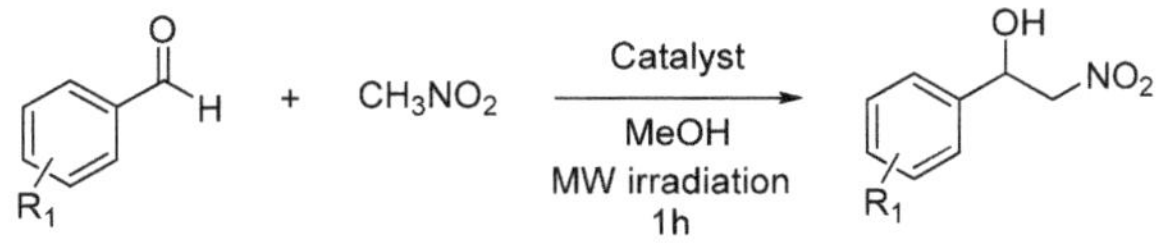

Entry	Aldehyde	Catalyst Loading	Yield (%)
1 [a]	*p*-NO_2-PhCHO	Zn (2% mol)	7
2 [a]	*p*-NO_2-PhCHO	7a·Zn (2% mol)	79
3 [a]	*p*-NO_2-PhCHO	7a·Zn (15% mol)	99
4 [a]	*p*-NO_2-PhCHO	7a·Zn (15% mol) + TEA (2% mol)	81
5 [a]	*p*-NO_2-PhCHO	7a·Cu (2% mol)	22
6 [a]	*p*-NO_2-PhCHO	7a·Cu (15% mol)	56
7	*p*-Br-PhCHO	7a·Zn (15% mol)	92
8	*p*-F-PhCHO	7a·Zn (15% mol)	91
9	*p*-CF_3-PhCHO	7a·Zn (15% mol)	94
10	*o*-NO_2-PhCHO	7a·Zn (15% mol)	81
11	2-naphthaldehyde	7a·Zn (15% mol)	88

[a] reactions were performed without the use of MW at RT for 24 h.

Later on, the best set-up was investigated to shorten the reaction time, testing classical heating against microwave irradiation. Under the optimized reaction conditions, namely **7a·Zn** 15% mol, 80 °C in MeOH for 1 h under microwave irradiation, a screening was performed using different aromatic aldehydes as substrates to exploit the scope of the reaction. The best results (Table 4, entries 7–11) were obtained with electron-poor aldehydes, whereas aliphatic and EDG aldehydes led to unsatisfactory yields.

Most notably, the efficiency of this reaction set-up was also retained with different nitro-compounds; for instance, when nitropropane was used instead of nitromethane in the best conditions (Table 4, entry 3), the product was achieved in good yield with the same substrate (Scheme 6).

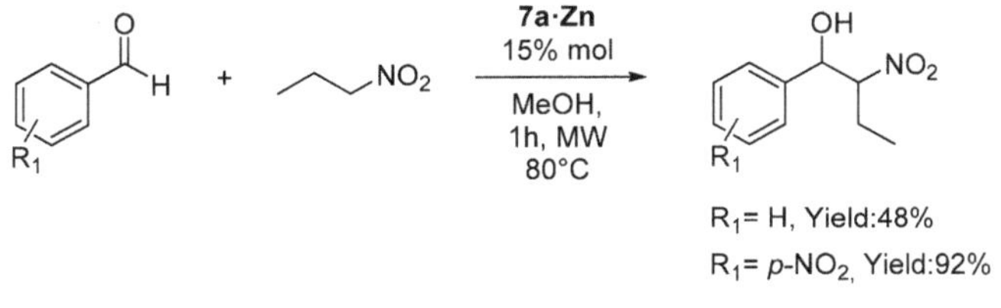

Scheme 6. Henry reaction with nitropropane. Conditions: aldehyde (1 eq), nitropropane (5 eq), **7a·Zn** (15% mol), methanol (0.2 M), 1 h, 80 °C, MW irradiation.

3. Conclusions

The [3.3.1]-diazabicyclo core of bispidines plays a crucial role in defining their properties as ligands. Moreover, the substituents bound to it greatly influence their effectiveness as coordinating agents for various metal cations. In this work, a library of triazole bispidines bearing diverse substituents was designed and synthesized to explore additional chelation points with respect to known bispidines. In order to investigate the coordination chemistry of these distinct systems with different metals, the results obtained from structural, spectroscopic, and computational methods were compared, revealing a notable consistency between experimental observations and theoretical calculations. As expected from our previous work [6], where the presence of pyridine rings strongly stabilized the formation of metal complexes with the bispidine, the introduction of the triazole ring enables a strong coordination. Nevertheless, the further addition of pyridines to the triazole rings does not promote further coordination in those positions, as the pyridine nitrogens are distant from the chelation center. Interesting chelating properties were discovered for mono-triazole bispidines; in this respect, SC-XRD data of 8a allowed to obtain a 3D picture of the ligands in the solid state. The metal complexes were deeply characterized using ESI-MS spectrometry to calculate the molecular mass, and NMR titration to verify the formation of the complex in solution as well as its stoichiometry. The catalytic ability of the metal complexes was investigated in established C-C bond-forming reactions; in detail, the Henry reaction achieved excellent results with zinc-based bispidines as catalysts under microwave irradiation.

4. Materials and Methods

4.1. General Remarks

Chemicals and solvents were purchased from Merck KGaA (Darmstadt, Germany) and used without further purifications. Microwave reactions were conducted in a Biotage® Initiator+ (Uppsala, Sweden). Reactions were monitored mostly by thin-layer chromatography (TLC), performed on Merck Kieselgel 60 F_{254} plates (Merck KGaA, Darmstadt, Germany). Visualization was accomplished by UV irradiation at 254 nm and subsequently by treatment with the alkaline $KMnO_4$ reactant or with a phosphomolybdic reagent. GC-MS analyses were performed on an Agilent HP 6890 gas chromatograph equipped with a HP-5MS column (30 m × 0.25 mm × 0.25 μm), with injection temperature = 250 °C, injecting 1 μL of solution, and using He as a carrier gas (1.0 mL·min^{-1}). The method used for the analyses was: 60 °C (1 min)/6 °C/min/150 °C (1 min)/12 °C/min/280 °C (5 min). NMR spectra were recorded (^{1}H-NMR, 400 MHz; ^{13}C-NMR, 101 MHz) on a Bruker 400 spectrometer (Bruker Italia Srl, Milan, Italy) in deuterated solvents, using TMS as an internal standard; chemical shifts (δ) in the spectra are reported in ppm, the coupling constants *J* are reported in Hz. The ESI-MS spectra were recorded on a Bruker Esquire 3000 plus spectrometer (Bruker Italia Srl, Milan, Italy), whereas the melting points were measured on a Reichert apparatus, equipped with a Reichert microscope. Elemental analyses were performed on a Costech ECS mod.4010 instrument (Costech Analytical Technologies, Inc., Valencia, CA, USA).

4.2. Synthetic Procedures

1,5-Diphenyl-3,7-di(prop-2-yn-1-yl)-3,7-diazabicyclo[3.3.1]nonan-9-one (1)
Compound **3** (1 eq., 0.1 M) was dissolved in acetone with an excess of sodium carbonate (5 eq.) as a heterogeneous inorganic base; the mixture was cooled to 0 °C and 2.5 eq. of propargyl bromide was added dropwise under stirring. The reaction was left stirring at room temperature for 24 h. The solid was filtered off on a Buchner funnel, and the filtrate was dried under vacuum, affording the desired product **1**. Yield 95%. Yellow oil. ^{1}H-NMR (400 MHz, $CDCl_3$) δ (ppm) 7.43–7.14 (m, 10H, Ar-H), 3.61 (d, *J* = 10.8 Hz, 4H, CH_2-eq), 3.55 (d, *J* = 2.4 Hz, 4H, CH_2-propargyl), 3.32 (d, *J* = 10.8 Hz, 4H, CH_2-ax), 2.29 (t, *J* = 2.4 Hz, 2H, CH-propargyl). ^{13}C-NMR (101 MHz, $CDCl_3$) δ (ppm) 209.9 (1C, C=O), 142.3 (2C, Ph-*ipso*), 127.9 (4C, Ar), 126.9 (4C, Ar), 126.7 (2C, Ar), 78.2 (2C, propargyl), 73.7 (2C, propargyl),

64.0 (4C, CH_2-bispidine), 54.0 (2C, C-Ph bispidine), 46.4 (2C, CH_2-propargyl). Elemental analysis: $C_{25}H_{24}N_2O$: (368.48); calculated (%): C, 81.49; H, 6.57; N, 7.60; found (%): C, 81.98 H, 6.97; N, 7.23.

3,7-Dibenzyl-1,5-diphenyl-3,7-diazabicyclo[3.3.1]nonan-9-one (2)
Benzylamine (2 eq.) was dissolved in methanol and cooled to 0 °C. Acetic acid (2% vol/vol), 1,3-diphenyl-2-propanone (1 eq., 0.2 M) and paraformaldehyde (4 eq.) were added, and the mixture was refluxed for 12 h. The yellow solution was cooled to room temperature before filtering the white precipitate on a Buchner funnel and washing it with cold methanol. The pure product **2** was obtained without any further purification. Yield 84%. White solid. ^{1}H-NMR (400 MHz, $CDCl_3$) δ (ppm) 7.44–7.11 (m, 20H, Ar-H), 3.73 (s, 4H, CH_2-Bn), 3.54 (d, J = 10.8 Hz, 4H, CH_2-eq), 3.12 (d, J = 10.8 Hz, 4H, CH_2-ax). All the other data are in agreement with the literature (see Supplementary Materials for references).

1,5-Diphenyl-3,7-diazabicyclo[3.3.1]nonan-9-one (3) and 3-benzyl-1,5-diphenyl-3,7-diazabicyclo[3.3.1]nonan-9-one (4)
Compound **2** (2 g) was dissolved in ethyl acetate (100 mL). A catalytic amount of Pd/C was added to the reaction, and the mixture was stirred for 120 h at room temperature under hydrogen atmosphere. The work-up consisted of a filtration through a celite pad to remove the catalyst and washing with cold ethyl acetate and methanol. The liquid layer was collected in a round bottom flask to remove the solvent under vacuum. The crude was purified through column chromatography, starting from 1% of methanol in ethyl acetate, to 80% of methanol, to give the two compounds **3** and **4**.

3: Yield 63%. White solid. ^{1}H-NMR (400 MHz, $CDCl_3$) δ (ppm) 7.39–7.22 (m, 10H, Ar-H), 3.88 (d, J = 12.3 Hz, 4H, CH_2-eq), 3.71 (d, J = 12.1 Hz, 4H, CH_2-ax), 3.14 (br s, 2H, NH). All the other data are in agreement with the literature (see Supplementary Materials for references).

4: Yield 25%. Yellow oil. ^{1}H-NMR (400 MHz, $CDCl_3$) δ (ppm) 7.37–7.17 (m, 15H, Ar-H), 3.77 (d, J = 13.9 Hz, 2H, CH_2-eq), 3.59–354 (m, 7H, CH_2-eq, CH_2-Bn, CH_2-ax, NH), 3.11 (d, J = 13.9 Hz, 2H, CH_2-ax). ^{13}C-NMR (101 MHz, $CDCl_3$) δ (ppm) 208.5 (1C, C=O), 136.7 (2C, Ph-*ipso*), 136.3 (1C, PhBn-*ipso*), 127.8 (2C, Ar), 127.3 (2C, Ar), 127.0 (4C, Ar), 126.7 (2C, Ar), 126.3 (2C, Ar), 126.2 (1C, Ar), 64.9 (2C, CH_2-bispidine), 61.7 (2C, CH_2-bispidine), 61.2 (2C, CH_2-Bn), 54.6 (2C, C-Ph bispidine). Elemental analysis: $C_{26}H_{26}N_2O$: (382.51); calculated (%): C, 81.64; H, 6.85; N, 7.32; found (%): C, 81.21; H, 6.44; N, 7.62.

3-Benzyl-1,5-diphenyl-7-(prop-2-yn-1-yl)-3,7-diazabicyclo[3.3.1]nonan-9-one (5)
Compound **4** (1 eq., 0.1 M) was dissolved in acetone with an excess of sodium carbonate (5 eq.) as a heterogeneous inorganic base; the mixture was cooled to 0 °C, and 1.5 eq. of propargyl bromide were added dropwise under stirring. The reaction was left stirring at room temperature for 24 h. The solid was filtered off on a Buchner funnel, and the filtrate was dried under vacuum, affording the desired product **5**. Yield 82%. Yellow oil. ^{1}H-NMR (400 MHz, $CDCl_3$) δ (ppm) 7.49–7.16 (m, 15H, Ar-H), 3.72 (s, 2H, CH_2-Bn), 3.68 (d, J = 10.8 Hz, 2H, CH_2-eq), 3.58 (d, J = 2.4 Hz, 2H, CH_2-propargyl), 3.54 (d, J = 10.9 Hz, 2H, CH_2-eq), 3.27 (d, J = 10.8 Hz, 2H, CH_2-ax), 3.15 (d, J = 10.9 Hz, 2H, CH_2-ax), 2.34 (t, J = 2.4 Hz, 1H, CH-propargyl). ^{13}C-NMR (101 MHz, $CDCl_3$) δ (ppm) 210.4 (1C, C=O), 142.8 (2C, Ph-*ipso*), 139.6 (1C, PhBn-*ipso*), 128.7 (2C, Ar), 128.4 (2C, Ar), 127.7 (4C, Ar), 127.2 (2C, Ar), 127.0 (4C, Ar), 78.7 (1C, propargyl), 74.2 (1C, propargyl), 64.5 (2C, CH_2-bispidine), 64.3 (2C, CH_2-Bn), 61.6 (2C, CH_2-bispidine), 54.3 (2C, C-Ph bispidine), 46.8 (1C, CH_2-propargyl). Elemental analysis: $C_{29}H_{28}N_2O$: (420.56); calculated (%): C, 82.82; H, 6.71; N, 6.66; found (%): C, 82.21; H, 6.48; N, 6.62.

General procedure for the synthesis of azides (6a–6j)
An excess of sodium azide (15 eq.) was added to a mixture of alkyl or benzyl bromide (1 eq., 0.2 M) in *N*,*N*-dimethylformamide (DMF) and reacted under microwave irradiation at 100 °C for 15 min. The crude was extracted from ethyl acetate and water (5 times); the

organic phase was dried over anhydrous Na_2SO_4, filtered, and the liquid evaporated under vacuum to afford the azido-derivatives **6a–j** in quantitative yields.

6a: (Azidomethyl)benzene. ^{1}H-NMR (400 MHz, $CDCl_3$) δ (ppm) 7.34–7.19 (m, 5H, Ar), 4.27 (s, 2H, CH_2). All the other data are in agreement with the literature (see Supplementary Materials for references).

6b: 1-(Azidomethyl)-4-chlorobenzene. ^{1}H-NMR (400 MHz, $CDCl_3$) δ (ppm) 7.35 (d, *J* = 8.4 Hz, 2H, Ar), 7.24 (d, *J* = 8.4 Hz, 2H, Ar), 4.30 (s, 2H, CH_2). All the other data are in agreement with the literature (see Supplementary Materials for references).

6c: 1-(Azidomethyl)-4-nitrobenzene. ^{1}H-NMR (400 MHz, $CDCl_3$) δ (ppm) 8.25 (d, *J* = 8.8 Hz, 2H, Ar), 7.51 (d, *J* = 8.8 Hz, 2H, Ar), 4.51 (s, 2H, CH_2). All the other data are in agreement with the literature (see Supplementary Materials for references).

6d: 2-(Azidomethyl)pyridine. ^{1}H-NMR (400 MHz, $CDCl_3$) δ (ppm) 8.61 (d, *J* = 4.3 Hz, 1H, pyr), 7.72 (td, *J* = 7.7, 1.8 Hz, 1H, pyr), 7.35 (d, *J* = 7.8 Hz, 1H, pyr), 7.24 (d, 1H, pyr), 4.49 (s, 2H, CH_2). All the other data are in agreement with the literature (see Supplementary Materials for references).

6e: 4-(Azidomethyl)pyridine. ^{1}H-NMR (400 MHz, $CDCl_3$) δ (ppm) 8.63 (d, *J* = 7.5 Hz, 2H, pyr), 7.26 (d, *J* = 7.5 Hz, 2H, pyr), 4.41 (s, 2H, CH_2). All the other data are in agreement with the literature (see Supplementary Materials for references).

6f:1-Azidooctane. ^{1}H-NMR (400 MHz, $CDCl_3$) δ (ppm) 3.25 (t, *J* = 7.0 Hz, 2H, CH_2-N_3), 1.63–1.35 (m, 2H, alk), 1.33–1.27 (m, 10H, alk), 0.89 (t, *J* = 6.8 Hz, 3H, CH_3). All the other data are in agreement with the literature (see Supplementary Materials for references).

6g: 1-Azidoundecane. ^{1}H-NMR (400 MHz, $CDCl_3$) δ (ppm) 3.24 (t, *J* = 7.0 Hz, 2H, CH_2-N_3), 1.65–1.53 (m, 2H, alk), 1.40–1.21 (m, 16H, alk), 0.89 (t, *J* = 6.8 Hz, 3H, CH_3). All the other data are in agreement with the literature (see Supplementary Materials for references).

6h: 3-Azidopropan-1-ol. ^{1}H-NMR (400 MHz, $CDCl_3$) δ (ppm) 3.73 (m, 2H, CH_2-OH), 3.44 (t, *J* = 7.4 Hz, 2H, CH_2-N_3), 2.49 (br s, 1H, OH), 1.84 (q, *J* = 7.4 Hz, 2H, CH_2). All the other data are in agreement with the literature (see Supplementary Materials for references).

6i: 1,2-Bis(azidomethyl)benzene. ^{1}H-NMR (400 MHz, $CDCl_3$) δ (ppm) 7.37 (s, 4H, Ar-H), 4.43 (s, 4H, CH_2-N_3). All the other data are in agreement with the literature (see Supplementary Materials for references).

6j: 1,6-Diazidohexane. ^{1}H-NMR (400 MHz, $CDCl_3$) δ (ppm) 3.24 (t, *J* = 7.4 Hz, 4H, CH_2-N_3), 1.57–1.48 (m, 4H, alk), 1.36–1.31 (m, 4H, alk). All the other data are in agreement with the literature (see Supplementary Materials for references).

General procedure for the synthesis of bis-triazole-bispidines (7a–h)
Compound **1** (1 eq., 0.1 M) was dissolved in a 1:1 acetone-water mixture. Then, the appropriate azide (**6a–h**) (2.1 eq.), $CuSO_4$ (0.02 eq.), and sodium ascorbate (0.2 eq.) were added in sequence. The reaction was performed for 1 h under microwave (MW) irradiation at 50 °C. Then, acetone was removed under vacuum, and ethyl acetate was added to the aqueous medium to extract the desired compound in the organic phase. The complete removal of the copper catalyst was accomplished by washing the organic phase with a 1 M aqueous solution of ethylenediaminetetraacetic acid (EDTA). The organic phase was dried over anhydrous Na_2SO_4, filtered, and the liquid evaporated under vacuum. With this protocol, the desired product (**7a–h**) was obtained in good yield (73–95% yields, see Table 1).

7a: 3,7-Bis((1-benzyl-1*H*-1,2,3-triazol-4-yl)methyl)-1,5-diphenyl-3,7-diazabicyclo[3.3.1] nonan-9-one. Yield 95%. White solid. ^{1}H-NMR (400 MHz, $CDCl_3$) δ (ppm) 7.49 (s, 2H, triazole-H), 7.40–7.08 (m, 20 H, Ar-H), 5.52 (s, 4H, CH_2-Bn), 3.87 (s, 4H, CH_2-Bn), 3.50 (d, *J* = 10.8 Hz, 4H, CH_2-eq), 3.13 (d, *J* = 10.8 Hz, 4H, CH_2-ax). ^{13}C-NMR (101 MHz, $CDCl_3$) δ (ppm) 210.5 (1C, C=O), 145.1 (2C, triazole-*ipso*), 142.2 (2C, Ph-*ipso*), 135.5 (2C, Bn-*ipso*),

134.9 (2C, Ar), 129.3 (2C, Ar), 128.9 (2C, Ar), 128.8 (2C, Ar), 128.4 (2C, Ar), 128.3 (2C, Ar), 128.1 (2C, Ar), 128.0 (2C, Ar), 126.9 (2C, Ar), 126.8 (2C, Ar), 122.7 (2C, CH-triazole), 64.8 (4C, CH_2-bispidine), 54.3 (4C, CH_2-triazole + CH_2-Bn), 52.6 (2C, C-Ph bispidine). Elemental analysis: $C_{39}H_{38}N_8O$: (634.79); calculated (%): C, 73.79; H, 6.03; N, 17.65; found (%): C, 73.02; H, 5.97; N, 18.23; melting point: 271 °C.

7b: 3-((1-(3-Chlorobenzyl)-1*H*-1,2,3-triazol-4-yl)methyl)-7-((1-(4-chlorobenzyl)-1*H*-1,2,3-triazol-4-yl)methyl)-1,5-diphenyl-3,7-diazabicyclo[3.3.1]nonan-9-one. Yield 75%. White solid. ^{1}H-NMR (400 MHz, $CDCl_3$) δ (ppm) 7.52 (s, 2H, triazole-H), 7.36–7.08 (m, 18 H, Ar-H), 5.50 (s, 4H, CH_2-Bn), 3.88 (s, 4H, CH_2-Bn), 3.51 (d, *J* = 10.7 Hz, 4H, CH_2-eq), 3.13 (d, *J* = 10.7 Hz, 4H, CH_2-ax). ^{13}C-NMR (101 MHz, $CDCl_3$) δ (ppm) 210.4 (1C, C=O), 145.3 (2C, triazole-*ipso*), 142.1 (2C, Ph-*ipso*), 134.9 (2C, Bn-*ipso*), 133.4 (2C, Ar-Cl), 129.5 (4C, Ar), 129.4 (4C, Ar), 128.0 (4C, Ar), 126.9 (4C, Ar), 126.8 (2C, Ar), 122.7 (2C, CH-triazole), 64.9 (4C, CH_2-bispidine), 54.4 (2C, CH_2-triazole) 53.5 (2C, CH_2-Bn), 52.6 (2C, C-Ph bispidine). Elemental analysis: $C_{39}H_{36}Cl_2N_8O$: (703.67); calculated (%): C, 66.57; H, 5.16; N, 15.92; found (%): C, 67.00; H, 5.55; N, 16.21; melting point: 244 °C.

7c: 3-((1-(3-Nitrobenzyl)-1*H*-1,2,3-triazol-4-yl)methyl)-7-((1-(4-nitrobenzyl)-1*H*-1,2,3-triazol-4-yl)methyl)-1,5-diphenyl-3,7-diazabicyclo[3.3.1]nonan-9-one. Yield 78%. White solid. ^{1}H-NMR (400 MHz, $CDCl_3$) δ (ppm) 8.21 (d, *J* = 8.7 Hz, 4H, *o*-NO_2Ar), 7.64 (s, 2H, triazole-H), 7.41 (d, *J* = 8.6 Hz, 4H, *m*-NO_2Ar), 7.31–7.10 (m, 10H, Ar-H), 5.67 (s, 4H, CH_2-Bn), 3.92 (s, 4H, CH_2-Bn), 3.57 (d, *J* = 10.4 Hz, 4H, CH_2-eq), 3.16 (d, *J* = 10.4 Hz, 4H, CH_2-ax). ^{13}C-NMR (101 MHz, $CDCl_3$) δ (ppm) 210.2 (1C, C=O), 148.1 (2C, Ar-NO_2), 145.5 (2C, triazole-*ipso*), 141.8 (4C, Ph-*ipso* + Bn-*ipso*), 128.5 (2C, Ar), 127.9 (4C, Ar), 126.9 (4C, Ar), 126.8 (4C, Ar), 124.3 (4C, Ar), 123.0 (2C, CH-triazole), 64.8 (4C, CH_2-bispidine), 54.3 (2C, CH_2-triazole) 53.1 (2C, CH_2-Bn), 52.4 (2C, C-Ph bispidine). Elemental analysis: $C_{39}H_{36}N_{10}O_5$: (724.78); calculated (%): C, 64.63; H, 5.01; N, 19.33; found (%): C, 64.02; H, 4.87; N, 19.65; melting point: 267 °C.

7d: 1,5-Diphenyl-3,7-bis((1-(pyridin-2-ylmethyl)-1*H*-1,2,3-triazol-4-yl)methyl)-3,7-diazabicyclo[3.3.1]nonan-9-one. Yield 84%. White solid. ^{1}H-NMR (400 MHz, $CDCl_3$) δ (ppm) 8.58 (d, *J* = 4.3 Hz, 2H, CH-pyr), 7.73 (s, 2H, triazole-H), 7.65 (td, *J* = 7.7, 1.8 Hz, 2H, CH-pyr), 7.40–7.09 (m, 14H, Ar-H), 5.67 (s, 4H, CH_2-Bn), 3.92 (s, 4H, CH_2-Bn), 3.54 (d, *J* = 10.4 Hz, 4H, CH_2-eq), 3.15 (d, *J* = 10.4 Hz, 4H, CH_2-ax). ^{13}C-NMR (101 MHz, DMSO-d_6) δ (ppm) 211.2 (1C, C=O), 155.7 (2C, pyridine-*ipso*), 149.8 (2C, pyr), 143.9 (2C, triazole-*ipso*), 143.4, (2C, Ph-*ipso*), 128.2 (2C, Ar), 127.2 (4C, Ar), 126.8 (4C, Ar), 125.3 (2C, Ar), 123.6 (4C, Ar), 122.3 (2C, CH-triazole), 64.4 (4C, CH_2-bispidine), 54.8 (2C, CH_2-triazole) 54.5 (2C, CH_2-Bn), 51.9 (2C, C-Ph bispidine). Elemental analysis: $C_{37}H_{36}N_{10}O$: (636.76); calculated (%): C, 69.79; H, 5.70; N, 22.00; found (%): C, 70.59; H, 6.03; N, 22.14; melting point: 241 °C.

7e: 1,5-Diphenyl-3,7-bis((1-(pyridine-4-ylmethyl)-1*H*-1,2,3-triazol-4-yl)methyl)-3,7-diazabicyclo[3.3.1]nonan-9-one. Yield 83%. White solid. ^{1}H-NMR (400 MHz, $CDCl_3$) δ (ppm) 8.57 (dd, *J* = 4.5, 1.6 Hz, 2H, CH-pyr), 7.61 (s, 2H, triazole-H), 7.25–7.11 (m, 14H, Ar-H), 7.06 (d, *J* = 6.0 Hz, 2H, CH-pyr), 5.53 (s, 4H, CH_2-Bn), 3.91 (s, 4H, CH_2-Bn), 3.55 (d, *J* = 10.4 Hz, 4H, CH_2-eq), 3.15 (d, *J* = 10.4 Hz, 4H, CH_2-ax). ^{13}C-NMR (101 MHz, $CDCl_3$) δ (ppm) 210.2 (1C, C=O), 150.6 (4C, pyr), 145.4 (2C, pyridine-*ipso*), 143.7 (2C, triazole-*ipso*), 141.9 (2C, Ph-*ipso*), 127.9 (4C, Ar), 126.8 (6C, Ar), 123.1 (4C, Ar), 122.0 (2C, CH-triazole), 64.8 (4C, CH_2-bispidine), 54.3 (2C, CH_2-triazole) 52.7 (2C, CH_2-Bn), 52.4 (2C, C-Ph bispidine). Elemental analysis: $C_{37}H_{36}N_{10}O$: (636.76); calculated (%): C, 69.79; H, 5.70; N, 22.00; found (%): C, 70.53; H, 6.12; N, 22.11; melting point: 257 °C.

7f: 3,7-Bis((1-octyl-1*H*-1,2,3-triazol-4-yl)methyl)-1,5-diphenyl-3,7-diazabicyclo[3.3.1] nonan-9-one. Yield 86%. Yellow oil. ^{1}H-NMR (400 MHz, $CDCl_3$) δ (ppm) 7.56 (s, 2H, triazole-H), 7.29–7.15 (m, 10H, Ar-H), 4.35 (t, *J* = 7.3 Hz, 4H, alk-CH_2-triazole), 3.91 (s, 4H, N-CH_2-triazole), 3.56 (d, *J* = 10.8 Hz, 4H, CH_2-eq), 3.16 (d, *J* = 10.8 Hz, 4H, CH_2-ax), 1.98–1.82 (m, 4H, alk), 1.37–1.19 (m, 20H, alk), 0.86 (t, *J* = 6.7 Hz, 6H, alk). ^{13}C-NMR (101 MHz, $CDCl_3$) δ (ppm) 210.4 (1C, C=O), 144.5 (2C, triazole-*ipso*), 142.3 (2C, Ph-*ipso*), 127.8

(4C, Ar), 126.8 (4C, Ar), 126.6 (2C, Ar), 122.4 (2C, CH-triazole), 64.7 (4C, CH_2-bispidine), 54.3 (2C, CH_2-triazole), 52.5 (2C, C-Ph bispidine), 50.4 (2C, alk), 31.7 (2C, alk), 30.3 (2C, alk), 29.0 (2C, alk), 28.9 (2C, alk), 26.5 (2C, alk), 22.5 (2C, alk), 14.0 (2C, alk). Elemental analysis: $C_{41}H_{58}N_8O$: (678.97); calculated (%): C, 72.53; H, 8.61; N, 16.50; found (%): C, 72.91; H, 8.11; N, 15.99.

7g: 1,5-Diphenyl-3,7-bis((1-undecyl-1*H*-1,2,3-triazol-4-yl)methyl)-3,7-diazabicyclo[3.3.1] nonan-9-one. Yield 73%. Yellow oil. ^{1}H-NMR (400 MHz, DMSO-d$_6$) δ (ppm) 8.13 (s, 2H, triazole-H), 7.36–7.07 (m, 10H, Ar-H), 4.35 (t, *J* = 6.9 Hz, 4H, alk-CH_2-triazole), 3.85 (s, 4H, N-CH_2-triazole), 3.50 (d, *J* = 10.8 Hz, 4H, CH_2-eq), 3.03 (d, *J* = 10.7 Hz, 4H, CH_2-ax), 1.82 (m, 4H, alk), 1.26–1.11 (m, 32H, alk), 0.85 (t, *J* = 6.9 Hz, 6H, alk). ^{13}C-NMR (101 MHz, DMSO-d$_6$) δ (ppm) 211.1 (1C, C=O), 143.8 (2C, triazole-*ipso*), 143.4 (2C, Ph-*ipso*), 128.1 (4C, Ar), 127.2 (4C, Ar), 126.7 (2C, Ar), 124.15 (2C, CH-triazole), 64.45 (4C, CH_2-bispidine), 54.53 (2C, CH_2-triazole), 52.02 (2C, C-Ph bispidine), 49.76 (2C, alk), 31.75 (2C, alk), 29.38 (6C, alk), 29.31 (2C, alk), 29.13 (2C, alk), 28.84 (2C, alk), 26.27 (2C, alk), 22.54 (2C, alk), 14.39 (2C, alk). Elemental analysis: $C_{47}H_{70}N_8O$: (763.13); calculated (%): C, 73.97; H, 9.25; N, 14.68; found (%): C, 73.09; H, 8.99; N, 14.18.

7h: 3,7-Bis((1-(3-hydroxypropyl)-1*H*-1,2,3-triazol-4-yl)methyl)-1,5-diphenyl-3,7-diazabicyclo[3.3.1]nonan-9-one. Yield 85%. White solid. ^{1}H-NMR (400 MHz, $CDCl_3$) δ (ppm) 7.68 (s, 2H, triazole-H), 7.32–7.10 (m, 10H, Ar-H), 4.52 (t, *J* = 6.6 Hz, 4H, alk-CH_2-triazole), 3.90 (s, 4H, N-CH_2-triazole), 3.60–3.56 (m, 4H, -CH_2-OH), 3.54 (d, *J* = 10.9 Hz, 4H, CH_2-eq), 3.14 (d, *J* = 10.8 Hz, 4H, CH_2-ax), 2.96 (br s, 2H, OH), 2.14–2.06 (m, 4H, alk-CH_2). ^{13}C- NMR (101 MHz, $CDCl_3$) δ (ppm) 210.5 (1C, C=O), 144.5 (2C, triazole-*ipso*), 142.0 (2C, Ph-*ipso*), 128.0 (4C, Ar), 127.0 (4C, Ar), 126.9 (2C, Ar), 123.8 (2C, CH-triazole), 64.8 (4C, CH_2-bispidine), 58.4 (2C, CH_2-OH), 54.3 (2C, CH_2-triazole), 52.4 (2C, C-Ph bispidine), 47.0 (2C, alk), 32.7 (2C, alk). Elemental analysis: $C_{31}H_{38}N_8O_3$: (570.70); calculated (%): C, 65.24; H, 6.71; N, 19.63; found (%): C, 65.87; H, 625; N, 19.18; melting point: 275 °C.

General procedure for the synthesis of mono-triazole-bispidines (8a and 8b)
Compound **5** (1 eq., 0.1 M) was dissolved in a 1:1 acetone-water mixture. Then, azide **6a** or **6g** (1.1 eq.), $CuSO_4$ (0.02 eq.), and sodium ascorbate (0.2 eq.) were added in sequence. The reaction was performed under microwave irradiation for 1 h at 50 °C. Then, the mixture was dissolved in ethyl acetate and washed with 1 M aqueous ammonia solution to accomplish the complete removal of the copper catalyst. The organic phase was dried over anhydrous Na_2SO_4, filtered, and the liquid evaporated under vacuum to give the desired pure product.

8a: 3-Benzyl-7-((1-benzyl-1*H*-1,2,3-triazol-4-yl)methyl)-1,5-diphenyl-3,7-diazabicyclo[3.3.1]nonan-9-one. Yield 91%. White solid. ^{1}H-NMR (400 MHz, $CDCl_3$) δ (ppm) 8.21 (s, 1H, triazole-H), 7.41–7.08 (m, 20H, Ar-H), 5.63 (s, 2H, triazole-CH_2-Bn), 3.89 (s, 2H, CH_2-Bn), 3.71 (s, 2H, N-CH_2-triazole), 3.55 (d, *J* = 10.7 Hz, 2H, CH_2-eq), 3.45 (d, *J* = 10.6 Hz, 2H, CH_2-eq), 3.06 (d, *J* = 10.6 Hz, 2H, CH_2-ax), 2.97 (d, *J* = 10.6 Hz, 2H, CH_2-ax). ^{13}C-NMR (101 MHz, DMSO-d$_6$) δ (ppm) 211.2 (1C, C=O), 143.8 (1C, triazole-*ipso*), 143.4 (1C, Ph-*ipso*), 138.6 (1C, Ph-*ipso*), 136.7 (1C, Ph-*ipso*), 129.3 (4C, Ar), 129.1 (2C, Ar), 128.7 (2C, Ar), 128.5 (2C, Ar), 128.1 (4C, Ar), 127.6 (2C, Ar), 127.2 (2C, Ar), 126.8 (2C, Ar), 124.6 (1C, CH-triazole), 64.5 (4C, CH_2-bispidine), 61.1 (1C, N-CH_2-triazole), 60.2 (1C, CH_2 bispidine), 54.5 (1C, CH_2-Bn), 53.2 (1C, CH_2-triazole), 51.9 (2C, C-Ph bispidine). Elemental analysis: $C_{36}H_{35}N_5O$: (553.71); calculated (%): C, 78.09; H, 6.37; N, 12.65; found (%): C, 78.97; H, 6.81; N, 12.99; melting point: 259 °C.

8b: 3-Benzyl-1,5-diphenyl-7-((1-undecyl-1*H*-1,2,3-triazol-4-yl)methyl)-3,7-diazabicyclo[3.3.1]nonan-9-one. Yield 94%. Yellow oil. ^{1}H-NMR (400 MHz, DMSO-d$_6$) δ (ppm) 8.13 (s, 1H, triazole-H), 7.42–7.11 (m, 15H, Ar-H), 4.36 (t, *J* = 6.9 Hz, 2H, alk-CH_2-triazole), 3.88 (s, 2H, CH_2-Bn), 3.72 (s, 2H, N-CH_2-triazole), 3.54 (d, *J* = 10.8 Hz, 2H, CH_2-eq), 3.46 (d, *J* = 10.8 Hz, 2H, CH_2-eq), 3.05 (d, *J* = 10.8 Hz, 2H, CH_2-ax), 2.99 (d, *J* = 10.8 Hz, 2H, CH_2-ax), 1.82 (dd, *J* = 14.1, 7.0 Hz, 2H, alk), 1.17 (d, *J* = 14.3 Hz, 16H, alk), 0.84 (t, *J* = 6.8 Hz, 3H, alk). ^{13}C-NMR (101 MHz, DMSO-d$_6$) δ (ppm) 211.2 (1C, C=O), 143.4 (1C, triazole-*ipso*), 143.3

(1C, Ph-*ipso*), 138.6 (1C, Ph-*ipso*), 129.3 (4C, Ar), 128.7 (2C, Ar), 128.1 (2C, Ar), 127.6 (4C, Ar), 127.2 (2C, Ar), 126.7 (1C, Ar), 124.2 (1C, CH-triazole), 64.6 (2C, CH_2-bispidine), 64.4 (2C, CH_2-bispidine), 61.1 (1C, N-CH_2-triazole), 54.5 (2C, CH_2-Bn + CH_2-triazole), 51.9 (1C, C-Ph bispidine), 49.7 (1C, alk), 31.7 (1C, alk), 30.2 (1C, alk), 29.3 (2C, alk), 29.1 (3C, alk), 28.8 (1C, alk), 26.2 (1C, alk), 22.5 (1C, alk), 14.4 (1C, alk). Elemental analysis: $C_{40}H_{51}N_5O$: (617.88); calculated (%): C, 77.76; H, 8.32; N, 11.33; found (%): C, 78.26; H, 8.70; N, 11.67.

General procedure for the synthesis of the bispidine-metal complexes
The 1:1 bispidine–metal complexes were prepared by stirring at room temperature a 0.1 M solution of the ligand in acetonitrile with a stoichiometric amount of the salt for 24 h. The resulting precipitate was filtered off on a Buchner funnel and submitted to ESI-MS analysis and NMR in CD_3CN.

Henry reaction's optimized procedure
Aldehyde (1 eq, 0.2 M) was dissolved in methanol; 15% mol **7a·Zn** catalyst was added, and then nitromethane (5 eq) was slowly dripped into the mixture. The reaction was left stirring for 1 h at 80 °C under microwave irradiation; the crude was then filtered, and the liquid phase submitted to GC-MS analysis for the conversion quantification.

4.3. Crystallographic Data

Poor-quality crystals of **8a** were obtained as transparent plates by the slow evaporation of an acetone/ethanol 1:1 solution at room temperature. Diffraction data were collected on a Bruker-AXS CCD-based three circle diffractometer, working at 150 K with graphite-monochromatized Mo-Kα X-radiation (λ = 0.7107 Å), employing a 0.55 × 0.22 × 0.02 mm crystal. The structure was solved by direct method via SIR-2014 [30] and completed by iterative cycles of full-matrix least squares refinement on F_o^2 and ΔF synthesis using SHELXL-2019/3 [31] on the WinGX v2021.3 suite [32]. H atoms were generated stereochemically and refined by a riding model; $U_{iso}(H)$ was defined as 1.2 Ueq of the parent carbon atom for phenyl and methylene residues. The analyzed crystal was a two-component pseudo-merohedral twin in the monoclinic system, found using the TwinRotMat routine in PLATON [22]. Twin law [−1 0 0 0 −1 0 1 0 1] reduced the R1 residual [I > 2σ(I)] from 0.103 to 0.0629, and the mass ratio of the twin components was refined to 0.894(5):0.106.

Crystal data for **8a**. Formula: $C_{36}H_{35}N_5O_1$; MW = 553.69 g/mol; Bravais lattice: monoclinic; Space group: Cc (n° 9); Z = 4; Cell parameters: *a* = 15.354(2) Å, *b* = 15.453(2) Å, *c* = 51.948(10) Å, β = 98.65(3)°; V = 12185(4) Å^3; D_{calc} =1.207 Mg/m^3; T = 150(2)K; μ = (MoKα) 0.074 mm^{-1}; $2\theta_{min}$ = 1.189°; $2\theta_{max}$ = 25.850°; Limiting indices = $-17 \leq h \leq 17$, $-18 \leq k \leq 18$, $-63 \leq l \leq 61$; Crystal size: 0.55 × 0.22 × 0.02 mm; F(000) = 4704; R_{int} = 0.0422; Data/restraints/parameters: 17072/5/1514; R = 0.0629 for 13880 reflections with I > 2σ(I) (R = 0.0885 for all 17072 unique/27192 collected reflections); wR2 = 0.1009 for reflections with I > 2σ(I) (wR2 = 0.1110 for all unique reflections); GOOF: 1.139; Residual positive and negative electron densities in the final map: 0.226 and −0.268 eÅ^{-3}.

Supplementary Materials: The following are available online at https://www.mdpi.com/article/10.3390/molecules28176351/s1, Figures S1–S25: NMR data for the characterization of the synthesized products. Figures S26–S29: NMR titration spectra of bispidine-metal complexes. Figures S30–S33: Comparison of the experimental ESI-MS spectra of bispidine-metal complexes and the simulation of the isotopic pattern for the elemental composition. Table S1: Comparison of the free ligands **7a,b,d,h** and their metal complexes: list of the Δδ in the ^{1}H-NMR spectra. CCDC-2063528 contains the supplementary crystallographic data for this paper.

Author Contributions: Conceptualization, A.S. and A.R.; investigation, A.R. and G.C.D.; X-ray data curation, M.M., C.C. and F.M.; supervision, A.S.; writing—original draft preparation, A.R., G.C.D., F.M. and A.S.; writing—review and editing, all authors. All authors have read and agreed to the published version of the manuscript.

Funding: The authors thank the University of Milan and the Polytechnic University of Milan for financial support.

Institutional Review Board Statement: Not applicable.

Informed Consent Statement: Not applicable.

Data Availability Statement: CCDC-2063528 contains the supplementary crystallographic data for this paper. These data can be obtained free of charge via https://www.ccdc.cam.ac.uk/structures/ (accessed on 13 July 2023) or by e-mailing data_request@ccdc.cam.ac.uk, or by contacting The Cambridge Crystallographic Data Centre, 12 Union Road, Cambridge CB2 1EZ, UK; fax: +44(0)1223-336033.

Conflicts of Interest: The authors declare no conflict of interest.

Sample Availability: Not available.

References

1. Comba, P.; Haaf, C.; Wadepohl, H. Novel Bispidine Ligands and Their First-Row Transition Metal Complexes: Trigonal Bipyramidal and Trigonal Prismatic Geometries. *Inorg. Chem.* **2009**, *48*, 6604–6614. [CrossRef]
2. Sacchetti, A.; Rossetti, A. Synthesis of Natural Compounds Based on the [3,7]-Diazabicyclo[3.3.1]nonane (Bispidine) Core. *Eur. J. Org. Chem.* **2021**, 1491–1507. [CrossRef]
3. Black, D.S.C.; Deacon, G.B.; Rose, M. Synthesis and metal complexes of symmetrically N-substituted bispidinones. *Tetrahedron* **1995**, *51*, 2055–2076. [CrossRef]
4. Comba, P.; Hunoldt, S.; Morgen, M.; Pietzsch, J.; Stephan, H.; Wadepohl, H. Optimization of pentadentate bispidines as bifunctional chelators for 64Cu positron emission tomography (PET). *Inorg. Chem.* **2013**, *52*, 8131–8143. [CrossRef] [PubMed]
5. Comba, P.; Jermilova, U.; Orvig, C.; Patrick, B.O.; Ramogida, C.F.; Rück, K.; Schneider, C.; Starke, M. Octadentate Picolinic Acid-Based Bispidine Ligand for Radiometal Ions. *Chem. Eur. J.* **2017**, *23*, 15945–15956. [CrossRef]
6. Rossetti, A.; Landoni, S.; Meneghetti, F.; Castellano, C.; Mori, M.; Colombo Dugoni, G.; Sacchetti, A. Application of chiral bi- and tetra-dentate bispidine-derived ligands in the copper(ii)-catalyzed asymmetric Henry reaction. *New J. Chem.* **2018**, *42*, 12072–12081. [CrossRef]
7. Lippi, M.; Wadepohl, H.; Comba, P.; Cametti, M. A Bispidine Based CuII/ZnII Heterobimetallic Coordination Polymer. *Eur. J. Inorg. Chem.* **2022**, *2022*, e202200221. [CrossRef]
8. Mori, M.; Fumagalli, E.; Castellano, C.; Tresoldi, A.; Sacchetti, A.; Meneghetti, F. Synthesis and characterization of a tetradentate bispidine-based ligand and its zinc(II) complex. *Inorganica Chim. Acta* **2022**, *538*, 120968. [CrossRef]
9. Gao, F.; Sihver, W.; Bergmann, R.; Walther, M.; Stephan, H.; Belter, B.; Neuber, C.; Haase-Kohn, C.; Bolzati, C.; Pietzsch, J.; et al. Radiochemical and radiopharmacological characterization of a 64Cu-labeled α-MSH analog conjugated with different chelators. *J. Label. Compd. Radiopharm.* **2019**, *62*, 495–509. [CrossRef]
10. Bleher, K.; Comba, P.; Kass, D.; Ray, K.; Wadepohl, H. Reactivities of iron(IV)-oxido compounds with pentadentate bispidine ligands. *J. Inorg. Biochem.* **2023**, *241*, 112123. [CrossRef]
11. Rossetti, A.; Lippi, M.; Martí-Rujas, J.; Sacchetti, A.; Cametti, M. Highly Dynamic and Tunable Behavior of 1D Coordination Polymers Based on the Bispidine Ligand. *Chem. Eur. J.* **2018**, *24*, 19368–19372. [CrossRef]
12. Grosshauser, M.; Comba, P.; Kim, J.Y.; Ohto, K.; Thuéry, P.; Lee, Y.H.; Kim, Y.; Harrowfield, J. Ferro- and antiferromagnetic coupling in a chlorido-bridged, tetranuclear Cu(ii) complex. *Dalt. Trans.* **2014**, *43*, 5662–5666. [CrossRef]
13. Nonat, A.M.; Roux, A.; Sy, M.; Charbonnière, L.J. 2,4-Substituted bispidines as rigid hosts for versatile applications: From κ-opioid receptor to metal coordination. *Dalt. Trans.* **2019**, *48*, 16476–16492. [CrossRef]
14. Kolb, H.C.; Finn, M.G.; Sharpless, K.B. Click Chemistry: Diverse Chemical Function from a Few Good Reactions. *Angew. Chem. Int. Ed.* **2001**, *40*, 2004–2021. [CrossRef]
15. Eremina, O.E.; Kapitanova, O.O.; Medved'ko, A.V.; Zelenetskaya, A.S.; Egorova, B.V.; Shekhovtsova, T.N.; Vatsadze, S.Z.; Veselova, I.A. Plier Ligands for Trapping Neurotransmitters into Complexes for Sensitive Analysis by SERS Spectroscopy. *Biosensors* **2023**, *13*, 124. [CrossRef]
16. Dalinger, A.I.; Medved'ko, A.V.; Balalaeva, A.I.; Vatsadze, I.; Dalinger, I.L.; Vatsadze, S.Z. Synthesis of Novel Azides and Triazoles on the Basis of 1*H*-Pyrazole-3(5)-Carboxylic Acids. *Chem. Heterocycl. Compd.* **2020**, *56*, 180–191. [CrossRef]
17. Vatsadze, S.Z.; Medved'ko, A.V.; Bodunov, A.A.; Lyssenko, K.A. Bispidine-based bis-azoles as a new family of supramolecular receptors: The theoretical approach. *Mendeleev Commun.* **2020**, *30*, 344–346. [CrossRef]
18. Elliott, P.I.P. Chapter 1 Organometallic complexes with 1,2,3-triazole-derived ligands. In *Organometallic Chemistry*; The Royal Society of Chemistry: London, UK, 2014; Volume 39, pp. 1–25, ISBN 978-1-84973-583-4.
19. Creary, X.; Chormanski, K.; Peirats, G.; Renneburg, C. Electronic Properties of Triazoles. Experimental and Computational Determination of Carbocation and Radical-Stabilizing Properties. *J. Org. Chem.* **2017**, *82*, 5720–5730. [CrossRef] [PubMed]

20. Bulygina, L.A.; Kagramanov, N.D.; Khrushcheva, N.S.; Lyssenko, K.A.; Peregudov, A.S.; Sokolov, V.I. Unsymmetrical pincer CNN palladium complex of 7-ferrocenylmethyl-3-methyl-3,7-diazabicyclo[3.3.1]nonane. *J. Organomet. Chem.* **2017**, *846*, 169–175. [CrossRef]
21. Bulygina, L.A.; Khrushcheva, N.S.; Peregudov, A.S.; Sokolov, V.I. Cyclopalladate complex of 3-benzyl-7-methyl-3,7-diazabicyclo[3.3.1]nonane. *Russ. Chem. Bull.* **2016**, *65*, 2479–2484. [CrossRef]
22. Spek, A.L. Single-crystal structure validation with the program platon. *J. Appl. Crystallogr.* **2003**, *36*, 7–13. [CrossRef]
23. MacRae, C.F.; Sovago, I.; Cottrell, S.J.; Galek, P.T.A.; McCabe, P.; Pidcock, E.; Platings, M.; Shields, G.P.; Stevens, J.S.; Towler, M.; et al. Mercury 4.0: From visualization to analysis, design and prediction. *J. Appl. Crystallogr.* **2020**, *53*, 226–235. [CrossRef] [PubMed]
24. Cremer, D.; Pople, J.A. General definition of ring puckering coordinates. *J. Am. Chem. Soc.* **1975**, *97*, 1354–1358. [CrossRef]
25. Luzzio, F.A. The Henry reaction: Recent examples. *Tetrahedron* **2001**, *57*, 915–945. [CrossRef]
26. Noboru, O. *The Nitro Group in Organic Synthesis*; Wiley Online Books: Hoboken, NJ, USA, 2001; ISBN 9780471224488.
27. Ballini, R. Synthesis of natural products via aliphatic nitroderivatives. In *Structure and Chemistry (Part E)*; Atta-ur-Rahman, B.T.-S.N.P.C., Ed.; Elsevier: Amsterdam, The Netherlands, 1996; Volume 19, pp. 117–184, ISBN 1572-5995.
28. Murugavel, G.; Sadhu, P.; Punniyamurthy, T. Copper(II)-Catalyzed Nitroaldol (Henry) Reactions: Recent Developments. *Chem. Rec.* **2016**, *16*, 1906–1917. [CrossRef]
29. Saranya, S.; Harry, N.A.; Ujwaldev, S.M.; Anilkumar, G. Recent Advances and Perspectives on the Zinc-Catalyzed Nitroaldol (Henry) Reaction. *Asian J. Org. Chem.* **2017**, *6*, 1349–1360. [CrossRef]
30. Burla, M.C.; Caliandro, R.; Carrozzini, B.; Cascarano, G.L.; Cuocci, C.; Giacovazzo, C.; Mallamo, M.; Mazzone, A.; Polidori, G. Crystal structure determination and refinement via SIR2014. *J. Appl. Crystallogr.* **2015**, *48*, 306–309. [CrossRef]
31. Sheldrick, G.M. Crystal structure refinement with SHELXL. *Acta Crystallogr. Sect. C Struct. Chem.* **2015**, *71*, 3–8. [CrossRef] [PubMed]
32. Farrugia, L.J. WinGX and ORTEP for Windows: An update. *J. Appl. Crystallogr.* **2012**, *45*, 849–854. [CrossRef]

molecules

Article

Magnetic Aerogels for Room-Temperature Catalytic Production of Bis(indolyl)methane Derivatives

Nicola Melis [1], Danilo Loche [2], Swapneel V. Thakkar [3,†], Maria Giorgia Cutrufello [3], Maria Franca Sini [3], Gianmarco Sedda [3], Luca Pilia [1], Angelo Frongia [3,*] and Maria Francesca Casula [1,*]

1 Department of Mechanical, Chemical and Materials Engineering, University of Cagliari, 09123 Cagliari, Italy
2 Nanostructures & Biotech Laboratory, Biological and Environmental Science and Engineering (BESE) Division, King Abdullah University of Science and Technology, Thuwal 23955-6900, Saudi Arabia
3 Department of Chemical and Geological Sciences, University of Cagliari, 09042 Monserrato, Italy
* Correspondence: afrongia@unica.it (A.F.); mariaf.casula@unica.it (M.F.C.)
† Current address: Tronox, Research Center Thann, 95 Rue du Général de Gaulle, 68800 Thann, France.

Abstract: The potential of aerogels as catalysts for the synthesis of a relevant class of bis-heterocyclic compounds such as bis(indolyl)methanes was investigated. In particular, the studied catalyst was a nanocomposite aerogel based on nanocrystalline nickel ferrite ($NiFe_2O_4$) dispersed on amorphous porous silica aerogel obtained by two-step sol–gel synthesis followed by gel drying under supercritical conditions and calcination treatments. It was found that the $NiFe_2O_4/SiO_2$ aerogel is an active catalyst for the selected reaction, enabling high conversions at room temperature, and it proved to be active for three repeated runs. The catalytic activity can be ascribed to both the textural and acidic features of the silica matrix and of the nanocrystalline ferrite. In addition, ferrite nanocrystals provide functionality for magnetic recovery of the catalyst from the crude mixture, enabling time-effective separation from the reaction environment. Evidence of the retention of species involved in the reaction into the catalyst is also pointed out, likely due to the porosity of the aerogel together with the affinity of some species towards the silica matrix. Our work contributes to the study of aerogels as catalysts for organic reactions by demonstrating their potential as well as limitations for the room-temperature synthesis of bis(indolyl)methanes.

Keywords: aerogel; ferrite; nanocomposite; catalyst; organic synthesis; bis(indolyl)methanes

Citation: Melis, N.; Loche, D.; Thakkar, S.V.; Cutrufello, M.G.; Sini, M.F.; Sedda, G.; Pilia, L.; Frongia, A.; Casula, M.F. Magnetic Aerogels for Room-Temperature Catalytic Production of Bis(indolyl)methane Derivatives. *Molecules* **2024**, *29*, 2223. https://doi.org/10.3390/molecules29102223

Academic Editors: Fabio Ganazzoli and Giuseppina Raffaini

Received: 31 March 2024
Revised: 5 May 2024
Accepted: 6 May 2024
Published: 9 May 2024

1. Introduction

Unique features of aerogel materials such as their extremely high and open porosity, the controlled and tunable composition and purity, as well as the ability to stabilize highly dispersed active metal-based nanocrystals, make them ideal candidates as catalysts [1–3].

The use of aerogels in heterogeneous catalysis dates back to pioneering work by Pajonk, where simple and mixed oxide aerogels were applied to selective oxidation, hydrogenation, and reduction reactions, taking advantage of the high thermal and time-on-stream stability of oxide aerogels [4–6]. Since then, aerogels have been used as catalysts and supports for catalytic active phases for a broad range of processes, including biocatalysis [7].

Current trends in silica-based materials, which rank among the most investigated aerogels, have been recently reviewed and include nanofiber-reinforced and silica-hybridized cellulose for targeted applications such as thermal insulation [8–10]. In particular, advances in the production of aerogel composites have enabled the preparation of catalysts where the catalytically active nanocrystalline phase is finely dispersed over a highly porous silica matrix. Such nanocomposite aerogels have been demonstrated to be active as heterogeneous catalysts for a wide range of gas-phase reactions relevant for energy and technological applications, such as the Fischer–Tropsch process, the Catalytic Chemical Vapor Deposition production of carbon nanotubes, and the Water–Gas Shift reaction [11–14]. Together with the peculiar textural features of aerogels, which may confer improved catalytic performance as compared to the corresponding xerogels, a major advantage associated with the dispersion of catalytically active nanocrystals into highly porous aerogel matrices is that sintering is prevented during operating conditions, retaining the catalytic performance [12,15].

Molins and coworkers have investigated the use of silica-based and carbon-based nanocomposite aerogels as catalysts for organic reactions such as Mizoroki–Heck coupling and Biginelli condensation reactions [16,17]. This innovative approach offers the opportunity to explore the potential of novel aerogel-based catalysts as an alternative to conventional homogeneous catalysts used for organic processes. Among the advantages of using a solid catalyst, major aspects relate to the ease of separation of the catalyst from the reaction mixture, enabling therefore a more cost- and time-effective process and opening the way for catalyst reuse. In particular, together with filtration, magnetic separation of the catalyst from the reaction mixture can be easily performed by using magnetic solid catalysts. In addition, by taking advantage of the fine tuning enabled by sol–gel chemistry, the catalyst performance can be optimized by combining optimized features of the matrix and supported phase, as demonstrated by the design of alkylation catalysts based on metal halide supported on acidic silica-alumina aerogel matrix [18].

In this work, we investigate, to the best of our knowledge for the first time, the use of nanocomposite magnetic aerogels as catalysts for the synthesis of bis(indolyl)methanes starting from indole and aromatic aldehydes.

Bis(indolyl)methanes (BIMs) rank among the natural bis-heterocyclic compounds whose relevance is related to their broad occurrence in terrestrial and marine sources as well as to their biological role as metabolites [19]. Synthetic BIMs represent relevant organic intermediates for the pharmaceutical and chemical industry, with potential areas of applications ranging from colorimetric ion detection to dietary supplements [20]. Recently, BIMs have attracted great interest due to their prospective pharmacological properties such as antiproliferative and anti-cancer activity [21,22].

The wide range of applications in the synthesis of organic derivatives, as well as potential applications in the detection, sensing, biological, and pharmaceutical fields, have motivated the research on synthetic approaches to BIMs. BIMs are usually obtained by acid-catalyzed electrophilic substitution reaction of indole with a carbonyl compound such as an aldehyde or a ketone. The overall process implies a reaction between indole **1** and an aromatic aldehyde **2** leading to the formation of the corresponding alcohol **A** and, upon dehydration, of the corresponding azafulven intermediate **B**, as shown in Figure 1. This intermediate undergoes the subsequent addition of a second indole molecule to yield the final BIM derivative. In this classic approach, both Lewis and Brønsted acids have been proved to act as effective catalysts of the reaction.

Alternative strategies include synthetic protocols starting from intermediate **A** or **B**. In particular, based on such a methodology, the synthesis of asymmetric BIMs was reported by Bergman [23]. Moreover, BIMs have been produced through photochemical-induced methods [24–26], and ultrasound and microwave irradiation [27,28], with the aim to establish green and health-caring approaches.

Nevertheless, the standard method remains the most straightforward and versatile approach for access to BIM derivatives. In fact, the reaction has been extensively studied using a wide variety of Brønsted and Lewis acids in solution and several solids with acid behaviour for heterogeneous catalysis. Mineral acids (such as HCl, HBr, or H_2SO_4) and organic acids (such as formic or acetic acids [29–32], sulfamic acid [33–36], or p-Toluenesulfonic acid [37]) have been successfully employed as catalysts in this method. Furthermore, tests of a wide selection of Lewis acids (such as chlorides, oxides, and other salts of transition metals such as Fe, Cu [38–42], Zn [43,44], Al [45,46], Ti [47–49], and Zr [50], along with different examples of rare earth salts) have been reported in the literature. Among other examples, Wang and co-workers studied with an extensive screening the effect of the nature of the Lewis acids used as catalytic species in the reaction between indole and benzaldehyde [51].

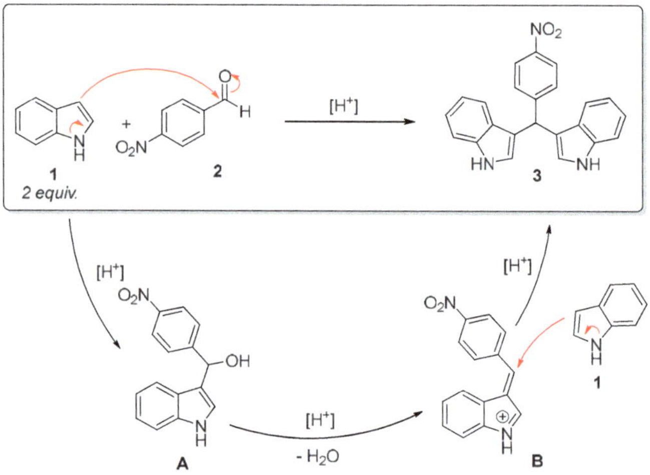

Figure 1. Mechanism for the formation of bis(indolyl)methane **3** from indole **1** and 4-nitrobenzaldehyde **2**. Red arrows suggest possible electron rearrangements.

As an alternative to the synthesis under homogeneous catalysis, different approaches based on heterogeneous catalysis have been proposed, including those based on HY and ZnY zeolites [52–54], polystyrene-based resins [55], amberlyst [56–58], PEG-supported sulfonic acid [59], lanthanide resins [60], and montmorillonite clay K-10 catalysts [61].

Nanocrystalline catalysts such as semiconducting CdS nanorods have also been proposed for the synthesis of bis(indolyl)methanes in different media at reflux temperature [62], opening the way to greener approaches such as solvent-free reaction at 80 °C mediated by magnetically recoverable γ-Fe_2O_3 nanocatalysts [63]. Indeed, the advantages of a magnetic functionality in catalyst separation, recovery, and reuse has been reported for diverse organic reactions, ranging from the synthesis of heterocycle building blocks (spiropyrans) to the reduction of environmental contaminants (dyes, drugs) [64–66]. Nanocrystals, however, may suffer from aggregation under reaction conditions, and novel nanocomposite materials based on the immobilization of catalytically active phases on supports such as carbon nanotubes and graphene oxide aerogels have been proposed [67,68].

In this work, we made use of nanocomposite aerogels which combine the features of iron-based magnetic nanocrystals and of highly porous silica to address the catalytic synthesis of 3,3′-((4-nitrophenyl)methylene)bis(1*H*-indole). The investigated catalysts were highly porous $NiFe_2O_4/SiO_2$ aerogel nanocomposites containing ferrite nanocrystal with narrow size distribution around 10 nm. The investigated materials were effective catalysts for the synthesis of BIMs at room temperature, demonstrating the potential of nanocomposite aerogels for the catalytic production of relevant heterocyclic compounds.

2. Results

2.1. Catalyst Preparation and Characterization

The aerogel catalysts were prepared by a sol–gel procedure followed by supercritical drying and thermal treatments, as depicted in Figure 2. The synthetic approach is based on a protocol established in our laboratories which enables the production of multicomponent silica-based gels by a two-step acid-base urea-mediated catalysis of metal and silica precursors. Aerogels are produced by a high-temperature supercritical drying, and finally the MFe_2O_4/SiO_2 nanocomposite aerogels are obtained by thermal treatment to promote the formation of the ferrite nanocrystals dispersed on porous amorphous silica. The formation of the desired nanocrystalline phase for this work, $NiFe_2O_4$, was assessed by X-ray powder diffraction (see Supplementary Materials, Figure S1) which showed the occurrence of the ferrite spinel phase superimposed to the broad halo due to amorphous silica. XRD peak broadening indicates an average nanocrystalline domain size around 8 nm for the $NiFe_2O_4$ phase. In the multicomponent aerogels as obtained right after supercritical drying, the dispersed metals occur in poorly ordered nanophases which are non-magnetic or poorly magnetic, depending on the composition of the composite. On the other hand, upon calcination, highly magnetic nanocrystalline substituted ferrites which readily respond to an external magnet are obtained. Thermal treatments also affect the surface properties of the aerogels. In particular, the aerogels as produced by high-temperature supercritical drying are hydrophobic as surface silanols undergo esterification by ethoxy functional groups during the drying process. When the aerogel is treated in air, the ethoxy groups are removed and, as a consequence of surface silanols, the aerogel becomes hydrophilic [2,69].

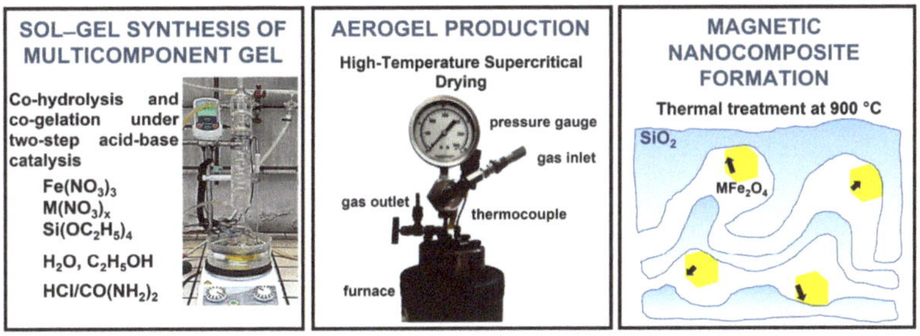

Figure 2. Schematic of the production procedure of the aerogel catalysts: (**a**) sol–gel synthesis of the multicomponent gel by co-hydrolysis and co-gelation of the metal and silica precursors; (**b**) aerogel production by high-temperature supercritical drying of the multicomponent gel; (**c**) thermal treatments to promote the formation of magnetic $NiFe_2O_4/SiO_2$ nanocomposite aerogel catalysts.

The nickel-based composite aerogel, as shown in Figure 3a, is extremely lightweight and homogeneous. Scanning electron microscopy and energy-filtered images, acquired in order to assess compositional homogeneity, showed that the distribution of the present elements is quite homogeneous within the aerogel, as demonstrated by representative micrographs shown in Figure 3b–f. It is found that Si and O are relatively more intense as compared to Ni and Fe, as expected based on the gel composition which was adjusted in order to achieve a ferrite loading of 10 wt%, and in particular that Ni and Fe are correlated, suggesting that the two metals are associated in the same phase. Thermal treatment up to 900 °C promotes the formation of the ferrite nanocrystals, which appear as round-shaped darker spots superimposed to the silica matrix under transmission electron microscopy imaging, as shown in Figure 3g,h. TEM images clearly point out that the nanocrystals have an average size around 8 nm in the Ni-CAT and are well dispersed in the silica matrix, as is desirable for prospective use in catalysis. TEM observations (see also Figure S1) indicate that, despite the thermal treatment at 900 °C, and thanks to the very high porosity of the starting aerogel, the $NiFe_2O_4/SiO_2$ nanocomposite still exhibits the typical texture of aerogels with high and open porosity.

The textural features of the $NiFe_2O_4/SiO_2$ aerogel catalysts were investigated, together with that of corresponding plain SiO_2 aerogel, by N_2 physisorption analysis at 77 K, which indicated (Figure S2) the occurrence of a porous texture dominated by large mesopores. In particular, the isotherm of SiO_2 can be described as a type IVa isotherm with a narrow H1 hysteresis lying at high relative pressures, suggesting the occurrence of large mesopores with relatively uniform diameter. The nanocomposite aerogel exhibits a similar physisorption isotherm of IIb type, suggesting the occurrence of a very similar texture typical of aerogel structures, associated to interconnected nearly cylindrical mesopores with large sizes [70]. The relevant textural parameters of the aerogel catalysts as obtained by physisorption data analysis are summarized in Table 1, where the porosity of the nanocomposite aerogels can be mainly ascribed to the occurrence of mesopores, while the micropore contribution is negligible. On the other hand, a contribution arising from macropores, which cannot be directly detected by N_2 physisorption, cannot be ruled out and seems to be suggested by TEM observations.

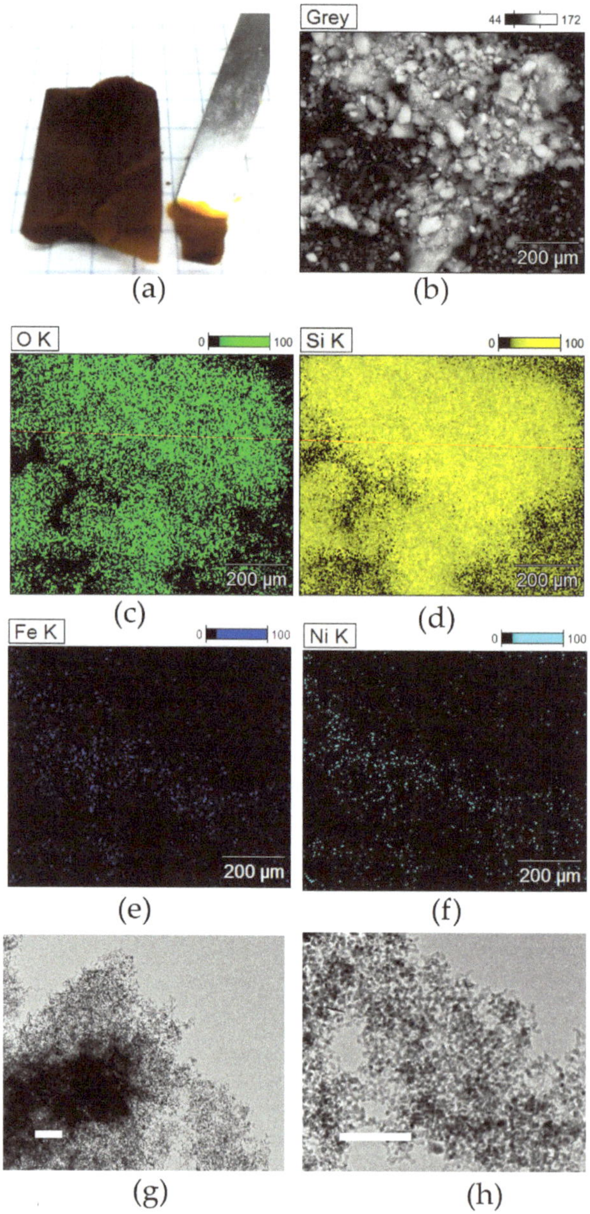

Figure 3. Representative images of the aerogel catalyst at different stages of nanocomposite preparation: (**a**) optical image of a highly porous nickel-containing composite aerogel as obtained after supercritical drying; (**b**) corresponding SEM image and (**c**–**f**) energy-filtered images showing oxygen distribution (**c**), silicon distribution (**d**), Fe distribution (**e**), and nickel distribution (**f**). TEM images (scale bar is 100 nm) of the $NiFe_2O_4/SiO_2$ aerogel catalyst as obtained by calcination at 900 °C (**g**,**h**).

Table 1. List of aerogel catalysts and corresponding relevant textural features. Thermal treatment was performed under static air atmosphere.

Aerogel Label	Processing Conditions	Composition (10 wt% Loading MFe_2O_4)	Surface Area ($m^2 \cdot g^{-1}$)	Pore Volume ($cm^3 \cdot g^{-1}$)
Ni-CAT	900 °C 1 h	$NiFe_2O_4/SiO_2$	405	2.09
SiO_2-CAT	900 °C 1 h	SiO_2	373	1.36

2.2. Catalytic Activity Evaluation

The potential of the $NiFe_2O_4/SiO_2$ nanocomposite aerogels as acid catalysts for the synthesis of a relevant class of heterocyclic compounds such as BIMs was investigated. In particular, the studied reaction is represented in Table 2 and involves the formation of 3,3′-((4-nitrophenyl)methylene)bis(1*H*-indole) **3** by reaction of two equivalents of indole **1** with 4-nitro-benzaldehyde **2**.

Table 2. Catalytic tests.

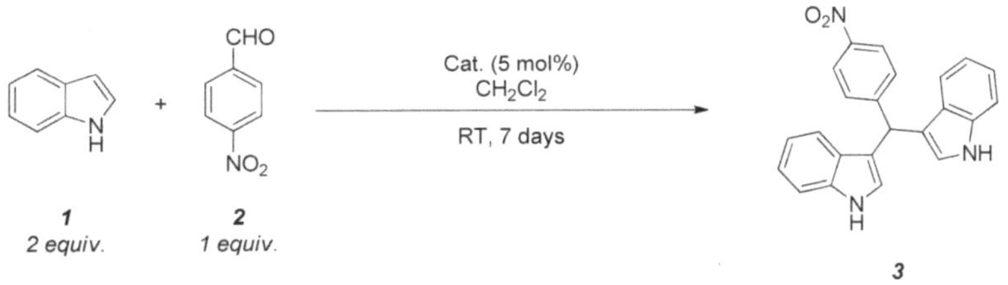

Catalyst	1:2:3 Ratio [1]	2:3 Ratio [1]
None	44:48:8	86:14
SiO_2	7:37:56	40:60
$NiFe_2O_4$-SiO_2	4:2:94	2:98

[1] All ratios were calculated by crude ^1H NMR analysis and are normalized by the reaction stoichiometry.

The reaction was carried out, under stirring, over 1 week at room temperature using 5 mol% of $NiFe_2O_4/SiO_2$ nanocomposite aerogel (Ni-CAT) in CH_2Cl_2 and in the presence of plain SiO_2 (SiO_2-CAT) as well as without any catalyst. The reaction was monitored by ^1H NMR analysis of the crude mixture (see Supplementary Materials, Figures S3 and S4) [21,71].

Figure 4 shows a comparison of the reaction mixtures as obtained with the Ni-CAT, and with a SiO_2-CAT and without catalyst as a reference in a relevant spectral range.

It was found that when the reaction is carried out without the use of any catalyst, after 1 week the desired BIM product **3** represents only 8% of the final reaction mixture. When SiO_2-CAT is used, a very significant increase in the product formation is observed, up to 60% of the final reaction mixture, while using Ni-CAT leads to 94% of the desired product, together with an almost complete consumption of the aldehyde **2**. The results demonstrate that SiO_2-CAT is already active towards the investigated reaction, as a result of its high porosity (Table 1) and expected surface features. The occurrence of the nanocrystalline nickel substituted ferrites improves the yield of the product **3** and leads to an almost quantitative consumption of the aldehyde **2**. These results were highly encouraging when taking into account that the reaction was carried out at room temperature. The **1**:**2** ratio in the reaction mixture does not agree with the expected stoichiometry; the observed differences could be due both to the fact that the reaction does not take place in a single step, as described earlier, as well as to interactions of the species involved in the reaction with the porous aerogel matrix, as will be discussed later on.

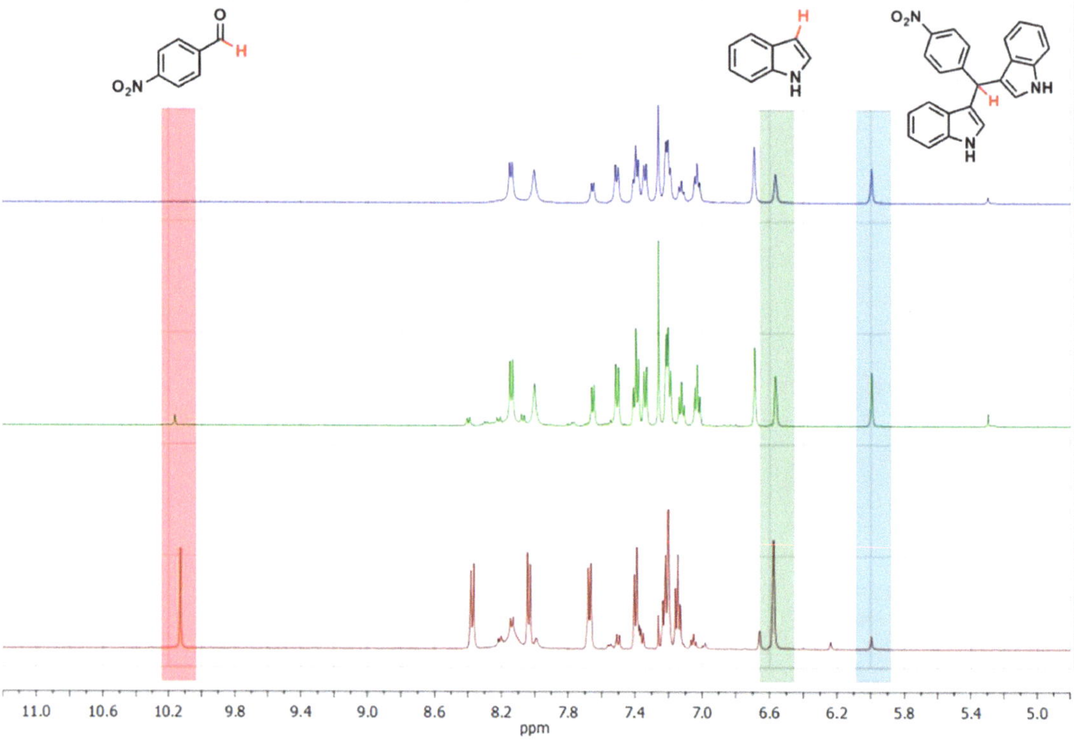

Figure 4. ^{1}H NMR spectra of the reaction mixture as obtained without catalyst (red bottom curve); with the use of plain SiO_2 aerogel catalyst (green intermediate curve); and with the use of $NiFeO_2$-SiO_2 aerogel catalyst (top blue curve). Significant spectral ranges with corresponding attribution are included as a guide (catalyst amount: 5 mol %; run time: 1 week; solvent: CH_2Cl_2; reaction temperature: RT).

It should be noted that Ni-CAT offers the advantage of an easy and effective separation procedure of the catalyst from the reaction mixture by the use of an external magnet which selectively separates the catalyst. On the other hand, when the reaction was performed by using SiO_2-CAT, a filtration process was required to separate and remove the catalyst from the reaction mixture. Screening of the reaction in other solvents, using Ni-CAT, gave considerably poorer yields of **3** (see Table S1). Based on these results, CH_2Cl_2 was used for further experiments.

For practical applicability of a heterogeneous catalyst, recyclability is a very important factor. Therefore, we investigated the Ni-CAT aerogel in repeated cycles of reaction. Figure 5 shows that Ni-CAT aerogel, which can be recovered by magnetic separation from the reaction mixture, is still effective in catalyzing BIM synthesis after three repeated runs, although a decreased efficiency is progressively observed.

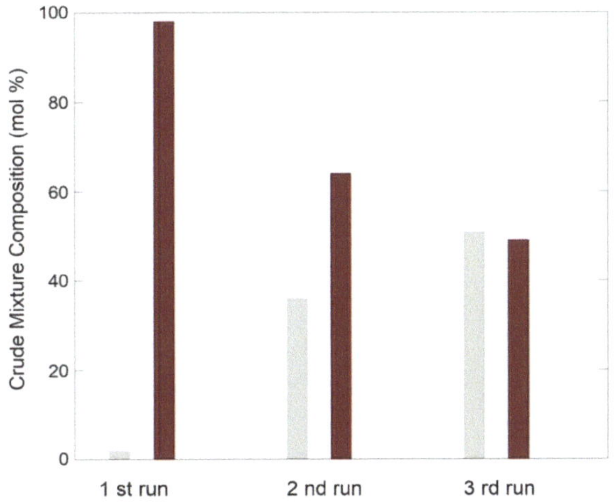

Figure 5. BIMs synthesis catalyzed by Ni-CAT aerogel catalysts (catalyst amount: 5 mol %; run time: 1 week; solvent: CH_2Cl_2; reaction temperature: RT): the composition of the resulting reaction mixture is represented as relative amounts of reactant **2** (grey bars) and product **3** (brown bars).

As a matter of fact, characterization of the aerogels after catalytic runs by scanning and transmission electron microscopy do not provide strong evidence of significant changes in the morphology and microstructure of aerogel after the catalytic runs (see Supplementary Materials, Figure S5-1). However, the XRD pattern of the Ni-CAT after catalysis (Figure S5-2) shows the occurrence of a peak around $2\theta \approx 18^\circ$ which was not present in the original nanocomposite aerogel. Although the observed pattern does not enable us to identify unambiguously the additional phase present, there are some similar features in the pattern of the BIM product. The same peak was observed when a nanocomposite aerogel catalyst prepared under similar conditions but with different ferrite composition ($MnFe_2O_4/SiO_2$) was used as a catalyst, supporting the idea that the observed feature is not related to nickel-based phases. In addition, elemental (CHN) analysis of the Ni-CAT aerogel after use suggests the occurrence of C, H, N (11.78% C; 0.48% H; 1.23% N) but there is no match with any of the three species involved.

These findings suggest that, although the Ni-CAT aerogel was isolated from the reaction mixture by magnetic separation, and washed repeatedly with CH_2Cl_2, it is likely that some of the species involved in the reaction were trapped in the aerogel. The Ni-CAT aerogel after one catalytic run and after three catalytic runs was therefore treated with hot methanol and the corresponding extract was analyzed by ^{1}H NMR. Only compound **3** was observed and no traces of the corresponding starting materials **1** and **2** were detected, as illustrated in Figure 6. It should be pointed out, however, that the investigated reaction takes place with the formation of a transient polar intermediate such as **A** (see Figure 1); hence, its interaction with the porous support during the reaction, with subsequent trapping, cannot be completely ruled out. The extract from a catalyst used for three repeated runs does not show significant signals; hence, it is likely that the lower catalyst activity is associated with lower interaction and trapping of the reaction species. Overall, these observations (^{1}H NMR data together with insights from characterization of the catalyst after use) are consistent with the hypothesis that some reaction species (compound **3** and probably intermediate **A**) are trapped within the highly porous aerogel.

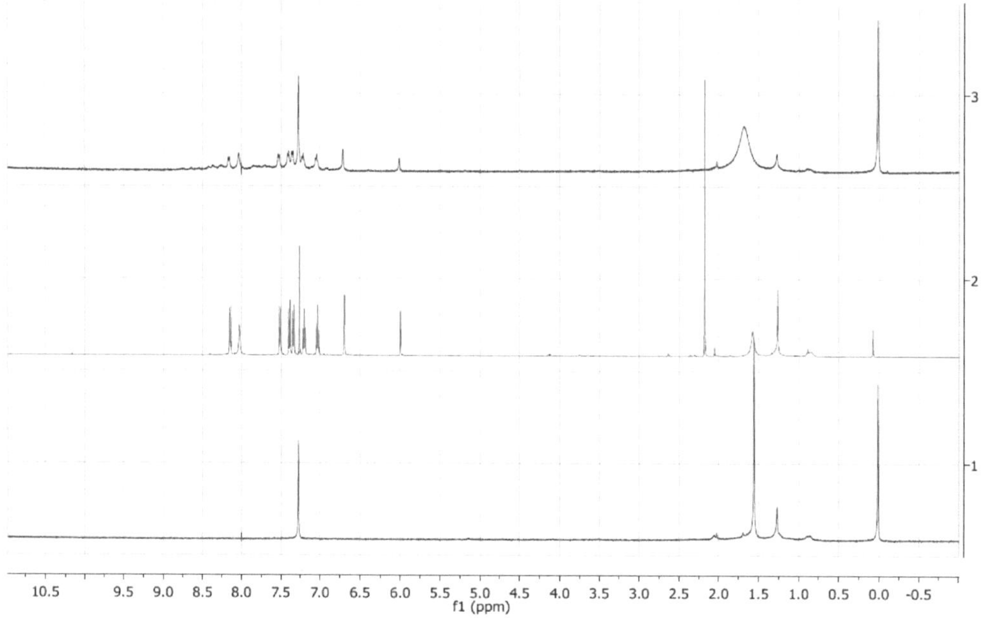

Figure 6. ^{1}H-NMR spectra of pure BIM (green line), and the extracts after 1 (blue line) and 3 (red line) catalytic runs.

3. Materials and Methods

3.1. Materials

Chemicals were purchased from the following providers and used without further purification. BIM synthesis: Indole (99+%, Aldrich, St. Louis, MO, USA); 4-Nitrobenzaldehyde (>99%, Aldrich); Dichloromethane (>99%, Aldrich); Acetone (>99.5%, Honeywell, Charlotte, NC, USA); Acetonitrile (>99.5%, puriss. p.a., ACS reagent, reag. Ph. Eur., Aldrich); Chloroform (99.8%, ACS, Alfa Aesar, Haverhill, MA, USA); Diethyl ether (RPE-For analysis-ACS, Carlo Erba Reagents, Cornaredo, Italy); Ethanol (96–97.2%, Honeywell); Ethyl Acetate (>99.7% Chromasolv, Sigma-Aldrich, St. Louis, MO, USA); 2-methyltetrahydrofuran (99%, Alfa Aesar); Toluene (>99.5% ACS Reagent, Sigma-Aldrich).

Aerogel catalyst synthesis: tetraethoxysilane (($Si(OC_2H_5)_4$, Aldrich 98%, TEOS); Urea ((NH_2CONH_2), Sigma-Aldrich (99.0–100.5%); Absolute Ethanol (CH_3CH_2OH, Carlo Erba); Nitric Acid (HNO_3, Carlo Erba); Iron (III) nitrate nonahydrate ($Fe(NO_3)_3{\cdot}9H_2O$, Sigma-Aldrich 98%); Manganese (II) nitrate hexahydrate $Mn(NO_3)_2{\cdot}6H_2O$, Sigma-Aldrich, ≥98%); Nickel (II) nitrate hexahydrate $Ni(NO_3)_2{\cdot}6H_2O$, Sigma-Aldrich, ≥97%).

3.2. Synthesis of Aerogel Catalysts

The aerogels were produced by a previously developed sol–gel procedure based on the co-hydrolysis and co-gelation of the metal and silica precursors as detailed in the Supplementary Materials [69,72].

Briefly, an ethanolic solution of TEOS is first pre-hydrolyzed under acidic catalysis by addition of an HCl hydroethanolic solution at 50 °C for 0.5 h. At this step, an ethanolic solution of metal precursors in stoichiometric amounts (divalent metal M precursor: Fe(III) precursor 1:2 molar ratio) is added under stirring. Basic catalysis is then promoted by the addition of an ethanolic solution of urea and kept under reflux for 2 h. Finally, the viscous sol is transferred in a container, sealed, and kept at 40 °C for gelation (20 to 40 h).

Aerogels are produced by high-temperature supercritical drying performed in an autoclave (Parr, Moline, IL, USA, 300 cm^3) filled with 70 mL of absolute ethanol and nitrogen and brought to around 330 °C and 70 atm, and finally vented and cooled down to room temperature. To obtain the MFe_2O_4/SiO_2 magnetic nanocomposites, the aerogels are first treated at 450 °C for 1 h in static air to remove synthesis residues and finally calcined in air at 900 °C for 1 h to promote the formation of nanocrystalline ferrite. In the case of pure iron oxide and of manganese ferrite, thermal treatment is performed under Ar flow (56 $mL \cdot min^{-1}$) to avoid further oxidation.

3.3. Catalytic Tests

The reaction was carried out starting from stoichiometric amounts of reactants (77.9 mg of **1** and 50.3 mg of **2**) in 2 mL CH_2Cl_2 at room temperature under stirring in a closed flask. The catalytic effect of the aerogel was tested by adding a 5 mol% amount to the reaction mixture. Reaction time was 1 week, after which 2 mL of CH_2Cl_2 was added and the catalyst was separated from the reaction mixture by magnetic separation. Briefly, a magnet was placed on the outer side of the flask containing the reaction mixture. The aerogel catalyst was readily attracted by the magnet and the reaction mixture was collected. Fresh CH_2Cl_2 was then added and the magnetic separation procedure was repeated. The crude was separated by evaporation of CH_2Cl_2 under reduced pressure under rotavapor. In the case of non-magnetic catalyst (silica), the catalyst was separated from the reaction mixture by filtration and further processed as described above.

In view of the characterization of the aerogel after use, as well as for further catalyst reuse, after recovery and washing as described above, aerogel drying at around 50 °C in static air was performed.

3.4. Characterization Techniques

^1H NMR spectra were recorded on a Varian 500 spectrometer (Palo Alto, CA, USA) at ambient temperature with $CDCl_3$ as solvent. Data are reported as follows: chemical shifts (δ), multiplicity, coupling constants, and integration. ^{13}C NMR spectra were recorded operating at 126 MHz at 27 °C with $CDCl_3$ as solvent.

Textural characterization was performed on a Micromeritics ASAP2020 (Norcross, GA, USA) by determining N_2 physisorption curves at −196 °C, after degassing the samples at 200 °C for 12 h. Surface areas were estimated using the Brunauer–Emmett–Teller (BET) model, whereas pore size and pore volumes were estimated by using the Barret–Joyner–Halenda (BJH) method.

Tian–Calvet heat flow equipment (Setaram, Lyon, France) was used for microcalorimetric measurements. Each sample was pretreated overnight at 400 °C under vacuum (10^{-3} Pa) before introducing ammonia as the probe gas for acidity. The adsorption temperature was maintained at 80 °C, in order to prevent physisorption. The equilibrium pressure relative to each adsorbed amount was measured by means of a differential pressure gauge (Datametrics, Plymouth, MN, USA). The run was stopped at a final equilibrium pressure of 133.3 Pa.

Scanning electron microscopy (SEM) investigation was performed on an ESEM FEI Quanta 200 microscope (Hillsboro, OR, USA) operating at 25 KV and on a ZEISS microscope (Jena, Germany). The powdered samples were deposited on conductive carbon tape for observation.

TEM images were recorded on a Hitachi H-7000 (Tokyo, Japan) and on a JEM 1400 Plus instrument (JEOL, Akishima, Japan) running at 100 kV. Prior to observation, the samples were finely ground and deposited on a carbon-coated copper grid.

XRD patterns were acquired on a Panalytical Empyrean diffractometer (Malvern Panalytical, Malvern, UK) equipped with Cu Kα radiation, a graphite monochromator on the diffracted beam, and an X'Celerator linear detector (Malvern Panalytical). The average size of crystallite domains was calculated by using the Scherrer equation, by considering the full width at half-maximum of the diffraction peak corrected for instrumental broadening as determined by using a reference LaB_6 sample. Phase identification was performed by comparison to the Powder Diffraction Files database. Additional measurements were recorded on an X3000 Seifert diffractometer (GE Measurement and Control, Billerica, MA, USA).

Fourier Transform infrared (FT-IR) spectra in the Mid-IR range (4000–400 cm^{-1}) were recorded on a Bruker Tensor 27 spectrometer (Billerica, MA, USA) equipped with a Platinum-ATR accessory and a DTGS (deuterated triglycine sulfate) detector.

4. Discussion

Nanocomposites, where nanocrystalline magnetic nickel ferrite with crystal size around 10 nm is dispersed in porous silica aerogel, were tested for the catalytic synthesis of 3,3′-((4-nitrophenyl)methylene)bis(1*H*-indole) starting from indole and 4-nitro benzaldehyde. The $NiFe_2O_4$-SiO_2 nanocomposite exhibits high porosity and the occurrence of nanocrystals evenly distributed in the porous texture, exhibiting therefore promising textural and structural features for application in catalysis. Indeed, although some challenges remain in the reaction mixture characterization, it can be inferred that the Ni-CAT aerogel shows high activity towards the formation of BIMs even at room temperature, whereas the formation of the desired bis-heterocyclic product under catalyst-free conditions is nearly negligible. The activity of the nanocomposite catalyst can be ascribed both to the highly porous and interconnected texture typical of aerogels, and to the acidic features of the material (which seems to be due both to the occurrence of surface silanols as well as to the metal cations in the nanocrystals). Mechanistically, it is reasonable to assume that a contribution to the catalytic activity of the porous silica-based aerogels is associated with interactions, including hydrogen bonding/protonation, which are expected to be able to activate the electrophilic carbonyl of **2** (towards nucleophilic attack of **1**) in the first step of the reaction, leading to intermediate **A** as well as to promotion of the subsequent condensation reaction between **A** and a second equivalent of **1** via **B** (S_N1-type reaction, see Figure 1). To take into account the role of the catalyst composition in the overall acidity, microcalorimetric measurements were performed using ammonia as a probe molecule to determine the strength and number of acidic sites. Reporting (Figure S6) the differential heat of ammonia adsorption (Q_{diff}) as a function of the number of adsorbing sites per gram of catalyst (n_A), it was found that SiO_2-CAT is less acidic than the $NiFe_2O_4$-SiO_2 nanocomposite aerogel. The moderate acidity of silica as deduced by microcalorimetry, together with the observed catalytic activity, suggest the active role of the porous silica.

To corroborate this finding, we have compared the catalytic activity of the $NiFe_2O_4$-SiO_2 aerogel catalyst to the corresponding dry gel obtained by conventional thermal drying techniques (xerogel). In particular, $NiFe_2O_4$-SiO_2 composites were prepared in the form of xerogel (Ni-X-CAT) and compared to the corresponding aerogel discussed above; while the structural features as obtained by XRD pattern suggest a similar crystal structure, the textural features as obtained by TEM and N_2 physisorption suggest a significantly different texture (Figure S7). In particular, Ni-X-CAT exhibits a mainly microporous and fine texture, as compared to the meso- and macroporous morphology of the aerogel. Table 3 shows that, despite the same composition, $NiFe_2O_4$-SiO_2 nanocomposites exhibit a different catalytic behavior in the forms of aerogel and of xerogel, suggesting a relevant role for the textural features and a better performance for the aerogel catalysts. Collectively, these observations suggest that both the acidity due to silanols and the typical texture of porous silica aerogels are believed to contribute to the catalytic activity of these materials and may be responsible for the observed results.

Table 3. BIM synthesis [1] catalyzed by $NiFe_2O_4$-SiO_2 aerogel (Ni-CAT) and xerogel (Ni-X-CAT) nanocomposites (catalyst amount: 5 mol%; run time: 1 week; solvent: CH_2Cl_2; reaction temperature: RT).

Catalyst (5 mol%)	1:2:3 Ratio [1]	2:3 Ratio
Ni-X-CAT	20:34:46	43:57
Ni-CAT	4:2:94	2:98

[1] All ratios were calculated by crude ^1H NMR analysis.

In conclusion, our preliminary study investigates the potential of nanocomposite aerogels in the catalytic production of relevant organic compounds, as demonstrated for the synthesis of bis(indolyl)methanes. $NiFe_2O_4$-SiO_2 aerogels, as a consequence of their acidity combined with the typical texture of porous silica aerogels, enable the efficient synthesis of BIMs at room temperature. The high porosity and hydrophylic features of the silica matrix can also be responsible for the trapping of some species (including the intermediate or final product) involved during the reaction. The nanocrystalline ferrite provides magnetic properties for catalyst reusability in the development of cost-effective aerogel catalysts for the production of important heterocyclic compounds.

Supplementary Materials: The following supporting information can be downloaded at: https://www.mdpi.com/article/10.3390/molecules29102223/s1, Figure S1: XRD pattern of the $NiFe_2O_4/SiO_2$ nanocomposite aerogel catalyst; Figure S2: N_2 physisorption isotherms at 77 K of the $NiFe_2O_4/SiO_2$ and SiO_2 aerogel catalysts; Figure S3: ^{1}H NMR and FT-IR spectrum of pure compound **3**; Figure S4.1–16: ^{1}H NMR spectrum of crude reaction mixture under the different conditions tested; Table S1: Effect of solvent on the catalytic test; Table S2: Effect of catalyst reuse; Figure S5-1: TEM and SEM investigation of the Ni-CAT aerogel after catalysis; Figure S5-2: XRD pattern of the Ni-CAT aerogel after 3 runs of catalysis; Figure S6: Differential heat of adsorption of ammonia by the aerogels; Figure S7: TEM images, XRD pattern, and N_2 physisorption isotherm at 77 K of the $NiFe_2O_4/SiO_2$ nanocomposite xerogel catalyst (X-Ni-CAT).

Author Contributions: N.M., A.F., M.G.C. and M.F.C., conceptualization and original draft preparation; G.S., S.V.T., N.M. and M.F.S., experimental synthesis and investigation; N.M., D.L., M.G.C., L.P. and M.F.C., data validation and data analysis; All Authors, writing—review and editing. All authors have read and agreed to the published version of the manuscript.

Funding: The University of Cagliari is acknowledged for supporting this research.

Institutional Review Board Statement: Not applicable.

Informed Consent Statement: Not applicable.

Data Availability Statement: Data are contained within the article and Supplementary Materials.

Acknowledgments: We acknowledge the CeSAR (Centro Servizi d'Ateneo per la Ricerca) of the University of Cagliari, Italy, and in particular M. Marceddu and A. Ardu, respectively, for assistance in scanning electron microscopy experiments performed with an ESEM FEI Quanta 200 microscope and for the transmission electron microscopy measurements on a JEM 1400 Plus microscope. IREC is kindly acknowledged for access to a Zeiss SEM and the Centro Interdipartimentale NMR of the University of Cagliari for access to the NMR facility.

Conflicts of Interest: The authors declare no conflicts of interest.

References

1. Pierre, A.C.; Pajonk, G.M. Chemistry of Aerogels and Their Applications. *Chem. Rev.* **2002**, *102*, 4243–4266. [CrossRef] [PubMed]
2. Corrias, A.; Loche, D.; Casula, M.F. Aerogels Containing Metal, Alloy, and Oxide Nanoparticles Embedded into Dielectric Matrices. In *Springer Handbook of Aerogels*; Aegerter, M.A., Leventis, N., Koebel, M., Steiner, S.A., III, Eds.; Springer Handbooks; Springer Nature: Cham, Switzerland, 2023. [CrossRef]
3. Maleki, H.; Durães, L.; Portugal, A. An Overview on Silica Aerogels Synthesis and Different Mechanical Reinforcing Strategies. *J. Non Cryst. Solids* **2014**, *385*, 55–74. [CrossRef]
4. Pajonk, G.M. Aerogel Catalysts. *Appl. Catal.* **1991**, *72*, 217–266. [CrossRef]
5. Tleimat-Manzalji, R.; Manzalji, T.; Pajonk, G.M. Aerogels and Xerogels for Catalytic Applications. *J. Non Cryst. Solids* **1992**, *147–148*, 744–747. [CrossRef]
6. Gisler, A.; Bürgi, T.; Baiker, A. Epoxidation on Titania–Silica Aerogel Catalysts Studied by Attenuated Total Reflection Fourier Transform Infrared and Modulation Spectroscopy. *Phys. Chem. Chem. Phys.* **2003**, *5*, 3539–3548. [CrossRef]
7. Buisson, P.; Hernandez, C.; Pierre, M.; Pierre, A.C. Encapsulation of Lipases in Aerogels. *J. Non Cryst. Solids* **2001**, *285*, 295–302. [CrossRef]
8. Karamikamkar, S.; Abidli, A.; Aghababaei Tafreshi, O.; Ghaffari-Mosanenzadeh, S.; Buahom, P.; Naguib, H.E.; Park, C.B. Nanocomposite Aerogel Network Featuring High Surface Area and Superinsulation Properties. *Chem. Mater.* **2024**, *36*, 642–656. [CrossRef]

9. Liu, Y.; Bu, X.; Liu, R.; Feng, M.; Zhang, Z.; He, M.; Huang, J.; Zhou, Y. Construction of Robust Silica-Hybridized Cellulose Aerogels Integrating Passive Radiative Cooling and Thermal Insulation for Year-Round Building Energy Saving. *Chem. Eng. J.* **2024**, *481*, 148780. [CrossRef]
10. Niculescu, A.-G.; Tudorache, D.-I.; Bocioagă, M.; Mihaiescu, D.E.; Hadibarata, T.; Grumezescu, A.M. An Updated Overview of Silica Aerogel-Based Nanomaterials. *Nanomaterials* **2024**, *14*, 469. [CrossRef]
11. Loche, D.; Casula, M.F.; Corrias, A.; Marras, S.; Moggi, P. Bimetallic FeCo Nanocrystals Supported on Highly Porous Silica Aerogels as Fischer–Tropsch Catalysts. *Catal. Lett.* **2012**, *142*, 1061–1066. [CrossRef]
12. Marras, C.; Loche, D.; Carta, D.; Casula, M.F.; Schirru, M.; Cutrufello, M.G.; Corrias, A. Copper-Based Catalysts Supported on Highly Porous Silica for the Water Gas Shift Reaction. *Chempluschem* **2016**, *81*, 421–432. [CrossRef] [PubMed]
13. Vanyorek, L.; Loche, D.; Katona, H.; Casula, M.F.; Corrias, A.; Kónya, Z.; Kukovecz, Á.; Kiricsi, I. Optimization of the Catalytic Chemical Vapor Deposition Synthesis of Multiwall Carbon Nanotubes on FeCo(Ni)/SiO_2 Aerogel Catalysts by Statistical Design of Experiments. *J. Phys. Chem. C* **2011**, *115*, 5894–5902. [CrossRef]
14. Casula, M.F.; Concas, G.; Congiu, F.; Corrias, A.; Loche, D.; Marras, C.; Spano, G. Characterization of Stoichiometric Nanocrystalline Spinel Ferrites Dispersed on Porous Silica Aerogel. *J. Nanosci. Nanotechnol.* **2011**, *11*, 10136–10141. [CrossRef] [PubMed]
15. Cutrufello, M.G.; Rombi, E.; Ferino, I.; Loche, D.; Corrias, A.; Casula, M.F. Ni-Based Xero- and Aerogels as Catalysts for Nitroxidation Processes. *J. Solgel Sci. Technol.* **2011**, *60*, 324–332. [CrossRef]
16. Martínez, S.; Vallribera, A.; Cotet, C.L.; Popovici, M.; Martín, L.; Roig, A.; Moreno-Mañas, M.; Molins, E. Nanosized Metallic Particles Embedded in Silica and Carbon Aerogels as Catalysts in the Mizoroki–Heck Coupling Reaction. *New J. Chem.* **2005**, *29*, 1342. [CrossRef]
17. Martínez, S.; Meseguer, M.; Casas, L.; Rodríguez, E.; Molins, E.; Moreno-Mañas, M.; Roig, A.; Sebastián, R.M.; Vallribera, A. Silica Aerogel-Iron Oxide Nanocomposites: Recoverable Catalysts in Conjugate Additions and in the Biginelli Reaction. *Tetrahedron* **2003**, *59*, 1553–1556. [CrossRef]
18. Orlović, A.; Janaćković, D.; Skala, D. Alumina/Silica Aerogel with Zinc Chloride Alkylation Catalyst: Influence of Supercritical Drying Conditions and Aerogel Structure on Alkylation Catalytic Activity. *Catal. Commun.* **2002**, *3*, 119–123. [CrossRef]
19. Shiri, M.; Zolfigol, M.A.; Kruger, H.G.; Tanbakouchian, Z. Bis- and Trisindolylmethanes (BIMs and TIMs). *Chem. Rev.* **2010**, *110*, 2250–2293. [CrossRef]
20. Wang, Y.; Sang, R.; Zheng, Y.; Guo, L.; Guan, M.; Wu, Y. Graphene Oxide: An Efficient Recyclable Solid Acid for the Synthesis of Bis(Indolyl)Methanes from Aldehydes and Indoles in Water. *Catal. Commun.* **2017**, *89*, 138–142. [CrossRef]
21. Tocco, G.; Zedda, G.; Casu, M.; Simbula, G.; Begala, M. Solvent-Free Addition of Indole to Aldehydes: Unexpected Synthesis of Novel 1-[1-(1H-Indol-3-Yl) Alkyl]-1H-Indoles and Preliminary Evaluation of Their Cytotoxicity in Hepatocarcinoma Cells. *Molecules* **2017**, *22*, 1747. [CrossRef]
22. Grosso, C.; Cardoso, A.L.; Lemos, A.; Varela, J.; Rodrigues, M.J.; Custódio, L.; Barreira, L.; Pinho E Melo, T.M.V.D. Novel Approach to Bis(Indolyl)Methanes: De Novo Synthesis of 1-Hydroxyiminomethyl Derivatives with Anti-Cancer Properties. *Eur. J. Med. Chem.* **2015**, *93*, 9–15. [CrossRef] [PubMed]
23. Bergman, J.; Carlsson, R.; Misztal, S. The Reaction of Some Indoles and Indolines with 2,3-Dichloro-5,6-Dicyano-1,4-Benzoquinone. *Acta Chem. Scandinava B* **1976**, *30*, 853–862. [CrossRef]
24. D'Auria, M. Photochemical Synthesis of Diindolylmethanes. *Tetrahedron* **1991**, *47*, 9225–9230. [CrossRef]
25. Meng, J.-B.; Wang, W.-G.; Xiong, G.-X.; Wang, Y.-M.; Fu, D.-C.; Du, D.-M.; Wang, R.-J.; Wang, H.-G.; Koshima, H.; Matsuura, T. A Multistep Photoreaction of Aromatic Aldehydes with Heteroaromatics in the Solid State. *J. Photochem. Photobiol. A Chem.* **1993**, *74*, 43–49. [CrossRef]
26. Meng, J.-B.; Wang, W.-G.; Wang, H.-G.; Matsuura, T.; Koshima, H.; Sugimoto, I.; Ito, Y. Solid-State Photochemistry of Indoles with Naphtalese and Phenanthrene. *Photochem. Photobiol.* **1993**, *57*, 597–602. [CrossRef]
27. Wang, S.-Y.; Ji, S.-J.; Su, X.-M. A Meldrum's Acid Catalyzed Synthesis of Bis(Indolyl)Methanes in Water under Ultrasonic Condition. *Chin. J. Chem.* **2008**, *26*, 22–24. [CrossRef]
28. Chakrabarty, M.; Karmakar, S.; Harigaya, Y. First Isolation of Both Indolylcarbinols and Diindolylalkanes from Microwave-Assisted Acid (Clay)-Catalysed Reaction of Indoles with Diethyl Ketomalonate. *Heterocycles* **2005**, *65*, 37. [CrossRef]
29. Chakrabarty, M.; Khasnobis, S.; Harigaya, Y.; Konda, Y. Neat Formic Acid: An Excellent N-Formylating Agent for Carbazoles, 3-Alkylindoles, Diphenylamine and Moderately Weak Nucleophilic Anilines. *Synth. Commun.* **2000**, *30*, 187–200. [CrossRef]
30. Uhle, F.C.; Harris, L.S. The Synthesis and Cyclization of α-Methylamino-β-(4-Carboxy-3-Indole)-Propionic Acid. *J. Am. Chem. Soc.* **1957**, *79*, 102–109. [CrossRef]
31. Noland, W.E.; Venkiteswaran, M.R.; Richards, C.G. Cyclizative Condensations. I. 2-Methylindole with Acetone and Methyl Ethyl Ketone 1. *J. Org. Chem.* **1961**, *26*, 4241–4248. [CrossRef]
32. Freter, K. Synthesis and Reactions of 3-Indolyl.Beta. Ketones. *J. Org. Chem.* **1972**, *37*, 2010–2015. [CrossRef]
33. Li, W.; Lin, X.; Wang, J.; Li, G.; Wang, Y. A Mild and Efficient Synthesis of Bis-Indolylmethanes Catalyzed by Sulfamic Acid. *Synth. Commun.* **2005**, *35*, 2765–2769. [CrossRef]
34. An, L.-T.; Ding, F.-Q.; Zou, J.-P.; Lu, X.-H.; Zhang, L.-L. An Efficient and Solvent-Free Reaction for Synthesis of Bis(Indol-3-Yl)Methanes Catalyzed by Sulfamic Acid. *Chin. J. Chem.* **2007**, *25*, 822–827. [CrossRef]
35. Li, J.-T.; Dai, H.-G.; Xu, W.-Z.; Li, T.-S. An Efficient and Practical Synthesis of Bis(Indolyl)Methanes Catalyzed by Aminosulfonic Acid under Ultrasound. *Ultrason. Sonochem* **2006**, *13*, 24–27. [CrossRef] [PubMed]

36. Singh, P.R.; Singh, D.U.; Samant, S.D. Sulphamic Acid—A Mild, Efficient, and Cost-Effective Solid Acid Catalyst for the Synthesis of Bis(1H-indol-3-yl)Methanes. *Synth. Commun.* **2005**, *35*, 2133–2138. [CrossRef]
37. Raju, B.C.; Rao, J.M. P-TsOH-Catalyzed Efficient Synthesis of Bis(Indolyl)Methanes. *ChemInform* **2008**, *39*. [CrossRef]
38. Nasreen, A.; Varala, R.; Adapa, S.R. Copper Nitrate Trihydrate Catalyzed Efficient Synthesis of Bis(Indolyl)Methanes in Acetonitrile at Room Temperature. *J. Heterocycl. Chem.* **2007**, *44*, 983–987. [CrossRef]
39. Zhang, D.-M.; Tang, Q.-G.; Ji, C.-X.; Guo, C. 3,3′-(4-Bromophenylmethanediyl)Bis(5-Methoxy-1*H*-Indole). *Acta Crystallogr. Sect. E Struct. Rep. Online* **2007**, *63*, o81–o82. [CrossRef]
40. Guo, C.; Zhang, D.-M.; Tang, Q.-G.; Sun, H.-S. 5,5′-Dimethoxy-3,3′-(3-Nitrophenylmethanediyl)Bis(1*H*-Indole). *Acta Crystallogr. Sect. E Struct. Rep. Online* **2006**, *62*, o3994–o3995. [CrossRef]
41. Zhang, D.-M.; Tang, S.-G.; Wu, W.-Y.; Tang, Q.-G.; Guo, C. 3,3′-(4-Chlorophenylmethanediyl)Bis(5-Methoxy-1*H*-Indole). *Acta Crystallogr. Sect. E Struct. Rep. Online* **2006**, *62*, o5467–o5468. [CrossRef]
42. Tang, S.-G.; Zhang, D.-M.; Wu, W.-Y.; Shan, L.; Guo, C. 5,5′-Dimethoxy-3,3′-(3-Fluorophenylmethanediyl)Bis(1*H*-Indole). *Acta Crystallogr. Sect. E Struct. Rep. Online* **2006**, *62*, o4691–o4692. [CrossRef]
43. Hosseini-Sarvari, M. Synthesis of Bis(Indolyl)Methanes Using a Catalytic Amount of ZnO under Solvent-Free Conditions. *Synth. Commun.* **2008**, *38*, 832–840. [CrossRef]
44. Du, D.-M.; Meng, S.-M.; Wang, Y.-M.; Meng, J.-B.; Zhou, X.-Z. Solid State Reaction of Aromatic Ketones with Heteroaromatics. *Chin. J. Chem.* **1995**, *13*, 520–524. [CrossRef]
45. Firouzabadi, H.; Iranpoor, N.; Jafari, A.A. Aluminumdodecatungstophosphate (AlPW12O40), a Versatile and a Highly Water Tolerant Green Lewis Acid Catalyzes Efficient Preparation of Indole Derivatives. *J. Mol. Catal. A Chem.* **2006**, *244*, 168–172. [CrossRef]
46. Eisenberg, A.C.; Tanski, J.M.; Getzler, Y.D.Y.L. {2-[Bis(3-Methyl-1*H*-Indol-2-Yl)Methyl]Phenolato-κ*O* }dimethyl(Tetrahydrofuran-κ*O*)Aluminium(III). *Acta Crystallogr. Sect. E Struct. Rep. Online* **2009**, *65*, m1353. [CrossRef] [PubMed]
47. Hosseini-Sarvari, M. Titania (TiO_2)-Catalyzed Expedient, Solventless and Mild Synthesis of Bis(Indolyl)Methanes Scientific Paper. *Acta Chim. Slov.* **2007**, *54*, 354–359.
48. Rahimizadeh, M.; Bakhtiarpoor, Z.; Eshghi, H.; Pordel, M.; Rajabzadeh, G. TiO_2 Nanoparticles: An Efficient Heterogeneous Catalyst for Synthesis of Bis(Indolyl)Methanes under Solvent-Free Conditions. *Monatshefte Für Chem. Chem. Mon.* **2009**, *140*, 1465–1469. [CrossRef]
49. Thirupathi Reddy, Y.; Narsimha Reddy, P.; Sunil Kumar, B.; Rajitha, B. Efficient Synthesis of Bis(Indolyl)Methanes Catalyzed by $TiCl_4$. *Indian J. Chem.* **2005**, *44B*, 2393–2395.
50. Nagawade, R.R.; Shinde, D.B. Zirconium(IV) Chloride—Catalysed Reaction of Indoles: An Expeditious Synthesis of Bis(Indolyl)Methanes. *Bull. Korean Chem. Soc.* **2005**, *26*, 1962–1964. [CrossRef]
51. Zhang, Z.H.; Yin, L.; Wang, Y.M. An Efficient and Practical Process for the Synthesis of Bis(Indolyl)Methanes Catalyzed by Zirconium Tetrachloride. *Synthesis* **2005**, *2005*, 1949–1954. [CrossRef]
52. Reddy, A.V.; Ravinder, K.; Reddy, V.L.N.; Goud, T.V.; Ravikanth, V.; Venkateswarlu, Y. Zeolite Catalyzed Synthesis of Bis(Indolyl) Methanes. *Synth. Commun.* **2003**, *33*, 3687–3694. [CrossRef]
53. Karthik, M.; Magesh, C.J.; Perumal, P.T.; Palanichamy, M.; Arabindoo, B.; Murugesan, V. Zeolite-Catalyzed Ecofriendly Synthesis of Vibrindole A and Bis(Indolyl)Methanes. *Appl. Catal. A Gen.* **2005**, *286*, 137–141. [CrossRef]
54. Karthik, M.; Palanichamy, M.; Murugesan, V. A Mild, Eco-Friendly and Efficient Zeolite Catalyzed Synthesis of Vibrindole A and Bis(Indolyl)Methanes. In *Studies in Surface Science and Catalysis*; Elsevier: Amsterdam, The Netherlands, 2005; Volume 156, pp. 873–878.
55. Lin, Z.H.; Guan, C.J.; Feng, X.L.; Zhao, C.X. Synthesis of Macroreticular P-(ω-Sulfonic-Perfluoroalkylated)Polystyrene Ion-Exchange Resin and Its Application as Solid Acid Catalyst. *J. Mol. Catal. A Chem.* **2006**, *247*, 19–26. [CrossRef]
56. Ramesh, C.; Banerjee, J.; Pal, R.; Das, B. Silica Supported Sodium Hydrogen Sulfate and Amberlyst-15: Two Efficient Heterogeneous Catalysts for Facile Synthesis of Bis- and Tris(1H-Indol-3-Yl)Methanes from Indoles and Carbonyl Compounds1. *Adv. Synth. Catal.* **2003**, *345*, 557–559. [CrossRef]
57. Feng, X.; Guan, C.; Zhao, C. Ion Exchange Resin Catalyzed Condensation of Indole and Carbonyl Compounds—Synthesis of Bis -Indolylmethanes. *Synth. Commun.* **2004**, *34*, 487–492. [CrossRef]
58. Ke, B.; Qin, Y.; Wang, Y.; Wang, F. Amberlyst-Catalyzed Reaction of Indole: Synthesis of Bisindolylalkane. *Synth. Commun.* **2005**, *35*, 1209–1212. [CrossRef]
59. Sheng, S.R.; Wang, Q.Y.; Ding, Y.; Liu, X.L.; Cai, M.Z. Synthesis of Bis(Indolyl)Methanes Using Recyclable PEG-Supported Sulfonic Acid as Catalyst. *Catal. Lett.* **2009**, *128*, 418–422. [CrossRef]
60. Yu, L.; Chen, D.; Li, J.; Wang, P.G. Preparation, Characterization, and Synthetic Uses of Lanthanide(III) Catalysts Supported on Ion Exchange Resins. *J. Org. Chem.* **1997**, *62*, 3575–3581. [CrossRef]
61. Banerji, J.; Duttaa, U.; Basaka, B.; Saha, M.; BudzikiewiczC, H.; Chatterjeea, A. Electrophilic Substitution Reactions of Indole: Part XX-Use of Montmorillonite Clay K-LO. *Indian J. Chem.* **2001**, *40B*, 981–984.
62. Chhattise, P.K.; Arbuj, S.S.; Mohite, K.C.; Bhavsar, S.V.; Horne, A.S.; Handore, K.N.; Chabukswar, V.V. One Dimensional CdS Nanostructures: Heterogeneous Catalyst for Synthesis of Aryl-3,3′-Bis(Indol-3-Yl)Methanes. *RSC Adv.* **2014**, *4*, 28623–28627. [CrossRef]

63. Sobhani, S.; Jahanshahi, R. Nano N-Propylsulfonated γ-Fe_2O_3 (NPS-γ-Fe_2O_3) as a Magnetically Recyclable Heterogeneous Catalyst for the Efficient Synthesis of 2-Indolyl-1-Nitroalkanes and Bis(Indolyl)Methanes. *New J. Chem.* **2013**, *37*, 1009–1015. [CrossRef]
64. Huaccallo-Aguilar, Y.; Álvarez-Torrellas, S.; Martínez-Nieves, J.; Delgado-Adámez, J.; Gil, M.V.; Ovejero, G.; García, J. Magnetite-Based Catalyst in the Catalytic Wet Peroxide Oxidation for Different Aqueous Matrices Spiked with Naproxen–Diclofenac Mixture. *Catalysts* **2021**, *11*, 514. [CrossRef]
65. Wang, D.; Li, Y.; Wen, L.; Xi, J.; Liu, P.; Hansen, T.W.; Li, P. Ni-Pd-Incorporated Fe_3O_4 Yolk-Shelled Nanospheres as Efficient Magnetically Recyclable Catalysts for Reduction of N-Containing Unsaturated Compounds. *Catalysts* **2023**, *13*, 190. [CrossRef]
66. Hosseini Nasab, N.; Safari, J. Synthesis of a Wide Range of Biologically Important Spiropyrans and Spiroacenaphthylenes, Using $NiFe_2O_4$@SiO_2@Melamine Magnetic Nanoparticles as an Efficient, Green and Reusable Nanocatalyst. *J. Mol. Struct.* **2019**, *1193*, 118–124. [CrossRef]
67. Shaabani, A.; Afshari, R.; Hooshmand, S.E.; Tabatabaei, A.T.; Hajishaabanha, F. Copper Supported on MWCNT-Guanidine Acetic Acid@Fe_3O_4: Synthesis, Characterization and Application as a Novel Multi-Task Nanocatalyst for Preparation of Triazoles and Bis(Indolyl)Methanes in Water. *RSC Adv.* **2016**, *6*, 18113–18125. [CrossRef]
68. Kour, M.; Paul, S. Sulfonated Carbon/Nano-Metal Oxide Composites: A Novel and Recyclable Solid Acid Catalyst for Organic Synthesis in Benign Reaction Media. *New J. Chem.* **2015**, *39*, 6338–6350. [CrossRef]
69. Carta, D.; Casula, M.F.; Falqui, A.; Loche, D.; Mountjoy, G.; Sangregorio, C.; Corrias, A. A Structural and Magnetic Investigation of the Inversion Degree in Ferrite Nanocrystals MFe_2O_4 (M = Mn, Co, Ni). *J. Phys. Chem. C* **2009**, *113*, 8606–8615. [CrossRef]
70. Rouquerol, J.; Rouquerol, F.; Llewellyn, P.; Maurin, G.; Sing, K.S.W. *Adsorption by Powders and Porous Solids*; Elsevier: Amsterdam, The Netherlands, 2014; ISBN 9780080970356.
71. Chierotti, M.R.; Gaglioti, K.; Gobetto, R.; Barbero, M.; Nervi, C. Mechanism of the Solvent-Free Reactions between Indole Derivatives and 4-Nitrobenzaldehyde Studied by Solid-State NMR and DFT Calculations. *CrystEngComm* **2012**, *14*, 6732. [CrossRef]
72. Casula, M.F.; Loche, D.; Marras, S.; Paschina, G.; Corrias, A. Role of Urea in the Preparation of Highly Porous Nanocomposite Aerogels. *Langmuir* **2007**, *23*, 3509–3512. [CrossRef]

molecules

MDPI

Review

An Overview of the Sustainable Depolymerization/Degradation of Polypropylene Microplastics by Advanced Oxidation Technologies

Elisa I. García-López [1], Narimene Aoun [2] and Giuseppe Marcì [2,*]

[1] Department of Biological, Chemical and Pharmaceutical Sciences and Technologies (STEBICEF), University of Palermo, Viale delle Scienze, 90128 Palermo, Italy; elisaisabel.garcialopez@unipa.it

[2] Department of Engineering (DI), University of Palermo, Viale delle Scienze, 90128 Palermo, Italy; aoun.narimene95@gmail.com

* Correspondence: giuseppe.marci@unipa.it

Abstract: Plastics have become indispensable in modern society; however, the proliferation of their waste has become a problem that can no longer be ignored as most plastics are not biodegradable. Depolymerization/degradation through sustainable processes in the context of the circular economy are urgent issues. The presence of multiple types of plastic materials makes it necessary to study the specific characteristics of each material. This mini-review aims to provide an overview of technological approaches and their performance for the depolymerization and/or degradation of one of the most widespread plastic materials, polypropylene (PP). The state of the art is presented, describing the most relevant technologies focusing on advanced oxidation technologies (AOT) and the results obtained so far for some of the approaches, such as ozonation, sonochemistry, or photocatalysis, with the final aim of making more sustainable the PP depolymerization/degradation process.

Keywords: depolymerization; microplastics; advanced oxidation technologies (AOTs); sonochemistry; ozonation; photocatalysis

Citation: García-López, E.I.; Aoun, N.; Marcì, G. An Overview of the Sustainable Depolymerization/ Degradation of Polypropylene Microplastics by Advanced Oxidation Technologies. *Molecules* **2024**, *29*, 2816. https://doi.org/10.3390/molecules29122816

Academic Editors: Fabio Ganazzoli and Giuseppina Raffaini

Received: 18 April 2024
Revised: 3 June 2024
Accepted: 8 June 2024
Published: 13 June 2024

1. Introduction

The ubiquitous presence of solid plastics is an issue of growing environmental concern. A world without plastics seems today unimaginable, indeed, the increase in plastics production has been remarkable, surpassing most other manufactured materials, with the possible exception of steel or cement. The number of plastics in municipal solid waste was 1% in mass in 1960, increasing to more than 10% by 2015 [1]. Plastic waste is so ubiquitous in the environment that it has been suggested as a geological indicator of the proposed Anthropocene era [2]. The majority of the monomers used for the predominantly used plastics are derived from fossil hydrocarbons and they are not biodegradable; consequently, they accumulate in the natural environment [3]. Currently, the only strategy to permanently eliminate plastic wastes is combustion or pyrolysis. An amount of 14% of the plastic packaging is collected for recycling and 2% of all recovered plastic packaging waste returns to applications of the same or similar quality (primary recycling), whereas the remaining plastic packaging waste escapes into the environment during transport, use, or end-of-life collection failures [4]. Plastic debris has been found in all major ocean basins. The recycling of polymers necessitates different processes, such as the separation of impurities and the degradation of macromolecular structures, which influence the properties of the recycled materials (secondary recycling). A great challenge for polymer chemistry would be to develop stratagems where the wasted polymers could be transformed into their own starting materials, i.e., transform the current polymers, ubiquitously present as a waste, back into monomers, and purify them for re-polymerization. The transformation of polymers back into monomers (de-polymerization) is a process of great environmental value because the material recycled in this manner does not lose properties and would raise the ideal circular economy. Many research efforts are currently devoted to polymer recycling, although still, few investigations obtain successful results in which depolymerization gives rise to a monomer, or inferior fragments of the original polymer, possessing sufficient qualities to obtain the original polymer with the same initial properties, i.e., without suffering any loss of functionality. An alternative to reduce the environmental impact of plastic wastes is their degradation process, which should give rise to the complete breakage of C-C bonds in order to obtain H_2O and CO_2 as the final products. However, the potentially dangerous chemical substances released during the degradation of the polymers are aspects of huge environmental interest, and, consequently, their de-polymerization for the reinsertion in the cycle economy, as schematized in Figure 1, is preferable.

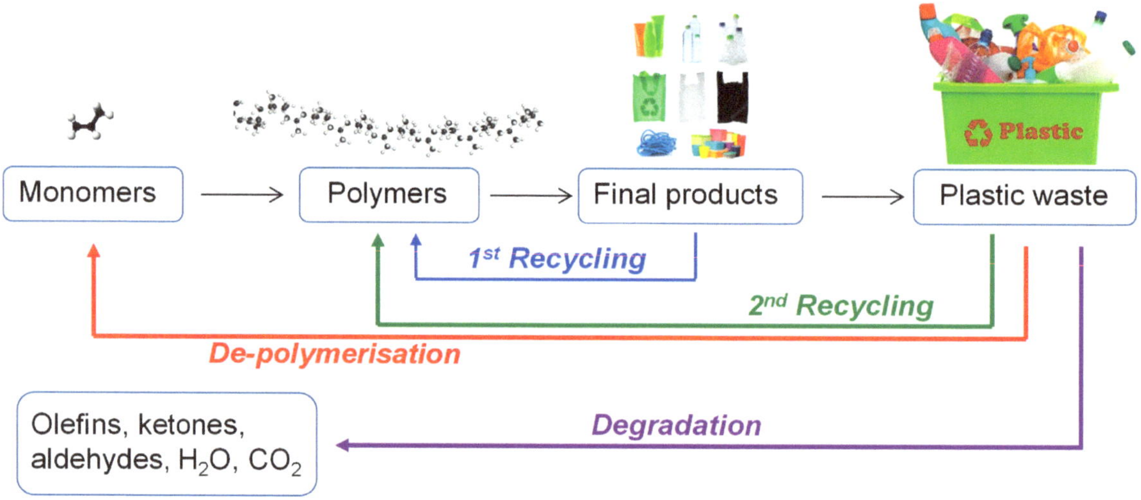

Figure 1. Scheme of the plastics waste recycling process or plastics degradation to obtain olefins, ketones, aldehydes with low molecular weight, and water and carbon dioxide.

Plastics are classified into seven categories based on the degree of hazard to humans and the environment, as well as considering their recyclability. The most commonly used plastic materials are reported in Scheme 1. Polyethylene terephthalate (PET) is one of the most produced types of plastic in the world. It is commonly used for packaging or beverage bottles. The second kind of plastic is polyethylene (PE), which is divided into two groups, i.e., HDPE (high density) and LDPE (low density). HDPE is a rigid plastic used for robust plastic packaging, such as laundry detergents, as well as construction applications or trash cans. LDPE is a transparent and flexible plastic used for plastic bags. It is highly flexible but presents low tensile strength. PE shows corrosion resistance. Another type of PE is the high molecular weight PE, which can be even stronger than steel, and it is mostly used in medical devices such as pelvic implants. Polyvinyl chloride (PVC) is a transparent and impact-resistant plastic, mostly used in construction and commercial applications such as plumbing, electrical wire insulation, and strong packaging. PVC is difficult to recycle and less than 1% is recycled. Polypropylene (PP) is a durable semi-transparent plastic with a low friction surface. It does not react with liquids and possesses good electrical resistance. The most widely used plastic on the market is PP due to its high flexibility and compatibility. Polystyrene (PS) is a versatile plastic applied in disposable tableware, building insulation, and as a transparent material or medical devices such as test tubes or Petri dishes. Finally, there are a series of polymers, indicated as type 7 in Scheme 1, which are polycarbonate (PC) and other plastics, such as polyoxymethylene (POM), polylactic acid, nylon (or polyamide), polymethyl methacrylate (PMMA), acrylonitrile butadiene styrene (ABS), among others [5,6].

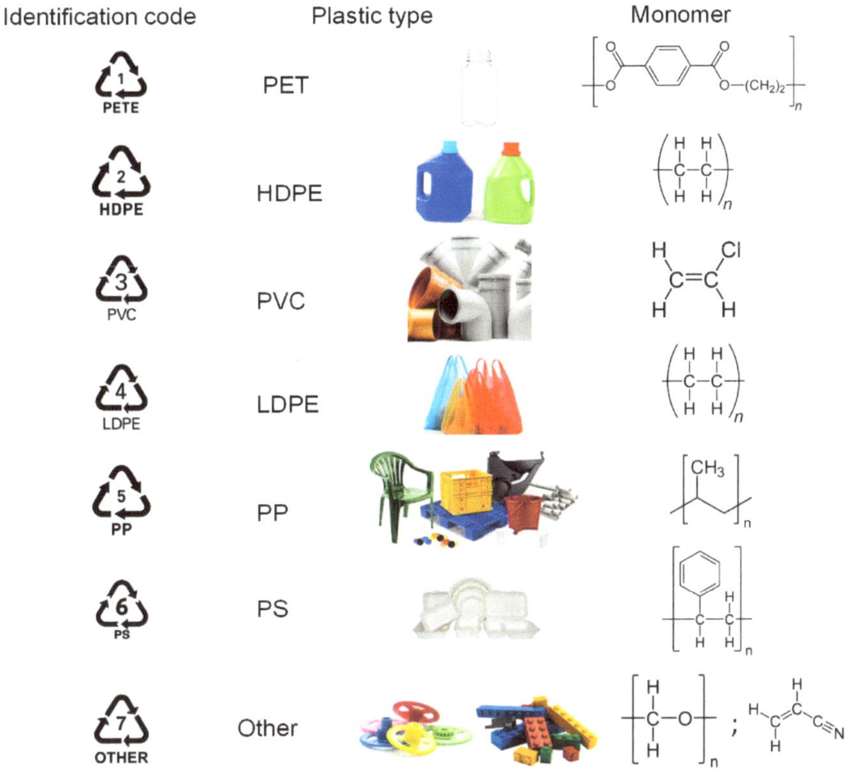

Scheme 1. List of most common plastics, their constitutive monomer, and identification code.

Polyethylene (PE) and polypropylene (PP) are the largest group of commercial synthetic plastics and by far the most important polymers. Its application in packaging is massive, as it is the second most used plastic in the world [7]. These materials are polyolefins, possessing the general formula (-CH_2CHR-)$_n$ where R is a hydrogen or a methyl group. PP emerges for its great mechanical resistance, lightness, excellent electrical insulation ability, and inertness to water. Both polyolefins are highly stable and do not readily degrade in the biosphere, so their massive waste quantities contaminate enormously. It is alarming to know that of the 8.3 billion metric tons of plastics manufactured since the 1950s, almost 80% have become waste [8]. The increased production and use of plastics gave rise to accumulation in marine, freshwater, and terrestrial ecosystems. Indeed, the serious problem is related to the presence of microplastics, which cause pollution by entering natural ecosystems. Microplastics (MPs) are plastic pieces measuring less than 5 mm whose variable composition has been individuated in many environments. The most common are PE, PP, and PVC [9]. For instance, the microplastics used in personal care products are generally PE and PP, present in municipal wastewater treatment plants and ultimately in the environment. Microplastics are categorized as primary microplastics, the raw materials used in domestic and personal care products, and secondary microplastics arising from the degradation of raw plastic particles by physical, chemical, and biological processes in the environment [10]. Long-term durability due to their polymeric structure and easy transport between different habitats make microplastics of high concern. According to biologist studies, PP microplastics are more toxic than PE [11]. For instance, Schiavo et al. have compared the polyethylene (PE), polystyrene (PS), and polypropylene (PP) microplastics impact on the inhibition of marine microalgae *Dunaliella tertiolecta* population growth, DNA damage, and oxidative stress (ROS production), and they have classified the toxicity of polymer as follows: PP > PS > PE [12]. Other authors found PP more toxic than polyvinyl chloride (PVC) as regards mice pulmonary toxicity [13].

Technologies for the elimination of MPs from water and wastewater are urgently needed. The concern is enormous because polyolefins are bio-inert, and they are highly resistant to degradation by microorganisms such as fungi and bacteria. The surfaces made from polyolefins are hydrophobic and thus restrain the growth of microorganisms on their surfaces [14]. Several reviews summarized the microorganisms that can degrade plastics as PP, PE, and others, reporting the kind of microorganisms and enzymes and the metabolic pathways for plastic degradation [15,16]. The bio-deterioration of PP utilizing bacterial strains and complex microbial populace; however, has been reported to be very slow [17]. Microorganisms capable of biodegrading microplastics can give rise to certain depolymerization of PP into monomers or oligomers, but they can enter into the cells, so further efforts are needed both to understand the process and to induce further degradation.

All atoms of PE and PP are connected through strong single C-C and C-H bonds, and the chemical inertness of polyolefins sets a difficulty for their depolymerization by low energy processes. PP is less stable than PE because it has tertiary carbons, which are more sensitive to oxygen attack [18]. Its exposure to sunlight and the related degenerations are important subjects that have attracted scientific interest. Severe molecular chain degradation in PP can be induced when it is irradiated within the active wavelength range of 310–350 nm, which means that photodegradation can occur in PP-based materials [19], as explained below.

2. Methodologies Used for Depolymerization and Degradation of Polyolefins

The polymerization process of polyolefins is an exergonic process and, by virtue of the kinetic efficiency of the Ziegler–Natta industrial catalysts, their polymerization is rather economical. The polymerizations are exothermic enough to provide their own heat, so not consuming external energy (Figure 2). Successful depolymerization must activate the polymer chain and create reactive species capable of depolymerization. For most polymers formed by addition through a C-C π bond, selective reactivation for chemical recycling into monomer is thermodynamically and kinetically demanding under moderate conditions, hence polyolefins, such as polyethylene (PE) or polypropylene (PP), are emblematic in solving this problem (Figure 2). The long chains of the polymer molecules can be cracked by chemical or physical (or biological) processes, giving rise to short units of lower molecular weight [20].

Depolymerization is an important strategy in the framework of the circular economy, as schematized in Figure 1. Depolymerization differs from degradation, which involves the reduction of the molecular weight of the polymer along with its partial oxidation or, in some cases, the complete destruction of the chemical structure of the substance. On the other hand, depolymerization concerns only the reduction of the molecular weight of the polymer without major changes in the chemical structure [21].

Degradation during mechanical reprocessing is common for plastics. Polyolefins degrade during the melting process due to radical reactions that lower the molecular weight of PP [22]. Unless advances in recycling [23,24] of nascent purification technologies [25,26] or other research innovations alter this dynamic, polyolefin waste will continue to grow in proportion to polymer production. Unfortunately, monomer chemical recycling is not energetically accessible for polyolefins; in fact, according to Coates et al., chemical recycling of monomer for the three polymers produced in larger volumes, PVC, PE, and PP, is either chemically impossible, as in the case of PVC, or extremely challenging, as for polyolefins as PP or PE, as shown in Figure 2 [27].

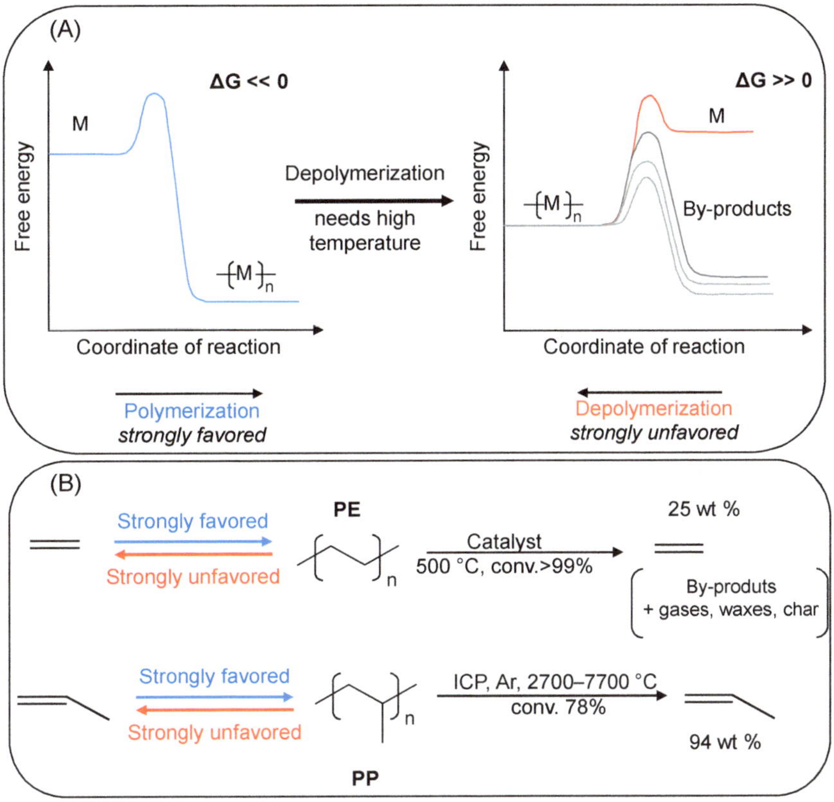

Figure 2. (**A**) Conceptual reaction profiles for a highly exergonic polymerization reaction and its corresponding depolymerization, where M represents the monomer. In these cases, the variation in Gibbs free energy is too negative for the reverse reaction of depolymerization. (**B**) Two representative examples of highly exergonic polymerizations, polyethylene (PE), and polypropylene (PP), and the correspondent depolymerization conditions and yield towards the original monomer [26].

Among the techniques investigated for polymer degradation, thermal, mechanical, photolytic, ultrasonic, microwave, biodegradation, oxidative, hydrolytic, and degradation by high-energy radiation are the most explored. Methodologies such as acid treatment, exposure to ionizing radiation, or enzymatic treatment suffer from major drawbacks such as higher treatment costs or uncontrolled reduction of the molecular weight, including changes in the chemical identity of the polymers [28]. Since all atoms in PP (and in PE) are linked via strong C-C and C-H single bonds, giving strong chemical inertness to the polyolefins, depolymerization by low-energy processes is a challenging procedure [29].

It can be mentioned that the generation of fuels from polyolefins has been extensively studied because of the absence of oxygen and the content of carbon and hydrogen in these materials, which, together with the absence of water in the polymer, confer the obtained fuels with a very high calorific value. Therefore, fuels produced from polyolefins possess similar combustible properties to fossil fuels and can become an alternative energy source [30].

The depolymerization of polyolefins in supercritical water has been also studied. This approach is a thermochemical process actuated at moderate temperature (>374 °C) and pressure (>22.129 MPa). Supercritical water gives rise to rapid, selective, and efficient reactions to convert organic waste into oil, compared to other depolymerization methods [31]. Recently, Chen et al. have converted polypropylene (PP) to oil in supercritical water for times in the range from 30 min to 6 h at 380–500 °C and 23 MPa [32]. A total of 91% of the weight of the PP was converted to oil at 425 °C in ca. 3 h or at 450 °C in ca. 1 h. At 425 °C, PP was rapidly (in ca. 30 min) decomposed into oligomers, and then the unsaturated aliphatics would be transformed into cyclics by cyclization. At the same time, small amounts of unsaturated aliphatics (olefins) can become saturated aliphatics (paraffins) and aromatics. Higher reaction temperatures (>450 °C) or longer reaction times (>4 h) lead to more gaseous products. About 80–90% of the oil components have the same boiling point range as naphtha (C_5–C_{11}) and heating values of 48–49 MJ·kg^{-1}. This conversion process is net energy positive and with higher energy efficiency and lower greenhouse gas emissions than incineration, mechanical recycling, or pyrolysis. Therefore, oil derived from PP has the potential to be used as gasoline blends or raw materials for other chemicals. The reaction pathway of the reaction process, as well as the main intermediates as proposed by Chen et al. [32], is reported in Figure 3.

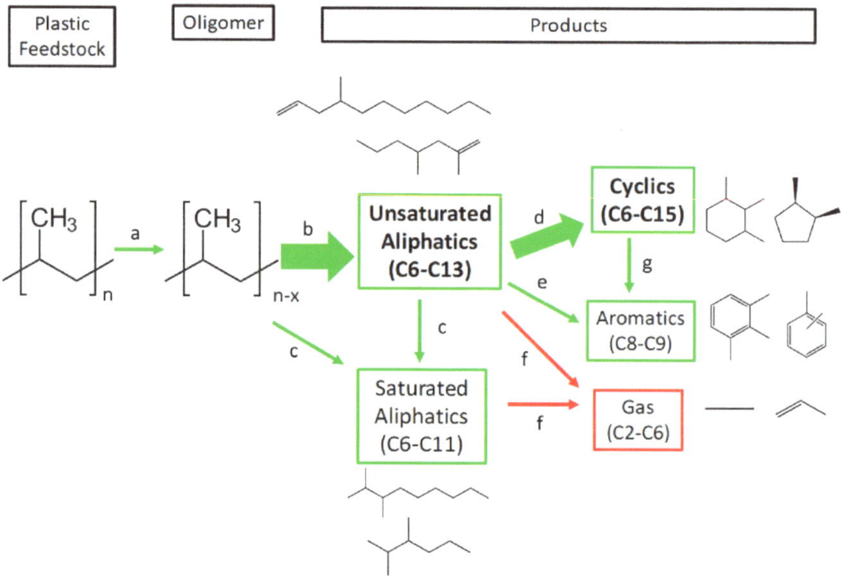

Figure 3. Scheme of the potential reaction of conversion of polypropylene by depolymerization process in supercritical water. A green box represents the oil phase products and a red box indicates the gas products. The thickness of the arrows represents the relative quantities of products. The letters on the arrows (a–g) indicate the evolution of the species. Reproduced from [32] with ACS permission.

2.1. *Advanced Oxidation Technologies (AOTs)*

Recently, effective results have been obtained by advanced oxidation technologies (AOTs). These methodologies are often used to mineralize organic pollutants and recalcitrant chemicals usually present in wastewater. AOTs utilize various oxidants such as H_2O_2, O_3, or Fe^{2+} to produce reactive oxidizing species (ROS). The photo-chemical methods to degrade pollutants, including also PP degradation, are based on the production of ROS ($^{\bullet}OH$, $^{\bullet}O_2^{-}$, $^{1}O_2$, and h^{+}) [33,34]. These species are strong oxidants and they can virtually oxidize any compound reacting unselectively with them once formed. The pollutant is speedily and efficiently fragmented and converted into small species. A series of processes can be considered AOTs, among them those summarized in Figure 4. The AOTs field has witnessed rapid development and, currently, Fenton, photo-Fenton, Electro-Fenton, and H_2O_2/UV systems as long as heterogeneous photocatalysis, particularly in the presence of TiO_2, have received extensive scrutiny [34].

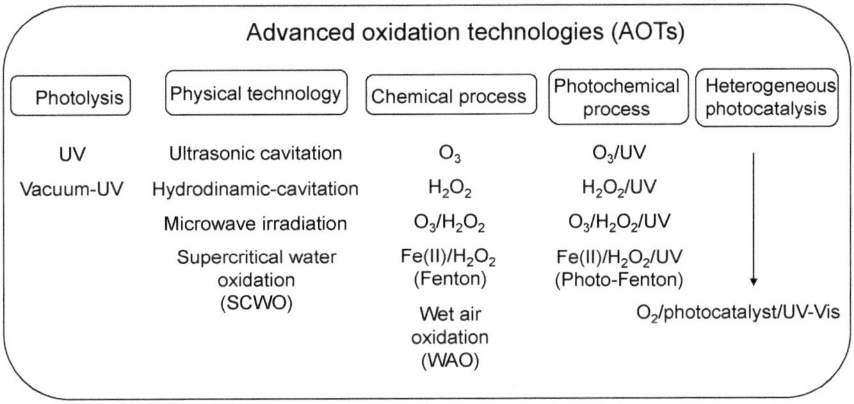

Figure 4. Different AOTs used for depolymerization/degradation of pollutants and chemicals recalcitrant to be depolluted.

2.1.1. Photolytic Degradation of Polymers

Degradation of plastic polymers in the natural environment can proceed by either abiotic or biotic pathways. Generally, abiotic degradation precedes biodegradation, and it is initiated thermally, hydrolytically, or by UV light [35]. PE and PP are susceptible to photo-initiated oxidative degradation, as schematized in Figure 5, which is believed to be their most important abiotic degradation pathway in aerobic outdoor environments [36]. Photodegradation in the absence of a catalyst (homogeneous) would be suitable to degrade polyolefins. This is the most important pathway of polyolefin abiotic degradation in aerobic external environments [37]. Photo-oxidation causes the oxygenation of the surface of the plastic, which increases the hydrophilicity of the polymer and improves the formation of the microbial biofilm on its surface. The reaction is divided into three main stages: initiation, propagation, and cessation. During the initiation phase, the chemical bonds of the polymer chain are cleaved by UV radiation to produce free radicals by breaking the C–H bonds. This process occurs only when polymers contain unsaturated chromophore groups that adsorb electromagnetic radiation, undergoing direct decomposition with bond dissociation upon ultraviolet [38]. As long as PP (and PE) does not contain unsaturated chromophore bonds, it is resistant to photo-initiated degradation. Nevertheless, the presence of impurities in the macromolecular structure can allow the photodegradation to proceed [38,39].

In the propagation phase, the polymeric radicals react with O_2 forming $^{\cdot}OOH$ radicals. In addition, further radical reactions give rise to the oxidation of the substrate [40]. Propagation eventually leads to chain splitting or crosslinking [41]. The combination of two radicals giving rise to inert species leads to the end of the reaction [42]. The oxidation gives rise to random chain cleavage producing oxygen-containing functional groups such as olefinic, ketone, and aldehyde compounds [39]. The formation of unsaturated double bonds during the process makes the molecules more susceptible to photodegradation. As the molecular weight of polymers decreases, the material becomes more susceptible to fragmentation through further reactions. For example, Albertsson et al. have studied the photodegradation of PE in an inert system for more than 10 years, showing that the degradation rate of PE is characterized by three phases. In the first stage, there is a rapid release of CO_2 and absorption of O_2 up to the equilibrium phase, while in the second stage, a decrease in the degradation rate is observed. Finally, a rapid deterioration of the surface structure and an increase in the degradation rate occurs [43].

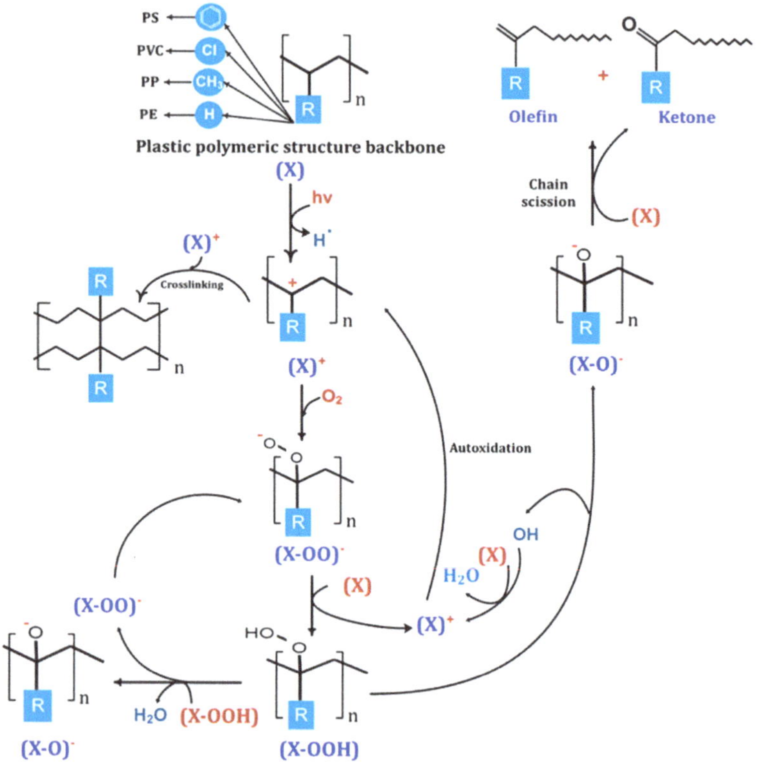

Figure 5. Mechanism of plastic UV photodegradation according to Ali et al. Reproduced with Elsevier permission from [37].

As mentioned, traces of impurities in PP allow the formation of radicals that react with oxygen giving rise to radical reactions making random chain scission and crosslinking feasible, leading predominantly to lower molecular weight fragments [44]. Also, functional groups such as carbonyl and hydroperoxides are formed. The final species are pentane, 2-methyl-1-pentene, and 2,4-dimethyl-1-heptene, among others [45]. The biodegradability of a molecule is in relation to its chemical structure and chain branching increases the resistance to aerobic biodegradation; consequently, due to the presence of a tertiary carbon of PP, the predisposition to microbial degradation diminished.

The degradation of PP in the presence of peroxide both with and without contemporary light irradiation has been also examined. The degradation of PP depends on the quantity of O_2, temperature, concentrations of both polymer and peroxide, and the radicals generated by the thermal decomposition of the peroxide [46]. Peroxides produce alkoxy radicals (highly reactive organic structures where the radicals are localized at the oxygen atom and singularly bound to an alkyl group) that abstract hydrogen atoms attached to tertiary carbons, and then the macro-radicals generated undergo β-fragmentation into alkenes and macro alkyl radicals (see Figure 6), which undergo further reactions.

Bertin et al. have observed that the extraction of H in the tertiary carbon is a minor process in the degradation of PP in the presence of peroxides in solution [46]; however, most of the literature reports the reaction pathway schematized in Figure 6. This is because the pathway depends very much on the experimental conditions and, in particular, on the presence of oxygen, the exclusion of which was difficult to achieve. Traces of oxygen increase PP degradation following the process schematized in Figure 7. Furthermore, degradation at high temperatures (about 300 °C) and the combination with cutting forces could also favor the fragmentation of the molecules. The reaction in the presence of peroxide radicals formed when O_2 is present in the reacting medium follows the oxidative scheme of Figure 7. After its formation, the peroxy radical can undergo various reactions that lead to the shortening of the polymer chain.

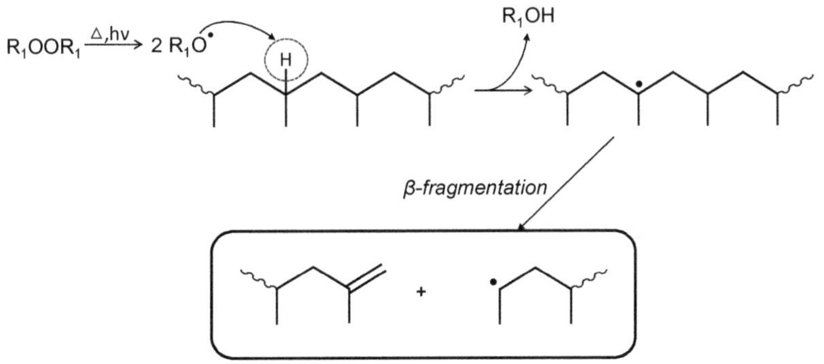

Figure 6. Polypropylene degradation in the presence of peroxide species by a β-fragmentation process.

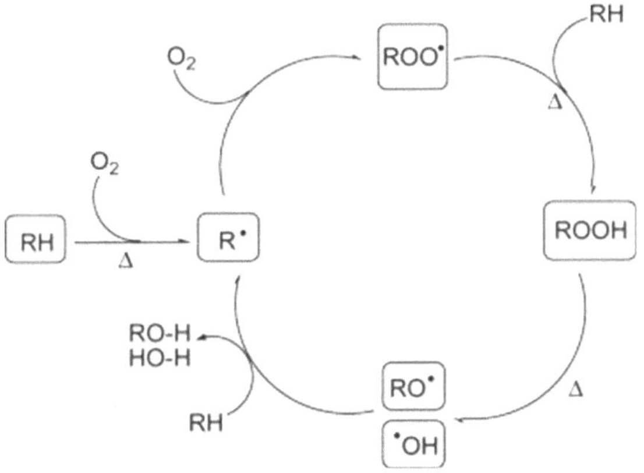

Figure 7. Oxidative cycle of polypropylene in the presence of oxygen, as proposed by Bertin et al. and reproduced with Elsevier permission [46].

The processes explained are also representative of the reactions that can be carried out in the laboratory in the presence of H_2O_2, O_3, light, or ultrasound irradiation, as well as in the presence of solid acid catalysts such as silica-alumina or Nb_2O_5. The latter can be activated by the light generating further radicals through photocatalytic processes [47]. The addition of salts such as peroxodisulfate ($S_2O_8{}^{-2}$) or Fenton reagent [48] can assist in the formation of ROS, which are extremely oxidant species, which will follow the same reactive pathway for PP degradation.

The influence of the temperature can be also considered because the thermal degradation of the plastic can be performed at temperatures above 100 °C, depending on the type and characteristics of the plastic polymer. The antioxidant additives incorporated through the manufacture of the plastic prevent thermal oxidation at low temperatures. Conversely, degradation due to thermal oxidation is accelerated by stress and exposure to reactive compounds such as O_3 or H_2O_2 generated by ROS. In general, the resistance to degradation depends on the chemical composition of the polymer, with PP, PVC, and polybutadiene (PBD) being the most susceptible to thermal degradation. Conversely, polymers such as polysulfone, polyether ketone, and polysiloxanes are thermally resistant due to the strong bonds in their backbone. Overall, the contribution of thermal degradation under normal environmental conditions is considered to be globally negligible, particularly in cold marine environments.

2.1.2. Ultrasound Irradiation (Sonochemistry)

Sonochemistry, based on the effect of ultrasound in forming acoustic cavitation in liquids, which results in a chemical activity has been extensively used for the degradation of pollutants, for instance, chlorinated organic compounds [49], or for the preparation of materials [50]. It is an eco-friendly green technology reported in many areas as organic chemistry, biomass valorization, electrochemistry, catalysis, environmental remediation, and also in polymer chemistry [51]. Ultrasound irradiation constitutes a valid alternative methodology for efficient depolymerization/degradation of PP [52]. It provides an accurate method to reduce the molecular weight of polymers in a targeted manner by carefully regulating both the rate of cleavage and the rate of polymerization. For the ultrasound-based approach, no chemicals are needed, so it offers a green alternative to other techniques; moreover, it can be modified by the presence of additives in combination with irradiation. Indeed, it has been reported that the use of additives and/or salts in combination with cavitation promotes the degradation of polymers [53].

The primary reactions that occur during sonication in water dispersion, which can be considered as the initiator of a series of radical reactions depending on the polymer species, are the following:

$$H_2O \rightarrow {}^{\bullet}OH + H^{\bullet} \quad (1)$$

$$H^{\bullet} + H^{\bullet} \rightarrow H_2 \quad (2)$$

$${}^{\bullet}OH + {}^{\bullet}OH \rightarrow H_2O_2 \quad (3)$$

$$H^{\bullet} + O_2 \rightarrow HO_2^{\bullet} \quad (4)$$

$$H^{\bullet} + HO_2^{\bullet} \rightarrow H_2O_2 \quad (5)$$

$$HO_2^{\bullet} + HO_2^{\bullet} \rightarrow H_2O_2 + O_2 \quad (6)$$

Sonication in water gives rise to the formation of strong oxidizing agents like ${}^{\bullet}OH$ and H· radicals, which subsequently form hydrogen peroxide (H_2O_2).

A lower polymer concentration increases the degradation rate and produces a lower-weight molecule in shorter times because the overlap of the polymer chains decreases; therefore, they are more susceptible to the hydrodynamic forces generated by the cavitation forces. In the case of the cavitation reactor, the operating reaction volume plays an essential role in the extent of degradation. The polymer degradation rate decreased with an increase in the reaction volume. Consequently, the operating parameters strongly influence the extent of polymer degradation to maximize intensification.

Ultrasound has been applied for the degradation of various polymeric compounds such as polypropylene (PP) [54,55].

For the cavitation processes, it has been determined that (i) low concentrations and low volumes favor the degradation; (ii) type of polymer, in particular the presence of substituents or functional groups on the polymer chain, plays a significant role in the extent of degradation; and (iii) a reduction of viscosity occurred by increasing ultrasound frequency and power density up to an optimal limit for soluble polymers while only physical changes are observed for insoluble polymers. An optimal temperature must be established since it influences the process of initiation of cavitation and also the generation of free radicals based on the collapse of the cavity contents. The type of solvent plays also a crucial role in the overall effectiveness of the degradation process. The degradation rate mainly depends on the physico-chemical properties of the solvent such as volatility and kinematic viscosity. The degradation degree decreases with the increase in vapor pressure and viscosity of the solvent.

The presence of additives increases the effectiveness of the degradation of the polymer; for instance, a reduction of the viscosity occurs by adding salt up to an optimal value, while the effect of the addition of surfactants depends on the nature of the polymer. Of course, the addition of further oxidizing additives, such as ozone, increases the generation of ·OH, which can significantly increase the degradation of the polymer.

Chakraborty investigated the ultrasonic degradation of isotactic polypropylene at 80, 90, 113, 133, and 155 °C using o-dichlorobenzene as a solvent, using a frequency of 25 kHz with a voltage of 180 V [56]. By increasing the vapor pressure of the solvent and reaction temperature, the degradation rate decreased, even by decreasing the viscosity of the solvent. Price et al. studied the effect of irradiation intensity (26.2 ± 1.3 W·cm^2) on solid polymer powder such as polypropylene suspended in water [57]. Particle fragmentation, deagglomeration, and surface modification resulted after the sonication treatment, and the extensions increased by increasing the irradiation intensity in a constant area of the transducer surface.

2.1.3. Ozonation

Ozonation can be used as a process for the degradation of polymers; indeed, a sufficient amount of ozone can have a great effect on the degradation rate of polymers. Moreover, a synergistic effect has been observed in the rate of degradation by coupling ozonization with other advanced oxidation methodologies.

It is interesting to know that, according to Gugumus et al., the concentration of O_3 in ambient air can range from 10 to 80 mg·m^{-3} in winter and summer, respectively [58], so a seasonal influence on thermal oxidation of PP can be attributed to changes in ozone concentration in the natural ambient. To investigate this hypothesis on the thermo-oxidative degradation of PP films, the effect of lower O_3 concentrations with respect to the environmental ones has been studied, concluding that an ozone concentration in the range of 100 to 200 mg·m^{-3} does not affect the degradation rate of PP at a temperature of 120 °C [59]. Also, experiments carried out under an O_3 flow twin-screw extruder with different polymer throughput and reaction temperatures demonstrate the ozone-thermal degradation of molten PP material on the reactive extrusion [60]. Ozone is introduced into the extruder to rapidly oxidize the molten PP within seconds. Oxidized PP had a higher melt flow index than the original PP, indicating a decrease in the molecular weight of PP. The ozone-induced degradation of PP may provide a way to produce PP with controlled rheology. These results indicate that O_3 and temperature have a synergistic effect on the PP degradation reaction. Due to the fact that ozone is only in contact with molten PP for a few seconds, this process has higher reaction efficiency than solid-state PP degradation in an ambient containing ozone. It is worth noting that no harmful by-products are reported to be produced from the ozonating reaction [60].

The mechanism scheme of the oxidative degradation process of PP is shown in Figure 8. Atomic oxygen abstracted hydrogen atoms from the tertiary carbon atoms producing radical carbon sites in the polymer chain. Then, molecular oxygen reacts with the tertiary carbon radical to form a radical peroxy group, which then, using the neighboring hydrogen, forms a hydroperoxide. Then, the β-chain scission of PP molecules occurs by forming an olefin end group at one chain end and a peroxyl radical at the other that is eventually rearranged into a ketone group. Consequently, the degradation of PP in the presence of ozone proceeds by the formation of olefin and, with further attacks to other tertiary carbon atoms in the polymer chains, giving rise to more olefin molecule formation.

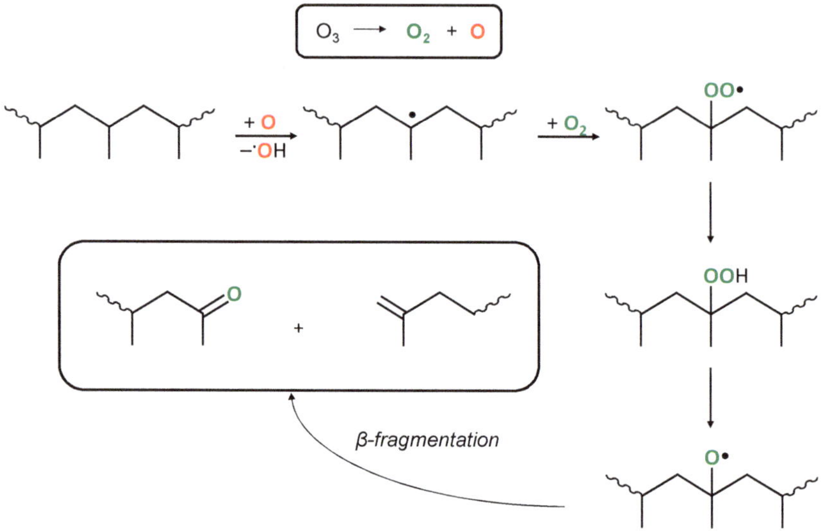

Figure 8. The mechanism of PP oxidative degradation with ozone.

2.1.4. Photocatalytic Technology for PP Degradation

The recently reviewed [34] study of the photolytic process, also called photoaging or photodegradation, is essential to understanding other strategies such as heterogeneous photocatalytic technology. Though many photochemical/UV reactions with ozone or hydrogen peroxide were carried out in some AOTs to remove organic pollutants, such as microplastics [61], the main disadvantage is the rise of harmful intermediates. This can be overcome by photocatalytic degradation. In photocatalytic degradation, organic pollutants present in wastewater are completely mineralized into carbon dioxide, water, and other non-toxic products. Nowadays, photocatalysts, which can enhance the degradation process under UV irradiation, are commonly used. The principle of photocatalysis involves the excitation of electrons from the valence band to the conduction band, thereby forming electron–hole pairs. Photogenerated electrons and holes are responsible for the reduction and oxidation reactions, respectively, occurring at the surface of the heterogeneous photocatalysts. Holes generated in the valence band react with $H_2O/OH^-/H_2O_2$ to form free radicals, which eventually lead to possible mineralization of organic pollutants. These species lead to an oxidizing environment through many parallel reactions, which will achieve the photodegradation of plastics. The process will result in the reduction of the plastic particle size and thus improve the suspension/solubility of plastics in the water and ultimately into the complete degradation.

Wastewater contaminated with hazardous chemicals, pesticides, phenols, chlorophenols, and other pollutants was effectively treated using photocatalysis. It also inactivates the viruses, bacteria, and protozoa residuals. Recently, photocatalysis has also been used to treat plastic waste material. To avoid the toxic by-products formed from other disposal methods, photocatalysis could be carried out to degrade the plastic waste with the help of a suitable catalyst.

Photocatalytic processes are seen as an efficient and eco-friendly method to convert plastics into value-added molecules [62]. Also, this technology has been demonstrated to be promising for PP treatment, among other plastics degradation. The sustainability, good performance, low cost, and soft conditions enforce the applicability of this strategy because it can exploit free and endless solar irradiation. Photocatalysis mineralizes contaminants to H_2O and CO_2 by the generation of ROS, i.e., $^{\bullet}OH$, $O_2^{\bullet -}$, and $^1O_2$, along with the holes (h^+) produced in the valence band of the semiconductor under UV-Vis irradiation.

Titanium dioxide is the most used photocatalyst because of its high oxido-reduction ability, chemical stability, high stability, cost-effectiveness, and environmental friendliness [63]. A report on the ability of TiO_2 as a photocatalyst for the degradation of polyolefins was published as early as 1974 [64]. The use of photocatalysis for the degradation and removal of different types of pollutants, including plastic, has been studied with increasing attention, although many problems, such as an electron–hole recombination, modulation of the band gap of the semiconductors, and slow kinetics of surface reactions, still remain to be solved [58]. An important issue to be focused on in the future is the chemicals generated during the photocatalytic degradation of plastics, which have not been studied from an environmental perspective [65].

A number of semiconductor oxides, such as TiO_2, ZrO_2, ZnO, BiOCl, and C_3N_4, among others, have been successfully used as photocatalysts to degrade polymers, including PP. TiO_2 has been recognized as the most efficient due to its excellent thermodynamical features, photogenerated carriers mobility, optical properties, non-toxicity, stability, and low cost.

A green bioinspired synthesis for C,N-TiO_2 photocatalysts has been explored, using the mussels' extrapallial fluid as a doping source for titania to be used as a photocatalyst for microplastic degradation. No photolytic deterioration of the MPs was observed in the reaction conditions utilized in this study, but photocatalytic degradation of primary HDPE MPs extracted from a commercial facial scrub was demonstrated. The result was evidenced by mass loss determination, degradation rate calculation, and microscope observations, among others [66]. In addition, after photocatalytic experiments, it was found that at pH = 3, hydrogen atoms were accessible as H^+ ions. Interestingly, increasing the concentration of H^+ enhanced the amount of hydroperoxy radical ($^{\bullet}OOH$), justifying the promoting degradation of the pollutant at pH 3. Photolysis at pH 3 does not result in plastic degradation due to the absence of hydroperoxides. The pH affects not just plastic breakdown but also the surface charge of TiO_2 particles (which possess a Point of Zero Charge (PZC) of ca. 6) and hence the electrostatic attraction of microplastics to the surface of the semiconductor. At pH 3, colloidal nanoparticles of titania showed a stronger contact with MPs, leading to a faster breakdown. The degradation of HDPE MPs at low temperatures (pH 3 and 0 °C) can be explained based on the photocatalytic system's specific properties. Microplastics, as extracted, and possessing sizes 240–725 times larger than those treated in the presence of C,N-TiO_2, make the adsorption on the semiconductor surface impossible, unlike in other photocatalytic systems with more frequent pollutants; consequently, this makes its degradation difficult because the photocatalytic process is efficient only on the surface of the photocatalyst.

The removal of nanoplastics utilizing three distinct TiO_2-based photocatalysts was examined to obtain fresh insights into the removal of polystyrene primary nanoplastics from aqueous solutions using UV light. The results were discussed by examining the turbidity of the suspensions. The use of the various TiO_2 architectures resulted in substantial deterioration of the target organic polymer [67]. The most effective structure gave optimal transfer and separation of the photogenerated charge carriers, as well as the most efficient polystyrene photodegradation.

According to Asghar et al. during the photodegradation, the polyethylene coated with TiO_2 forming the composite film (PE-TiO_2 film) achieves a more efficient degradation rate compared to pure PE film under UV and artificial light irradiation [68]. The presence of oxidant species such as peroxydisulfate ($S_2O_8^{2-}$) in the presence of TiO_2 enhances the photocatalytic degradation of the plastic [69]. Similarly, the polystyrene (PS) TiO_2 composite photodegradation process was faster than that of the photolysis of pure polymer samples. During this photodegradation, there is no dioxin or other component released. Bandara et al. have compared TiO_2 and ZrO_2 suspensions for PE and PP photocatalytic degradation under natural or simulated solar irradiation, concluding that ZrO_2 showed higher degradation than TiO_2 at the same experimental conditions [70].

ZnO has also been used in organic polymer photocatalytic degradation due to its suitable optical properties, excellent redox ability, great electron mobility, and non-toxicity. Tofa et al. prepared ZnO via spray pyrolysis that was used for the photocatalytic degradation of a specimen plate of low-density polyethylene (LDPE) film sized 1 cm^2. The experiment was carried out for 175 h in a Petri dish containing the photocatalyst and deionized water. The results reveal that heterogeneous photocatalysis enhances the formation of carbonyl and vinyl groups, thus indicating the degradation of the polymeric film [71]. As a result, the photocatalytic degradation of the polymer gave rise to its oxidation, producing low-molecular-weight molecules and leading to brittleness, wrinkles, cracks, and cavities on the LDPE surface. Additionally, increasing catalyst surface area improves polymer breakdown. The use of Pt enhances more than 15% of the degradation of the plastic under visible light due to plasmon absorption and also by lowering the electron–hole recombination on ZnO [72]. Authors claim that superoxides and hydroxyl radicals formed during photocatalysis are the oxidant species responsible for plastic degradation. Uheida et al. presented a sustainable and green solution approach to eliminate microplastics using visible light by trapping low-density particles of plastics like polypropylene (PP) on glass fiber substrates, while also supporting the photocatalyst material [73]. This study shows that visible light irradiation of zinc oxide nanorods (ZnO NRs) mounted on glass fiber substrates can degrade PP microplastics floating in water in a flow-through system. Irradiating PP microplastics with visible light for two weeks resulted in a 65% reduction in average particle volume.

Other semiconductors such as Cu_xO have been also developed via anodization for analogous scope. The anodization procedure gave rise to Cu_2O/CuO semiconductors with varying morphologies and a bandgap of 1.6 to 2 eV [74]. Results revealed that photocatalysis using visible light irradiation was able to obtain the polymer chain scission up to 23%, six times more than the degradation achieved by photolysis. In addition, a mineralization of up to 15% was accomplished. BiOCl has been also used for the degradation of polystyrene nanoplastics by preparing polystyrene-based nano-composites with flower- and disk-shaped BiOCl nanoparticles. The photocatalytic degradation of the films under visible irradiation was tested by mechanical, morphological, and optical properties. The deterioration of the films was remarkable [75]. $NiAl_2O_4$ prepared via co-precipitation and hydrothermal methodologies was used for the degradation of commercially available polyethylene (PE) bags by photocatalysis [76]. The results obtained from FTIR analysis carried out after the degradation process in the presence of the spinel confirmed that the polyethylene sheet was degraded in 5 h showing a weight loss of ca. 12%. The degradation of a low-density polyethylene (LDPE) film was studied by using Au nanoparticles as a photocatalyst. The photoinduced degradation of the LDPE@Au nanocomposite film was higher than that of the pure LDPE film. The weight loss of LDPE@Au with 1 wt% of Au reached ca. 52% after 240 h of solar light irradiation, compared with the 9% photodegradation of the polymer in the absence of Au. The solid maintains its activity even after five consecutive cycles of photocatalytic runs [77].

Photocatalytic degradation of plastic materials can be performed in an integrated process in which contemporaneously to the oxidation of polymers dispersed in water also hydrogen is formed. The next paragraph will discuss this interesting novel approach by considering polypropylene as the polymer to be degraded. It is worth noting that, however, the number of scientific reports in this field is increasing, there are currently still few publications dedicated to this topic, and, in particular, those reporting the use of PP as the substrate to be oxidized simultaneously with the generation of hydrogen.

3. Polypropylene (PP) Waste as Source of Green Hydrogen in Photoreforming

Plastic recycling has been handled in three ways: depolymerization, partial oxidation, or cracking. Depolymerization via reversible synthesis reactions (i.e., alcoholysis, glycolysis, and hydrolysis) works well for polyamides and polyesters (e.g., nylons and polyethylene terephthalate (PET)), but requires harsh conditions as high temperature and pressure [78]; nonetheless, it is ineffective for polypropylene, and, consequently, the oxidative vias in coordination with the obtaining of H_2 in the same process seems particularly appealing.

Hydrogen production by photocatalysis in the presence of light is a versatile and environmentally benign manner to obtain energy. Photoreforming (see Figure 9) is the reaction able to transform an organic, which can be a waste, into a valuable chemical and at the same time to obtain clean H_2 fuel [79]. Hydrogen can be produced at room temperature and atmospheric pressure by a simple, efficient, low-cost, and sustainable process, with the use of a heterogeneous photocatalyst using a waste material that can be biomass or plastic, light, and water [80]. Photoreforming involves the splitting of water to generate H_2 by a reduction reaction and the simultaneous oxidation of an organic species to obtain other molecules with higher added value or, simply, to completely oxidize (mineralize) organics to CO_2 and H_2O.

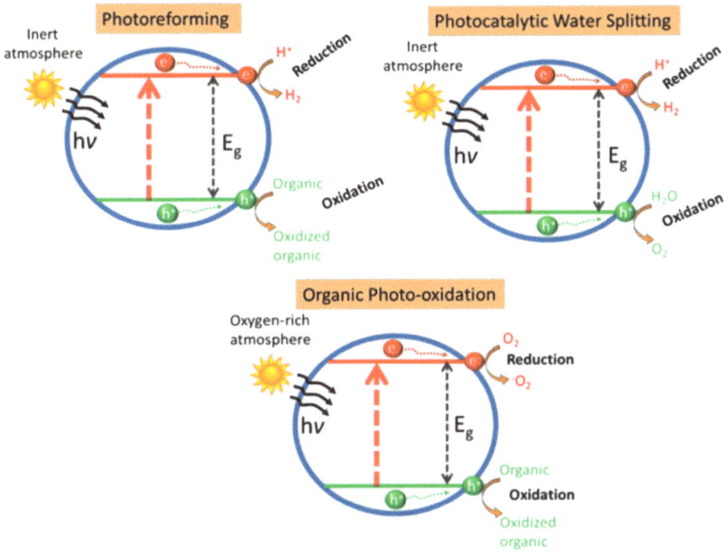

Figure 9. Mechanism of the photoreforming reaction along with the photocatalytic water splitting and the oxidation of an organic molecule in the presence of oxygen; from [81].

As we have mentioned before, PP possesses C-C bonds in its backbone and it is susceptible to light-induced oxidative degradation, which is the most effective abiotic degradation route of plastic in outdoor environments [82] involving a radical mechanism. The initiatory degradation step, in which light leads to cleavage of the chemical bonds in the backbone chain of the polymer, is favored by the presence in the chain of unsaturated chromophore groups that can absorb light giving rise to the formation of free radicals [83]. Unfortunately, this mechanism cannot be applied to all synthetic polymers as most of them, like PP, do not possess chromophores capable of absorbing UV light. Consequently, in the case of PP, which does not present unsaturated chromophores or double bonds it is more difficult to generate free radicals [84]. However, in the case of photoreforming, which must be considered as a photocatalytic process there is always the formation of radical species like $^{\bullet}OH$, $O_2^{\bullet -}$ (see Section 2.1.4) that are capable of initiating the degradation of the polymer chain as already discussed in Sections 2.1.1 and 2.1.3 (see also Figures 6–8). PP has tertiary carbon atoms while PE has secondary carbon atoms; for this reason, PP has lower stability, which makes it more susceptible to abiotic attacks. However, regarding the mechanism of degradation, it is quite similar for PP and PE, leading to low-molecular-weight fragments. In addition to the decrease in molecular weight, new functional groups such as carbonyl groups are formed, which leads to products, including pentene, 2-methyl-1-pentene, and 2,4-dimethyl-1-heptene. Plastics containing a C-C bond in the main structure can be used as hole scavengers in the process of photoreforming, giving rise to oxidized products, possibly into fine chemicals with the concomitant formation of H_2 gas by the reduction of H_2O at room temperature. This reaction has been reported to occur with some semiconductor oxides [85].

Recently, Liang et al. have reviewed the new results on the conversion of plastic into fuels, fine chemicals, and materials [86], concluding that the photocatalytic processes are more environmentally friendly and sustainable than thermo-catalysis under harsh conditions. These technologies for plastic upcycling are still in their early stages and there is still a huge space to improve the efficiency for practical production and real applications. Particularly, very limited work has been devoted to the upcycling of plastics in photoreforming reactions. The literature is very limited in this area and it is in great augment.

Polyethylene terephthalate was used as a hole scavenger in photoreforming using SiC-g-C_3N_4 composites as photocatalysts. The presence of the heterojunction produced by small amounts of g-C_3N_4 on the surface of SiC enhances the separation of the photoproduced electron and holes and yields H_2 with a rate of 18 μmol per gram of catalysts and hour of reaction. The polymer oxidation gave intermediates such as ethylene glycol, which further enhanced the photoreforming effectiveness. It is worth noting the strong basicity of the suspension (pH = 13) that was essential to pre-treat the polymer and that favors the interaction between the reactants and the surface of the heterogeneous photocatalyst [87].

Xu et al. have treated plastic PE bags, PP boxes, and PET bottles, which were mineralized to CO and H_2, i.e., syngas, in the presence of H_2O by the Co-Ga_2O_3 nanosheets. The H_2 and CO formation rates were approx. 648 and 158 μmol g^{-1} h^{-1} ca. double the amount of that obtained with bare Ga_2O_3. The weight losses of PE bags, PP boxes, and PET bottles were ca. 81, 78, and 72% after 48 h irradiation in the presence of Co-Ga_2O_3 [88]. Cao et al. have developed an effective photoreforming process in which the H_2 production was combined with PET microplastic degradation in the presence of MXene/$Zn_xCd_{1-x}S$ [89]. The highest photocatalytic H_2 evolution rate reached 14 mmol $g^{-1}\cdot h^{-1}$ in alkaline polymer solution. PET was transformed into glycolate, acetate, and ethanol. C_3N_4 was also tested for alkaline PET solution degradation giving rise to a H_2 evolution rate of 600 mmol g^{-1} h^{-1} [90]. A Z-scheme heterostructure of V-substituted phosphomolybdic acid and C_3N_4 has also been tested in the upcycling of various plastics. The optimal composite exhibits a remarkable formic acid production rate of 55 μmol $g^{-1}\cdot h^{-1}$ for the upcycling of polyethylene, which is 262-fold higher than that of pristine C_3N_4 [91]. In a slightly different approach, Jiao et al. propose the selective conversion of waste plastics, such as polyethylene, polypropylene, and PVC, in the presence of Nb_2O_5. Polyethylene was photodegraded completely into CO_2, which was then photoreduced into acetic acid [92].

4. Conclusions

Inefficient disposal of plastic materials represents a serious environmental problem; therefore, scientific studies regarding possible strategies dedicated to their treatments can contribute to mitigating the pollution linked to the uncontrolled release of these materials into the environment. The slow kinetics of the natural degradation of polymers and in particular of the most used ones, such as polypropylene (PP), makes it necessary to use advanced oxidation processes, which are technologies capable of offering a strategy for the treatment of this type of waste. Through these processes, various organic pollutants and recalcitrant chemicals are effectively removed from both water and wastewater. Processes such as ozonation, catalysis in the presence of UV radiation, hydrogen peroxide, and/or heterogeneous photocatalytic processes generate intermediates that can act on the degradation of polymers and implement their introduction in a circular economy framework. This mini-review provides an overview of the strategies that can be implemented in this framework. Emerging aspects for the treatment of these recalcitrant pollutants are examined with particular attention to the degradation of polypropylene, chosen as an example of a material widely present in the environment as a recalcitrant pollutant when dispersed in soil or water. In fact, the presence of micro and nanoplastics is well known as a serious cause of threat to human health and the environment. The mini-review describes economical and efficient methods for polymer degradation. The chemical recycling of polypropylene (PP) can be addressed through its depolymerization to obtain polymers with a lower molecular weight that may be suitable for returning to the original material preparation cycle or which could be used as fuels to support the process itself. This overview gives an account of the results obtained by applying these technologies and studying the different operating parameters.

Funding: This research received no external funding.

Institutional Review Board Statement: Not applicable.

Informed Consent Statement: Not applicable.

Data Availability Statement: No new data were created.

Conflicts of Interest: The authors declare no conflicts of interest.

References

1. Jambeck, J.R.; Geyer, R.; Wilcox, C.; Siegler, T.R.; Perryman, M.; Andrady, A.; Narayan, R.; Law, K.L. Plastic waste inputs from land into the ocean. *Science* **2015**, *347*, 768–771. [CrossRef] [PubMed]
2. Zalasiewicz, J.; Waters, C.N.; Ivar do Sul, J.; Corcoran, P.L.; Barnosky, A.D.; Cearreta, A.; Edgeworth, M.; Gałuszka, A.; Jeandel, C.; Leinfelder, R.; et al. The geological cycle of plasticsand their use as a stratigraphic indicator of the Anthropocene. *Anthropocene* **2016**, *13*, 4–17. [CrossRef]
3. Barnes, D.K.A.; Galgani, F.; Thompson, R.C.; Barlaz, M. Accumulation and fragmentation of plastic debris in global environments. *Philos. Trans. R. Soc. B* **2009**, *364*, 1985–1998. [CrossRef] [PubMed]
4. Ellen MacArthur Foundation. The New Plastics Economy: Rethinking the Future of Plastics & Catalysing Action. 2017. Available online: https://www.ellenmacarthurfoundation.org/the-new-plastics-economy-rethinking-the-future-of-plastics-and-catalysing (accessed on 7 June 2024).
5. Lesli, O.M.; Melissa, C.C.; Ive, H. The Use of Heterogeneous Catalysis in the Chemical Valorization of Plastic Waste. *ChemSusChem* **2020**, *13*, 5808–5836.
6. Yu, M.; Annette von, J.; Alexandre, Y. Current Technologies in Depolymerization Process and the Road Ahead. *Polymers* **2021**, *13*, 449. [CrossRef] [PubMed]
7. Plastics Europe. Plastics Europe–Annual Review 2017–2018. 2018. Available online: https://www.plasticseurope.org/en/resources/publications/498-plasticseurope-annual-review-2017-2018 (accessed on 7 June 2024).
8. Geyer, R.; Jambeck, J.R.; Law, K.L. Production, use, and fate of all plastics ever made. *Sci. Adv.* **2017**, *3*, 1700782. [CrossRef] [PubMed]
9. Padervand, M.; Lichtfouse, E.; Robert, D.; Wang, C. Removal of microplastics from the environment. A review. *Environ. Chem. Lett.* **2000**, *18*, 807–828. [CrossRef]
10. Galgani, F.; Hanke, G.; Werner, S.; De Vrees, L. Marine litter within the European marine strategy framework directive. *ICES J. Mar. Sci.* **2013**, *70*, 1055–1064. [CrossRef]
11. Au, S.Y.; Bruce, T.F.; Bridges, W.C.; Klaine, S.J. Responses of Hyalella azteca to acute and chronic microplastic exposures. *Environ. Toxicol. Chem.* **2015**, *34*, 2564–2572. [CrossRef]
12. Schiavo, S.; Oliviero, M.; Chiavarini, S.; Dumontet, S.; Manzo, S. Polyethylene, Polystyrene, and Polypropylene leachate impact upon marine microalgae Dunaiella tertiolecta. *J. Toxicol. Environ. Health A* **2021**, *84*, 249–260. [CrossRef]
13. Danso, I.K.; Woo, J.H.; Lee, K. Pulmonary Toxicity of Polystyrene, Polypropylene, and Polyvinyl Chloride Microplastics in Mice. *Molecules* **2022**, *27*, 7926. [CrossRef] [PubMed]
14. Li, C.; Kong, X.Y.; Lyu, M.; Tay, X.T.; Đokić, M.; Chin, K.F.; Yang, C.T.; Lee, E.K.X.; Zhang, J.; Tham, C.Y.; et al. Upcycling of non-biodegradable plastics by base metal photocatalysis. *Chem* **2023**, *9*, 2683–2700. [CrossRef]
15. Wróbel, M.; Szymańska, S.; Kowalkowski, T.; Hrynkiewicz, K. Selection of microorganisms capable of polyethylene (PE) and polypropylene (PP) degradation. *Microbiol. Res.* **2023**, *267*, 127251. [CrossRef] [PubMed]
16. Ru, J.; Huo, Y.; Yang, Y. Microbial degradation and valorization of plastic wastes. *Front. Microbiol.* **2020**, *11*, 442. [CrossRef] [PubMed]
17. Rana, A.K.; Thakur, M.K.; Saini, A.K.; Mokhta, S.K.; Moradi, O.; Rydzkowski, T.; Alsanie, W.F.; Wang, O.; Grammatikos, S.; Thakur, V.K. Recent developments in microbial degradation of polypropylene: Integrated approaches towards a sustainable environment. *Sci. Total Environ.* **2022**, *826*, 154056. [CrossRef] [PubMed]
18. Weber, R.; Watson, A.; Forter, M.; Oliaei, F. Persistent organic pollutants and landfills—A review of past experiences and future challenges. *Waste Manag. Res.* **2011**, *29*, 107–121. [CrossRef]
19. Allen, N.S.; Edge, M. *Fundamentals of Polymer Degradation and Stabilization*; Elsevier Applied Science: London, UK, 1992; Chapter 4.
20. Guo, X.; Wang, J. The chemical behaviors of microplastics in marine environment: A review. *Mar. Pollut. Bull.* **2019**, *142*, 1–14. [CrossRef] [PubMed]

21. Desai, V.; Shenoy, M.A.; Gogate, P.R. Ultrasonic degradation of low-density polyethylene. *Chem. Eng. Process. Process Intensif.* **2008**, *47*, 1451–1455. [CrossRef]
22. Hinsken, H.; Moss, S.; Pauquet, J.R.; Zweifel, H. Degradation of polyolefins during melt processing. *Polym. Degrad. Stab.* **1991**, *34*, 279–293. [CrossRef]
23. Eagan, J.M.; Xu, J.; Di Girolamo, R.; Thumber, C.M.; Macosko, C.W.; Lapointe, A.M.; Bates, F.S.; Coates, G.W. Combining polyethylene and polypropylene: Enhanced performance with PE/iPP multiblock polymers. *Science* **2017**, *355*, 814–816. [CrossRef]
24. García, J.M.; Robertson, M.L. The future of plastics recycling. *Science* **2017**, *358*, 870–872. [CrossRef] [PubMed]
25. Layman, J.M.; Gunnerson, M.; Bond, E.B.; Schonemann, H.; Williams, K. Reclaimed Polypropylene Composition. U.S. Patent WO/2017/003800 A1, 5 January 2017.
26. Layman, J.M.; Collias, D.I.; Gunnerson, M.; Schonemann, H.; Williams, K. Method for Purifying Reclaimed Polymers. U.S. Patent Application 2018/0171096 A1, 5 November 2019.
27. Coates, G.W.; Getzler, Y.D.Y.L. Chemical recycling to monomer for an ideal, circular polymer economy. *Nat. Rev. Mater.* **2020**, *5*, 501–516. [CrossRef]
28. Kumar, A.P.; Depan, D.; Tomer, N.S.; Singh, R.P. Nanoscale particles for polymer degradation and stabilization—Trends and future perspectives. *Prog. Polym. Sci.* **2009**, *34*, 479–515. [CrossRef]
29. Scheirs, J.; Kaminsky, W. *Feedstock Recycling and Pyrolysis of Waste Plastics*; John Wiley & Sons Ltd.: Hoboken, NJ, USA, 2006; pp. 709–728.
30. Sharma, B.K.; Moser, B.R.; Vermillion, K.E.; Doll, K.M.; Rajagopalan, N. Production, characterization and fuel properties of alternative diesel fuel from pyrolysis of waste plastic grocery bags. *Fuel Process. Technol.* **2014**, *122*, 79–90. [CrossRef]
31. Kraft, S.; Vogel, F. Estimation of binary diffusion coefficients in supercritical water: Mini review. *Ind. Eng. Chem. Res.* **2017**, *56*, 4847–4855. [CrossRef]
32. Chen, W.T.; Jin, K.; Wang, N.H.L. Use of supercritical water for the liquefaction of polypropylene into oil. *ACS Sustain. Chem. Eng.* **2019**, *7*, 3749–3758. [CrossRef]
33. Duan, J.J.; Li, Y.; Gao, J.N.; Cao, R.Z.; Shang, E.X.; Zhang, W. ROS-mediated photoaging pathways of nano- and micro-plastic particles under UV irradiation. *Water Res.* **2022**, *216*, 118320. [CrossRef] [PubMed]
34. Oturan, M.A.; Aaron, J.J. Advanced Oxidation Processes in Water/Wastewater Treatment: Principles and Applications. A Review. *Crit. Rev. Environ. Sci. Technol.* **2014**, *44*, 2577–2641. [CrossRef]
35. Andrady, A.L. Microplastics in the marine environment. *Mar. Pollut. Bull.* **2011**, *62*, 1596–1605. [CrossRef]
36. Hu, K.; Tian, W.; Yang, Y.; Nie, G.; Zhou, P.; Wang, Y.; Duan, X.; Wang, S. Microplastics remediation in aqueous systems: Strategies and technologies. *Water Res.* **2021**, *198*, 117144. [CrossRef]
37. Ali, S.S.; Elsamahy, T.; Koutra, E.; Kornaros, M.; El-Sheekh, M.; Abdelkarima, E.A.; Zhu, D.; Sun, J. Degradation of conventional plastic wastes in the environment: A review on current status of knowledge and future perspectives of disposal. *Sci. Total Environ.* **2021**, *771*, 144719. [CrossRef] [PubMed]
38. Gijsman, P.; Meijers, G.; Vitarelli, G. Comparison of the UV-degradation chemistry of polypropylene, polyethylene, polyamide 6 and polybutylene terephthalate. *Polym. Degrad. Stab.* **1999**, *65*, 433–441. [CrossRef]
39. Scott, G. *Degradable Polymers Principles and Applications*; Springer: Dordrecht, The Netherlands, 2002.
40. Singh, B.; Sharma, N. Mechanistic implications of plastic degradation. *Polym. Degrad. Stab.* **2008**, *93*, 561–584. [CrossRef]
41. Tolinski, M. *Additives for Polyolefins Getting the Most out of Polypropylene, Polyethylene and TPO*; William Andrew Pub.: Oxford, UK, 2009.
42. Peacock, A.J. *Handbook of Polyethylene: Structures, Properties and Applications*; Marcel Dekker: New York, NY, USA, 2000.
43. Albertsson, A.C.; Karlsson, S. The three stages in degradation of polymers-polyethylene as a model substance. *J. Appl. Polym. Sci.* **1988**, *35*, 1289–1302. [CrossRef]
44. Shyichuk, A.V.; Stavychna, D.Y.; White, J.R. Effect of tensile stress on chain scission and crosslinking during photo-oxidation of polypropylene. *Polym. Degrad. Stab.* **2001**, *72*, 279–285. [CrossRef]
45. Gewert, B.; Plassmann, M.M.; MacLeod, M. Pathways for degradation of plastic polymers floating in the marine environment. *Environ. Sci. Process. Impacts* **2015**, *17*, 1513–1521. [CrossRef] [PubMed]
46. Bertin, D.; Leblanc, M.; Marque, S.R.A.; Siri, D. Polypropylene degradation: Theoretical and experimental investigations. *Polym. Degrad. Stab.* **2010**, *95*, 782–791. [CrossRef]
47. Su, K.; Liu, H.; Gao, Z.; Fornasiero, P.; Wang, F. Nb_2O_5-Based Photocatalysts. *Adv. Sci.* **2021**, *8*, 2003156. [CrossRef] [PubMed]
48. Litter, M.I.; Slodowicz, M. An overview on heterogeneous Fenton and photo-Fenton reactions using zerovalent iron materials. *J. Adv. Oxid. Technol.* **2017**, *20*, 20160164. [CrossRef]
49. González-García, J.; Sáez, V.; Tudela, I.; Díez-Garcia, M.I.; Esclapez, M.D.; Louisnard, O. Sonochemical Treatment of Water Polluted by Chlorinated Organocompounds: A Review. *Water* **2010**, *2*, 28–74. [CrossRef]
50. Pokhrel, N.; Vabbina, P.K.; Pala, N. Sonochemistry: Science and Engineering. *Ultrason. Sonochem.* **2016**, *29*, 104–128. [CrossRef]
51. Chatel, G. How sonochemistry contributes to green chemistry? *Ultrason. Sonochem.* **2018**, *40*, 117–122. [CrossRef] [PubMed]
52. Gogate, P.R.; Prajapat, A.L. Depolymerization using sonochemical reactors: A critical review. *Ultrason. Sonochem.* **2015**, *27*, 480–494. [CrossRef] [PubMed]
53. Ashokkumar, M.; Hodnett, M.; Zeqiri, B.; Grieser, F.; Price, G.J. Acoustic emission spectra from 515 kHz cavitation in aqueous solutions containing surfaceactive solutes. *J. Am. Chem. Soc.* **2007**, *129*, 2250–2258. [CrossRef]

54. Hernández-Fernández, J.; Pérez-Mendoza, J.; Ortega-Toro, R. Quantification of Irgafos P-168 and Degradative Profile in Samples of a Polypropylene/Polyethylene Composite Using Microwave, Ultrasound and Soxhlet Extraction Techniques. *J. Compos. Sci.* **2024**, *8*, 156. [CrossRef]
55. Desai, V.; Shenoy, M.A.; Gogate, P.R. Degradation of polypropylene using ultrasound-induced acoustic cavitation. *Chem. Eng. J.* **2008**, *140*, 483–487. [CrossRef]
56. Chakraborty, J.; Sarkar, J.; Kumar, R.; Madras, G. Ultrasonic degradation of polybutadiene and isotactic polypropylene. *Polym. Degrad. Stab.* **2004**, *85*, 555–558. [CrossRef]
57. Price, G.J.; White, A.J.; Andrew Clifton, A. The effect of high-intensity ultrasound on solid polymers. *Polymer* **1995**, *36*, 4919–4925. [CrossRef]
58. Gugumus, F. Novel role for tropospheric ozone in initiation of auto-oxidation. *Polym. Degrad. Stab.* **1998**, *62*, 403–406. [CrossRef]
59. Meijers, G.; Gijsman, P. Influence of environmental concentrations of ozone on thermo-oxidative degradation of PP. *Polym. Degrad. Stab.* **2001**, *74*, 387–391. [CrossRef]
60. He, G.J.; Zheng, T.T.; Ke, D.M.; Cao, X.H.; Yin, X.C.; Xu, B.P. Impact of rapid ozone degradation on the structure and properties of polypropylene using a reactive extrusion process. *RSC Adv.* **2015**, *5*, 44115–44120. [CrossRef]
61. Kim, S.; Sin, A.; Nam, H.; Park, Y.; Lee, Y.; Han, C. Advanced oxidation processes for microplastics degradation: A recent trend. *Chem. Eng. J. Adv.* **2022**, *9*, 100213. [CrossRef]
62. Chu, S.; Zhang, B.; Zhao, X.; Soo, H.S.; Wang, F.; Xiao, R.; Zhang, H. Photocatalytic Conversion of Plastic Waste: From Photodegradation to Photosynthesis. *Adv. Energy Mater.* **2022**, *12*, 2200435. [CrossRef]
63. García-López, E.I.; Palmisano, L. *Materials Science in Photocatalysis*, 1st ed.; Elsevier: Amsterdam, The Netherland, 2021.
64. Allen, N.S.; McKellar, J.F.; Phillips, G.O.; Wood, D.G.M. Effect of titanium dioxide pigments on the phosphorescence from polyolefins. *Polym. J. Sci. Polym. Lett.* **1974**, *12*, 241–245. [CrossRef]
65. Ouyang, Z.; Yang, Y.; Zhang, C.; Zhu, S.; Qin, L.; Wang, W.; He, D.; Zhou, Y.; Luo, H.; Qin, F. Recent advances in photocatalytic degradation of plastics and plastic-derived chemicals. *J. Mater. Chem. A* **2021**, *9*, 13402–13441. [CrossRef]
66. Ariza-Tarazona, M.C.; Villarreal-Chiu, J.F.; Hernández-López, J.M.; Rivera De la Rosa, J.; Barbieri, V.; Siligardi, C.; Cedillo-González, E.I. Microplastic pollution reduction by a carbon and nitrogen-doped TiO_2: Effect of pH and temperature in the photocatalytic degradation process. *J. Hazard. Mater.* **2020**, *395*, 122632. [CrossRef]
67. Domínguez-Jaimes, L.P.; Cedillo-González, E.I.; Luévano-Hipólito, E.; Acuña-Bedoya, J.D.; Hernández-López, J.M. Degradation of primary nanoplastics by photocatalysis using different anodized TiO_2 structures. *J. Hazard. Mater.* **2021**, *413*, 125452. [CrossRef]
68. Asghar, W.; Qazi, I.A.; Ilyas, H.; Khan, A.A.; Awan, M.A.; Aslam, M.R. Comparative solid phase photocatalytic degradation of polythene films with doped and undoped TiO. *J. Nanomater.* **2011**, *8*, 461930.
69. Phonsy, P.D.; Yesodharan, S.; Yesodharan, E.P. Enhancement of semiconductor mediated photocatalytic removal of polyethylene plastic wastes from the environment by oxidizers. *Res. J. Recent Sci.* **2015**, *4*, 105–112.
70. Bandara, W.R.L.N.; de Silva, R.M.; de Silva, K.M.N.; Dahanayake, D.; Gunasekar, S.; Thanabalasingam, K. Is nano ZrO_2 a better photocatalyst than nano TiO_2 for degradation of plastics? *RSC Adv.* **2017**, *7*, 46155–46163. [CrossRef]
71. Tofa, T.S.; Kunjali, K.L.; Paul, S.; Dutta, J. Visible light photocatalytic degradation of microplastic residues with zinc oxide nanorods. *Environ. Chem. Lett.* **2019**, *17*, 1341–1346. [CrossRef]
72. Tofa, T.S.; Ye, F.; Kunjali, K.L.; Dutta, J. Enhanced Visible Light Photodegradation of Microplastic Fragments with Plasmonic Platinum/Zinc Oxide Nanorod Photocatalysts. *Catalysts* **2019**, *9*, 819. [CrossRef]
73. Uheida, A.; Giraldo Mejía, H.; Abdel-Rehim, M.; Hamd, W.; Dutta, J. Visible light photocatalytic degradation of polypropylene microplastics in a continuous water flow system. *J. Hazard. Mater.* **2021**, *406*, 124299. [CrossRef] [PubMed]
74. Acuña-Bedoya, J.D.; Luévano-Hipólito, E.; Cedillo-González, E.I.; Patricia Domínguez-Jaimes, L.P.; Martínez Hurtado, a.; Hernández-López, J.M. Boosting visible-light photocatalytic degradation of polystyrene nanoplastics with immobilized Cu_xO obtained by anodization. *J. Environ. Chem. Eng.* **2021**, *9*, 106208. [CrossRef]
75. Sarwan, B.; Acharya, A.D.; Kaur, S.; Pare, B. Visible light photocatalytic deterioration of polystyrene plastic using supported BiOCl nanoflower and nanodisk. *Eur. Polym. J.* **2020**, *134*, 109793. [CrossRef]
76. Venkataramana, C.; Botsa, S.M.; Shyamala, P.; Muralikrishna, R. Photocatalytic degradation of polyethylene plastics by $NiAl_2O_4$ spinels-synthesis and characterization. *Chemosphere* **2021**, *265*, 129021. [CrossRef] [PubMed]
77. Olajire, A.A.; Mohammed, A.A. Bio-directed synthesis of gold nanoparticles using Ananas comosus aqueous leaf extract and their photocatalytic activity for LDPE degradation. *Adv. Powder Technol.* **2021**, *32*, 600–610. [CrossRef]
78. Panda, A.K.; Singh, R.K.; Mishra, D.K. Thermolysis of waste plastics to liquid fuel: A suitable method for plastic waste management and manufacture of value added products-A world prospective. *Renew. Sustain. Energy Rev.* **2010**, *14*, 233–248. [CrossRef]
79. García-López, E.I.; Palmisano, L.; Marcì, G. Overview on Photoreforming of Biomass Aqueous Solutions to Generate H_2 in the Presence of g-C_3N_4-Based Materials. *ChemEngineering* **2023**, *7*, 11. [CrossRef]
80. Ashraf, M.; Ullah, N.; Khan, I.; Tremel, W.; Ahmad, S.; Tahir, M.N. Photoreforming of Waste Polymers for Sustainable Hydrogen Fuel and Chemicals Feedstock: Waste to Energy. *Chem. Rev.* **2023**, *123*, 4443–4509. [CrossRef]
81. Samage, A.; Gupta, P.; Halakarni, M.A.; Nataraj, S.K.; Sinhamahapatra, A. Progress in the Photoreforming of Carboxylic Acids for Hydrogen Production. *Photochemistry* **2022**, *2*, 580–608. [CrossRef]

82. Canopoli, L.; Coulon, F.; Wagland, S.T. Degradation of Excavated Polyethylene and Polypropylene Waste from Landfill. *Sci. Total Environ.* **2020**, *698*, 134125. [CrossRef] [PubMed]
83. Allen, N.S. Photoinitiators for UV and visible curing of coatings: Mechanisms and properties. *J. Photochem. Photobiol. A* **1996**, *100*, 101–107. [CrossRef]
84. Calvert, P.D. *Polymer Degradation and Stabilization*; John Wiley & Sons, Ltd.: Hoboken, NJ, USA, 1986; Volume 18, p. 278.
85. Qi, M.Y.; Conte, M.; Anpo, M.; Tang, Z.R.; Xu, Y.J. Cooperative Coupling of Oxidative Organic Synthesis and Hydrogen Production over Semiconductor-Based Photocatalysts. *Chem. Rev.* **2021**, *121*, 13051–13085. [CrossRef] [PubMed]
86. Liang, X.; Li, X.; Dong, O.; Gao, T.; Cao, M.; Zhao, K.; Lichtfouse, E.; Otavio, A.; Patrocinio, T.; Wang, C. Photo- and electrochemical processes to convert plastic waste into fuels and high-value chemicals. *Chem. Eng. J.* **2024**, *482*, 148827. [CrossRef]
87. Armeli Iapichino, M.T.; Fiorenza, R.; Patamia, V.; Floresta, G.; Gulino, A.; Condorelli, M.; Impellizzeri, G.; Compagnini, G.; Sciré, S. H_2 production by solar photoreforming of plastic materials using SiC-g-C_3N_4 composites. *Catal. Commun.* **2024**, *187*, 106850.
88. Xu, J.; Jiao, X.; Zheng, K.; Shao, W.; Zhu, S.; Li, X.; Zhu, J.; Pan, Y.; Sun, Y.; Xie, Y. Plastics-to-syngas photocatalysed by Co–Ga_2O_3 nanosheets. *Natl. Sci. Rev.* **2022**, *9*, nwac011.
89. Cao, B.; Wan, S.; Wang, Y.; Guo, H.; Ou, M.; Zhong, Q. Highly-efficient visible-light-driven photocatalytic H_2 evolution integrated with microplastic degradation over MXene/$Zn_xCd_{1-x}S$ photocatalyst. *J. Colloid Interface Sci.* **2022**, *605*, 311–319. [CrossRef] [PubMed]
90. Liu, X.; Yang, Y.; Wan, S.; Li, S.; Ou, M.; Song, F.; Fan, X.; Zhong, Q. Tuning the surface hydrophilicity of a C_3N_4 nanosheet for efficient photocatalytic H_2 evolution coupled with microplastic degradation. *Int. J. Hydrogen Energy* **2023**, *48*, 27599–27610. [CrossRef]
91. Xing, C.; Yu, G.; Zhou, J.; Liu, Q.; Chen, T.; Liu, H.; Li, X. Solar energy-driven upcycling of plastic waste on direct Z-scheme heterostructure of V-substituted phosphomolybdic acid/g-C_3N_4 nanosheets. *Appl. Catal. B-Environ.* **2022**, *315*, 121496. [CrossRef]
92. Jiao, X.; Zheng, K.; Chen, Q.; Li, X.; Li, Y.; Shao, W.; Xu, J.; Zhu, J.; Pan, Y.; Sun, Y. Photocatalytic Conversion of Waste Plastics into C2 Fuels under Simulated Natural Environment Conditions. *Angew. Chem. Int. Ed.* **2020**, *59*, 15497–15501. [CrossRef] [PubMed]

molecules

MDPI

Article

Graphene Quantum Dots from Agricultural Wastes: Green Synthesis and Advanced Applications for Energy Storage

Pierfrancesco Atanasio [1], Rubia Y. S. Zampiva [1], Luca Buccini [1], Corrado Di Conzo [2], Anacleto Proietti [1], Francesco Mura [1,3], Annalisa Aurora [4], Andrea G. Marrani [5], Daniele Passeri [1,3], Marco Rossi [1,3], Mauro Pasquali [1,3] and Francesca A. Scaramuzzo [1,*]

[1] Department of Basic and Applied Sciences for Engineering (SBAI), Sapienza University of Rome, Via A. Scarpa 14, 00161 Rome, Italy; pierfrancesco.atanasio@uniroma1.it (P.A.); rubia.zampiva@uniroma1.it (R.Y.S.Z.); luca.buccini@uniroma1.it (L.B.); anacleto.proietti@uniroma1.it (A.P.); francesco.mura@uniroma1.it (F.M.); daniele.passeri@uniroma1.it (D.P.); marco.rossi@uniroma1.it (M.R.); mauro.pasquali@uniroma1.it (M.P.)

[2] Department of Applied Science and Technology (DISAT), Polytechnic of Turin, Corso Castelfilardo 39, 10129 Torino, Italy; corrado.diconzo@polito.it

[3] Research Centre for Nanotechnology Applied to Engineering, Sapienza University of Rome (CNIS), Piazzale A. Moro 5, 00185 Rome, Italy

[4] Department of Energy Technologies and Renewable Sources C.R. ENEA Casaccia, Via Anguillarese 301, 00123 Rome, Italy; annalisa.aurora@enea.it

[5] Department of Chemistry, Sapienza University of Rome, Piazzale A. Moro 5, 00185 Rome, Italy; andrea.marrani@uniroma1.it

* Correspondence: francesca.scaramuzzo@uniroma1.it

Abstract: Carbon nanostructures are highly promising materials for applications in a variety of different fields. Besides their interesting performances, the possibility to synthesize them from biowaste makes them an eco-friendly resource widely exploitable within a circular economy context. The present work deals with the green, one-pot synthesis of graphene quantum dots (GQDs) from carbon aerogels (CAs) derived from rice husk (RH). After having obtained CAs upon purification of RH, followed by gelification and carbonization of the resulting cellulose, the one-pot solventless production of GQDs was obtained by ball milling. This method determined the formation of crystalline nanostructures with a diameter of around 20 nm, which were analyzed via scanning electron microscopy, transmission electron microscopy, atomic force microscopy, X-ray diffraction, and Raman spectroscopy to obtain a full morphological and structural characterization. GQDs were used as electrode materials for supercapacitors and Li-ion batteries, showing the ability to both accumulate charges over the surface and intercalate lithium-ions. The reported results are a proof of principle of the possibility of exploiting GQDs as support material for the development of advanced systems for energy storage.

Keywords: graphene quantum dots; rice husk; supercapacitors; Li-ion batteries; nanomaterials; energy storage; waste-to-energy

Citation: Atanasio, P.; Zampiva, R.Y.S.; Buccini, L.; Di Conzo, C.; Proietti, A.; Mura, F.; Aurora, A.; Marrani, A.G.; Passeri, D.; Rossi, M.; et al. Graphene Quantum Dots from Agricultural Wastes: Green Synthesis and Advanced Applications for Energy Storage. *Molecules* **2024**, *29*, 5666. https://doi.org/10.3390/molecules29235666

Academic Editors: Fabio Ganazzoli and Giuseppina Raffaini

Received: 31 August 2024
Revised: 8 November 2024
Accepted: 15 November 2024
Published: 29 November 2024

1. Introduction

Carbon nanomaterials derived from biowaste are being extensively explored as eco-friendly resources in the pursuit of sustainable technological advancements [1]. Together with industrial waste [2], biowaste often serves as a source to produce graphitic structures, following the principles of circular economy and waste valorization [3]. Among the biowaste sources, rice husk (RH) has garnered significant research interest in both academic and industrial contexts due to its abundant availability at minimal cost and its substantial potential for conversion into high-quality graphene [4,5]. Studies involving RH have shown a significant increase since 2020 and continue to rise, with no indication of a slowdown [5].

Current rice production worldwide is estimated to be 515.83 million metric tons (milled basis) [6,7]. RH is a by-product of the rice milling process, accounting for 20 wt% to 33 wt% of dried rough rice. Between 30 wt% to 50 wt% of the RH composition is organic carbon [8,9]. With the ongoing focus on the environment, the random disposal and open burning of RH have been drastically reduced, and various alternative uses for this biowaste are being developed. RH can be found as a heavy metal adsorbent, an insulator in refractory brick and steel industries, and a filler in pigments, rubber, cement, and concrete [9,10]. It is also utilized in the electronic industries, solar grade, and energy fields [11].

On the energy storage field, the most popular commercially available systems are Li-ion batteries, characterized by robustness and safety. Depending on the application, the cathode can be made of oxides or salts like $LiCoO_2$ or $LiFePO_4$, while graphite is generally used as material for the anode [12]. However, the rapid development of electronic tools creates a continuous need for increasingly high-performance energy storage devices. Consequently, research on new electrode materials is currently among the hot topics in the field [13–16]. Moreover, lithium is a critical raw material, and it is consequently necessary to go beyond lithium technology, exploring the possibility of using different systems like lithium–sulfur batteries, Na-ion batteries, and supercapacitors [17–19].

Supercapacitors have gained attention in the scientific community due to their high-power density, long cycle life, outstanding cycling stability, and low cost [20]. However, the broad utilization of these devices has been challenging because of their relatively low energy density. Currently, multiple research groups are working on producing high-energy-density supercapacitors by either improving specific capacitance or increasing the voltage window [21,22]. Therefore, the type and nature of electrode materials have a critical impact on the electrochemical properties of supercapacitors [23].

One promising approach to producing electrodes for supercapacitors is the utilization of the organic carbon content present in RH. As indicated in the literature, various graphitic structures can be derived from RH biomass [5,24], including carbon-based materials classified as zero-dimensional (0D), such as graphene quantum dots (GQDs). GQDs are formed by highly crystalline and few-atom-thick graphene with sp2-hybridized carbon and dimensions under 100 nm. The thickness of the GQD structure is close to the single atom [25]. Therefore, unique properties deriving from strong quantum confinement and edge effects of quantum dots are expected. GQDs present photoluminescence, high conductivity, chemical inertness, excellent stability, and low toxicity. These dots contain energy band gaps and delocalized charge carriers within their nanoscale structure. There are also plenty of edge sites for functionalization, resulting in additional properties with a high specific surface area and excellent ionic transporting ability [26–28]. Current research on these structures involves both top-down and bottom-up synthesis approaches and the applications can range across a wide set of topics like sensors, solar cells, bio imaging, catalysis, and optoelectronic devices [29–31].

Considering the abovementioned GQDs' properties, it is reasonable to expect them to be highly functional as supercapacitor electrode material with elevated capacitance and stability. Furthermore, as for the supercapacitors, those properties make GQDs interesting for application as electrodes in various electrochemical devices [32,33].

Based on the presented information, this study proposes the utilization of RH as a precursor for synthesizing high-purity GQDs and their application in energy storage. The literature outlines various routes for the production of GQDs from biomass in general [34,35] and specifically from RH [10,36,37]. However, these methods typically involve rigorous chemical treatments and often more than one passage at high temperature. The processing of RH includes a step in which amorphous carbon is obtained through a purification process that removes silicon and other impurities inherent to the natural material, and the resulting carbonaceous material typically undergoes a second step, which frequently involves additional elevated temperatures and chemical treatments to produce GQDs [4].

With a focus on eco-sustainability, a top-down synthesis route based on two simple steps for producing high-purity GQDs by recycling RH is presented in this paper. The first step consists of the formation of a carbon aerogel (CA) after cellulose purification and gelification. The second step involves a mechanical-energy-based process, during which the obtained CA is subjected to ball milling, resulting in the production of GQDs with an approximate size of 20 nm. This approach utilizes a recyclable source and employs a green synthesis passage, ensuring that product quality remains uncompromised. Ball milling further proved to be a non-toxic, pollution-free technique which can be extended to a wide variety of starting matrices to obtain nanostructured materials.

To investigate the potential of the obtained GQDs in electrochemical devices, and given the well-known importance of obtaining a complete morphological and structural characterization to fully exploit the potential of materials for energy applications [38,39], the nanostructures were analyzed by different techniques, e.g., scanning electron microscopy (SEM), atomic force microscopy (AFM), transmission electron microscopy (TEM), X-ray diffraction (XRD), Raman spectroscopy, Fourier transform infrared spectroscopy (FTIR), X-ray photoelectron spectroscopy (XPS), and thermal gravimetric analysis (TGA). Finally, as a proof of principle, the synthesized 0D materials were used as carbonaceous electrodes for supercapacitors and lithium-ion batteries. Despite GQDs being more often coupled with a second active material component, the shown physico-chemical properties and morphology suggest that GQDs produced via the proposed method could demonstrate superior performance compared to those reported in the literature for single-component GQD electrodes. The production of high-quality single-component GQD electrodes enables the optimization of a starting material, which can still subsequently be treated or combined with various solutions to achieve maximum performance.

2. Results

2.1. GQD Characterization

The CAs obtained from RH and used as precursors for the synthesis of GQDs were characterized by carbonized cellulose in the shape of interconnected networks of both fibers and thin platelets, whose typical SEM appearance is shown in Figure 1.

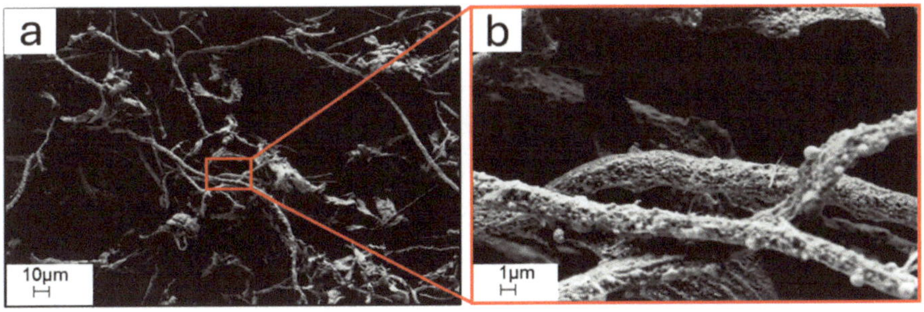

Figure 1. (**a**) SEM micrography 1k× magnification of starting CAs; (**b**) corresponding 10k× magnification of the area selected in red.

Upon the facile one-step synthesis of GQDs, i.e., ball milling of CAs, about a 10% increase in sample mass was observed. Since the synthesis step occurs in the air, such an increase is probably due to a reaction with environmental oxygen induced by the high-energy impacts of the ball milling spheres against the carbonaceous substrate. Such a process may be considered responsible for the formation of oxygen-rich groups along the particles' surfaces. This hypothesis is supported by SEM-EDX data acquired on bulk aggregate powder, which gave information about the qualitative and quantitative elemental composition of GQDs. Upon comparison with the starting CAs, reported in Figure 2, the change in morphology is coupled with an increase in the oxygen percentage, rising from an average of 2.5% up to more than 15%.

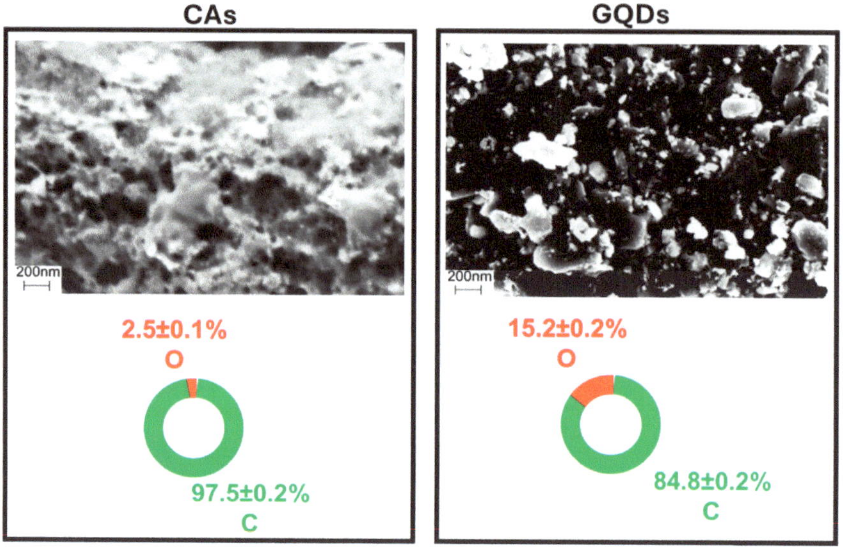

Figure 2. SEM-EDX of starting CAs and GCDs in bulk aggregate powder, pointing out the morphological and compositional differences in terms of carbon and oxygen between precursor and final product.

Besides as a bulk aggregate powder, GQDs were also observed using SEM-EDX upon dispersion over a silicon wafer substrate after suspension in water, to properly observe single nanoparticles and to accurately determine their diameter distribution. As observable in Figure 3, GQDs appear to have an irregular almost circular shape, while an average diameter of 27 ± 9 nm was estimated for them by ImageJ software.

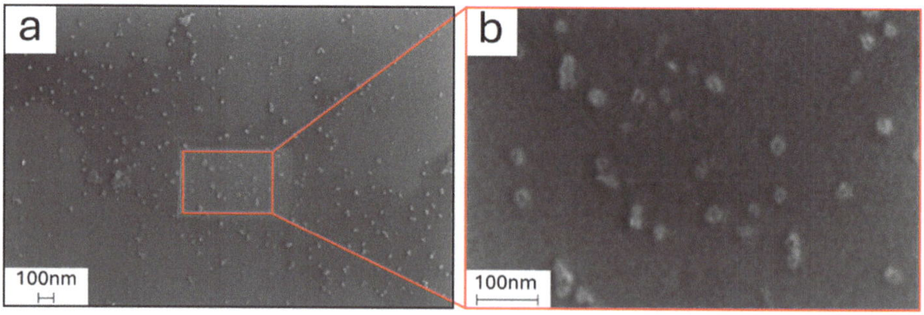

Figure 3. (**a**) SEM micrographs of graphene quantum dots dispersed on a silicon wafer after dilution in water at 100k× magnification and (**b**) 400k× magnification.

The morphology and dimension of graphene quantum dots were also investigated using atomic force microscopy. The typical topography and phase-recorded images of the diluted sample dispersed on a Si wafer are shown in Figure 4. In good agreement with SEM, the AFM of dispersed graphene quantum dots confirms the irregular shape of the nanostructures, with an average diameter estimated using ImageJ to be around 30 ± 6 nm. According to a *t*-test performed on the two sets of data collected with SEM and AFM, the estimated average diameters are statistically identical; however, the slightly higher values obtained by AFM are reasonable, considering the tip-sample convolution due to the interaction during the scan.

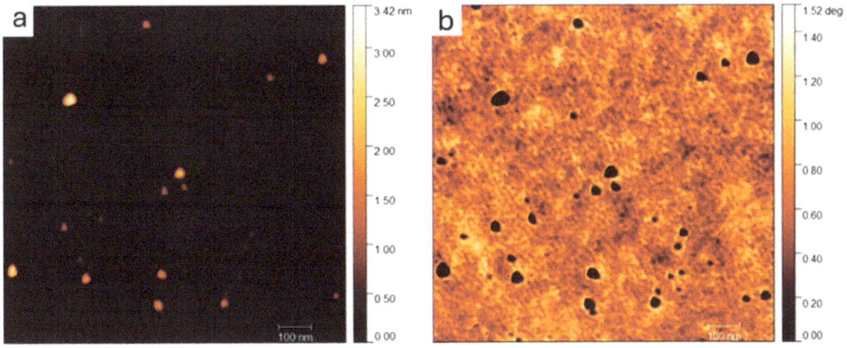

Figure 4. (**a**) Typical topography and (**b**) phase 1 µm × 1 µm AFM images of GQDs deposited on Si wafer from a diluted suspension in water.

To further validate the identification of the observed sample as GQDs and obtain additional information about their morphology and crystallinity, HRTEM measurements were performed on a highly diluted suspension (1:106). As observable in Figure 5, HRTEM shows nanostructures with irregular circular shapes and visible crystalline planes (insert b). Based on HRTEM data, an average diameter of 22 ± 1 nm was calculated for the dots. This value is slightly lower than the values obtained with SEM and AFM analysis but is still in good agreement with them. This is reasonable, considering the abovementioned tip-sample convolution for AFM and the low sensibility of SEM at high magnification, which causes a blur in the imaging, while HRTEM is certainly a more accurate technique for particularly small carbon-based samples. By observing the crystalline plane distance, an average interplanar distance of 3.3 ± 0.2 Å was estimated, which is in good agreement with values in the literature for graphene plane distances in graphite (3.35 Å) [40,41]. However, despite being visible, the crystalline planes seem to show occasional interruptions and spots (i.e., the alternation of white and black lines that show the sample crystallinity is not totally regular), which could indicate some residual disorder and irregularities in the crystalline structure.

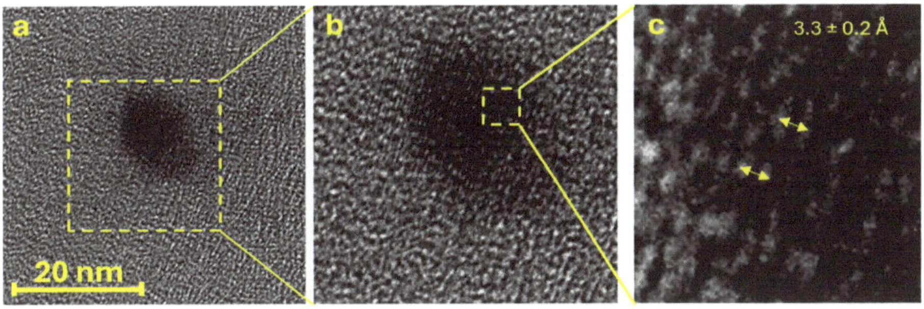

Figure 5. (**a**) HRTEM image of a GQD, (**b**) magnification on its crystalline planes, and (**c**) magnification on the interplanar distance among crystalline planes.

Aiming to more precisely evaluate sample crystallinity and amorphous content and collect structural information concerning both long- and short-range order, XRD and Raman spectroscopy were utilized. The obtained results were compared to the starting material (i.e., carbon aerogel) to evaluate modification during synthesis. According to XRD diffractograms shown in Figure 6, while the starting CAs showed no clear long-range order or structure, it is possible to observe a sharp peak at 26.57° in 2Θ, assigned to the (002) signal of graphite due to the repetition and stacking of graphene sheets. Such a clear change indicates that during ball milling, the impact between the powder and spheres not only promotes the formation of external oxygen-rich functional groups, but also induces crystallization of the resulting GQDs; therefore, the final material has a consistently higher crystalline structure compared to CAs. Moreover, by using Bragg's equation, it is possible to convert the 2Θ value of the peak in the interplanar distance, obtaining the value of 3.35 Å, which is exactly the reported interplanar distance in graphite and further validates the crystallinity and interplanar distance distribution observed by HRTEM. Despite having a higher crystallinity degree than CAs, GQD powder still shows a strong amorphous signal between 18° and 28°, thus indicating the presence of a disordered fraction in samples. Finally, the Scherrer analysis was applied to GQD diffractogram to estimate the average dimension of the crystalline grains according to the equation:

$$L = \frac{K\lambda}{FWHM\ \cos(\Theta)} \quad (1)$$

where L is the crystalline grain dimension, K is the shape coefficient (0.94 for spherical particles), λ is the wavelength of the copper radiation (1.54 Å), FWHM is the full width at half maximum of the main (002) in radiant, and Θ is the position of the peak. According to this calculation, the average size of the crystallites is around 18.1 nm. It is worth noting that the Scherrer equation has already been successfully used for graphene fragments [42], and our result is comparable to the value already reported in the literature for similar GQDs [43].

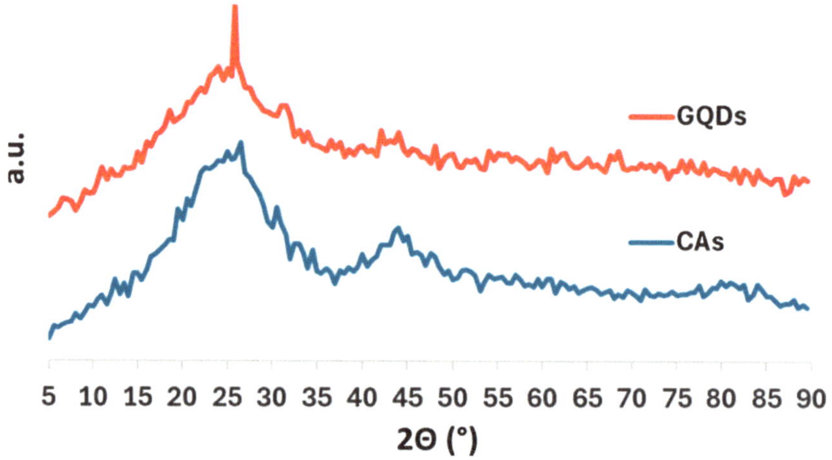

Figure 6. Diffractograms of starting carbon aerogels (red line) and graphene quantum dots (blue line).

The Raman spectra of starting CAs and obtained GQDs are reported in Figure 7. Both samples show the typical spectra of carbonaceous graphitic materials. However, there are differences in the band widths and both the D- and G-bands of starting CAs appear significantly broader, thus indicating a lower degree of disorder within graphene quantum dots compared to their precursor [44]. The position of the bands has been investigated with a four Gaussian fitting using Breit–Wigner–Fano lines [45]: according to the fitting, D- and G-band positions are, respectively, 1333 and 1587 cm^{-1} in GQDs, and 1307 and 1564 cm^{-1} in CAs (see Supplementary Information, Figures S1 and S2). Furthermore, the ratio between the intensity of the D-band and the G-band (i.e., I_D/I_G) decreases from 1.09 for CAs to 1.04 for GQDs. Based on the higher Raman shift in GQDs of G-band and its lower I_D/I_G around 1, the three-stage model [46] suggests a negligible percentage of sp^3 bonds and a more graphitic structure of GQDs, thus confirming the increase in crystallinity suggested by peak broadness, even though the hysteresis of the amorphization curve could potentially underestimate the percentage of sp^3 bonds in CAs.

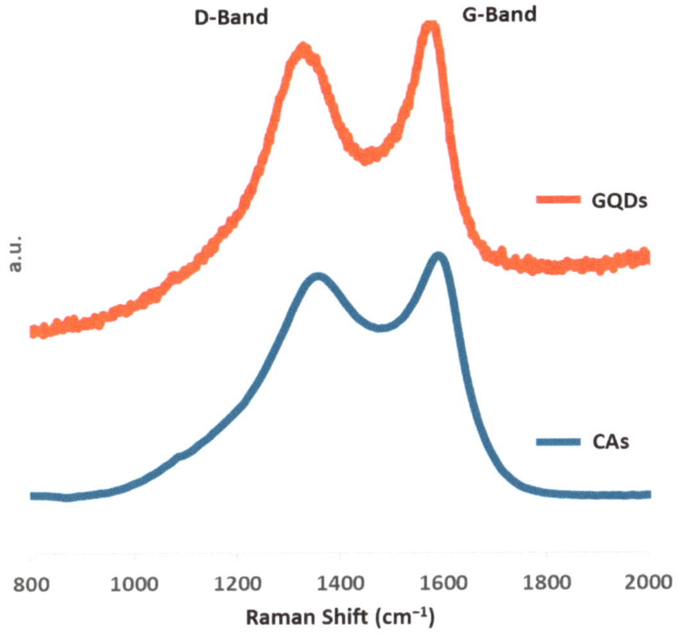

Figure 7. Raman spectra of starting CAs (blue line) and GQDs (red line).

The comparison of XRD and Raman data suggests that both samples shared the same short-range order. The phase transition during the reaction, i.e., the crystallization of GQDs into a more ordered graphite with a long-range order, seems to be still incomplete, leaving defects and irregularities among the graphene layers. The latter experimental evidence might confirm the irregularities and disordered spots shown in the crystalline planes observed in HRTEM imaging.

The samples' surfaces were also examined by FTIR spectroscopy (Figure 8). The spectra demonstrate an evident increase in oxygenated functional groups on the GQDs compared to the CA surface. This result is in accordance with the oxygen increase observed by EDX. Bands attributed to the C=O of carboxylic acid and carbonyl groups are shown at ~1753 and 645 cm^{-1} [47], while the bands at ~1263 and 1102 cm^{-1} belong to the stretching of C–O–C bonds [48] and C–OH vibrations [49], respectively. The band around 826 cm^{-1} is associated with the symmetric and asymmetric vibration modes of C–H groups [50]. C-H and C=O bands are also present in the CA spectrum, but with less intensity when compared to GQDs. Furthermore, a band at ~1640 cm^{-1} is also observed for both samples, with higher intensity in the GQD spectrum. This band can be associated with C=C stretching and indicates the formation of new sp^2–hybridized (graphitic) carbon bonds [48,49] for the ball-milled sample, in agreement with the results found by XRD and Raman spectroscopy. Both spectra present a similar band at 2360 cm^{-1} caused by CO_2 from the air [51].

XPS measurements were run on both CA and GQD samples in order to ascertain their chemical composition and the possible presence of oxygenated functional groups within the carbon atom network. XPS reported in Figure 9 shows the C 1s ionization region for both samples with the corresponding curve fitting results. In both cases, a common line shape can be identified, with a predominant peak at low binding energy (BE), followed by a series of weak contributions from various oxygenated functional groups. The lowest energy peak is located at 284.0 eV (red curves in Figure 9) and displays a moderate asymmetric tail towards high BEs. According to these features, this contribution can be assigned to C=C bonds within a network of conjugated π bonds, as those typical of graphitic materials [52–55]. The next contribution at 284.7 eV (blue curves) can be assigned to aliphatic defective sp^3 C atoms [56], whereas the higher BE peaks are representative of C atoms bound to oxygen, such as C–OH (hydroxyl, 286.2 eV, green curves), C=O (carbonyl, 288.0 eV, gray curves), and COOH (carboxyl, 288.8 eV, magenta curves) [54,55,57–59]. An additional broad and weak signal can also be detected around 290 eV, attributable to a π-π* shake-up satellite typical of π-conjugated systems.

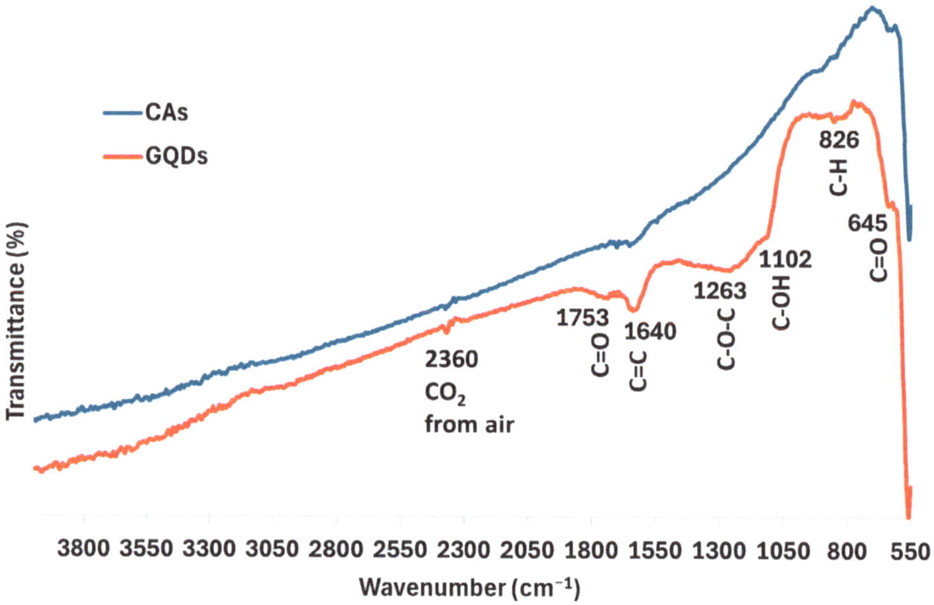

Figure 8. ATR-FTIR spectroscopy of the samples CAs (blue line) and GQDs (red line).

Despite having a common sequence of chemical contributions to the spectrum, the two samples displayed slightly different intensities in the oxygenated carbon atoms portion of the spectrum, with the GQD sample being more oxygen-rich than the CA sample, especially in the C-OH and COOH groups. The area of the peaks resulting from the curve fitting of the C 1s region allowed us to extract an atomic O/C ratio ($R_{O/C}$) through Equation (4) [52] (see Experimental), which resulted in 0.16 for CAs and 0.24 for GQDs. The higher amount of oxygenated functional groups in GQDs is in line with the SEM-EDX and FTIR findings, and can be traced back to a probable oxidation of the sample surface during the ball milling process.

TGA (Figure 10) shows that both samples have a slight weight loss due to adsorbed water before 100 °C (about 2.0% for CAs and 8.9% for GQDs) and a single decomposition step over 400 °C with a consistent weight loss. The CA curve shows a decomposition weight loss at the extrapolated onset temperature of 543.1 °C, which corresponds to a DTA exothermic peak with a maximum at 580.2 °C. GQD samples are more thermally unstable, and the weight loss starts slightly from 200 °C if compared with the CA curve. This phenomenon is associated with the increase of labile oxygen-containing functional groups in GQDs during the ball milling process [60]. For GQDs, the decomposition occurs at the onset temperature of 494.6 °C, and the corresponding DTA exothermic peak shows its maximum at 457 °C. The exothermic decomposition peaks for both samples are assigned to the combustion of the carbon skeleton of graphene oxide [60,61].

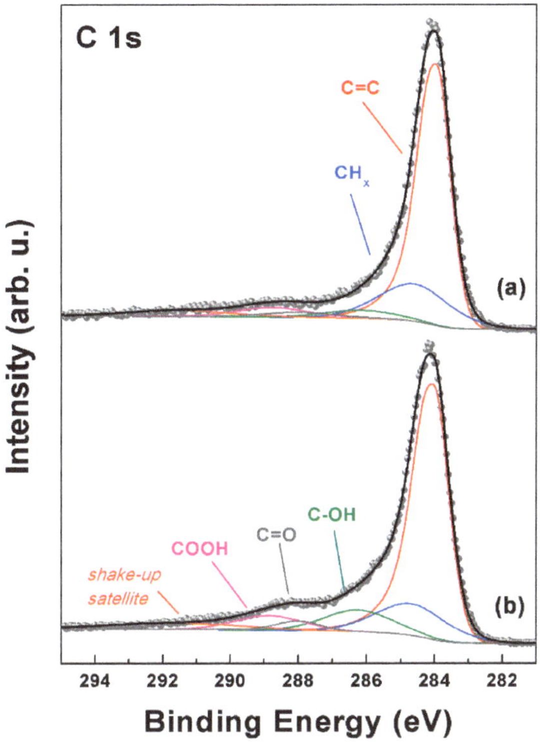

Figure 9. XPS C 1s ionization region of (**a**) CA and (**b**) GQD samples. Raw data are displayed with dots, while the curve fitting reconstruction is represented by continuous colored lines.

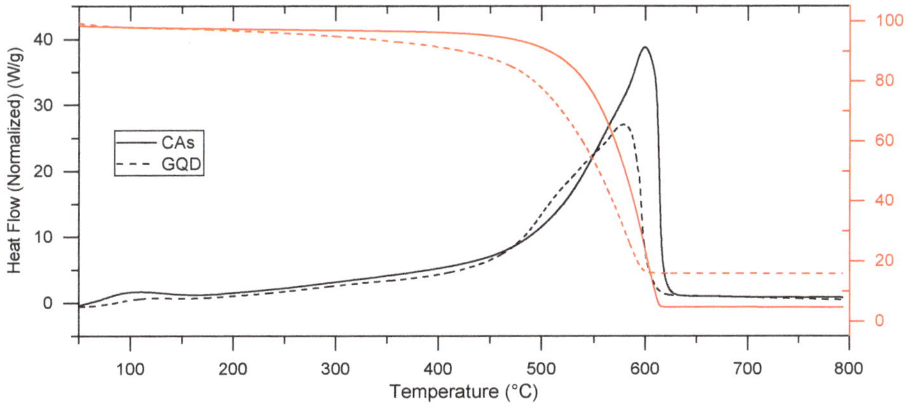

Figure 10. TGA-DTA curves of CAs (solid line) and GQDs (dashed line) carried out in technical air.

At 800 °C, the residue is 4.6% of the initial weight for CAs and 16.5% for GQDs. According to the above-presented chemical analysis, only carbon, oxygen, and hydrogen are present in the samples, and in this way, the remaining mass is attributed to graphitic carbon [61]. Those values indicate an increase of almost 28% in ordered graphitic carbon after the ball milling process.

2.2. GQD-Based Electrode Materials for Energy Storage

Graphene quantum dots have been studied as active material components in both supercapacitors and in lithium-ion devices in order to investigate the potential of 0D graphitic materials for electrochemical devices.

Cyclic voltammetry at different scan rates for symmetrical GQD electrode supercapacitors is shown in Figure 11a. At low scan rate values, the curves show a quasi-rectangular shape with no visible peak typical of supercapacitors, which seems almost lost at a high scan rate. In any case, the curves are symmetrical to the horizontal axis, and this can indicate a good reversibility of the charge accumulation. The absence of visible peaks indicates the absence of faradic reactions or side processes due to the functionalization of the surface during GQD synthesis, and the process appears totally capacitive with no transformations occurring in the device. Capacitance has been evaluated for different scan rates by CV using Equation (2):

$$C = \frac{\int IdV}{\varepsilon mV} \quad (2)$$

where C is the specific capacitance, I is the current, V is the potential window, m is the mass of the active material in the electrode, and ε is the scan rate.

Results are shown in Figure 11b, where the range of values goes from 10 Fg^{-1} at 50 mVs^{-1} to around 53 Fg^{-1} at 1 mVs^{-1}, with the material decreasing in capacitance when forced to work under more stressful conditions.

Galvanostatic cyclations were also performed: the trend of potential during the first cycle of discharge and charge at 0.1 Ag^{-1} is shown in Figure 11c. A quasi-triangular shape is maintained and confirms the absence of faradic reactions already proved during cyclic voltammetry. However, at the beginning of the charging process, there is a potential jump of almost 0.2 V, after which the potential increase is rather linear. This indicates a consistent irreversible loss of capacitance which could in principle hinder the device's life after many cycles.

In this case, the capacitance is calculated by using Equation (3):

$$C = \frac{I\Delta t}{mV} \quad (3)$$

where C is the specific capacitance, I is the constant discharging current density, Δt is the discharging time, m is the mass of active material in the electrode, and ΔV is the potential window in the galvanostatic discharge curves. Capacitance has also been observed at different currents applied and it can be seen in Figure 11d that performance is not hindered by higher currents applied.

The capacitance trend over the charge/discharge galvanostatic cycle, i.e., the supercapacitor life cycle of a device with a GQD-based electrode cycling at 0.1 Ag^{-1} current density, is reported for a thousand cycles in Figure 11e. From this plot, the effect of the abovementioned irreversible capacitance loss is clearly visible: after outstanding values in the first cycle (over 100 Fg^{-1}), capacitance fades until it reaches a stable trend in the range between the 50th and the 200th cycles around 55 Fg^{-1}. Moreover, a second fast decrease in capacitance occurs, and after 1000 cycles, the sample reaches a performance of around 5.2 Fg^{-1}. Although it is clear that our GQDs, as tested under experimental settings, are not suitable for commercial applications, the results obtained in galvanostatic cyclations are definitely comparable, and even superior, to those reported in the literature for single-component GQD electrodes with a similar average particle size [62]. Çolak et al. [62], using a bottom-up synthesized material from citric acid, only obtained a capacitance of 32.08 Fg^{-1} at 0.1 Ag^{-1} with an electrode made using only carbon dots as the active material. Similarly, and both using a top-down synthesis, Dharmalingam et al. [63] only obtained a maximum capacitance of around 30.5 Fg^{-1} at 0.1 Ag^{-1}, while Baslak et al. [64], using biomass (*Stachys euadenia*), managed to obtain carbon quantum dots of similar sizes compared to us (18–22 nm), but their performance in symmetric capacitors using KOH 6

M in cyclic voltammetry is significantly lower than our material (around 2 Fg^{-1}), with no crystalline order of the particles. A schematic comparison is reported in Table 1.

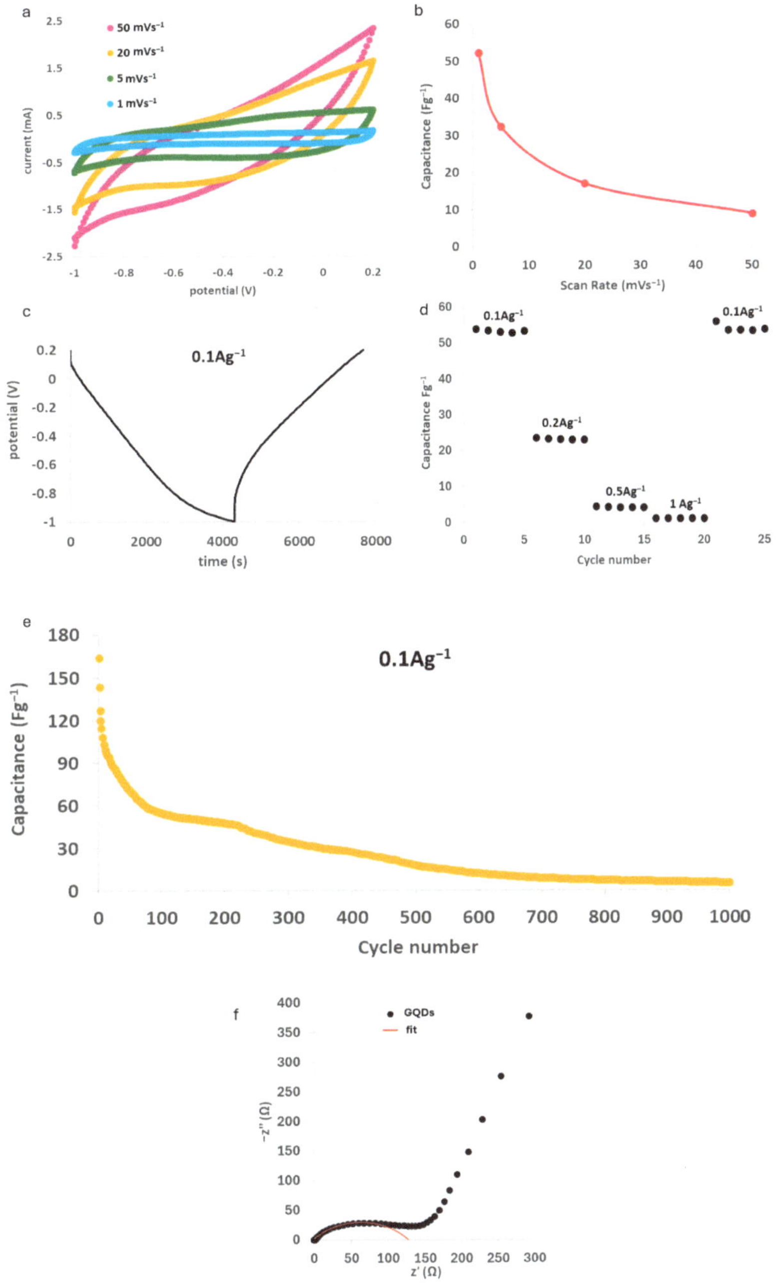

Figure 11. Electrochemical performance of GQDs in supercapacitors: (**a**) cyclic voltammetry at different scan rates; (**b**) capacitance evaluated by CV; (**c**) potential profile in time in galvanostatic cyclations; (**d**) capacitance values calculated at different currents; (**e**) device life; and (**f**) electrochemical impedance spectroscopy showing GQD behavior (black dots) and fitting curve (red line).

Table 1. Comparison of the material from the present work with the literature-reported electrodes made of 0D nano-dimensional carbon structures.

Materials	Capacitance [Fg^{-1}]	Authors
GQDS	55	Present work
CD	19.00	Ref. [62]
CD bis-16	17.64	Ref. [62]
CD bis-64	32.08	Ref. [62]
CDs	30.5	Ref. [63]
CQDs	2.12	Ref. [64]

It is worth noting that higher capacitance values reported in the literature for similar materials refer to systems in which the GQDs are coupled with other active carbonaceous components, e.g., carbon nanotubes or graphene oxide or even metallic compounds, giving rise to functional hybrid materials with enhanced performances. Therefore, the reported preliminary analysis demonstrates that the present system shows ample room for improvement, especially if coupled with other active materials. An example is in the work of Ji-Shi et al. [65], where various morphologies of composite material with $NiCo_2O_4$ were successfully prepared and stable capacitance above 800 Fg^{-1} were achieved even at currents above those examined in this paper.

Moreover, to further investigate the electrochemical behavior of GQDs, EIS analysis was applied and resistances around 0.6 Ω and 128.5 Ω were calculated by the fitting showed in Figure 11f.

GQDs were also tested in lithium-ion batteries to evaluate the efficacy of lithiation inside a 0D material with a high specific surface. GQDs alone typically do not exhibit high performance as anode materials due to the significant contact resistance between GQDs and their mismatch in volume concerning lithium intercalation [66].

Galvanostatic cyclations were performed at C/10 (assuming the material being comparable to graphite): the trend of potential in the first, second, fifth, and tenth cycles are shown in Figure 12a and performances at different currents are shown in Figure 12b. As can be noted, the first cycle is much longer than the others, likely due to the SEI formation occurring on the anode surface, and its discharging curve has a distinctly different shape in comparison to all the other cycles. More specifically, the decrease in potential at the beginning of the first cycle is less sharp than the decrease observed in the following cycles, in which the potential quickly fades around 1.5 V. SEI formation, however, still happens between 1.5 V and 1 V; therefore, we can conclude that there is a constant SEI formation during device operation. Considering their shape, the curves actually seem to indicate that different phenomena occur during the discharge, i.e., a first reaction below 1.5 V compatible with persistent SEI formation that decreases over cycling but never disappears, and a second reaction below 1 V compatible with lithiation of the small graphitic domain of graphene quantum dots. A possible explanation for this behavior could be a loss in cohesion of the active material and poor adhesion to the electrode. Despite having included a binder inside the electrode powder, GQDs apparently tend to detach from the rest of the material, thus exposing the underlying surface. This could lead to the irreversible formation of SEI even after the first cycle, which causes electrolyte consumption and a decrease in active surface, thus resulting in a continuous loss of capacity. The abovementioned considerations and experimental evidence have a direct effect on device life (Figure 12c). Even though the coulombic efficiency remains nearly constant at around 100%, the starting capacity, slightly below 120 $mAhg^{-1}$, instantly drops at 100 $mAhg^{-1}$. In the following cycles, the capacity fades linearly till around the 70th cycle, when the loss decreases: around the 100th cycle, the capacity tends to reach a plateau below 40 $mAhg^{-1}$, with a retention of 38.6%. The obtained results are of course far from the capacity value of graphite, which is currently the golden standard for commercial applications. However, as already mentioned for supercapacitors, similar GQDs are rarely used as such: in the literature, remarkable results have so far only been reported for boron- or nitrogen-doped GQDs, or for GQDs combined with other active materials in hybrid systems [66]. Consequently, the present results should be considered as a starting point to evaluate the potential of the GQDs we propose. Their capability of intercalating lithium-ions should actually be considered an excellent starting point for their exploitation as electrode material, upon improvement of its adhesion to the current collector and the coupling with a second active component.

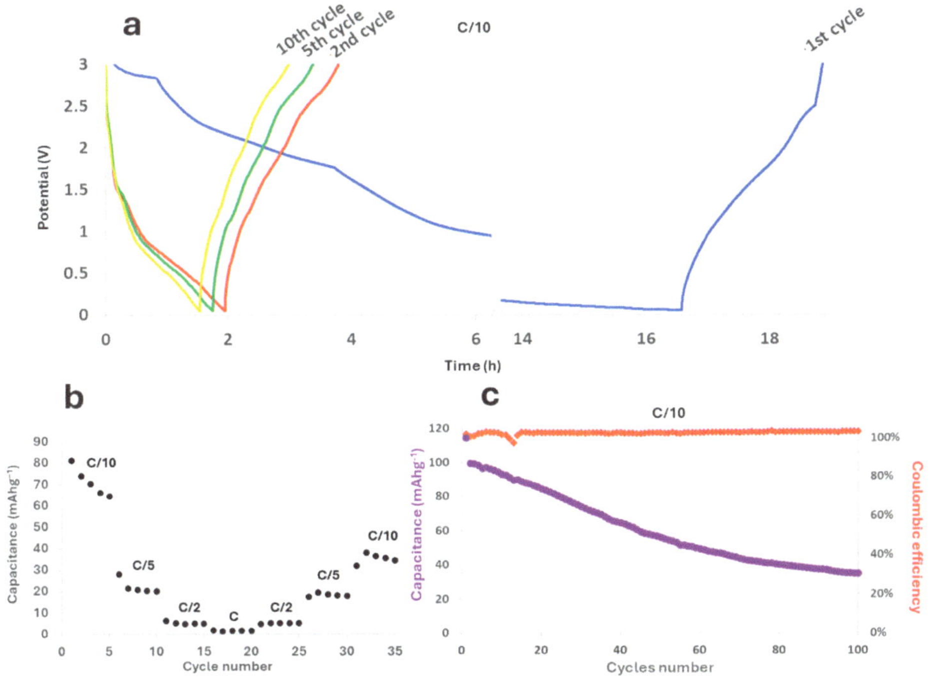

Figure 12. Electrochemical performance of GQDs as lithium-ions battery anodes: (**a**) potential profile in time in galvanostatic cyclations for cycles 1, 2, 5, and 10 at C/10; (**b**) capacitance calculated at different currents at C/10, C/5, C/2, C, and then back to C/10; (**c**) device life and coulombic efficiency.

In order to prove this statement, both post-mortem SEM analysis and electronic impedance spectroscopy were performed, and the results are shown in Figure 13. SEM micrographs were taken after charging and show that, by moving from a pristine electrode (inserts a and b) to a post-cycled electrode after 50 cycles (inserts c and d), an inhomogeneous SEI is formed. There are regions where, due to gas formation during electrolyte degradation, SEI assumes a bubble-like morphology that covers the material underneath and other regions where the particles of GQDs visible in pristine samples are covered by a film. However, this non-uniform film seems to leave some areas uncovered, which, when facing the subsequent process of discharge, will serve as active sites for new SEI degradation.

The inhomogeneous formation of SEI and the continuous discovery of the underneath surface during cyclations is also confirmed by EIS spectroscopy, where EIS is collected on pristine device (cycle 0) and at four different moments, i.e., after the first, the second, the fifth, and the fifteenth cycles, as shown in Figure 13e. Before cyclations, the material shows a singular semicircle due to charge transfer phenomena, and right after the first cycle, when SEI is formed, a second semicircle appears, demonstrating the formation of a new layer above the electrode surface. This semicircle gets bigger after another cycle but it remains stable up to the fifth cycle, which means resistance is still kept low after a few cyclations; however, after this moment, due to the exposure of active material as shown by SEM post-mortem analysis, there is a further increase in resistance as the semicircle diameters become bigger after the fifteenth cycle. This increase in charge transfer phenomena resistance causes the capacitance to quickly fade.

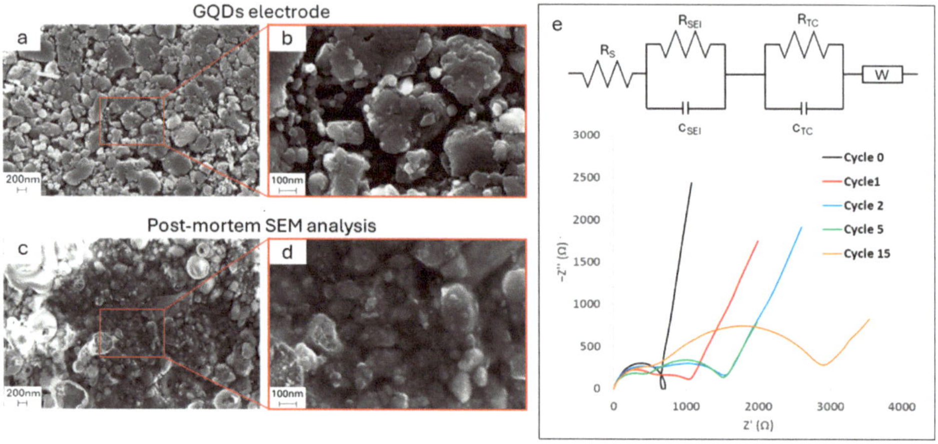

Figure 13. SEM micrographs of pristine GQDs at (**a**) 50k× and (**b**) 200k× magnification; SEM micrographs of post-mortem GQDs at (**c**) 50k and (**d**) 200k× magnification; (**e**) EIS analysis on GQD electrodes.

Resistance values calculated using the equivalent circuit shown as a fitting model are shown in the Supplementary Materials (Table S1).

3. Materials and Methods

Rice husk was purchased by LD Carlson Co. (Kent, OH, USA) and was finely ground before use. All other chemicals were purchased from Sigma Aldrich (St. Louis, MO, USA) and were employed as is, without any further purification.

GQDs were synthesized starting from carbon aerogels (CAs) obtained by RH via an innovative synthesis already developed in our group [67]. Basically, RH underwent a bleaching in a 1.7% wt sodium chlorite and acetic acid aqueous solution (pH 3) to remove lignin and part of hemicellulose, followed by digestion in NaOH 1M at reflux temperature to remove silica and other inorganic impurities, together with the residual part of hemicellulose. The obtained cellulose pulp was dissolved into a 7% wt NaOH and 12% wt urea aqueous solution in an ice bath to obtain a final concentration of 7% wt of cellulose and aged at 50 °C until a stable cellulose gel was formed. Regeneration in water, freeze-drying, and carbonization in Ar atmosphere at 800 °C finally resulted in the formation of a carbon aerogel.

CA samples were ball-milled at 500 rpm for 1 h for 5 times and the final GQD powder was collected using pure water to rinse the ball milling jar.

Morphological characterization was performed using field emission scanning electron microscopy (FESEM) and atomic force microscopy (AFM). FESEM images were acquired by using a ZEISS Auriga platform (Oberkochen, Germany) equipped with energy-dispersive X-ray spectroscopy (EDX). FESEM analysis was performed both on freshly prepared materials and electrodes along with post-mortem samples after cyclations in lithium-ion devices. AFM analysis was performed in tapping mode air by using a BRUKER Dimension Icon (Bremen, Germany) and RTESP-300 BRUKER tips (300 kHz frequency, 40 N/m spring constant and nominal radius of 8 nm). Suitable samples were prepared by depositing a few drops of a diluted suspension (1:104 starting from a 0.4 g/L solution) of graphene quantum dots in water over a (100) crystalline silicon wafer and drying the wafer in air.

The recorded images were postprocessed for background removal and leveling using the software Gwyddion version 2.62.

A F200 JEOL Multipurpose (Tokyo, Japan) transmission electron microscope (TEM) was used in high-resolution (HRTEM) mode to further investigate the morphology and crystalline structure with a higher accuracy. Analysis was conducted at 80 kV with an emission current of 134.7 mA. The camera used was a Gatan Rio16 model (Pleasanton, CA, USA). Suitable samples were prepared by depositing a few drops of a diluted suspension (1:106 starting from a 0.4 g/L solution) of graphene quantum dots in water over a dedicated TEM grid.

Dimensional distributions in SEM, AFM, and TEM were evaluated using ImageJ software, version 1.54j.

X-ray Diffraction (XRD) for structural analysis was performed using a Rigaku Miniflex diffractometer (Cedar Park, TX, USA) with Cu-Kα radiation (λ 1.54 Å) in 2θ range 8–40°, at 30 kV voltage and 15 mA of current. Raman spectroscopy was performed with a Renishaw (Wotton-under-Edge, UK) inVia Raman confocal Microscope using a green lamp (532.1 nm, output power 50 mW) and 100× lens, in the Raman shift range between 800 and 2200 cm^{-1}. FTIR analysis was performed using a Bruker Lumos II micro-FTIR ATR equipped with Ge crystal with 4 cm^{-1} resolution and 2048 data points scan.

X-ray photoelectron spectroscopy (XPS) measurements were carried out using an Omicron (Uppsala, Sweden) NanoTechnology Multiprobe MXPS system equipped with a monochromatic Al Kα (hν = 1486.7 eV) X-ray source (Omicron XM-1000), operating the anode at 14 kV and 16 mA. The C 1s photoionization region was acquired using an analyzer pass energy of 20 eV. A take-off angle of 21° with respect to the sample surface normal was adopted. CA and GQD powders were spread onto double-sided conductive scotch tape attached to the XPS sample holder. The experimental spectra were theoretically reconstructed by fitting the secondary electron background to a Shirley function and the elastic peaks to pseudo-Voigt functions described by a common set of parameters: position, full width at half maximum (FWHM), and the Gaussian–Lorentzian ratio. The oxygen content was determined through the $R_{O/C}$ ratio obtained after the curve fitting of the C 1s region, by means of the following equation:

$$R_{O/C} = \frac{A_{C-OH} + 1/2A_{C-O-C} + A_{C=O} + 2A_{COOH}}{A_{C=C} + A_{C-OH} + A_{C-O-C} + A_{C=O} + A_{COOH}} \quad (4)$$

where the terms A_x represent the OFG peak areas obtained by curve fitting.

Simultaneous thermogravimetric (TG-DTA) curves were registered using the TA Instruments Q650 system analyzer (Waters, Milford, MA, USA) thermal analysis equipment. The temperature was calibrated using the nickel Curie point as a reference, and the DTA baseline was calibrated using sapphire. Samples of about 8 mg in weight were placed in a high-purity alumina crucible and tested with a thermal profile consisting of a heating ramp from room temperature to 800 °C, at a heating rate of 10 °C min^{-1}. Measurements were performed in technical air at a gas flow rate of 100 mL min^{-1}. Exothermic peaks are conventionally up.

Electrochemical performances of graphene quantum dots were evaluated using a multichannel VMP potentiostat by Perkin Elmer Instruments (Waltham, MA, USA). Electrode powder was obtained upon mixing GQDs with PVDF and acetylene black in a proportion of 80:10:10 *w*/*w*. The electrodes were prepared upon suspending the powder in a slurry of N-Methyl-2-pyrrolidone (NMP) and drop-casting it either over platinum (for supercapacitor) or copper (for Li-ion batteries) current collectors. The chosen electrolytes were 6 M aqueous KOH for supercapacitors and $LiPF_6$ in EC:DMC 1:1 for lithium-ion batteries. Two-electrode T-shaped cells were assembled in a symmetric configuration for supercapacitors, and in a half-cell configuration for Li-ion batteries. Galvanostatic cyclations and cyclic voltammetry tests for supercapacitors were performed in −1.0–0.2 V potential window, respectively, at different currents (0.1–1.0 Ag^{-1}) and potential scan rates (1–50 mVs^{-1}). In the case of Li-ion batteries, galvanostatic cyclations were performed in the range 0.04–3 V. Electrochemical impedance spectroscopy (EIS) was performed in the range of frequency from 1 MHz to 1 mHz with 10 mV of amplitude.

4. Conclusions

An efficient one-step way to produce graphene quantum dots from carbon aerogels was developed, and the final result was a fine powder of graphene quantum dots with an average diameter of around 20 nm as shown by TEM analysis. The GQD surface seemed functionalized due to the air atmosphere where the synthetic process occurred, while their structure in long and short range appeared to be made of short domains of graphitic nature generated by a crystallization process happening during synthesis. A preliminary study concerning the application of GQDs as both supercapacitor electrodes and lithium-ion anodes showed that the material has quickly fading performances probably due to poor contact with the rest of the electrode mixture and the current collector. However, graphene quantum dots proved to be able to both accumulate charges over the surface and intercalate ions, thus resulting in a promising 0D material worth deeper study in hybrid compounds.

Supplementary Materials: The following supporting information can be downloaded at: https://www.mdpi.com/article/10.3390/molecules29235666/s1, Figure S1: Gaussian fitting of the Raman spectrum of CAs; Figure S2: Gaussian fitting of the Raman spectrum of GQDs; Table S1: Evaluated resistance values obtained by fitting EIS spectra for lithium-ion batteries electrodes.

Author Contributions: Conceptualization, P.A.; methodology, P.A.; formal analysis, P.A., D.P. and F.A.S.; investigation, P.A., R.Y.S.Z., L.B., C.D.C., A.P., F.M., A.A. and A.G.M.; writing—original draft preparation, P.A., R.Y.S.Z. and F.A.S.; writing—review and editing, M.R., M.P. and F.A.S.; visualization, P.A. and F.A.S.; supervision, M.R. and M.P.; funding acquisition, M.R., M.P. and F.A.S. All authors have read and agreed to the published version of the manuscript.

Funding: This research was funded by (i) Project Infrastructure for Energy Transition and Circular Economy @ EuroNanoLab (iENTRANCE@ENL); (ii) ENEA (Agenzia nazionale per le nuove tecnologie, l'energia e lo sviluppo economico sostenibile) within the three-year 2022–2024 plan of research on national electric systems (PIANO TRIENNALE DI REALIZZAZIONE 2022–2024 DELLA RICERCA DI SISTEMA ELETTRICO NAZIONALE).

Institutional Review Board Statement: The present study did not require ethical approval.

Informed Consent Statement: Not applicable.

Data Availability Statement: No new data were created.

Acknowledgments: Sergio Brutti, Department of Chemistry, Sapienza University of Rome, is kindly acknowledged for FTIR availability.

Conflicts of Interest: The authors declare no conflicts of interest. The funders had no role in the design of the study; in the collection, analyses, or interpretation of data; in the writing of the manuscript; or in the decision to publish the results.

References

1. Sharma, S.; Kumar, R.; Kumar, K.; Thakur, N. Sustainable Applications of Biowaste-Derived Carbon; Dots in Eco-Friendly Technological Advancements: A Review. *Mater. Sci. Eng. B* **2024**, *305*, 117414. [CrossRef]
2. Dell'Era, A.; Pasquali, M.; Tarquini, G.; Scaramuzzo, F.A.; De Gasperis, P.; Prosini, P.P.; Mezzi, A.; Tuffi, R.; Cafiero, L. Carbon. Powder Material Obtained from an Innovative High Pressure Water Jet Recycling Process of Tires Used as Anode in Alkali Ion (Li, Na) Batteries. *Solid State Ion.* **2018**, *324*, 20–27. [CrossRef]
3. Kartick, B.; Srivastava, S.K.; Srivastava, I. Green Synthesis of Graphene. *J. Nanosci. Nanotechnol.* **2013**, *13*, 4320–4324. [CrossRef] [PubMed]
4. Mahmoud, M.E.; Fekry, N.A.; Abdelfattah, A.M. A Novel Nanobiosorbent of Functionalized Graphene Quantum Dots from Rice Husk with Barium Hydroxide for Microwave Enhanced Removal of Lead (II) and Lanthanum (III). *Bioresour. Technol.* **2020**, *298*, 122514. [CrossRef]
5. Othman, F.E.C.; Nordin, N.A.H.M.; Ismail, N.; Zakria, H.S.; Junoh, H.; Aziz, M.H.A. A Review on Sustainable Graphene Production from Rice Husks: Strategies and Key Considerations. *Chem. Eng. J.* **2024**, *497*, 154408. [CrossRef]
6. Childs, N.; Lebeau, B. *Rice Outlook: December 2023*; USDA, Economic Research Service: Washington, DC, USA, 2023.

7. Lim, J.S.; Abdul Manan, Z.; Hashim, H.; Wan Alwi, S.R. Towards an Integrated, Resource-Efficient Rice Mill Complex. *Resour. Conserv. Recycl.* **2013**, *75*, 41–51. [CrossRef]
8. Omrani, E.; Menezes, P.L.; Rohatgi, P.K. State of the Art on Tribological Behavior of Polymer Matrix Composites Reinforced with Natural Fibers in the Green Materials World. *Eng. Sci. Technol. Int. J.* **2016**, *19*, 717–736. [CrossRef]
9. Singh, B. Rice Husk Ash. In *Waste and Supplementary Cementitious Materials in Concrete: Characterisation, Properties and Applications*; Elsevier: Amsterdam, The Netherlands, 2018; pp. 417–460, ISBN 9780081021569.
10. Jessy Mercy, D.; Kiran, V.; Thirumalai, A.; Harini, K.; Girigoswami, K.; Girigoswami, A. Rice Husk Assisted Carbon Quantum Dots Synthesis for Amoxicillin Sensing. *Results Chem.* **2023**, *6*, 101219. [CrossRef]
11. Soltani, N.; Bahrami, A.; Pech-Canul, M.I.; González, L.A. Review on the Physicochemical Treatments of Rice Husk for Production of Advanced Materials. *Chem. Eng. J.* **2015**, *264*, 899–935. [CrossRef]
12. Deng, D. Li-Ion Batteries: Basics, Progress, and Challenges. *Energy Sci. Eng.* **2015**, *3*, 385–418. [CrossRef]
13. Dell'Era, A.; Scaramuzzo, F.A.; Stoller, M.; Lupi, C.; Rossi, M.; Passeri, D.; Pasquali, M. Spinning Disk Reactor Technique for the Synthesis of Nanometric Sulfur TiO_2 Core-Shell Powder for Lithium Batteries. *Appl. Sci.* **2019**, *9*, 1913. [CrossRef]
14. Roy, K.; Banerjee, A.; Ogale, S. Search for New Anode Materials for High Performance Li-Ion Batteries. *ACS Appl. Mater. Interfaces* **2022**, *14*, 20326–20348. [CrossRef] [PubMed]
15. Dell'Era, A.; Pasquali, M.; Bauer, E.M.; Vecchio Ciprioti, S.; Scaramuzzo, F.A.; Lupi, C. Synthesis, Characterization, and Electrochemical Behavior of $LiMn_xFe_{(1-x)}PO_4$ Composites Obtained from Phenylphosphonate-Based Organic-Inorganic Hybrids. *Materials* **2018**, *11*, 56. [CrossRef] [PubMed]
16. Mohamed, N.; Allam, N.K. Recent Advances in the Design of Cathode Materials for Li-Ion Batteries. *RSC Adv.* **2020**, *10*, 21662–21685. [CrossRef] [PubMed]
17. Tarquini, G.; Dell'Era, A.; Prosini, P.P.; Scaramuzzo, F.A.; Lupi, C.; Pasquali, M. Polysulfide Solution Effects on LiS Batteries Performances. *J. Electroanal. Chem.* **2020**, *870*, 114239. [CrossRef]
18. Chayambuka, K.; Mulder, G.; Danilov, D.L.; Notten, P.H.L. From Li-Ion Batteries toward Na-Ion Chemistries: Challenges and Opportunities. *Adv. Energy Mater.* **2020**, *10*, 2001310. [CrossRef]
19. Zhong, M.; Zhang, M.; Li, X. Carbon Nanomaterials and Their Composites for Supercapacitors. *Carbon Energy* **2022**, *4*, 950–985. [CrossRef]
20. Dissanayake, K.; Kularatna-Abeywardana, D. A Review of Supercapacitors: Materials, Technology, Challenges, and Renewable Energy Applications. *J. Energy Storage* **2024**, *96*, 112563. [CrossRef]
21. Tyagi, A.; Joshi, M.C.; Shah, A.; Thakur, V.K.; Gupta, R.K. Hydrothermally Tailored Three-Dimensional Ni-V Layered Double Hydroxide Nanosheets as High-Performance Hybrid Supercapacitor Applications. *ACS Omega* **2019**, *4*, 3257–3267. [CrossRef]
22. Yadav, K.K.; Singh, H.; Rana, S.; Sunaina; Sammi, H.; Nishanthi, S.T.; Wadhwa, R.; Khan, N.; Jha, M. Utilization of Waste Coir Fibre Architecture to Synthesize Porous Graphene Oxide and Their Derivatives: An Efficient Energy Storage Material. *J. Clean. Prod.* **2020**, *276*, 124240. [CrossRef]
23. Xiao, J.; Momen, R.; Liu, C. Application of Carbon Quantum Dots in Supercapacitors: A Mini Review. *Electrochem. Commun.* **2021**, *132*, 107143. [CrossRef]
24. Jin, H.; Wu, S.; Li, T.; Bai, Y.; Wang, X.; Zhang, H.; Xu, H.; Kong, C.; Wang, H. Synthesis of Porous Carbon Nano-Onions Derived from Rice Husk for High-Performance Supercapacitors. *Appl. Surf. Sci.* **2019**, *488*, 593–599. [CrossRef]
25. Kalluri, A.; Dharmadhikari, B.; Debnath, D.; Patra, P.; Kumar, C.V. Advances in Structural Modifications and Properties of Graphene Quantum Dots for Biomedical Applications. *ACS Omega* **2023**, *8*, 21358–21376. [CrossRef] [PubMed]
26. Tajik, S.; Dourandish, Z.; Zhang, K.; Beitollahi, H.; Van Le, Q.; Jang, H.W.; Shokouhimehr, M. Carbon and Graphene Quantum Dots: A Review on Syntheses, Characterization, Biological and Sensing Applications for Neurotransmitter Determination. *RSC Adv.* **2020**, *10*, 15406–15429. [CrossRef]
27. Zhang, S.; Sui, L.; Dong, H.; He, W.; Dong, L.; Yu, L. High-Performance Supercapacitor of Graphene Quantum Dots with Uniform Sizes. *ACS Appl. Mater. Interfaces* **2018**, *10*, 12983–12991. [CrossRef]
28. Michenzi, C.; Scaramuzzo, F.; Salvitti, C.; Pepi, F.; Troiani, A.; Chiarotto, I. Photo-Activated Carbon Dots as Catalysts in Knoevenagel Condensation: An Advance in the Synthetic Field. *Photochem* **2024**, *4*, 361–376. [CrossRef]
29. Chen, W.; Lv, G.; Hu, W.; Li, D.; Chen, S.; Dai, Z. Synthesis and Applications of Graphene Quantum Dots—A Review. *Nanotechnol. Rev.* **2018**, *7*, 157–185. [CrossRef]
30. Bak, S.; Kim, D.; Lee, H. Graphene Quantum Dots and Their Possible Energy Applications: A Review. *Curr. Appl. Phys.* **2016**, *16*, 1192–1201. [CrossRef]
31. Khaleghi Abbasabadi, M.; Azarifar, D. β-Alanine-Functionalized Magnetic Graphene Oxide Quantum Dots: An Efficient and Recyclable Heterogeneous Basic Catalyst for the Synthesis of 1H-Pyrazolo [1,2-b]Phthalazine-5,10-Dione and 2,3-Dihydroquinazolin-4(1H)-One Derivatives. *Appl. Organomet. Chem.* **2020**, *34*, e5872. [CrossRef]
32. Zahir, N.; Magri, P.; Luo, W.; Gaumet, J.J.; Pierrat, P. Recent Advances on Graphene Quantum Dots for Electrochemical Energy Storage Devices. *Energy Environ. Mater.* **2022**, *5*, 201–214. [CrossRef]
33. Liu, W.; Li, M.; Jiang, G.; Li, G.; Zhu, J.; Xiao, M.; Zhu, Y.; Gao, R.; Yu, A.; Feng, M.; et al. Graphene Quantum Dots-Based Advanced Electrode Materials: Design, Synthesis and Their Applications in Electrochemical Energy Storage and Electrocatalysis. *Adv. Energy Mater.* **2020**, *10*, 2001275. [CrossRef]

34. Adaikalapandi, S.; Thangadurai, T.D.; Manjubaashini, N.; Nataraj, D.; Babu, T.G.S.; Kumar, S.M. Bamboo Stem Biomass Waste-Derived Excitation-Dependent Carbon Dots for Nanomolar Detection of Fungicide Dodine in Real Samples and Their PH-Sensitive Bacterial Interaction Studies. *Diam. Relat. Mater.* **2024**, *141*, 110692. [CrossRef]
35. Rajkishore, S.K.; Devadharshini, K.P.; Moorthy, P.S.; Kalyan, V.S.R.K.; Sunitha, R.; Prasanthrajan, M.; Maheswari, M.; Subramanian, K.S.; Sakthivel, N.; Sakrabani, R. Novel Synthesis of Carbon Dots from Coconut Wastes and Its Potential as Water Disinfectant. *Sustainability* **2023**, *15*, 10924. [CrossRef]
36. Dhongde, N.R.; Das, N.K.; Banerjee, T.; Rajaraman, P.V. Synthesis of Carbon Quantum Dots from Rice Husk for Anti-Corrosive Coating Applications: Experimental and Theoretical Investigations. *Ind. Crops Prod.* **2024**, *212*, 118329. [CrossRef]
37. Gaayathri, K.H.; Debnath, R.; Roy, M.; Saha, M. Sustainable Production of Graphene Quantum Dots from Rice Husk for Photo-Degradation of Organochlorine Pesticides. *Mater. Sci. Eng. Technol.* **2024**, *55*, 487–495. [CrossRef]
38. Dini, D.; Cognigni, F.; Passeri, D.; Scaramuzzo, F.A.; Pasquali, M.; Rossi, M. Review—Multiscale Characterization of Li-Ion Batteries through the Combined Use of Atomic Force Microscopy and X-ray Microscopy and Considerations for a Correlative Analysis of the Reviewed Data. *J. Electrochem. Soc.* **2021**, *168*, 126522. [CrossRef]
39. Cognigni, F.; Pasquali, M.; Prosini, P.P.; Paoletti, C.; Aurora, A.; Scaramuzzo, F.A.; Rossi, M. X-ray Microscopy: A Non-Destructive Multi-Scale Imaging to Study the Inner Workings of Batteries. *ChemElectroChem* **2023**, *10*, e202201081. [CrossRef]
40. Palser, A.H.R. Interlayer Interactions in Graphite and Carbon Nanotubes. *Phys. Chem. Chem. Phys.* **1999**, *1*, 4459–4464. [CrossRef]
41. Hod, O. Graphite and Hexagonal Boron-Nitride Have the Same Interlayer Distance. Why? *J. Chem. Theory Comput.* **2012**, *8*, 1360–1369. [CrossRef]
42. Lim, D.J.; Marks, N.A.; Rowles, M.R. Universal Scherrer Equation for Graphene Fragments. *Carbon N. Y.* **2020**, *162*, 475–480. [CrossRef]
43. Batool, M.; Hussain, D.; Akrem, A.; Najam-ul-Haq, M.; Saeed, S.; Zaka, S.M.; Nawaz, M.S.; Buck, F.; Saeed, Q. Graphene Quantum Dots as Cysteine Protease Nanocarriers against Stored Grain Insect Pests. *Sci. Rep.* **2020**, *10*, 3444. [CrossRef] [PubMed]
44. Cuesta, A.; Dhamelincourt, P.; Laureyns, J.; Martinez-Alonso, A.; Tascòn, J.M.D. Raman Microprobe Studies On Carbon Materials. *Carbon* **1994**, *32*, 1523–1532. [CrossRef]
45. Shimodaira, N.; Masui, A. Raman Spectroscopic Investigations of Activated Carbon Materials. *J. Appl. Phys.* **2002**, *92*, 902–909. [CrossRef]
46. Ferrari, A.C.; Robertson, J. Interpretation of Raman Spectra of Disordered and Amorphous Carbon. *Phys. Rev. B* **2000**, *61*, 14095. [CrossRef]
47. Suneetha, R.B. Spectral, Thermal and Morphological Characterization of Biodegradable Graphene Oxide-Chitosan Nanocomposites. *J. Nanosci. Technol.* **2018**, *4*, 342–344. [CrossRef]
48. Wang, H.; Qi, C.; Yang, A.; Wang, X.; Xu, J. One-Pot Synthesis of Bright Blue Luminescent N-Doped GQDs. *Nanomaterials* **2021**, *11*, 2798. [CrossRef]
49. Sudesh; Kumar, N.; Das, S.; Das, S.; Bernhard, C.; Varma, G.D. Effect of Graphene Oxide Doping on Superconducting Properties of Bulk MgB2. *Supercond. Sci. Technol.* **2013**, *26*, 095008. [CrossRef]
50. Bello, R.H.; Coelho, L.A.F.; Becker, D. Role of Chemical Functionalization of Carbon Nanoparticles in Epoxy Matrices. *J. Compos. Mater.* **2018**, *52*, 4. [CrossRef]
51. Hayyan, M.; Abo-Hamad, A.; AlSaadi, M.A.H.; Hashim, M.A. Functionalization of Graphene Using Deep Eutectic Solvents. *Nanoscale Res. Lett.* **2015**, *10*, 324. [CrossRef]
52. Marrani, A.G.; Coico, A.C.; Giacco, D.; Zanoni, R.; Scaramuzzo, F.A.; Schrebler, R.; Dini, D.; Bonomo, M.; Dalchiele, E.A. Integration of Graphene onto Silicon through Electrochemical Reduction of Graphene Oxide Layers in Non-Aqueous Medium. *Appl. Surf. Sci.* **2018**, *445*, 404–414. [CrossRef]
53. Kovtun, A.; Jones, D.; Dell'Elce, S.; Treossi, E.; Liscio, A.; Palermo, V. Accurate Chemical Analysis of Oxygenated Graphene-Based Materials Using X-ray Photoelectron Spectroscopy. *Carbon* **2019**, *143*, 268–275. [CrossRef]
54. Larciprete, R.; Lacovig, P.; Gardonio, S.; Baraldi, A.; Lizzit, S. Atomic Oxygen on Graphite Chemical Characterization and Thermal Reduction. *J. Phys. Chem. C* **2012**, *116*, 18. [CrossRef]
55. Lin, C.Y.; Cheng, C.E.; Wang, S.; Shiu, H.W.; Chang, L.Y.; Chen, C.H.; Lin, T.W.; Chang, C.S.; Chien, F.S.S. Synchrotron Radiation Soft X-ray Induced Reduction in Graphene Oxide Characterized by Time-Resolved Photoelectron Spectroscopy. *J. Phys. Chem. C* **2015**, *119*, 23. [CrossRef]
56. Estrade-Szwarckopf, H. XPS Photoemission in Carbonaceous Materials: A "Defect" Peak beside the Graphitic Asymmetric Peak. *Carbon* **2004**, *42*, 1713–1721. [CrossRef]
57. Briggs, J.D.; Seah, M.P. Practical Surface Analysis. In *Auger and X-ray Photoelectron Spectroscopy*; John Wiley Sons: Chichester, UK, 1990; Volume 1.
58. Tiberio, F.; Amato, F.; Desiderio, C.; Vincenzoni, F.; Perini, G.; Moretti, I.; Augello, A.; Friggeri, G.; Cui, L.; Giaccari, L.; et al. The Osteoconductive Properties of Graphene-Based Material Surfaces Are Finely Tuned by the Conditioning Layer and Surface Chemistry. *Mater. Adv.* **2024**, *5*, 4772–4785. [CrossRef]
59. Amato, F.; Ferrari, I.; Motta, A.; Zanoni, R.; Dalchiele, E.A.; Marrani, A.G. Assessing the Evolution of Oxygenated Functional Groups on the Graphene Oxide Surface upon Mild Thermal Annealing in Water. *RSC Adv.* **2023**, *13*, 29308–29315. [CrossRef]

60. Morais, A.; Alves, J.P.C.; Lima, F.A.S.; Lira-Cantu, M.; Nogueira, A.F. Enhanced Photovoltaic Performance of Inverted Hybrid Bulk-Heterojunction Solar Cells Using TiO 2 /Reduced Graphene Oxide Films as Electron Transport Layers. *J. Photonics Energy* **2015**, *5*, 057408. [CrossRef]
61. Farivar, F.; Lay Yap, P.; Karunagaran, R.U.; Losic, D. Thermogravimetric Analysis (TGA) of Graphene Materials: Effect of Particle Size of Graphene, Graphene Oxide and Graphite on Thermal Parameters. *C* **2021**, *7*, 41. [CrossRef]
62. Özge Alaş Çolak, M.; Güngör, A.; Akturk, M.B.; Erdem, E.; Genç, R. Unlocking the Full Potential of Citric Acid-Synthesized Carbon Dots as a Supercapacitor Electrode Material via Surface Functionalization. *Nanoscale* **2023**, *16*, 719–733. [CrossRef]
63. Dharmalingam, P.; Ramanan, V.; Karthikeyan, G.G.; Palani, N.S.; Ilangovan, R.; Ramamurthy, P. A Study on the Electrochemical Performance of Nitrogen and Oxygen Co-Doped Carbon Dots Derived from a Green Precursor for Supercapacitor Applications. *J. Mater. Sci. Mater. Electron.* **2017**, *28*, 18489–18496. [CrossRef]
64. Baslak, C.; Demirel, S.; Dogu, S.; Ozturk, G.; Kocyigit, A.; Yıldırım, M. Green Synthesis Capacitor of Carbon Quantum Dots from Stachys Euadenia. *Env. Prog. Sustain. Energy* **2024**, *43*, e14340. [CrossRef]
65. Wei, J.S.; Ding, H.; Zhang, P.; Song, Y.F.; Chen, J.; Wang, Y.G.; Xiong, H.M. Carbon Dots-$NiCo_2O_4$ Nanocomposites with Various Morphologies for High Performance Supercapacitors. *Small* **2016**, *12*, 5927–5934. [CrossRef] [PubMed]
66. Song, T.B.; Huang, Z.H.; Niu, X.Q.; Liu, J.; Wei, J.S.; Chen, X.B.; Xiong, H.M. Applications of Carbon *Dots in Next-Generation Lithium-Ion Batteries. ChemNanoMat* **2020**, *6*, 1421–1436. [CrossRef]
67. Atanasio, P.; Zampiva, R.Y.S.; Fornari, A.; Mancini, C.; Rossi, M.; Pasquali, M.; Scaramuzzo, F.A. Innovative and green synthesis of Carbon aerogels for advanced *supercapacitors*. 2024, *submitted*.

molecules

MDPI

Article

Enrichment of Trypsin Inhibitor from Soybean Whey Wastewater Using Different Precipitating Agents and Analysis of Their Properties

Yongsheng Zhou, Siyun Zhou, Cuiwen Lu, Yihao Zhang * and Haiyan Zhao *

College of Food and Biochemical Engineering, Guangxi Science & Technology Normal University, Laibin 546199, China
* Correspondence: zhangyihao@gxstnu.edu.cn (Y.Z.); zhaohaiyan@gxstnu.edu.cn (H.Z.)

Abstract: Recovering valuable active substances from the by-products of agricultural processing is a crucial concern for scientific researchers. This paper focuses on the enrichment of soybean trypsin inhibitor (STI) from soybean whey wastewater using either ammonium sulfate salting or ethanol precipitation, and discusses their physicochemical properties. The results show that at a 60% ethanol content, the yield of STI was 3.983 mg/mL, whereas the yield was 3.833 mg/mL at 60% ammonium sulfate saturation. The inhibitory activity of STI obtained by ammonium sulfate salting out (A-STI) was higher than that obtained by ethanol precipitation (E-STI). A-STI exhibited better solubility than E-STI at specific temperatures and pH levels, as confirmed by turbidity and surface hydrophobicity measurements. Thermal characterization revealed that both A-STI and E-STI showed thermal transition temperatures above 90 °C. Scanning electron microscopy demonstrated that A-STI had a smooth surface with fewer pores, while E-STI had a rough surface with more pores. In conclusion, there was no significant difference in the yield of A-STI and E-STI ($p < 0.05$); however, the physicochemical properties of A-STI were superior to those of E-STI, making it more suitable for further processing and utilization. This study provides a theoretical reference for the enrichment of STI from soybean whey wastewater.

Keywords: trypsin inhibitor; soybean whey; ethanol precipitation

Citation: Zhou, Y.; Zhou, S.; Lu, C.; Zhang, Y.; Zhao, H. Enrichment of Trypsin Inhibitor from Soybean Whey Wastewater Using Different Precipitating Agents and Analysis of Their Properties. *Molecules* **2024**, *29*, 2613. https://doi.org/10.3390/molecules29112613

Academic Editors: Giuseppina Raffaini and Fabio Ganazzoli

Received: 7 May 2024
Revised: 29 May 2024
Accepted: 30 May 2024
Published: 2 June 2024

1. Introduction

Soybean, renowned for its rich oil and protein content, is a significant source of protein and fat nutrients for humans [1]. It is commonly called the "king of beans" due to its abundant nutrients and high nutritional value, making it highly sought after worldwide [1]. In 2020, the worldwide market value of soybean reached USD 127.81 billion and is expected to reach approximately USD 162 billion by 2027 [2]. Soybean protein isolate (SPI) is a deep-processing product derived from defatted soybean meal. Due to its excellent nutritional profile, functional properties, and health benefits, SPI exhibits significant potential as a valuable food ingredient [3]. SPI is typically obtained through alkali extraction-acid precipitation, involving the extraction of defatted soybean meal under alkaline conditions (pH 7.5~pH 8.5), followed by precipitation under acidic conditions (pH 4.5) [3]. The production of SPI results in the generation of significant quantities of soybean whey by-products [4]. On average, 20 tons of soybean whey are generated per ton of SPI produced [4]. Soybean whey contains various nutrients, including monosaccharides, oligosaccharides, and soybean whey protein [5]. As soybean whey is rich in sugars, proteins, minerals, and various nutrients, it is prone to microbial growth and can develop an unpleasant odor when stored under natural conditions [6]. Consequently, the timely disposal or management of soybean whey becomes necessary. The direct discharge or traditional biochemical treatment of soybean whey can adversely affect the environment and waste valuable resources, which is incompatible with sustainability strategies [6,7]. Directly discharging soybean whey into water can lead to eutrophication. This nutrient-rich wastewater promotes the rapid growth of algae and bacteria, which, in turn, depletes the oxygen levels in the water. Consequently, this can create anaerobic conditions, harming aquatic animals and plants and potentially causing large-scale death. This process ultimately degrades the water quality of the river and adversely affects the surrounding ecological environment [6]. Consequently, the adoption of an appropriate strategy for the integrated utilization of soybean whey becomes of paramount importance. By doing so, we can contribute to environmental preservation, resource conservation, and cost reduction for companies. Tu et al. conducted a study utilizing water kefir grains for fermenting soybean whey to transform it into novel functional food ingredients through microbial fermentation or enzyme-catalyzed reactions [8]. The findings demonstrated a significant increase in total flavonoids, total phenols, and isoflavone glycosides in soybean whey following fermentation. Moreover, fermentation resulted in the generation of numerous new aromatic volatile compounds, thereby enhancing the sensory attributes of soybean whey [8]. Dai et al. also used *Cordyceps militaris* SN-18 to ferment soybean whey. The fermentation increased the content of essential amino acids, total phenolics, flavonoids, and isoflavone glycosides while reducing oligosaccharides [9]. In addition, the recovery of valuable compounds from soybean whey, such as soybean oligosaccharides, soybean whey protein, soybean isoflavones, and polyphenols, represents an advantageous approach for energy conservation and emission reduction. However, significant challenges persist due to the high cost and inadequate motivation to recover organic substances.

Soybean whey protein is an acid-soluble protein, mainly composed of 2S protein and 7S protein, accounting for approximately 9.0% to 15.3% of the total soybean seed protein. It contains various components such as soybean trypsin inhibitor (STI), including Kunitz trypsin inhibitor (KTI) and Bowman–Birk trypsin inhibitor (BBI), soybean lectin, lipid oxidase, β-amylase, and other fractions [10]. Enriching STI from soybean whey wastewater can reduce organic matter and minimize environmental pollution. Moreover, STI exhibits specific physiological functions, such as anti-cancer, anti-inflammatory, and anti-bacterial activities, thereby possessing significant development potential in the health food and biopharmaceutical markets [11–13].

Currently, the main methods for crude protein separation are the isoelectric point method, salting out, and organic solvent precipitation [14]. The isoelectric point precipitation method relies on the principle that when the pH of an amphoteric electrolyte reaches its isoelectric point, the electrostatic charge on the molecular surface becomes zero. This leads to the weakening or destruction of the stable double-electric layer and hydration film, resulting in increased intermolecular attraction and decreased solubility. As a result, proteins aggregate and precipitate out [15]. Soybean whey wastewater is a by-product obtained from the precipitation of SPI using the isoelectric point method [3]. Moreover, the isoelectric point of STI closely resembles that of SPI. Consequently, the conventional isoelectric point precipitation method proves ineffective for the recovery of STI from soybean whey wastewater. An alternative approach known as the "salting out method" involves the introduction of inorganic salts into the protein solution. This addition leads to the mutual neutralization of salt ions and protein molecules' surface charges, reducing the electrostatic interactions between the proteins. On the other hand, salt ions mediate the hydrophobic interaction of the proteins, reducing their solubility and leading to the aggregation and precipitation of proteins. The organic solvent precipitation method uses organic solvents to reduce the dielectric constant of aqueous solutions, thereby increasing the attraction between two oppositely charged groups. This process destroys the hydrophobic membrane of proteins, reducing their hydrophilicity and resulting in the aggregation and precipitation of protein molecules [16]. Organic solvent precipitation is a commonly used and scalable method for protein separation. The discriminatory capacity of this method is higher than that of salinization, as precipitation does not require desalination, filtration is easier, the conditions are mild and inexpensive, and the process is simple. Nevertheless, it is essential to acknowledge that protein solutions treated with organic solvents may cause the irreversible denaturation of proteins and the loss of their original functional properties. Consequently, carefully selecting an appropriate precipitating agent to recover STI from soybean whey is potentially instructive.

In this paper, soybean trypsin inhibitor (STI) was enriched from soybean whey wastewater using two different methods: ammonium sulfate salting out and ethanol precipitation. We compared these enrichment methods to determine the most effective extraction technique for STI from soybean whey wastewater, providing a scientific basis for selecting the optimal method. Subsequently, we examined the physicochemical properties of the obtained STI, including solubility, thermal properties, and surface morphology, which are critical for its application and further processing. The results of this study offer a valuable theoretical reference for the efficient enrichment of STI from soybean whey wastewater.

2. Results and Discussion

2.1. Analysis of Yield and Protein Recovery Rate

Soybean whey powder was obtained after soybean whey freeze-drying (Table 1). In total, 24.90 mg of soybean whey powder was obtained per 100 mL of soybean whey. The analysis of the freeze-dried samples showed that the protein content accounted for 17.19% of the total solids.

Table 1. The yield of STI and protein recovery rate.

Precipitation Agent	Yield (mg/mL)	Protein Content (%)	Recovery Rate (%)
Soybean whey	24.90 ± 0.15	17.19 ± 0.44	100.00
Ammonium sulfate (%)			
20	0.317 ± 0.047 ^{g}	95.33 ± 0.48 ^{b}	7.06 ± 0.28 ^{e}
30	0.950 ± 0.041 ^{f}	98.00 ± 0.55 ^{a}	21.75 ± 0.69 ^{d}
40	2.900 ± 0.071 ^{c}	94.84 ± 0.84 ^{b}	64.27 ± 0.57 ^{c}
50	3.567 ± 0.131 ^{b}	93.24 ± 0.37 ^{b}	77.71 ± 0.11 ^{b}
60	3.833 ± 0.332 ^{a}	93.11 ± 0.75 ^{b}	83.39 ± 0.03 ^{a}
Ethanol (%)			
20	1.533 ± 0.062 ^{e}	94.00 ± 2.36 ^{b}	33.67 ± 0.85 ^{e}
30	2.517 ± 0.085 ^{d}	97.89 ± 0.65 ^{a}	57.57 ± 0.44 ^{d}
40	2.933 ± 0.062 ^{c}	93.12 ± 0.44 ^{b}	63.81 ± 0.30 ^{c}
50	3.317 ± 0.062 ^{b}	92.69 ± 0.77 ^{b}	71.83 ± 0.64 ^{b}
60	3.983 ± 0.340 ^{a}	93.70 ± 0.27 ^{b}	87.20 ± 0.25 ^{a}

Results are presented as mean values ± standard deviation (n = 3). Different letters on the same column indicate significant differences ($p < 0.05$) among the different conditions.

Inorganic salt ammonium sulfate and organic solvent ethanol were used to enrich STI from soybean whey. The results, as presented in Table 1, demonstrated a gradual increase in the yields of STI with an increase in ammonium sulfate saturation or ethanol percentage. In all cases, the obtained STI exhibited a high protein content, exceeding 90%. The yield of STI was found to be 0.317 mg/mL with a minimum protein recovery of 7.06% at 20% ammonium sulfate saturation and 3.983 mg/mL with a maximum protein recovery of 87.02% at 60% ethanol content. Notably, at 60% ammonium sulfate saturation, the yield of STI was 3.833 mg/mL, and the protein recovery was 83.39%. At this point, no significant difference was observed in the yield of STI enriched using the ethanol precipitation method compared to the ammonium sulfate salting out method.

2.2. STI Composition Analysis

STI was analyzed by SDS-PAGE, and the results are shown in Figure 1. The SDS-PAGE analysis revealed that the STI was mainly composed of proteins with molecular weights smaller than 35 kDa. As shown in Figure 1a, when the ammonium sulfate saturation was below 40%, the grayness of the bands corresponding to a molecular weight less than 20 kDa gradually deepened as the ammonium sulfate saturation increased, indicating that the purity of the STI increased [17]. However, when the ammonium sulfate saturation was higher than 40%, with the increase in the ammonium sulfate saturation, several bands with a molecular weight greater than 25 kDa appeared, while the protein bands with a molecular weight less than 20 kDa did not significantly deepen in grayness, indicating that exceeding 40% ammonium sulfate saturation might lead to a decrease in the STI purity. Furthermore, Figure 1b displays the effect of increasing ethanol percentage on STI composition. As the ethanol percentage increased, the grayness of protein bands with molecular weights less than 20 kDa gradually decreased. Conversely, bands with molecular weights greater than 25 kDa exhibited increased intensity and deep grayness. These observations indicated that an elevated ethanol percentage might lead to a reduction in STI purity.

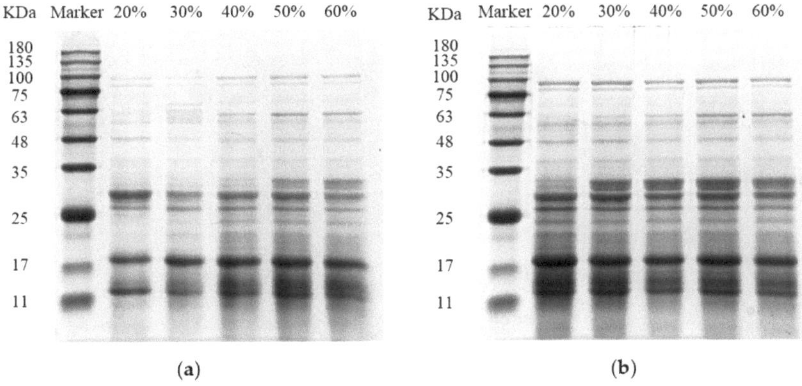

Figure 1. Electrophoretic diagram of precipitated protein with different ammonium sulfate saturation (**a**) and ethanol content (**b**).

2.3. *STI Purity Analysis*

Gel filtration chromatography is a separation technique based on the size and shape of proteins, often used for further purification of crudely isolated proteins [18]. Figure 2 shows the chromatograms of the samples dissolved in 0.2 M phosphate-buffered solution, passing through a Superdex 75 Increase 10/300 gel filtration pre-load column. Figure 2a shows the gel filtration chromatograms of KTI (sigma, T9128), BBI (sigma, T9777), and A-STI. The results indicated that the peak of KTI (20 kDa) appeared at 22 min (11 mL mobile phase elapsed) and diminished after 26 min (13 mL mobile phase), while the peak of BBI (8 kDa) appeared at 28 min (14 mL mobile phase) and disappeared after 30 min (15 mL mobile phase). Therefore, based on the retention time of the KTI and BBI peaks, the purity of the STI obtained with different ammonium sulfate saturation levels can be tentatively determined. As shown in Table 2, the purity of A-STI was above 68%. When the ammonium sulfate saturation was 40%, there was 81.77% STI and 18.23% hetero protein, with the highest purity of STI found in the concentrate; this result is consistent with the SDS-PAGE results. Figure 2b shows the gel filtration chromatograms of KTI, BBI, and E-STI. The results demonstrate that the total peak area of STI gradually decreased with the increase in the ethanol percentage, indicating that less STI was soluble in the 0.2 M phosphate-buffered solution. This observation may be related to the structural changes in the STI caused by ethanol, impacting the solubility, and the high ethanol concentration leading to protein denaturation [19]. A high concentration of ethanol solution can induce the exposure of hydrophobic groups, thus decreasing the solubility of proteins. Moreover, we observed that the total peak area of the E-STI chromatogram was generally smaller than that of A-STI, indicating that the solubility of the protein precipitated by ethanol precipitation may be inferior to that of the protein obtained by ammonium sulfate precipitation. Table 2 indicates that the purity of E-STI was consistently above 60%. When the ethanol percentage was 60%, the highest purity of STI was 78.79%. However, this contrasts with the results of

SDS-PAGE, possibly because, after treatment with a high ethanol percentage, larger protein molecules (>20 kDa) aggregated together, leading to their exclusion from the mobile phase after passing through the 0.22 μm filter membrane. This phenomenon contributes to the high purity of STI, corresponding to the small total peak area of E-STI.

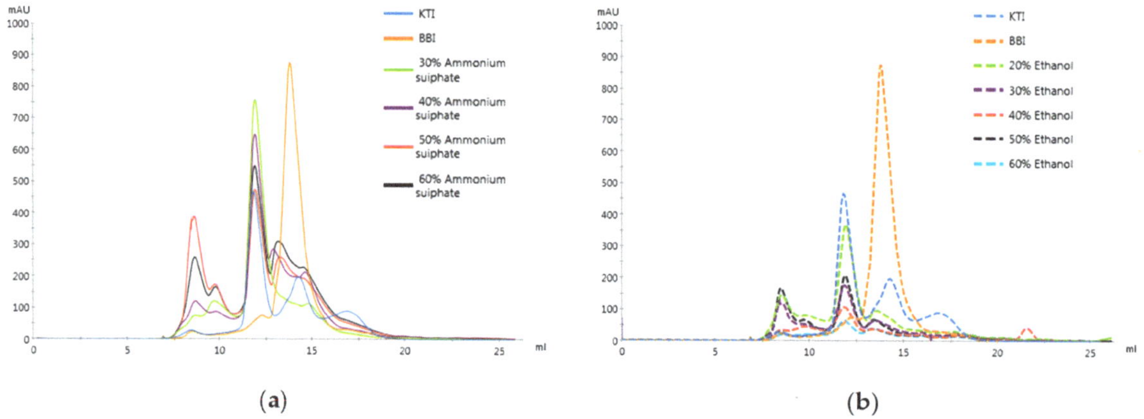

Figure 2. Gel filtration chromatogram of precipitated protein with different ammonium sulfate saturation (**a**) and ethanol content (**b**).

Table 2. Gel filtration chromatogram peak areas for precipitated protein with different ammonium sulfate saturation (A) and ethanol content (E).

Sample	Peak 1 Area (%)	Peak 2 Area (%)	Peak 3 Area (%)
KTI	0	53.95	46.05
BBI	0	0	100.00
A-30%	18.23	57.00	24.77
A-40%	14.08	49.48	36.44
A-50%	31.84	33.04	35.13
A-60%	24.07	31.82	46.57
E-20%	27.99	43.96	28.05
E-30%	31.23	36.30	32.47
E-40%	27.20	38.30	34.50
E-50%	36.60	36.40	27.01
E-60%	21.78	29.72	49.07

2.4. Analysis of STI Activity

As shown in Figure 3, the trypsin-inhibitory activity of A-STI was found to be stronger than that of E-STI. Figure 3a illustrates that the trypsin inhibitory activity of STI initially increased and then decreased with increasing ammonium sulfate saturation. A-STI exhibited a maximum trypsin inhibitory activity of 1129 U/mg at 40% ammonium sulfate saturation, possibly attributed to its highest purity level. This result aligns with the findings of the electrophoresis and gel filtration chromatography. Figure 3b shows that the inhibitory activity of STI showed a fluctuating trend (decreasing, then increasing, and then decreasing) as the percentage of ethanol increased. This result may be related to ethanol changing the protein structure. It was shown that the increase in ethanol content would lead to irreversible changes in protein spatial structure, consequently impacting their physicochemical properties and diminishing or even eliminating their original physiological and functional attributes [19].

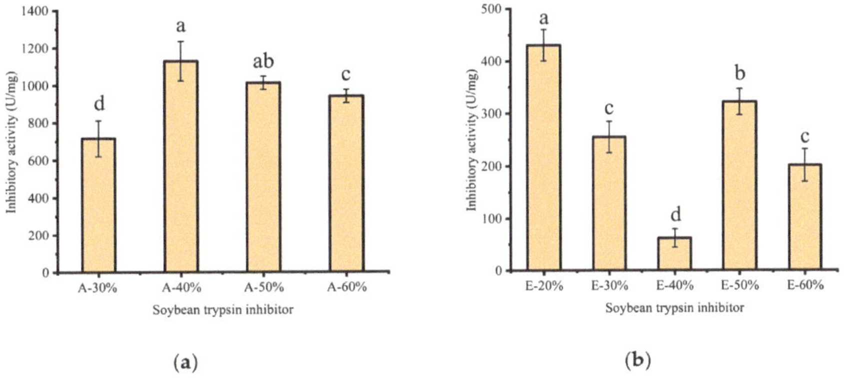

Figure 3. Analysis of STI activity from different methods (A: ammonium sulfate; E: ethanol); Inhibitory activity of STI obtained with different ammonium sulfate saturation (**a**); Inhibitory activity of STI obtained with different ethanol content (**b**); Different lowercase letters indicate significant differences ($p < 0.05$) among the different conditions.

2.5. Effect of Temperature and pH on the Solubility of STI

Solubility is a physical property of substances forming solutions and refers to the ability of a substance to dissolve in a particular solvent. Proteins, as organic macromolecular compounds, exist in a dispersed state (colloidal state) in water. Therefore, the concept of the solubility of proteins in water becomes more nuanced, referring to the degree or extent of protein dispersion within the aqueous medium [20]. The protein solubility characteristics are significant in practical applications, particularly in the context of the extraction, separation, and purification of natural proteins. Changes in protein solubility behavior can also serve as indicators of protein denaturation, in addition to the fact that the application of proteins in beverages is directly related to their solubility properties. As a direct consequence, understanding the solubility of STI holds crucial importance in their isolation and purification and in comprehending their structural and functional properties [21,22].

Figure 4 shows the solubility curves of A-STI and E-STI under different pH and temperature conditions. In Figure 4a, the solubility of A-STI exhibited a characteristic trend of first decreasing and then increasing with the increase in pH within the pH range of 3.0 to 10.0. Notably, the minimum solubility of A-STI occurred at pH 5.0, measuring 67.70%, while the maximum solubility was achieved at pH 10.0, reaching 100%. Similarly, the solubility curves of E-STI showed the same trend as that of A-STI, with decreasing and then increasing patterns. The solubility of E-STI reached its minimum at pH 4.0, measuring 14.59%, and reached its peak at pH 10.0, attaining 75.77%. In summary, the results indicated that the solubility of A-STI was higher than that of E-STI at the same pH value within the pH range of 3.0 to 10.0. This disparity in solubility could be attributed to protein denaturation induced by the high ethanol content. Moreover, A-STI exhibited its lowest solubility at pH 5.0, while E-STI exhibited the lowest solubility at pH 4.0, a phenomenon potentially related to the isoelectric point of STI, which typically corresponds to a protein's lowest solubility state [20].

Protein activity is generally weak at low temperatures; the lower the temperature, the weaker the activity. Increasing the temperature within an appropriate range can significantly enhance protein activity [23]. However, it is essential to note that higher temperatures may induce changes in protein structure, potentially affecting the physicochemical properties of the protein. Figure 4b shows the effect of temperature on the solubility of STI. The results indicated that the solubility of A-STI decreased with the increase in temperature (25 °C→45 °C) and then stabilized (45 °C→85 °C), followed by a subsequent decrease (85 °C→95 °C). Throughout the process, a slight overall reduction in solubility was observed with increasing temperature. In contrast, the solubility of E-STI exhibited an initial increase (25 °C→35 °C) followed by stabilization (35 °C→95 °C). Although the effect of temperature on the solubility of both A-STI and E-STI is not particularly significant, it is evident that temperature does influence their solubility characteristics.

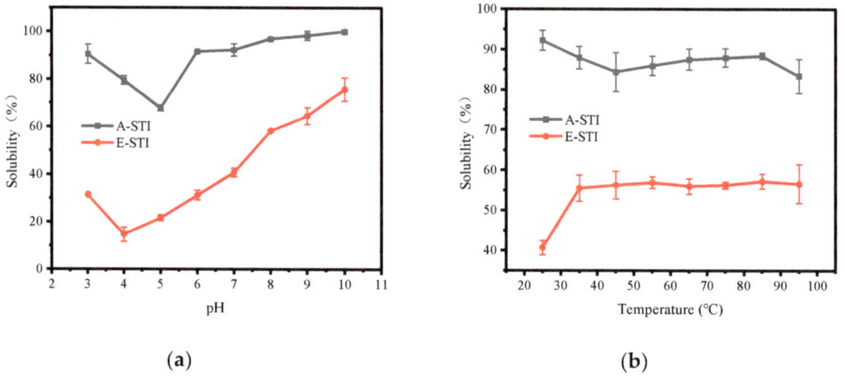

Figure 4. Effect of temperature and pH on the solubility of STI: (**a**) effect of pH on solubility of STI; (**b**) effect of temperature on solubility of STI.

2.6. *Effect of Temperature and pH on the Turbidity of STI*

Turbidity indicates the degree of obstruction caused by suspended particles to light transmission in water [24]. When proteins are dispersed in water, their particle size, shape, and surface area affect light transmission. Therefore, the turbidity value can visually reflect the state of the protein in water. Figure 5 shows the turbidity curves of A-STI and E-STI under various pH and temperature conditions. Figure 5a shows that the absorbance values of both A-STI and E-STI initially increased and then decreased within the pH range of 3.0 to 10.0, reaching their maximum at pH 5.0. This phenomenon indicates that STI at pH 5.0 exhibited excellent particle density, leading to increased light obstruction and, consequently, reflecting its lower solubility, which aligns with the results in Section 3.5. Figure 5b shows that the absorbance value of A-STI gradually increased with the temperature increase from 25 °C to 95 °C, indicating that temperature affects the particle size of STI. Higher temperatures result in reduced light transmission through the protein solution, indicating a decline in STI solubility, which is consistent with the findings presented in Section 3.5. On the other hand, the absorbance value of E-STI showed a trend of increasing and then decreasing with the increase in temperature, indicating that the appropriate increase in temperature can lead to enhanced particle size reduction in E-STI and improved solubility. However, these results are inconsistent with the results in Section 3.5, possibly because the increase in temperature accelerates the aggregated precipitation of particles, altering the absorbance value of STI. When comparing the turbidity of A-STI and A-STI, we find that the absorbance value of A-STI is larger than that of E-STI. This observation may be attributed to A-STI's smaller but more numerous particles, whereas E-STI exhibits larger particles and reduced dispersion, rendering it more prone to precipitation.

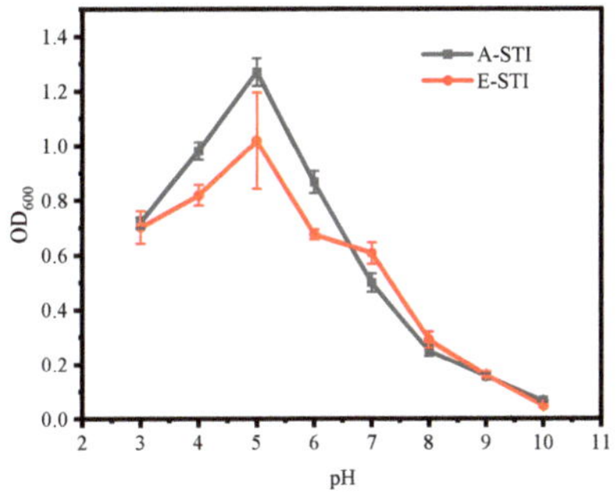

(**a**)

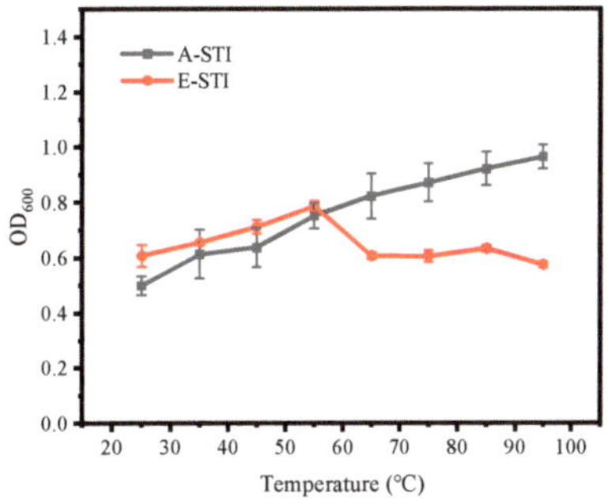

(**b**)

Figure 5. Effect of temperature and pH on the turbidity of STI: (**a**) effect of pH on the turbidity of STI; (**b**) effect of temperature on the turbidity of STI.

2.7. Surface Hydrophobicity Analysis of STI

When the conditions of excitation intensity, wavelength, solvent, and temperature are fixed, the intensity of the emitted light of a substance is proportional to its concentration in solution within a specific concentration range, making it suitable for quantitative analysis. Hydrophobicity is the repulsive force between a non-polar substance and a polar environment. Thermodynamically, it represents the high or low energy required to dissolve a non-polar substance in water or the tendency of the substance to self-aggregate in the aqueous phase, and the greater the tendency for self-aggregation, the stronger the hydrophobicity [25].

Surface hydrophobicity is an essential property of proteins, indicating the physical property of mutual repulsion between protein molecules and water. This characteristic is pivotal in maintaining protein stability, influencing their conformation, and determining their functional activity [26]. Moreover, protein solubility is linked to its surface hydrophobicity, wherein increased hydrophobicity corresponds to reduced protein solubility and vice versa [25]. Therefore, determining the surface hydrophobicity of proteins helps in understanding the interactions between protein molecules, between proteins and other non-protein molecules, and in comprehending the changes in protein properties in different solution environments. Figure 6a,b show the fluorescence intensity plots of A-STI and E-STI at different concentrations, respectively. The results demonstrated that the emission light intensity of both A-STI and E-STI gradually decreased with the decrease in the STI concentration, exhibiting a proportional relationship. Notably, at the same concentration of STI, the emitted light intensity of A-STI was greater than that of E-STI. Figure 6c,d show the slope of the fluorescence intensity as a function of protein concentration for A-STI and E-STI, respectively. The results showed that the surface hydrophobicity index S1 of the A-STI was 528,143.1, while the surface hydrophobicity index S2 of the E-STI was 6,680,619.2. The higher value of S2 compared to S1 indicates that E-STI possesses a more elevated surface hydrophobicity than A-STI. This corresponds to the solubility of A-STI compared with that precipitated by ethanol precipitation. This observation aligns with the solubility characteristics of A-STI compared to that of E-STI, particularly in the context of ethanol precipitation.

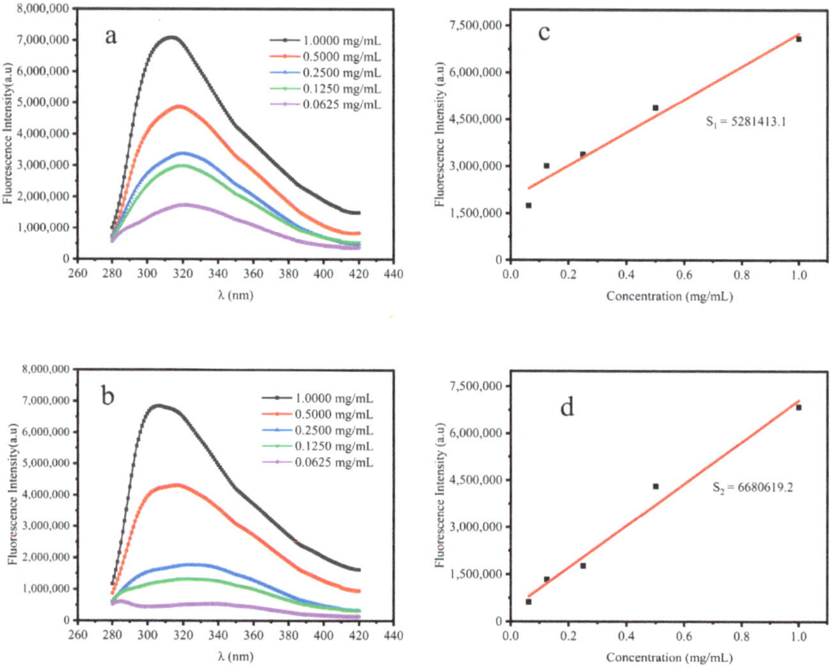

Figure 6. Surface hydrophobicity analysis of STI: (**a**) fluorescence intensity of A-STI; (**b**) fluorescence intensity of E-STI; (**c**) hydrophobicity index of A-STI; (**d**) hydrophobicity index of E-STI.

2.8. Thermal Characterization of STI

Differential Scanning Calorimetry is a widely used technique for assessing the heat absorption and exothermic processes of various materials. In the food field, DSC finds application in characterizing the thermal denaturation temperature of proteins. Figure 7 shows the thermal stability of STI. The results revealed that the thermal stability patterns of A-STI and E-STI exhibited negative single peaks, with both variants demonstrating similar behavior. The thermal transition temperature observed for A-STI was 92.01 °C, while E-STI displayed a slightly higher thermal transition temperature of 93.38 °C. These findings collectively indicate that both A-STI and E-STI possess elevated thermal stability. Moreover, it is noteworthy that the thermal stability of E-STI appears slightly superior to that of A-STI.

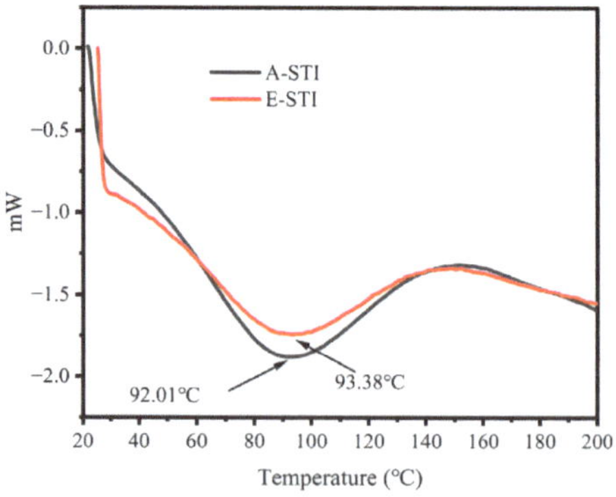

Figure 7. Thermal properties of A-STI and E-STI.

2.9. Surface Structure Analysis of STI

Figure 8 presents the schematic scanning electron microscopy images of STI obtained from soybean whey wastewater using different precipitating agents. Among these images, Figure 8a-1 (A-STI) and Figure 8b-1 (E-STI) show that the STI obtained by different precipitating agents were observed in general agreement at a field of view of 200× magnification, and the microstructure of STI appeared fragmented. However, at a higher magnification of 20,000×, discrepancies in the observed results become apparent. The A-STI (Figure 8a-2) exhibited a smooth surface structure with relatively fewer pores, while the E-STI (Figure 8b-2) displayed a rough surface structure and more pores.

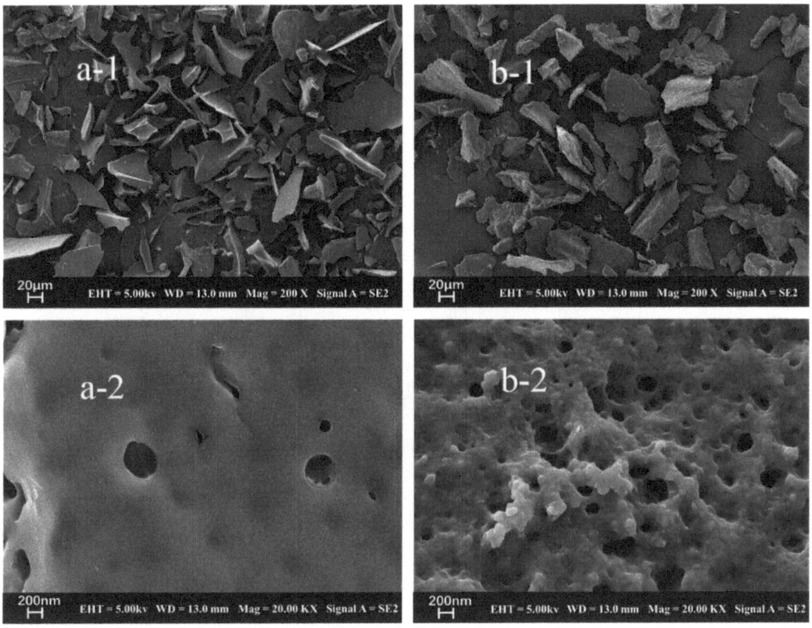

Figure 8. SEM micrographs of A-STI ((**a-1**): 200×, (**a-2**): 20,000×) and E-STI ((**b-1**): 200×, (**b-2**): 20,000×).

3. Materials and Methods

3.1. Feedstocks and Reagents

The Yuwang Ecological Food Industry Co., Ltd. (Dezhou, China) provided a cooled, defatted soybean meal stored at 0~4 °C. The protein marker and loading buffer were obtained from Beijing Solarbio Technology Co., Ltd. (Beijing, China). The trypsin (BAEE > 10,000 Units/mg) was purchased from Shanghai Macklin Biochemical Co., Ltd. (Shanghai, China). The benzoyl-l-arginine-p-nitroaniline (BAPA), KTI (T9128), and BBI (T9777) were obtained from Sigma Chemical Co., Ltd. (St. Louis, MO, USA). All other reagents were of analytical grade.

3.2. Preparation of the Soybean Whey

Soybean whey was prepared according to previous procedures with some modifications [3]. The detailed steps were as follows: Mixing the defatted soybean meal with deionized water at a ratio of 1:10 (*w*/*v*), using 1 M NaOH to adjust the pH of the mixture to 7.5, extracting in a constant temperature water bath at 50 °C for 50 min, and centrifuging at 4000 rpm for 20 min to achieve solid/liquid separation. The supernatant was adjusted to pH 4.5 using 20% HCl and centrifuged to obtain the soybean whey.

3.3. *Preparation of Soybean Whey Concentrate*

The soybean whey obtained from Section 2.2 was added into a rotary evaporation flask and evaporated at 40 °C. Part of the water was removed to obtain the soybean whey concentrate. The obtained soybean whey concentrate volume was 1/3 of the original soybean whey.

3.4. *Enrichment of STI by Ammonium Sulfate Precipitation*

Ammonium sulfate was slowly added to the soybean whey concentrate to achieve different saturation levels: 20%, 30%, 40%, 50%, and 60%, respectively. After standing for 120 min at 4 °C, the solid–liquid separation was performed by centrifuging the mixture at 4000 rpm for 20 min. The resulting precipitate was dissolved using deionized water. The solutions were then dialyzed overnight with dialysis bags with a molecular weight cutoff (MwCO) of 1000 Da (MYM biological technology company limited, Chicago, IL, USA). During dialysis, the deionized water was replaced 2–3 times. The dialysate was freeze-dried and weighed, and the precipitates obtained from each saturation level were marked as A-20%, A-30%, A-40%, A-50%, and A-60%, respectively [3].

3.5. *Enrichment of STI by Ethanol Precipitation Method*

Anhydrous ethanol was slowly added to the soybean whey concentrates to achieve different ethanol content percentages: 20%, 30%, 40%, 50%, and 60% (v/v), respectively. After standing for 120 min at 4 °C, the solid–liquid separation was performed by centrifugation at 4000 rpm for 20 min. The resulting precipitate was dissolved using deionized water. The solutions were then dialyzed overnight using dialysis bags. During dialysis, the deionized water was replaced 2–3 times. The dialysate was freeze-dried and weighed, and the precipitates obtained from each ethanol content level were marked as E-20%, E-30%, E-40%, E-50%, and E-60%, respectively [27,28].

3.6. *Analytical Method*

3.6.1. Calculation of STI Yield

$$\text{Yield (mg/mL)} = \frac{\text{m}}{\text{v}} \times 100\%$$

where m: the mass (mg) of the soybean trypsin inhibitors; v: the volume (mL) of the soybean whey.

3.6.2. Determination of STI Protein Content

The total crude protein of STI was evaluated using automatic Kjeldahl analysis equipment (Kjeltec™ 8400, FOSS, Hillerød, Denmark) and calculated using a protein conversion factor of 5.71 [29].

3.6.3. Analysis of STI Composition by SDS-PAGE

The analysis of STI composition was performed using SDS-PAGE under reducing conditions on a mini-vertical electrophoresis system (Bio-Rad, Hercules, CA, USA) [3,30]. Here, 15% separation gel and 5% concentrated gel were prepared. The different samples were loaded onto the gel at 40 µg. After electrophoresis, a Coomassie brilliant blue G-250 solution was used for staining, and the decolorizing solution was used to remove excess stain. The samples were scanned using a gel electrophoresis imager system (Bio-Rad, Hercules, CA, USA).

3.6.4. Analysis of STI Purity by Gel Filtration Chromatography

STI purity was analyzed using an AKTA protein purification system (Marlborough, MA, USA) [28]. Superdex 75 Increase 10/300 gel filtration pre-loaded columns were equilibrated with three column volumes of 0.2 M phosphate buffer at pH 7.4. STI was re-dispersed in 0.2 M phosphate buffer at a concentration of 2.0 mg/mL. The sample solution was passed over a 0.22 μm aqueous membrane and slowly injected into the AKTA protein purifier with a syringe. The AKTA protein purifier operated at a flow rate of 0.5 mL/min for elution with a detection wavelength of 220 nm.

3.6.5. Determination of the Trypsin Inhibitory Activity

The prepared sample solution (1 mL) and Tris-HCl buffer solution (1 mL) were pipetted into 15 mL tubes. After incubation in a water bath at 37 °C for 10 min, 2.5 mL of a BAPA solution at a concentration of 0.4 mg/mL was added to each tube and mixed, followed by the addition of 1.0 mL of trypsin solution at a concentration of 20 μg/mL. The mixture was allowed to react at 37 °C for exactly 10 min, after which 0.5 mL of acetic acid (30% *v*/*v*) was added to terminate the reaction. A negative control was prepared by adding trypsin only after adding acetic acid [3]. The trypsin inhibitor activity was then calculated by using the following equation:

$$Trypsin\ inhibitor\ activity/(TIU) = [(Ar - Abr) - (As - Abs)] \times \frac{F}{0.02}$$

where *Ar* is the absorbance of the standard solution, *Abr* is the absorbance of the standard blank solution, *As* is the absorbance of the sample solution, *Abs* is the absorbance of the sample blank solution, and *F* is the dilution multiple.

3.6.6. Determination of Solubility

STI solubility was measured using a previously described method with slight modifications [30]. STI (100 mg) was dispersed into 10 mL of deionized water. The pH was adjusted using HCl or NaOH, and the sample suspensions were thoroughly mixed using a magnetic stirring device at different temperatures for 2 h. Temperature (25, 35, 45, 55, 65, 75, 85, 95 °C) and pH (3, 4, 5, 6, 7, 8, 9, 10) were considered. The suspension was centrifuged at 4000 rpm for 10 min to separate the insoluble residues. The protein content of the supernatant was determined using the BCA protein assay kit.

3.6.7. Determination of Turbidity

STI (100 mg) was dispersed into 10 mL of deionized water. The pH was adjusted using HCl or NaOH, and the sample suspensions were thoroughly mixed using a magnetic stirring device at different temperatures for 2 h. Temperature (25, 35, 45, 55, 65, 75, 85, 95 °C) and pH (3, 4, 5, 6, 7, 8, 9, 10) were considered. The suspensions were diluted 5-fold with deionized water and measured by ultraviolet spectrophotometer (Agilent, Santa Clara, CA, USA) at OD600 [31].

3.6.8. Determination of Surface Hydrophobicity

STI samples were serially diluted with 20 mM phosphate buffer at pH 7.4 to obtain different concentrations (0.0625, 0.1250, 0.2500, 0.5000, 1.0000 mg/mL). Then, 20 μL of 8-Anilino-1-naphthalenesulfonic acid (ANS) solution (8 mM ANS in 20 mM phosphate buffer) was added to 4 mL of each sample and shaken for 3 min in the dark. The slope of the fluorescence intensity as a function of protein concentration was used as an index indicating the hydrophobicity surface of the protein using an FS5 fluorescence spectrometer (Edinburgh Instruments, Livingston, UK) with a slit of 1 nm, an excitation wavelength of 260 nm, and an emission wavelength range of 280 nm~420 nm [29,32].

3.6.9. Thermal Characteristics of STI by Differential Scanning Calorimetry

STI (5 mg) was placed in a solid sample crucible while a blank crucible was prepared. The blank crucible was placed on the left side, and the sample crucible containing STI was placed on the right side for DSC analysis with an initial temperature of 40 °C, ramped up at 10 °C/min, and ending at 200 °C.

3.6.10. Morphology of STI by Scanning Electron Microscopy (SEM)

The microstructure of STI was observed using the field-emission SEM (Zeiss Merlin Compact, Jena, Germany) [31]. The samples were sprayed with gold for 45 s using an Oxford Quorum SC7620 sputter coater, followed by a Zeiss Merlin Compact scanning electron microscope to photograph the sample morphology with an accelerating voltage of 3 kV during morphology.

3.7. Data Analysis

SPSS Statistics 19 software (IBM, Chicago, IL, USA) was used for data processing. The experimental data were expressed as "X $\pm$ SD". Significant differences between measurements were set at $p < 0.05$. Origin 2021 software was used for data visualization.

4. Conclusions

In this study, two methods, namely, ammonium sulfate salting out and ethanol precipitation, were successfully employed for enriching STI from soybean whey wastewater. The yield of STI demonstrated a gradual increase with the increase in ammonium sulfate saturation or ethanol content. At 60% ammonium sulfate saturation and 60% ethanol content, the yield of STI surpassed 3.80 mg/mL, with a protein recovery rate exceeding 80%. Regarding purity and trypsin inhibitory activity, the highest levels were achieved at 40% ammonium sulfate saturation. Comparing the solubility of the obtained STI variants, A-STI exhibited better solubility than E-STI. Both A-STI and E-STI exhibited high thermal stability, surpassing 90 °C. Microscopic analysis revealed that both A-STI and E-STI manifested as flakes. However, E-STI showed a rough surface structure with increased pores compared to A-STI.

In future research, we plan to optimize the ammonium sulfate salting out method to enhance the quality and yield of STI from soybean whey wastewater. Additionally, we will explore the potential applications of STI in the food industry.

Author Contributions: Conceptualization, methodology, investigation, formal analysis, software, writing—original draft: Y.Z. (Yongsheng Zhou); conceptualization, formal analysis: S.Z.; methodology, formal analysis: C.L.; resources, supervision, project administration, funding acquisition: Y.Z. (Yihao Zhang); methodology, supervision, writing original draft: H.Z. All authors have read and agreed to the published version of the manuscript.

Funding: This research was supported by the Basic Ability Enhancement Program for Young and Middle-aged Teachers in Guangxi Colleges and Universities, grant number: 2024KY0864.

Institutional Review Board Statement: Not applicable.

Informed Consent Statement: Not applicable.

Data Availability Statement: The data presented in this study are available on request from the corresponding author.

Conflicts of Interest: The authors declare no conflicts of interest.

References

1. Kumar, P.; Sharma, M.; Abubakar, A.A.; Nizam bin Hayat, M.; Ahmed, M.A.; Kaka, U.; Sazili, A.Q. Health implications of plant-based meat analogs. In *Handbook of Plant-Based Meat Analogs*; Academic Press: Cambridge, MA, USA, 2023; pp. 219–231. [CrossRef]
2. Singh, P.; Krishnaswamy, K. Sustainable zero-waste processing system for soybeans and soy by-product valorization. *Trends Food Sci. Technol.* **2022**, *128*, 331–344. [CrossRef]
3. Zhang, Y.; Zhang, Y.; Ying, Z.; Li, W.; Li, H.; Liu, X. Trypsin Inhibitor from Soybean Whey Wastewater: Isolation, Purification and Stability. *Appl. Sci.* **2022**, *12*, 10084. [CrossRef]
4. Jiang, C.; Wu, Z.; Li, R.; Liu, Q. Technology of protein separation from whey wastewater by two-stage foam separation. *Biochem. Eng. J.* **2011**, *55*, 43–48. [CrossRef]
5. Belén, F.; Sánchez, J.; Hernández, E.; Auleda, J.M.; Raventós, M. One option for the management of wastewater from tofu production: Freeze concentration in a falling-film system. *J. Food Eng.* **2012**, *110*, 364–373. [CrossRef]

6. Wang, Y.; Serventi, L. Sustainability of dairy and soy processing: A review on wastewater recycling. *J. Clean. Prod.* **2019**, *237*, 117821. [CrossRef]
7. Chua, J.-Y.; Liu, S.-Q. Soy whey: More than just wastewater from tofu and soy protein isolate industry. *Trends Food Sci. Technol.* **2019**, *91*, 24–32. [CrossRef]
8. Tu, C.; Tang, S.; Azi, F.; Hu, W.; Dong, M. Use of kombucha consortium to transform soy whey into a novel functional beverage. *J. Funct. Foods* **2019**, *52*, 81–89. [CrossRef]
9. Dai, Y.; Zhou, J.; Wang, L.; Dong, M.; Xia, X. Biotransformation of soy whey into a novel functional beverage by Cordyceps militaris SN-18. *Food Prod. Process Nutr.* **2021**, *3*, 13. [CrossRef]
10. Li, X.; Dong, D.; Hua, Y.; Chen, Y.; Kong, X.; Zhang, C. Soybean whey protein/chitosan complex behavior and selective recovery of kunitz trypsin inhibitor. *J. Agric. Food Chem.* **2014**, *62*, 7279–7286. [CrossRef]
11. Cruz-Huerta, E.; Fernandez-Tome, S.; Arques, M.C.; Amigo, L.; Recio, I.; Clemente, A.; Hernandez-Ledesma, B. The protective role of the Bowman-Birk protease inhibitor in soybean lunasin digestion: The effect of released peptides on colon cancer growth. *Food Funct.* **2015**, *6*, 2626–2635. [CrossRef]
12. Fang, E.F.; Wong, J.H.; Ng, T.B. Thermostable Kunitz trypsin inhibitor with cytokine inducing, antitumor and HIV-1 reverse transcriptase inhibitory activities from Korean large black soybeans. *J. Biosci. Bioeng.* **2010**, *109*, 211–217. [CrossRef] [PubMed]
13. de Siqueira Patriota, L.L.; Ramos, D.D.; e Silva, M.G.; dos Santos, A.C.; Silva, Y.A.; de Oliveira Marinho, A.; Coelho, L.C.; Paiva, P.M.; Pontual, E.V.; Mendes, R.L.; et al. The trypsin inhibitor from Moringa oleifera flowers (MoFTI) inhibits acute inflammation in mice by reducing cytokine and nitric oxide levels. *S. Afr. J. Bot.* **2021**, *143*, 474–481. [CrossRef]
14. Arrutia, F.; Binner, E.; Williams, P.; Waldron, K.W. Oilseeds beyond oil: Press cakes and meals supplying global protein requirements. *Trends Food Sci. Technol.* **2020**, *100*, 88–102. [CrossRef]
15. Benelhadj, S.; Gharsallaoui, A.; Degraeve, P.; Attia, H.; Ghorbel, D. Effect of pH on the functional properties of Arthrospira (Spirulina) platensis protein isolate. *Food Chem.* **2016**, *194*, 1056–1063. [CrossRef]
16. Liu, S.; Li, Z.; Yu, B.; Wang, S.; Shen, Y.; Cong, H. Recent advances on protein separation and purification methods. *Adv. Colloid. Interface Sci.* **2020**, *284*, 102254. [CrossRef]
17. Li, C.; Li, W.; Zhang, Y.; Simpson, B.K. Comparison of physicochemical properties of recombinant buckwheat trypsin inhibitor (rBTI) and soybean trypsin inhibitor (SBTI). *Protein. Expr. Purif.* **2020**, *171*, 105614. [CrossRef]
18. O'Fagain, C.; Cummins, P.M.; O'Connor, B.F. Gel-filtration chromatography. *Methods Mol. Biol.* **2011**, *681*, 25–33. [CrossRef]
19. Nikolaidis, A.; Moschakis, T. On the reversibility of ethanol-induced whey protein denaturation. *Food Hydrocoll.* **2018**, *84*, 389–395. [CrossRef]
20. Wouters, A.G.B.; Rombouts, I.; Fierens, E.; Brijs, K.; Delcour, J.A. Relevance of the Functional Properties of Enzymatic Plant Protein Hydrolysates in Food Systems. *Compr. Rev. Food Sci. Food Saf.* **2016**, *15*, 786–800. [CrossRef]
21. Srikar, L.N.; Reddy, G.V.S. Protein solubility and emulsifying capacity in frozen stored fish mince. *J. Sci. Food Agric.* **1991**, *55*, 447–453. [CrossRef]
22. Nguyen, Q.; Hettiarachchy, N.; Rayaprolu, S.; Seo, H.S.; Horax, R.; Chen, P.; Kumar, T.K. Protein-rich beverage developed using non-GM soybean (R08-4004) and evaluated for sensory acceptance and shelf-life. *J. Food Sci. Technol.* **2016**, *53*, 3271–3281. [CrossRef] [PubMed]
23. Bakwo Bassogog, C.B.; Nyobe, C.E.; Ngui, S.P.; Minka, S.R.; Mune Mune, M.A. Effect of heat treatment on the structure, functional properties and composition of Moringa oleifera seed proteins. *Food Chem* **2022**, *384*, 132546. [CrossRef]
24. Holtz, C.; Gastl, M.; Becker, T. Turbidity potentials of single long-chain fatty acids and gelatinised starch in synthetic lautering wort. *Int. J. Food Sci. Technol.* **2015**, *50*, 906–912. [CrossRef]
25. Li, N.; Wang, Y.; Gan, Y.; Wang, S.; Wang, Z.; Zhang, C.; Wang, Z. Physicochemical and functional properties of protein isolate recovered from Rana chensinensis ovum based on different drying techniques. *Food Chem.* **2022**, *396*, 133632. [CrossRef] [PubMed]
26. Zhang, Q.-T.; Tu, Z.-C.; Xiao, H.; Wang, H.; Huang, X.-Q.; Liu, G.-X.; Liu, C.-M.; Shi, Y.; Fan, L.-L.; Lin, D.-R. Influence of ultrasonic treatment on the structure and emulsifying properties of peanut protein isolate. *Food Bioprod. Process* **2014**, *92*, 30–37. [CrossRef]
27. Bartova, V.; Barta, J. Chemical composition and nutritional value of protein concentrates isolated from potato (Solanum tuberosum L.) fruit juice by precipitation with ethanol or ferric chloride. *J. Agric. Food Chem.* **2009**, *57*, 9028–9034. [CrossRef] [PubMed]
28. Nieto-Veloza, A.; Zhong, Q.; Kim, W.S.; D'Souza, D.; Krishnan, H.B.; Dia, V.P. Utilization of tofu processing wastewater as a source of the bioactive peptide lunasin. *Food Chem.* **2021**, *362*, 130220. [CrossRef] [PubMed]
29. Jiang, L.; Song, J.; Qi, M.; Suo, W.; Deng, Y.; Liu, Y.; Li, L.; Zhang, D.; Wang, C.; Li, H. Modification mechanism of protein in rice adjuncts upon extrusion and its effects on nitrogen conversion during mashing. *Food Chem.* **2023**, *407*, 135150. [CrossRef]
30. Zhu, L.; Li, X.; Song, X.; Li, Q.; Zheng, F.; Li, H.; Sun, J.; Huang, M.; Sun, B. Characterization of prolamin recycled from the byproduct of the Baijiu brewing industry (Jiuzao) by SDS-PAGE, multispectral analysis, and morphological analysis. *Food Biosci.* **2022**, *49*, 101854. [CrossRef]

31. Zhang, Y.; Liu, R.; Li, H.; Li, Y.; Liu, X. Interactions between Soybean Trypsin Inhibitor and Chitosan in an Aqueous Solution. *Polymers* **2023**, *15*, 1594. [CrossRef]
32. Cheng, J.H.; Li, J.; Sun, D.W. Effects of dielectric barrier discharge cold plasma on structure, surface hydrophobicity and allergenic properties of shrimp tropomyosin. *Food Chem.* **2023**, *409*, 135316. [CrossRef] [PubMed]

molecules

MDPI

Article

Glassy Powder Derived from Waste Printed Circuit Boards for Methylene Blue Adsorption

Saad Javaid [1], Alessandra Zanoletti [2,3], Angela Serpe [4,5], Elza Bontempi [2,3,*], Ivano Alessandri [1,3,6] and Irene Vassalini [1,3,6,*]

1 Sustainable Chemistry and Materials Laboratory, Department of Information Engineering, University of Brescia, Via Branze 38, 25123 Brescia, Italy; s.javaid@studenti.unibs.it (S.J.); ivano.alessandri@unibs.it (I.A.)
2 Chemistry for Technologies Laboratory, Department of Mechanical and Industrial Engineering, University of Brescia, Via Branze 38, 25123 Brescia, Italy; alessandra.zanoletti@unibs.it
3 Unit of National Interuniversity Consortium for Materials Science and Technology (INSTM), Research Unit of Brescia, Via Branze 38, 25123 Brescia, Italy
4 Department of Civil and Environmental Engineering and Architecture (DICAAR), INSTM Unit, Via Marengo 2, 09123 Cagliari, Italy; serpe@unica.it
5 National Research Council of Italy, Institute of Environmental Geology and Geoengineering (CNR-IGAG), Via Marengo 2, 09123 Cagliari, Italy
6 CNR-INO (National Research Council-National Institute of Optics), Research Unit of Brescia, Via Branze 38, 25123 Brescia, Italy
* Correspondence: elza.bontempi@unibs.it (E.B.); irene.vassalini@unibs.it (I.V.)

Abstract: Electronic waste (e-waste) is one of the fastest-growing waste streams in the world and Europe is classified as the first producer in terms of per capita amount. To reduce the environmental impact of e-waste, it is important to recycle it. This work shows the possibility of reusing glassy substrates, derived from the MW-assisted acidic leaching of Waste Printed Circuit Boards (WPCBs), as an adsorbent material. The results revealed an excellent adsorption capability against methylene blue (MB; aqueous solutions in the concentration range 10^{-5} M–2×10^{-5} M, at pH = 7.5). Comparisons were performed with reference samples such as activated carbons (ACs), the adsorbent mostly used at the industrial level; untreated PCB samples; and ground glass slides. The obtained results show that MW-treated WPCB powder outperformed both ground glass and ground untreated PCBs in MB adsorption, almost matching AC adsorption. The use of this new adsorbent obtained through the valorization of e-waste offers advantages not only in terms of cost but also in terms of environmental sustainability.

Keywords: methylene blue; adsorption; e-waste; recycling; printed circuit boards; glass fibers; water remediation

Citation: Javaid, S.; Zanoletti, A.; Serpe, A.; Bontempi, E.; Alessandri, I.; Vassalini, I. Glassy Powder Derived from Waste Printed Circuit Boards for Methylene Blue Adsorption. *Molecules* **2024**, *29*, 400. https://doi.org/10.3390/molecules29020400

Academic Editor: Stefano Salvestrini

Received: 18 December 2023
Revised: 10 January 2024
Accepted: 11 January 2024
Published: 13 January 2024

1. Introduction

Over the past few years, there has been a dramatic surge in electronic waste (e-waste) [1], primarily driven by the widespread consumption of electronic devices, and also due to the increased home activities, such as smart working, during COVID-19 [2].

In 2019, Norway led the world in per capita e-waste generation, with 28.5 kg per person, just slightly ahead of the United Kingdom and Denmark. During that year, the global e-waste generation surged to around 54 million tons (worldwide; 7.3 kg per capita), with 12 million tons produced in Europe and more than 1 million in Italy alone. Data are summarized in Figure 1 [3].

Moreover, the substantial annual waste generated is expected to continuously increase in the coming years, reaching a value of ~9 kg per capita in 2030, with a global production of about 75 Mt. Consequently, manufacturers have intensified their efforts in the electronics recycling sector, focusing on the production of reconditioned and recycled electronic devices. From 2022 to 2030, a substantial increase in the electronics recycling market is expected. If in 2022, this market's size stood at approximately 40 billion U.S. dollars, it is expected to attain a value of 110.6 billion U.S. dollars by 2030, with an annual growth rate of 13.6% [4].

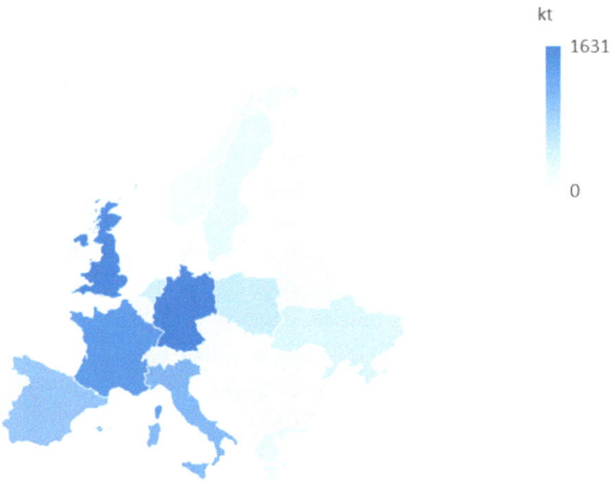

Figure 1. E-waste production in some European countries. Data taken from ref. [3].

Memory cards, such as SD cards, microSD cards, or compact flash cards are examples of e-waste of increasing interest in the recycling market. Unfortunately, they typically contain a combination of materials and units, making their recycling very complex and expensive. So, even if recycling e-waste and reusing their components, with a similar purpose to the original one, remain the preferred approaches, the recovery of all the components is often hindered by the intricate nature of electronic devices [5]. Extended activities in research and procedure optimization have been performed in this sense, leading to the development of specific recycling chains, after the preliminary steps of dismantling, sorting, and mechanical pretreatment (such as shredding and crushing) [6–8].

For example, memory cards, as well as other electronic waste, are often housed in plastic casings, which can be recycled and used in the production of new plastic products [9,10]. Similarly, any paper or plastic labels and printing on the memory card's surface can be separated, and the materials may be recycled or disposed of properly. Simultaneously, memory cards have various metal contact pins or connectors made of precious materials like gold or silver, which can be extracted and refined for reuse or resale [11,12]. Furthermore, memory cards have a small Printed Circuit Board (PCB) responsible for electrical interconnections among different elements. Also, PCBs have an intricate composition: for ~40% wt, they are composed of metals (mainly Cu, Sn, Fe, and Pb, with fractions of Au, Ag, and Pd used as contact materials or plating layers thanks to their electric conductivity and chemical stability); for ~30% wt, they are composed of polymers; while the remaining ~30% wt is made of ceramic–polymeric materials. For ~23% wt, this last component is made of a glassy plastic support, called fiberglass, composed of glass fibers included in an epoxy resin matrix [13]. As anticipated, up to now, the main focus of the recovery processes has been on precious metals that can be extracted from e-waste and recycled [14–17], but waste PCBs (WPCBs) can be repurposed more extensively as a reservoir of raw materials for diverse applications, following a circular economy approach. Considering that any electric and electronic device contains at least one PCB, and that PCBs represent ~8% of the weight of small electronic devices, their recycling is fundamental to reduce the amount of electronic waste. At the same time, they can be considered real "urban mining" sources, enabling the recovery of valuable resources and contributing to sustainability efforts [18]. For example, elastomeric components, such as rubbers or polyurethanes, can exhibit shape memory properties and can be reused in various applications [19], or epoxy resin and polymeric materials may be incinerated for energy recovery [20,21].

The packaging material usually also contains a high amount of silica, which can be easily converted into mesoporous silica and subsequently used as a template for the synthesis of mesoporous carbon [22]. The polymeric components are mainly thermoset resins and reinforcement materials, which can barely be recycled because their crosslinked structure makes their melting impossible using conventional processes. Traditionally, these materials are landfilled or incinerated, but recently their recovery and use as fillers for epoxy or polypropylene resin products, such as paints, adhesives, decorating agents, and building materials, have been proposed [8,23,24].

However, despite the continuous increase in the number of research activities devoted to recycling e-waste, there are only sporadic works focused on the recovery and reuse of glass fibers derived from WPCBs after the extraction of the most valuable components [25], especially in relation to their conversion into adsorbent materials. Furthermore, their field of application is limited to the removal of inorganic ions from water [26–30].

In this work, we aimed to investigate the possibility of valorizing fiberglass residual, converting it into an easily usable adsorbent for the removal of methylene blue (MB) from water. MB is a synthetic dye which is widely used in a large variety of sectors: it is used as a colorant for papers, wool, silk, and cotton, but it is also employed in the food, cosmetics, and pharmaceuticals industries. Although it can be used for some medical treatments, uncontrolled intake via contaminated water can expose humans to various ailments. Similarly, high concentrations of MB in water can create serious hazards to the whole ecosystem [31]. Unfortunately, MB has a strong affinity for water, and it (bio)degrades with difficultly, leading to its accumulation, especially in Asian countries, where the number of textile industries pouring contaminated effluents in natural watercourses is high. The same considerations are valid for various synthetic organic dyes. Their removal through conventional wastewater treatment is limited, and this fact has led the scientific community to devise innovative methods, such as electrocoagulation, photodegradation, biodegradation, or adsorption [32]. Among them, adsorption, consisting of the attraction and anchoring of solute molecules onto the surface of a solid, is one of the favorite strategies thanks to simplicity and affordability, and the high availability of low-cost adsorbent materials [33–35], frequently deriving from biomass or other waste materials [36,37]. In this context, developing high-added-value adsorbent materials from the so-far unexploited residuals of e-waste is an exciting area of study which enables researchers to find a common answer to a couple of environmental concerns: water pollution and waste disposal.

2. Results and Discussion

Waste Printed Circuit Boards (WPCBs) were collected and treated through acidic leaching assisted by microwave heating, as reported in the Materials and Methods section (Section 3), to obtain a solid fraction (MW-treated WPCBs) depleted of metal components and epoxydic resin. The obtained material was analyzed through X-ray diffraction and Raman Spectroscopy to obtain information about its specific chemical composition. As visible from Figure 2a, it was mainly composed of an amorphous fraction, ascribed to amorphous SiO_2 (glass), and crystalline Si, whose diffraction peaks were visible at $2\theta = 28.4°$, $47.3°$, and $56.1°$. A small contribution to the diffraction pattern came also from quartz (crystallin SiO_2), with a small peak centered at $2\theta = 26.6°$.

In Figure 2b, the Raman spectrum is reported, confirming the presence of crystalline Si (Raman peak centered ad 520 cm^{-1}), while no impurities deriving from additional original components of PCBs were detected. These data demonstrated that the grinding and MW-assisted acidic digestion with HNO_3, HCl, and H_2O_2 enabled the removal of the epoxy resin originally contained in the fiberglass substrate (together with glass fibers) and almost all the metallic components (Au, Cu, Ag, Ni, Fe, Al, Mn, Pb, Pb, Sn, Cr, and Zn) previously contained in the WPCBs, in accordance to that reported in [16]. The permanence of crystalline Si, instead, was due to the fact that HF was not used during the leaching process. The obtained powder was also investigated through optical and electronic microscopy, which enabled us to confirm the presence of Si residues and proved the presence of the morphology typical of glass fibers (Figure 2c,d). In Section S1 of the Supplementary Materials, the corresponding energy-dispersive X-ray spectroscopy analysis is reported, which elucidated the presence of minor metallic impurities corresponding to Al, Ti, Cr, and Fe, together with C, F, Ca, and Cl.

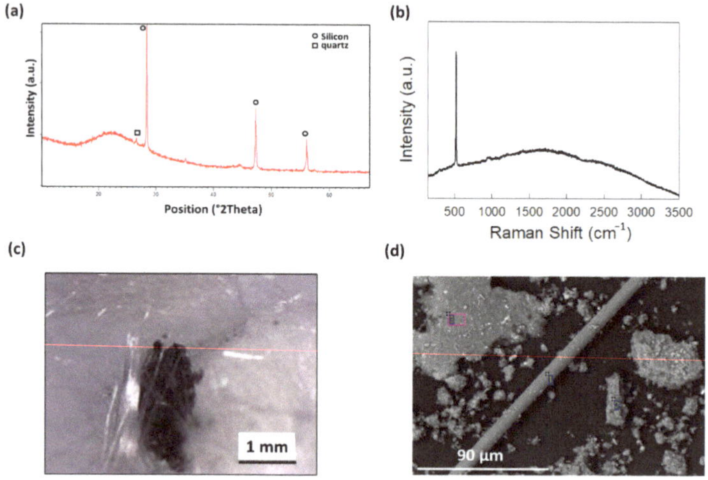

Figure 2. Characterization of MW-treated WPCB samples: (**a**) X-ray diffraction pattern; (**b**) Raman spectrum; (**c**) Stereoscopic Optical Microscopy; (**d**) Scanning Electron Microscopy.

The MW-treated WPCB samples were tested as adsorbents for the removal of organic dyes from mineral water (see Table S1 for water chemical analysis) by putting known amounts of solid samples in contact with 5 mL of methylene blue (MB) 10^{-5} M solutions (measured pH = 7.5) and evaluating the variation in the absorption spectra of the dye solution over the time, as schematized in Figure 3a. The procedure for the adsorption process was kept simple on purpose (no pH variation or buffering, simple agitation by means of magnetic stirring, no heating) in order to match conditions easily applicable in the real world.

Initially, the effect of the granulometry of the MW-treated WPCB samples on the adsorption efficiency was investigated by comparing the adsorption percentage of MB achieved using 3 mg of comminuted MW-treated WPCBs or 3 mg of pulverized MW-treated WPCBs (dosage of adsorbent = 0.6 mg/mL). The results reported in Figure 3b clearly show that further grinding and pulverization after MW acidic treatment of WPCBs was a fundamental step to achieve high adsorption percentages. In fact, in the case of macroscopic fragments (size~0.3 cm^2), the removal of MB, even after 24 h of contact and stirring, was very low (limited to 16%), while it significantly increased up to 89% after proper grinding through a ball mill, obtaining a powder with a granulometry lower than 500 µm. The enhancement of adsorption was evident immediately, just after the first intervals of contact: the pulverized sample was able to outperform the adsorption percentage achieved in 24 h using the coarse-grained samples in less than 1 min (removal efficiency of 38.7%). The reason for this behavior is linked to the fact that smaller granulometry entailed a higher specific surface area, which is an ideal condition for adsorption processes. For this reason, all the subsequent adsorption tests were performed on pulverized MW-treated WPCB samples.

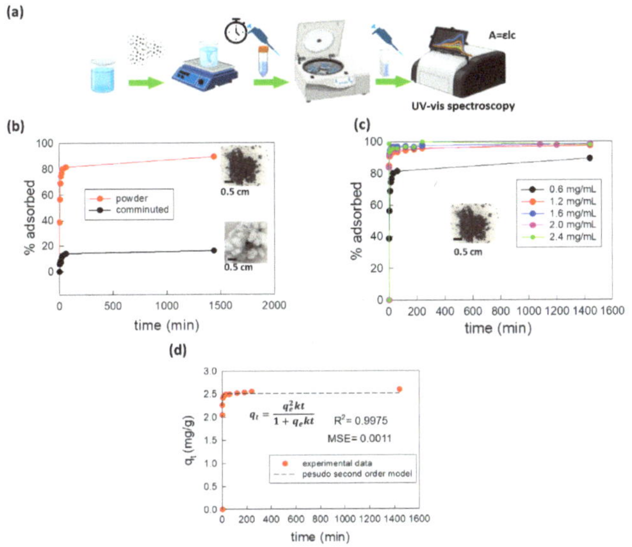

Figure 3. Investigation of the adsorption process of MB (10^{-5} M) on MW-treated WPCB samples at pH = 7.5: (**a**) schematic representation of the adsorption experiments, in accordance with what is described in the Materials and Methods section (Section 3); (**b**) comparison between the percentages of adsorbed MB 10^{-5} M in the time interval 0–24 h, using as the adsorbent MW-treated WPCB samples with different granulometry: comminuted fragments of 0.3 cm^2 (blackline) or fine powder with granulometry <500 µm (red line); (**c**) comparison between the percentages of adsorbed MB 10^{-5} M in the time interval 0–24 h using different amounts of powder derived from MW-treated WPCBs; (**d**) variation in the adsorption capacity of the powder derived from MW-treated WPCBs at the dosage of 1.2 mg/L as a function of soaking time inside the MB 10^{-5} M solution. Points represent the experimental data, while the dashed line represents the results of the fitting using the non-linearized form of the pseudo-second-order model. The high value of the correlation coefficient (R^2) and the low value of the mean sum of squares error (MSE) indicate the goodness of the fit. All the experiments were conducted in triplicate; error bars are included inside dots' size. Figure 3a was created with BioRender.com, accessed on 10 January 2024.

Adsorption could also be enhanced by increasing the amount of adsorbent material, as illustrated in Figure 3c, where the % of removed MB achieved by adding 3, 6, 8, 10, or 12 mg in 5 mL of solution are compared. The most significant difference was observed when passing from a dosage of adsorbent material of 0.6 mg/mL (3 mg in 5 mL of MB solution) to 1.2 mg/mL (6 mg in 5 mL of MB solution), while further dosage increments led to almost un-noticeable adsorption variations: small variations were limited to the first minutes of the adsorption process, while the equilibrium value reached after 24 h remained constant (MB removal efficiency ~98%). For these reasons, all further experiments were conducted considering the adsorbent dose of 1.2 mg/mL.

The obtained data were used for the calculation of the adsorption capacity of the powder derived from MW-treated WPCBs, q_t, corresponding to the amount (mg) of MB adsorbed on their surface over time and normalizing it towards the amount of adsorbent material (g). The variation in q_t as a function of the contact time between the powder and the dye solution is reported in Figure 3d, showing that most of MB was adsorbed in the first 5 min, after which q_t tended to plateau, thanks to an equilibrium being reached between the adsorption of MB molecules on the powder surface and their desorption into the surrounding solution. These features are typical of adsorption processes characterized by a kinetic of the pseudo-second order. Further details regarding the fitting of the adsorption data of MW-treated WPCB powder according to different kinetic models are reported in Section S3 of the Supplementary Materials.

From these results, it was evident that the powder derived from MW-treated WPCBs enabled almost complete MB removal in very easy experimental conditions: no pH buffering, no addition of chemicals, room temperature, and simple agitation. We tried to extend the application of these adsorbents to a higher MB concentration, doubling their value to 2×10^{-5} M (Figure S3). Also in this case, very satisfactory results were obtained: after 1 min of contact and stirring, the powder enabled the removal of 77.5% of the initial MB (in the case of MB 10^{-5} M, the % removed in the first minute was 84.8%), which rapidly increased up to 89.9% at 5 min and reached the equilibrium value of 98.9% after 24 h, even surpassing the value obtained in the case of MB 10^{-5} M solution). Again, the adsorption process followed a kinetic of the pseudo-second order. Interestingly, the obtained value for the equilibrium adsorption capacity (5.27 ± 0.007 mg/g) was more than double the adsorption capacity obtained in the case of MB 10^{-5} M solution ($2 \times 2.59 = 5.18$ mg/g), suggesting that the MW-treated WPCB powder could adsorb an even higher amount of MB.

The adsorption performances of the MW-treated WPCB powder against MB 10^{-5} M were compared with reference samples: commercial activated carbons (ACs), untreated PCBs, and glass. All the samples were considered in the form of powder (untreated PCBs and glass were ground, as described in the Materials and Methods section (Section 3)), and all the experimental conditions (MB concentration, not-buffered pH (pH = 7.5), mineral water, room temperature, stirring at 700 rpm, adsorbent dosage of 1.2 mg/mL) were maintained constant.

Activated carbons were selected because they can be considered the commercial standard for industrial adsorption processes; untreated PCBs were selected to verify if the performed MW treatment and acidic leaching influenced the adsorption process; glass was selected as reference material with a chemical composition similar to that of MW-treated WPCB samples.

The obtained results in terms of q_t are reported in Figure 4a, while the correlated percentage of adsorbed MB 10^{-5} M for selected significant time intervals is reported in Figure 4b.

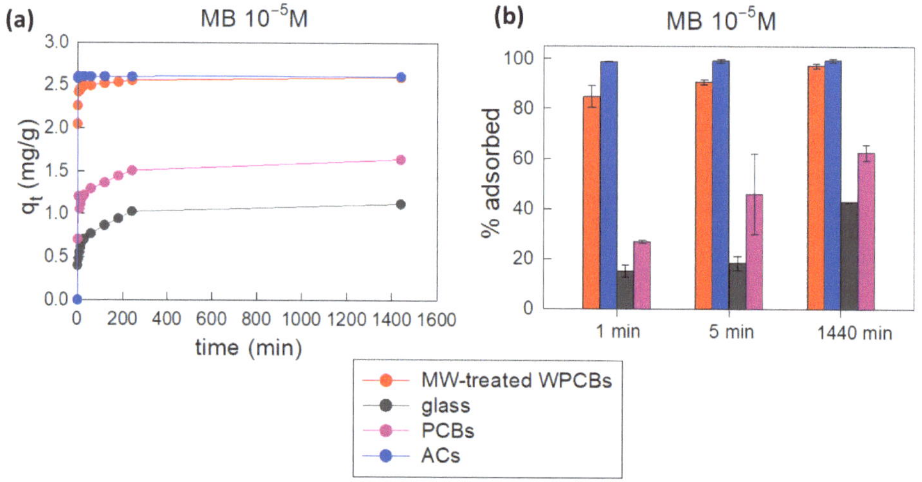

Figure 4. Comparison between the adsorption capacity of MW-treated WPCB powder and those of reference materials (ACs, glass powder, and ground untreated PCBs) during the adsorption of MB (10^{-5} M): (**a**) variation in adsorption capacities as a function of time in relation to MB 10^{-5} M; (**b**) comparison between the percentage of adsorbed MB 10^{-5} M at selected time intervals. All the experiments were conducted in triplicate, where non-visible error bars are included inside dots' size.

From these data, it is evident that the MW-treated WPCB powder outperformed both ground glass and ground untreated PCBs in MB adsorption, almost matching ACs. It seems that Si and other minor impurities contaminating the glass matrix in the MW-treated WPCBs sample, as well as the fiber morphology, enabled a better interaction with MB in comparison to simple glass. In particular, the morphological effect has already been observed by Chakrabarti and Dutta [38], who showed that glass fibers contain microcracks capable of harboring MB molecules, leading to higher adsorption in comparison to borosilicate glass.

Data reported in Figure 4a,b also suggest that metal leaching through MW acidic treatment was fundamental to maximize MB adsorption, probably thanks to an increase in the material porosity and surface area, as well as a reduction in positive charges on the adsorbent surface due to metals. During this process, various metals were removed from the fiberglass substrate, leaving empty spaces and enabling more direct contact between the dye molecules in the solution and silica, which is the primary constituent of glass. Considering that at pH = 7.5 MB is a cationic dye and silica is negatively charged at pH > 3 (pzc of SiO_2 2–4 [39]), the above-described conditions are ideal for enhancing MB adsorption. However, it was quite surprising that the powder derived from the MW-treated WPCBs was able to almost match the adsorption performances of ACs: even if ACs were characterized by a slightly faster adsorption process in the first minutes, the two types of materials reached the same equilibrium values of q_t (2.59 $\pm$ 0.02 mg/g for MW-treated WPCBs and 2.61 $\pm$ 0.02 mg/g for ACs) and percentages of adsorbed MB (97.3 $\pm$ 0.9% for MW-treated WPCBs and 99 $\pm$ 1% for ACs) in 24 h. Given that the MW-treated WPCB powder was obtained from a waste material, it can be considered a very promising alternative to commercial adsorbents, characterized by lower price and higher environmental sustainability. Additionally, ACs and MW-treated PCBs seemed to be characterized by the same kinetic behavior, since their experimental data can be satisfactorily fitted following a pseudo-second-order kinetic model (see Figure S4a): very fast adsorption occurred in the first few minutes, followed by a prolonged process of continuous adsorption/desorption of MB molecules, leading to a dynamic equilibrium being reached. In the case of glass and untreated PCBs, adsorption instead occurred more gradually and the best kinetic model for the fitting of the experimental data resulted to be the Elovich model (Figure S4b,c).

In view of these promising results, we investigated the possibility of using MW-treated WPCB powder for the adsorption of methylene orange (MO), and we compared its activity with that of ACs, glass powder, and not-treated PCB powder. The same experimental conditions were considered: adsorbent materials at the dosage of 1.2 mg/mL, room temperature, no pH buffering (pH = 7.5), dye concentration equal to 10^{-5} M, and mineral water. The obtained results are reported in Figure S5a (variation in q_t as a function of time) and S5b (comparison between the percentage of MO adsorbed at selected time intervals). It is clearly visible that in this case, the MW-treated WPCB powder was able to remove only a limited percentage of the dye and had a significantly lower adsorption capacity in comparison to commercial ACs.

While MB is a cationic dye, MO is characterized by a negative charge at approximately neutral pH (experimental pH of dye solutions was 7.5). One of the reasons for the different behavior of the MW-treated WPCB powder could be linked to the fact that it adsorbed dye mainly through electrostatic interactions, thanks to the presence of a net electrostatic charge on its surface. We measured the surface charge of ground MW-treated WPCBs through Dynamic Light Scattering, and it resulted to be slightly negative, equal to -23 ± 6 mV, in line with the value reported by Tsai and Horng [40] in relation to waste fiberglass. Consequently, they should be capable of adsorbing cationic dyes, like MB, while they would not be ideal for the interaction and removal of anionic dyes, such as MO. We also measured the surface charge of Acs, which resulted to be negative too (-26 ± 1 mV). However, ACs are composed of piled stacks of 2–10 small aromatic and graphitic layers with a size of about 1 nm combined with disorganized carbon units, mainly aliphatic chains, which are present in the periphery of the aromatic layers and work as cross-linkage structures.

This "turbostratic structure" was confirmed in the batch of ACs we used as reference, as demonstrated by the XRD pattern reported in Figure S6a, and was characterized by the presence of two broad peaks centered at 25°, corresponding to the (002) set of planes, and at around 44°, which corresponds to the (100/101) set of planes [41]. Each of the piled stacks was mainly characterized by a graphitic structure, as visible in the associated Raman spectrum reported in Figure S6b, which shows only the peaks ascribable to the typical D (associated with sp^3 carbon atoms and defects in a graphene layer) and G bands (associated with the sp^2 carbon atoms forming the graphene skeleton), centered at 1350 cm^{-1} and 1600 cm^{-1}, respectively, with no contribution from other organic functional groups, in accordance with previous studies [42].

The above-described organic structure with a high number of aromatic units enables the interaction with and adsorption of various organic dyes and pollutants, independently from their charge, thanks to the insurrection of π-π interactions. This fact, together with the well-known enhanced specific surface area, can justify the higher performance of ACs, as regards both MB and MO.

From Figure S5, it is visible that both glass powder and the powder obtained from untreated PCBs were able to absorb a slightly higher percentage of MO in comparison to MW-treated WPCBs. Even if their adsorption capabilities were significantly lower than that of ACs, after 24 h glass removed ~12% of MO, and untreated PCBs removed ~23% of MO, leading to adsorption efficiencies higher than the ~5% achieved by the MW-treated WPCB samples. As reported in Figure S7a, the X-ray diffractogram of untreated PCBs was characterized by the presence of peaks representative of crystallin copper, aluminum silicate, and $FeAl_2$, in addition to the features typical of quartz and amorphous silica, also maintained in the samples which underwent the MW treatment. The presence of these components at the atomic level at a higher concentration in comparison to the MW-treated WPCBs was also confirmed through SEM and EDX analysis (Figure S7c). Furthermore, the MW treatment enabled the removal of the epoxy resin, which, together with glass fibers, constituted the fiberglass substrate. Its presence, instead, was clearly visible in the Raman spectrum reported in Figure S7b, which was characterized by the presence of peaks centered at 690 cm^{-1} (aromatic C-H out-of-plane deformation), 770 cm^{-1} (C3-C2 skeletal), 1220 and 1290 cm^{-1} (C-O stretching, 1450 cm^{-1} due to $-CH_3$ bending), and 1550 cm^{-1} (stretching of C=C bonds of the aromatic rings) [43].

It is probable that this organic component was responsible for the increased MO adsorption in the case of untreated PCB samples. Similarly to what happened in the case of ACs, it could improve π-π interactions between the solid and the organic dye in solution, facilitating its adsorption. However, untreated PCBs also did not enable a complete removal of MO, maintaining performance values well under those achieved by employing commercial adsorbents. Further studies will be performed to extend the activity of MW-treated WPCBs to the adsorption of anionic dyes, such as MO, or other classes of water contaminants, and to test the possibility of subsequent degradation of adsorbed pollutants, but these promising results related to MB adsorption pave the way for the development of systems capable of environmental remediation starting from e-waste.

3. Materials and Methods

3.1. MW-Treated WPCB Samples' Preparation and Characterization

The MW-treated WPCB samples represent the non-metal fraction deriving from waste Random Access Memory (RAM) electronic boards obtained as a solid residue of their acidic digestion. This fraction counts for the 40% wt of the starting material. Specifically, 200 g of RAMs of different origin were roughly milled for 24 h in a stainless-steel jar by means of hard metal balls (Ø 6 mm, 1.4 kg) in a planetary apparatus (4-stage Retsch mill, 300 rpm) in the presence of Carbsyn 110 (250 mL), as described in [16]. The final slurry was separated from the hard metal balls using sieves with grates of 4 mm. Then, Carbsyn was recovered via distillation, and the milled sample was collected and dried. Aliquots of the comminuted sample were weighed and then digested under microwaves into TFM vessels containing a mixture of HNO_3 (65%, 2 mL), HCl (37%, 6 mL), and H_2O_2 (30%, 0.5 mL). The treatment was performed using a Milestone Ethos 1 Microwave digester (Milestone srl, Sorisole (BG), Italy), equipped with an HPR1000/10S high-pressure segmented rotor, an ATC-400CE automatic temperature control, and a Terminal 640 with easy-CONTROL software, applying a microwave program consisting of two steps lasting 10 and 20 min, respectively, at a temperature of 220 °C and microwave power up to 1000 W. Digested samples were washed three times with Milli-Q water and once with acetone, and left to dry.

The obtained comminuted fraction was characterized by a granulometry of about 0.3 cm^2, and it was further ground through ball milling (MM400, Retsch, Haan, Germany) until reaching a fine powder: 2–4 mL of samples corresponding to ~25 mg of MW-treated WPCB fragments were inserted in a stainless-steel jar (total volume: 10 mL) together with 7 steel balls (Ø 7 mm) and the instrument was activated at a frequency of 25 Hz for 3 min. The obtained powder was sieved with grates of 500 μm.

The crystallographic structure and chemical composition of the obtained powder were investigated usin X-ray diffraction (Panalytical (Malvern, UK) diffractometer using Cu Ka (1.5406 Å) radiation and operating at 40 kV and 40 mA) and Raman Spectroscopy (Labram HR-800 spectrophotometer (Horiba/Jobin Yvon, Kyoto, Japan) equipped with a He−Ne laser source (λ = 632.8 nm); the acquisition time was 10 s, laser power was attenuated to 0.3 mW (10% filter)). Its morphology was investigated through Stereoscopic Microscopy (Leica MZ 16 A coupled with software Leica Qwin (Leica, Wetzlar, Germany) and Scanning Electron Microscopy (FEI NOVA 600 (FEI, currently Thermofisher, Eindhoven, The Netherlands)).

The surface charge was measured through Dynamic Light Scattering (DLS, Nanolink S900, Linkoptik (Zhuhai, China)).

3.2. *Reference Adsorbents Preparation and Characterization*

The adsorption performances of the MW-treated WPCB powder were compared with those of commercial activated carbon (DARCO, Sigma Aldrich, St. Louis, MO, USA) and powders obtained from not-treated PCBs and glass slides. In particular, a glass slide and a PCB sample were manually fragmented and subjected to ball mill fragmentation: ~2 mL of each sample (~100 mg) was inserted in a stainless-steel jar (total volume: 10 mL) together with 7 steel balls (Ø 7 mm), and the instrument was activated at a frequency of 25 Hz. The grinding process lasted for 3 min in the case of glass, while it was extended up to 9 min in the case of PCB samples. Both the obtained powders were sieved with grates of 500 μm. Their characterization was performed similarly to what is reported in the previous section in relation to the MW-treated WPCBs.

3.3. *Adsorption Experiments*

Known amounts (3, 6, 8, 10, 12 mg) of MW-treated WPCB samples were added to 5 mL of methylene blue (MB) or methyl orange (MO) solutions with a concentration of 10^{-5} M prepared using mineral water (chemical analysis reported in Table S1), and they were left under stirring at 700 rpm for at least 24 h. In the case of MB, concentration 2×10^{-5} M was also tested. After regular time intervals (1, 5, 10, 15, 20, 30, 60, 120, 180, 240, and 1440 min), each sample was centrifuged at 9000 rpm for 4 min at 22 °C (Neya 16R centrifuge) to separate the solid from the liquid phase, which was analyzed through UV-vis spectroscopy (QE 65000 Ocean Optics Spectrometer, Orlando, FL, USA).

Absorption spectra were recorded and the changes in the absorbance intensity at 660 nm for MB and at 460 nm for MO were measured.

The percentage of adsorbed pollutant was calculated as follows:

$$\%\, Adsorbed = \frac{A_0 - A_t}{A_0} \times 100$$

where A_0 corresponds to value of absorbance of the starting solution of MB or MO and A_t corresponds to the absorbance measured at time t, after the addition of the adsorbent material. The obtained data were used for the calculation of q_t, which represents the amount of adsorbed MB or MO per gram of adsorbent (mg g^{-1}) at any time t (min). At the end of the adsorption test, it was possible to calculate the value of q_e (mg g^{-1}), which corresponds to the equilibrium adsorption capacity.

The experimental data were fitted using the Solver add-in program of Excel using the not-linearized equations of the pseudo-first-order model, pseudo-second-order model, Elovich model, and intraparticle diffusion model [44]. Further details can be found in Section S3 of the Supplementary Materials.

The adsorption performances of the powder derived from MW-treated WPCBs were compared with the adsorption capacity of analogous powders obtained from not-treated PCBs, glass slides, and commercial activated carbon (DARCO), keeping all the experimental parameters constant (room temperature, sampling times, mineral water, 10^{-5} M dye concentration, no pH adjustment, adsorbent dose of 1.2 mg/mL).

All the experiments were performed in triplicate.

The pH of the solutions was measured by means of the SI Analytics, Lab 845, pH meter and resulted to be 7.5.

4. Conclusions

In this work, we demonstrated that by performing acidic digestion assisted by MW heating it was possible to leach metals and epoxy resin from waste PCBs, leading to the production of a Si-enriched glassy substrate. After its grinding into a powder with a granulometry lower than 500 μm, it was possible to achieve a powder characterized by an excellent adsorption capability against MB (in the concentration range 10^{-5} M–2×10^{-5} M, pH = 7.5). Although its adsorption performance was limited to cationic dye, it was able to match the activity of commercial activated carbons during MB removal, significantly outperforming similar powders obtained from the grinding of glass slides or un-treated PCB samples. The here-developed adsorbent was characterized by an intrinsic low cost, since it was obtained through the valorization of wastes, limiting not only the costs of raw materials but also those of the disposal of the original waste, with clear advantages in comparison to commercial activated carbons (~250 EUR/kg). Furthermore, following this approach based on the principles of circular economy, it was possible to limit the CO_2 emissions linked to the conventional disposal of PCBs in landfills, paving the way for the development of highly sustainable adsorbents and extending the potential sectors in which e-waste can find application through appropriate recycling processes.

Supplementary Materials: The following supporting information can be downloaded at https://www.mdpi.com/article/10.3390/molecules29020400/s1, Section S1: EDX analysis of MW-treated WPCBs; Section S2: Chemical analysis of mineral water used for the preparation of dye solutions; Section S3: Identification of the best kinetic model for the fitting of MB adsorption data of MW-treated PCBs; Section S4: Adsorption of MB at various concentrations; Section S5: Fitting of MB adsorption data obtained using different adsorbent materials; Section S6: Adsorption of MO 10^{-5} M; Section S7: Structural and chemical characterization of activated carbons, used as reference material; Section S8: Structural and chemical characterization of powder derived from untreated PCBs, used as reference material.

Author Contributions: Conceptualization, I.V. and I.A.; methodology, I.V. and A.Z.; formal analysis, S.J., A.Z. and I.V.; investigation, S.J., A.Z. and I.V.; data curation, I.V.; writing—original draft preparation, I.V.; writing—review and editing, S.J., A.Z., A.S., E.B., I.A. and I.V.; visualization, I.V. and A.Z.; supervision, E.B., I.A. and I.V.; project administration, A.S. and E.B.; funding acquisition, A.S. and E.B. All authors have read and agreed to the published version of the manuscript.

Funding: This research was founded by the Italian Ministry of the Ecological Transition, in the framework of the project "Sustainable MAterials Recycling Technology for Printed Circuits Boards-SMART PCBs"—CUP F57G20000050001.

Institutional Review Board Statement: Not applicable.

Informed Consent Statement: Not applicable.

Data Availability Statement: The data are reported within the article and in the Supplementary Materials.

Acknowledgments: The authors thank Leonardo Lauri for the SEM analysis and Serena Ducoli for assisting during DLS measurements. Graphical abstract and Figure 3a were created with BioRender.com, accessed on 10 January 2024.

Conflicts of Interest: The authors declare no conflicts of interest.

References

1. Liu, K.; Tan, Q.; Yu, J.; Wang, M. A global perspective on e-waste recycling. *Circ. Econ.* **2023**, *2*, 100028. [CrossRef]
2. Zanoletti, A.; Cornelio, A.; Bontempi, E. A post-pandemic sustainable scenario: What actions can be pursued to increase the raw materials availability? *Environ. Res.* **2021**, *202*, 111681. [CrossRef] [PubMed]
3. Forti, V.; Baldé, C.P.; Kuehr, R.; Bel, G. *The Global E-waste Monitor 2020: Quantities, Flows, and the Circular Economy Potential*; United Nations University/United Nations Institute for Training and Research, International Telecommunication Union, and International Solid Waste Association: Bonn, Germany; Geneva, Switerland; Rotterdam, The Netherlands, 2020.
4. Research and Markets. *Electronics Recycling—Global Strategic Business Report*; Research and Markets: Dublin, Ireland, 2023.
5. Mir, S.; Dhawan, N. A comprehensive review on the recycling of discarded printed circuit boards for resource recovery. *Resour. Conserv. Recycl.* **2022**, *178*, 106027. [CrossRef]
6. Niu, B.; Shanshan, E.; Xu, Z.; Guo, J. How to efficient and high-value recycling of electronic components mounted on waste printed circuit boards: Recent progress, challenge, and future perspectives. *J. Clean. Prod.* **2023**, *415*, 137815. [CrossRef]
7. Wang, J.; Xu, Z. Disposing and recycling waste printed circuit boards: Disconnecting, resource recovery, and pollution control. *Environ. Sci. Technol.* **2015**, *49*, 721–733. [CrossRef] [PubMed]
8. Tembhare, S.P.; Bhanvase, B.A.; Barai, D.P.; Dhoble, S.J. E-waste recycling practices: A review on environmental concerns, remediation and technological developments with a focus on printed circuit boards. *Environ. Dev. Sustain.* **2022**, *24*, 8965–9047. [CrossRef]
9. Grigorescu, R.M.; Grigore, M.E.; Iancu, L.; Ghioca, P.; Ion, R.M. Waste electrical and electronic equipment: A review on the identification methods for polymeric materials. *Recycling* **2019**, *4*, 32. [CrossRef]
10. Elvinger, J.; Preiss, I.; Törneling, C.; Markus, R.; Roessing, E.; Coelho, J.; Williams, A.; Meisenzahl, M. *EU Actions and Existing Challenges on E-Waste Review*; European Court of Auditors: Luxembourg, 2021.
11. Do Nascimento, J.D.R.V.; Wohnrath, K.; Garcia, J.R. Synthesis of gold nanoparticles using recovered gold from electronic waste. *Orbital Electron. J. Chem.* **2021**, *13*, 153–159. [CrossRef]
12. Lu, Y.; Xu, Z. Recycling non-leaching gold from gold-plated memory cards: Parameters optimization, experimental verification, and mechanism analysis. *J. Clean. Prod.* **2017**, *162*, 1518–1526. [CrossRef]
13. Luda, M.P. Recycling of Printed Circuit Boards. In *Integrated Waste Management—Volume II*; Kumar, S., Ed.; InTech: London, UK, 2011; pp. 285–298. ISBN 978-953-307-447-4.
14. Ulman, K.; Ghose, A.; Maroufi, S.; Mansuri, I.; Sahajwalla, V. Disentanglement of random access memory cards to regenerate copper foil: A novel thermo-electrical approach. *Waste Manag.* **2018**, *81*, 138–147. [CrossRef]
15. Hu, M.; Wang, J.; Xu, Z. Pyrolysis-Based Technology for Recovering Copper from Transistors on Waste Printed Circuit Boards. *ACS Sustain. Chem. Eng.* **2017**, *5*, 11354–11361. [CrossRef]
16. Rigoldi, A.; Trogu, E.F.; Marcheselli, G.C.; Artizzu, F.; Picone, N.; Colledani, M.; Deplano, P.; Serpe, A. Advances in Recovering Noble Metals from Waste Printed Circuit Boards (WPCBs). *ACS Sustain. Chem. Eng.* **2019**, *7*, 1308–1317. [CrossRef]
17. Barragan, J.A.; Ponce De León, C.; Alemán Castro, J.R.; Peregrina-Lucano, A.; Gómez-Zamudio, F.; Larios-Durán, E.R. Copper and Antimony Recovery from Electronic Waste by Hydrometallurgical and Electrochemical Techniques. *ACS Omega* **2020**, *5*, 12355–12363. [CrossRef]
18. Hadi, P.; Xu, M.; Lin, C.S.K.; Hui, C.W.; McKay, G. Waste printed circuit board recycling techniques and product utilization. *J. Hazard. Mater.* **2015**, *283*, 234–243. [CrossRef] [PubMed]
19. Reghunadhan, A.; Jibin, K.P.; Kaliyathan, A.V.; Velayudhan, P.; Strankowski, M.; Thomas, S. Shape memory materials from rubbers. *Materials* **2021**, *14*, 7216. [CrossRef]
20. Sahle-Demessie, E.; Mezgebe, B.; Dietrich, J.; Shan, Y.; Harmon, S.; Lee, C.C. Material recovery from electronic waste using pyrolysis: Emissions measurements and risk assessment. *J. Environ. Chem. Eng.* **2021**, *9*, 104943. [CrossRef] [PubMed]
21. Shen, Y.; Chen, X.; Ge, X.; Chen, M. Chemical pyrolysis of E-waste plastics: Char characterization. *J. Environ. Manag.* **2018**, *214*, 94–103. [CrossRef]
22. Liou, T.H.; Jheng, J.Y. Synthesis of High-Quality Ordered Mesoporous Carbons Using a Sustainable Way from Recycling of E-waste as a Silica Template Source. *ACS Sustain. Chem. Eng.* **2018**, *6*, 6507–6517. [CrossRef]
23. Zheng, Y.; Shen, Z.; Cai, C.; Ma, S.; Xing, Y. The reuse of nonmetals recycled from waste printed circuit boards as reinforcing fillers in the polypropylene composites. *J. Hazard. Mater.* **2009**, *163*, 600–606. [CrossRef]
24. Wang, Q.; Zhang, B.; Yu, S.; Xiong, J.; Yao, Z.; Hu, B.; Yan, J. Waste-Printed Circuit Board Recycling: Focusing on Preparing Polymer Composites and Geopolymers. *ACS Omega* **2020**, *5*, 17850–17856. [CrossRef]

25. Zheng, Y.; Shen, Z.; Ma, S.; Cai, C.; Zhao, X.; Xing, Y. A novel approach to recycling of glass fibers from nonmetal materials of waste printed circuit boards. *J. Hazard. Mater.* **2009**, *170*, 978–982. [CrossRef] [PubMed]
26. Hadi, P.; Barford, J.; McKay, G. Toxic heavy metal capture using a novel electronic waste-based material—Mechanism, modeling and comparison. *Environ. Sci. Technol.* **2013**, *47*, 8248–8255. [CrossRef] [PubMed]
27. Hadi, P.; Barford, J.; McKay, G. Selective toxic metal uptake using an e-waste-based novel sorbent-Single, binary and ternary systems. *J. Environ. Chem. Eng.* **2014**, *2*, 332–339. [CrossRef]
28. Hadi, P.; Gao, P.; Barford, J.P.; McKay, G. Novel application of the nonmetallic fraction of the recycled printed circuit boards as a toxic heavy metal adsorbent. *J. Hazard. Mater.* **2013**, *252–253*, 166–170. [CrossRef]
29. Xu, M.; Hadi, P.; Chen, G.; McKay, G. Removal of cadmium ions from wastewater using innovative electronic waste-derived material. *J. Hazard. Mater.* **2014**, *273*, 118–123. [CrossRef]
30. Mariyam, S.; Zuhara, S.; Al-Ansari, T.; Mackey, H.; McKay, G. Novel high capacity model for copper binary ion exchange on e-waste derived adsorbent resin. *Adsorption* **2022**, *28*, 185–196. [CrossRef]
31. Oladoye, P.O.; Ajiboye, T.O.; Omotola, E.O.; Oyewola, O.J. Methylene blue dye: Toxicity and potential elimination technology from wastewater. *Results Eng.* **2022**, *16*, 100678. [CrossRef]
32. Samsami, S.; Mohamadi, M.; Sarrafzadeh, M.H.; Rene, E.R.; Firoozbahr, M. Recent advances in the treatment of dye-containing wastewater from textile industries: Overview and perspectives. *Process Saf. Environ. Prot.* **2020**, *143*, 138–163. [CrossRef]
33. Vassalini, I.; Ribaudo, G.; Gianoncelli, A.; Casula, M.F.; Alessandri, I. Plasmonic hydrogels for capture, detection and removal of organic pollutants. *Environ. Sci. Nano* **2020**, *7*, 3888–3900. [CrossRef]
34. Vassalini, I.; Gjipalaj, J.; Crespi, S.; Gianoncelli, A.; Mella, M.; Ferroni, M.; Alessandri, I. Alginate-Derived Active Blend Enhances Adsorption and Photocatalytic Removal of Organic Pollutants in Water. *Adv. Sustain. Syst.* **2020**, *4*, 1900112. [CrossRef]
35. Vassalini, I.; Maddaloni, M.; Depedro, M.; De Villi, A.; Ferroni, M.; Alessandri, I. From Water for Water: PEDOT: PSS-Chitosan Beads for Sustainable Dyes Adsorption. *Gels* **2024**, *10*, 37. [CrossRef]
36. Zanoletti, A.; Vassura, I.; Venturini, E.; Monai, M.; Montini, T.; Federici, S.; Zacco, A.; Treccani, L.; Bontempi, E. A new porous hybrid material derived from silica fume and alginate for sustainable pollutants reduction. *Front. Chem.* **2018**, *6*, 60. [CrossRef] [PubMed]
37. Rafatullah, M.; Sulaiman, O.; Hashim, R.; Ahmad, A. Adsorption of methylene blue on low-cost adsorbents: A review. *J. Hazard. Mater.* **2010**, *177*, 70–80. [CrossRef] [PubMed]
38. Chakrabarti, S.; Dutta, B.K. On the adsorption and diffusion of Methylene Blue in glass fibers. *J. Colloid Interface Sci.* **2005**, *286*, 807–811. [CrossRef] [PubMed]
39. Kosmulski, M. The pH dependent surface charging and points of zero charge. VIII. Update. *Adv. Colloid Interface Sci.* **2020**, *275*, 102064. [CrossRef]
40. Tsai, C.K.; Horng, J.J. Transformation of glass fiber waste into mesoporous zeolite-like nanomaterials with efficient adsorption of methylene blue. *Sustainability* **2021**, *13*, 6207. [CrossRef]
41. Girgis, B.S.; Temerk, Y.M.; Gadelrab, M.M.; Abdullah, I.D. X-ray Diffraction Patterns of Activated Carbons Prepared under Various Conditions. *Carbon Sci.* **2007**, *8*, 95–100. [CrossRef]
42. Shimodaira, N.; Masui, A. Raman spectroscopic investigations of activated carbon materials. *J. Appl. Phys.* **2002**, *92*, 902–909. [CrossRef]
43. Chike, K.E.; Myrick, M.L.; Lyon, R.E.; Angel, S.M. Raman and near-infrared studies of an epoxy resin. *Appl. Spectrosc.* **1993**, *47*, 1631–1635. [CrossRef]
44. Wang, J.; Guo, X. Adsorption kinetic models: Physical meanings, applications, and solving methods. *J. Hazard. Mater.* **2020**, *390*, 122156. [CrossRef]

molecules

MDPI

Article

Selective Co(II) and Ni(II) Separation Using the Trihexyl(tetradecyl)phosphonium Decanoate Ionic Liquid

Anđela Kovačević [1], José Alejandro Ricardo García [1], Marilena Tolazzi [1], Andrea Melchior [1,*] and Martina Sanadar [2]

[1] Chemical Technologies Laboratories, Polytechnic Department of Engineering, University of Udine, Via Cotonificio 108, 33100 Udine, Italy; kovacevic.andela@spes.uniud.it (A.K.); ricardogarcia.josealejandro@spes.uniud.it (J.A.R.G.); marilena.tolazzi@uniud.it (M.T.)

[2] Centre de Biophysique Moléculaire, CNRS, UPR 4301, Université d'Orléans, Rue Charles Sadron, 45071 Orléans, Cedex 2, France; martina.sanadar@cnrs-orleans.fr

* Correspondence: andrea.melchior@uniud.it

Abstract: The room temperature ionic liquid trihexyl(tetradecyl)phosphonium decanoate ([P_{66614}][Dec]) was employed in the liquid-liquid extraction of Co(II) from hydrochloric acid solutions in the presence of Ni(II). The extraction performance in liquid-liquid separations showed a strong dependence on the acid content of the feed aqueous solution. The best performance in terms of extracted cobalt and selectivity was obtained when the feed contained a HCl concentration above 6 M On the contrary, when the experiment was performed in absence of HCl, a lower extraction and Co/Ni selectivity were obtained. This behavior has been rationalized by considering the protonation of the $[Dec]^-$ anion and the different Co(II)/Ni(II) speciation in HCl media. Moreover, polymer inclusion membranes (PIMs) were prepared using PVC and [P_{66614}][Dec] at different weight rations. Only the PIM formulated with a 30:70/PVC:[P_{66614}][Dec] weight ratio demonstrated effective extraction of Co(II) from the HCl solution. The extraction efficiency and selectivity of the PIM was comparable to that from biphasic liquid experiments at 8 M HCl. The results of this study constitute a promising background for further practical developments of carboxylate-based ILs applied in Co/Ni separations.

Keywords: ionic liquids; cobalt; nickel; separation; polymer inclusion membranes

Citation: Kovačević, A.; Ricardo García, J.A.; Tolazzi, M.; Melchior, A.; Sanadar, M. Selective Co(II) and Ni(II) Separation Using the Trihexyl(tetradecyl)phosphonium Decanoate Ionic Liquid. *Molecules* **2024**, *29*, 4545. https://doi.org/10.3390/molecules29194545

Academic Editors: Giuseppina Raffaini and Fabio Ganazzoli

Received: 23 August 2024
Revised: 17 September 2024
Accepted: 19 September 2024
Published: 25 September 2024

1. Introduction

It is estimated that more than 1.2 million tons of Li-ion batteries enter the European Union each year, with global demand predicted to grow considerably over the next five years [1]. As a result, the demand for Co(II), an essential element for manufacturing several types of Li-ion battery cathodes, is projected to increase 20 times by 2050 [2,3]. Over half of the global Co supply comes from the Democratic Republic of the Congo, where extraction is associated with significant social and political issues [4]. This steep increase in consumption is in turn projected to lead to corresponding waste generation, which needs to be addressed to protect the environment and to recover valuable critical raw materials (CRMs) [5,6].

Several types of extractive metallurgy still face a difficult challenge in separating Co(II) from Ni(II) due to the similarities in the chemical properties of these two elements [7]. The Co/Ni separation holds crucial importance for the production of these transition metals and their corresponding salts from primary ores, including Ni-Cu sulfides [8] and Ni laterite ores [9]. End-of-life battery recycling is also an area of active research because of the high material value and potential toxicity of the waste [10]. Recycling Co from spent Li-ion battery cathodes, such as nickel manganese cobalt oxide (NMC), could significantly reduce the pressure due to mining activity.

Hydrometallurgical processes [11] have the notable advantages of producing highly pure products and being much less energy intensive than pyrometallurgical processes [12]. However, the volatile organic compounds (VOCs) employed as solvents in combination with extracting ligands pose significant safety and environmental risks. Acidic extractants like organophosphorus acids (D2EHPA, PC88A, Cyanex 272, and Cyanex 302) [13,14] have been used for Co-Ni separations but exhibit low selectivity and require strict pH control [15–17]. Moreover, combined hydro/pyrometallurgical approaches have also been considered [18].

More recently, ionic liquids (ILs) have been proposed as a safer and more efficient media for metal ion extraction and selective separation [11,19,20]. Fluorinated hydrophobic ILs have been employed for solvent extraction [21–26]; however, these ILs do have certain disadvantages, including their high cost and persistence in the environment [27]. Such drawbacks could be reduced if the components of the ILs are derived from renewable biomaterials [28], thus being less expensive and more sustainable. In long-chain fatty acid ionic liquids (LCFA-ILs) the main physicochemical properties are strongly related to the alkyl chain length and the degree of saturation [29,30]. These ILs have been explored as green alternatives to conventional hydrophobic ILs in liquid–liquid extraction, where they have shown the ability to effectively extract metals [31,32] and phenols [33] from aqueous solutions. Furthermore, research has also indicated that these ILs possess antimicrobial properties [34].

Many applications of phosphonium-based ILs in metal separations have been reported in the literature. Mo(VI) with trihexyl(tetradecyl)phosphonium bromide, [P_{66614}][Br] [35], Pd(II) extraction as well as Fe(III) separation from Ni(II) with trihexyl(tetradecyl) phosphonium chloride, [P_{66614}][Cl] [36,37], extraction of Eu(III) and other rare-earth elements with trihexyl(tetradecyl)phosphonium nitrate, [P_{66614}][NO_3] [38], and Co(II) from Sm(III) using [P_{66614}][Cl] [39]. As far as the application of phosphonium-based ILs in Li-ion cathode battery recycling is concerned, several works have been published [40–42].

Besides the simple liquid-liquid separations, polymeric membranes can be employed in combination with ILs to fabricate composite systems (polymer inclusion membranes, PIMs). Among various membrane technologies, PIMs stand out as self-supported liquid membranes, gaining prominence due to their straightforward preparation, reusability [43,44], stability [44,45], and low toxicity [46–48]. The PIM is placed between the feed aqueous phase containing the metals and the receiving phase where the separated metals are stripped [49]. One notable advantage of PIMs is the reduced amount of IL employed with respect to liquid-liquid biphasic systems, which is important, as one of the main issues limiting industrial applications of ILs is their high cost. Moreover, in the membrane-based process, the extraction and stripping occur in a single stage.

In this framework, the aim of the present study is to assess the application of [P_{66614}][Dec] (trihexyl(tetradecyl)phosphonium decanoate, Figure 1) in the extraction of Co(II) from an aqueous phase and the separation from Ni(II). The carboxylate moiety can act as a complexing group and therefore allow extractions without the use of auxiliary ligands in the organic phase. Moreover, the decanoate anion can be considered as a model of a biomass-derived fatty acid which is more biocompatible than other anions employed in commercial hydrophobic ILs [28].

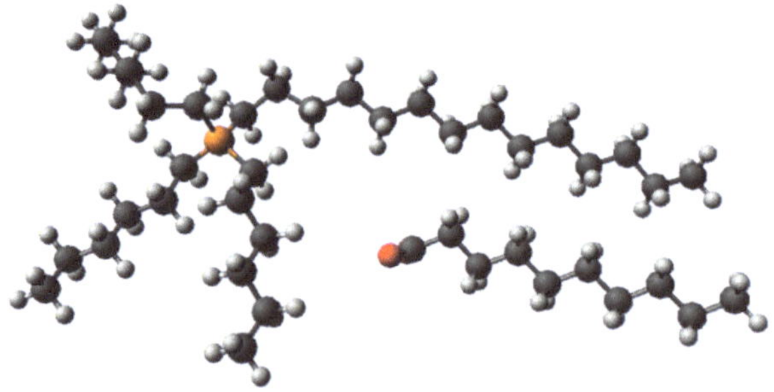

Figure 1. Structure of [P_{66614}][Dec].

While this IL has been previously mainly employed in the extraction of organic molecules from aqueous solutions [50–53], to date, only one study on metal ion extraction (La(III) and Yb(III) [54]) has been published.

In the present study, first the performance of the IL is studied in liquid-liquid extractions of Co(II) and Ni(II) from aqueous solutions containing different concentrations of HCl and NaCl with the aim of obtaining the conditions for best extraction and selectivity in separation. Then, a series of PIMs containing different weight fractions of [P_{66614}][Dec] are prepared, characterized, and tested for metal extractions.

2. Results and Discussion

2.1. Liquid-Liquid Extractions

This section examines how different HCl concentrations impact the extraction of Co(II) and Ni(II) using [P_{66614}][Dec]. Such acidic media have been selected as HCl is often used for leaching battery cathodes [55].

Different extraction efficiencies (E%) were obtained for Co(II) and Ni(II) as the HCl concentration was increased (Figure 2). The distribution coefficients (D) of metal ions between organic and aqueous phase are reported in Table S1.

The remarkable selectivity for Co(II) at 8 M HCl for [P_{66614}][Dec] is comparable to the data obtained previously with [P_{66614}][Cl] [56,57]. This result was not influenced by the presence of Ni(II), as can be deduced from Figure S3 where the E(%) for extractions are from solutions containing Co(II) only.

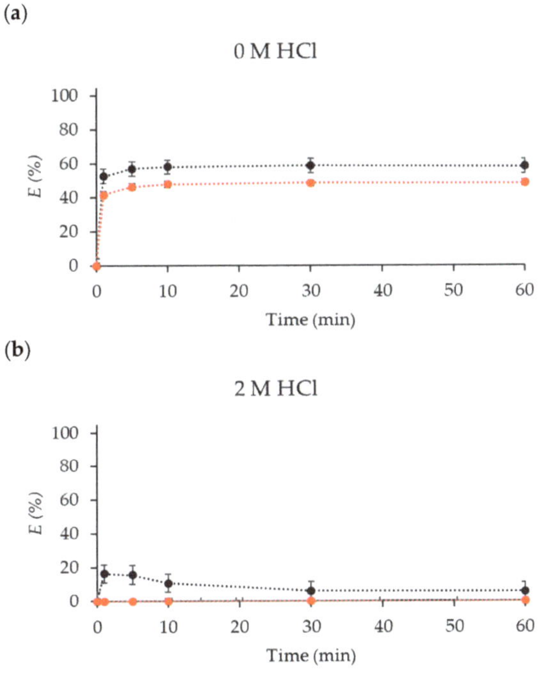

Figure 2. *Cont.*

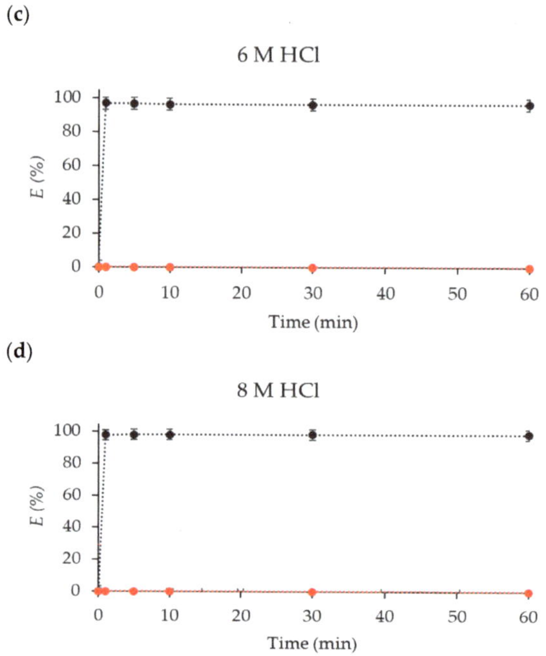

Figure 2. *E*(%) of Co(II) (black) and Ni(II) (red) in (**a**) 0 M HCl, (**b**) 2 M HCl, (**c**) 6 M HCl, and (**d**) 8 M HCl media at different times. Initial concentrations: $[Co]_{aq} = [Ni]_{aq} = 50$ mM.

The distinct extraction efficiencies of Co(II) and Ni(II) can be attributed to their different speciation in the aqueous phase [56,58–60]. It is well known that in concentrated chloride solutions Co(II) is able to form stable complexes with chloride anions, and different speciation models including up to 1:4 Co:Cl species [61–64]. Recent studies [65,66] suggest that in the HCl concentration range between 0 M and 11 M the dominant species in solution are the 1:1 $[CoCl]^+$ and the tetrahedral 1:4 $[CoCl_4]^{2-}$ (Figure 3). On the contrary, Ni(II) mainly forms one 1:1 species [67], $[NiCl]^+$, which retains the octahedral coordination mode in aqueous solutions (Figure S1).

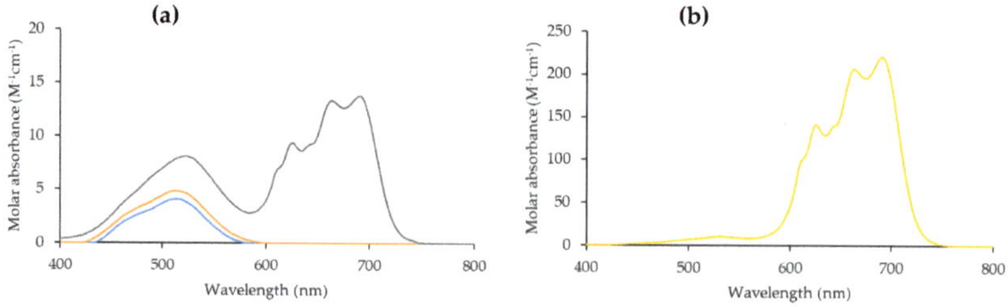

Figure 3. Absorption spectrum of Co(II) aqueous phase in (**a**) 0 M HCl (blue), 2 M HCl (orange), 6 M HCl (grey) and (**b**) 8 M HCl (yellow).

The UV-Vis absorption spectrum of the IL phase after extraction from 8 M HCl (Figure 4) corresponds to that of the $[CoCl_4]^{2-}$ complex, as it is nearly superimposable with that recorded after the extraction using $[P_{66614}][Cl]$ in the same conditions, where the coordination of tetrahedral Co(II) has been established previously [56].

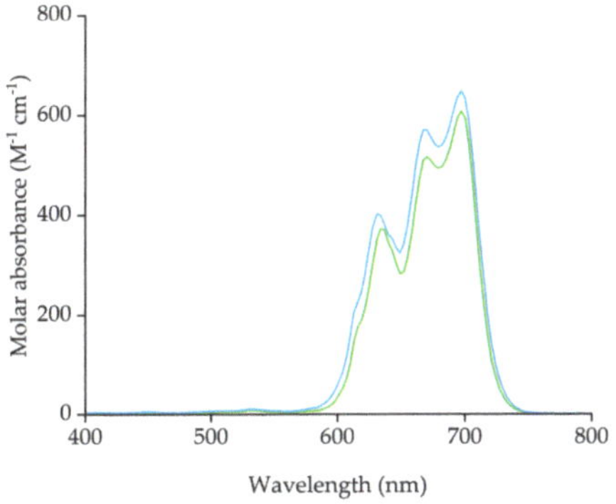

Figure 4. Absorption spectrum of the IL phase after extraction from 8 M HCl in $[P_{66614}][Dec]$ (blue) and $[P_{66614}][Cl]$ (green).

The extraction from an aqueous solution where $CoCl_2$ and $NiCl_2$ were dissolved in pure water (measured pH = 5.7) presents an extraction efficiency of 52.7% for Co(II) and 41.9% for Ni(II).

The spectra for the IL phase Co(II) (Figure 5) with a maximum absorption at λ = 573 nm (ε_{573} = 38.7 M^1 cm^{-1}), is intermediate between that of Co(II) in water (max. λ = 515 nm, ε_{515} = 5.14 M^{-1} cm^{-1}) and that of Co(II) acetate salt in anhydrous $[P_{66614}][Dec]$ (max. λ = 580 nm, ε_{580} = 201.9 M^{-1} cm^{-1}). The spectra of the extracted Ni(II) with $[P_{66614}][Dec]$ is depicted in Figure S2 (max. λ = 328 nm, ε_{328} = 15.9 M^{-1} cm^{-1}). It can therefore be proposed that in $[P_{66614}][Dec]$ both Co(II) and Ni(II) are extracted as octahedral species by coordination with the $[Dec]^-$ anions and water in their coordination spheres.

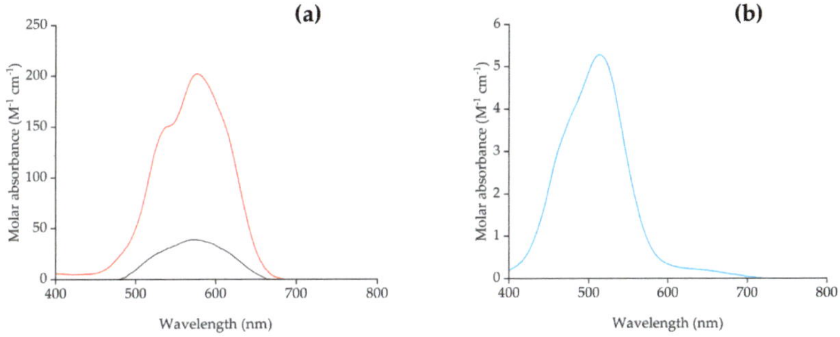

Figure 5. Absorption spectrum of (**a**) $CoCl_2$ extracted in $[P_{66614}][Dec]$ from aqueous solution (black) λ = 573 nm (ε_{573} = 38.7 M^{-1} cm^{-1}), and $Co(CH_3COO)_2$ in dry $[P_{66614}][Dec]$ (red) (max. λ = 580 nm, ε_{580} = 201.9 M^{-1} cm^{-1}); (**b**) $CoCl_2$ in water (blue) (max. λ = 515 nm, ε_{515} = 5.14 M^{-1} cm^{-1}).

On the basis of the above results, the extraction of Co(II) with $[P_{66614}][Dec]$ can be explained using different equilibria depending on the HCl concentration. In absence of chloride (0 M HCl) the extraction occurs through the equilibrium (1) as previously proposed for other phosphonium ILs [68]:

$$M^{2+} + 2Cl^- + \overline{2[P_{66614}][Dec]} \rightleftharpoons \overline{2[P_{66614}]Cl} + \overline{MDec_2} \quad (1)$$

M = Co, Ni

As in such conditions the extraction occurs through coordination of the metal ions, the low selectivity towards Co(II) can be explained by the similar affinity of the carboxylate group towards Co(II) and Ni(II).

On the contrary, in the conditions where Co(II) ions exist as anionic chloro-complexes, the following extraction equilibrium [68] can be proposed:

$$[CoCl_4]^{2-} + 2H^+ + \overline{2[P_{66614}][Dec]} \rightleftharpoons \overline{[P_{66614}]_2[CoCl_4]} + \overline{2DecH} \quad (2)$$

Unlike the extractions with $[P_{66614}][Br]$ and $[P_{66614}][Cl]$, which are based on an anion exchange mechanism [56,57,68–70] (i.e., the anion is transferred to the aqueous phase), for $[P_{66614}][Dec]$ the protonation/deprotonation state of the IL anion changes [68]. As discussed later (Section 2.3), in the stripping process with pure water, the protons are released to the aqueous phase.

Based on the equilibrium (2), the low extraction from 2 M HCl solution can be explained by the fact that in such condition a negligible amount of $[CoCl_4]^{2-}$ species is formed (if the model in ref. [65] is assumed), and decanoate anions are protonated due to the high acid concentration, hence the metal ion coordination by $[Dec]^-$ anion is suppressed.

Extraction experiments with NaCl (2 and 4 M) in the feed were also carried out (*D* values in Table S1). At higher concentrations (>5 M) NaCl is not completely soluble. It was found that extraction efficiency of Co(II) using $[P_{66614}][Dec]$ increased with increasing chloride concentration, but Ni(II) was also extracted at the same time (Figure 6). The spectra of the IL phase after extraction of Co(II) (Figure 7) suggests a mechanism similar to that from pure water. At higher concentrations of NaCl (>4 M), a colloidal phase is formed [71].

(**a**)

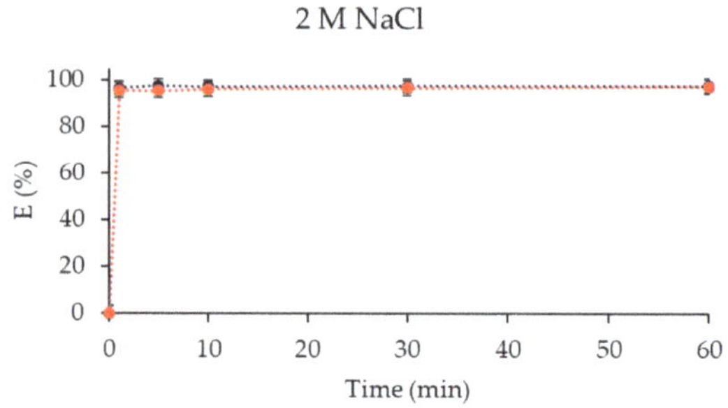

(**b**)

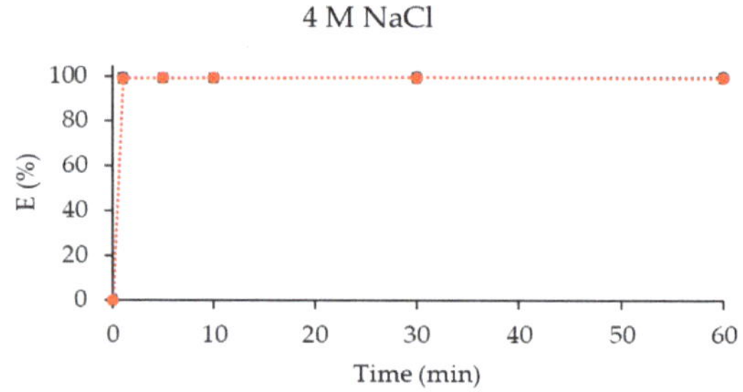

Figure 6. Co(II) (black) and Ni(II) (red) *E*(%) from aqueous NaCl solutions; (**a**) 2 M NaCl, (**b**) 4 M NaCl. $[Co]_{aq} = [Ni]_{aq} = 50$ mM.

Interestingly, the spectrum of the IL phase after extraction from 2 M NaCl (Figure 7) indicates that an octahedral Co(II) species is formed, and suggests that the process proceeds through the complexation of the metal ion by decanoate. The fact that the extraction from 2M NaCl is higher than that from water could be assigned to the salting out effect [56].

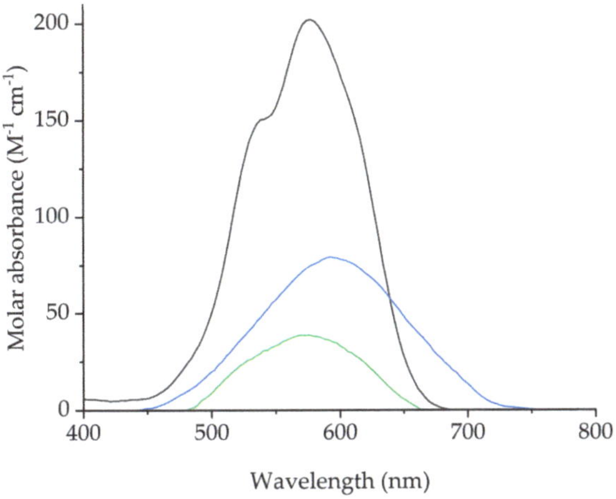

Figure 7. Absorption spectrum of $CoCl_2$ extracted in $[P_{66614}][Dec]$ from aqueous solution (0 M HCl, green) λ = 573 nm (ε_{573} = 38.7 M^{-1} cm^{-1}), $Co(CH_3COO)_2$ in dry $[P_{66614}][Dec]$ (black) (max. λ = 580 nm, ε_{580} = 201.9 M^{-1} cm^{-1}), and of the $[P_{66614}][Dec]$ IL phase after extraction of Co(II) in 2 M NaCl solution (blue) (max. λ = 595 nm, ε_{595} = 79 M^{-1} cm^{-1}).

2.2. *Effect of Temperature*

The extraction of Co(II) was performed at six different temperatures (15–65 °C) from pure water and 6 M HCl (Figure 8).

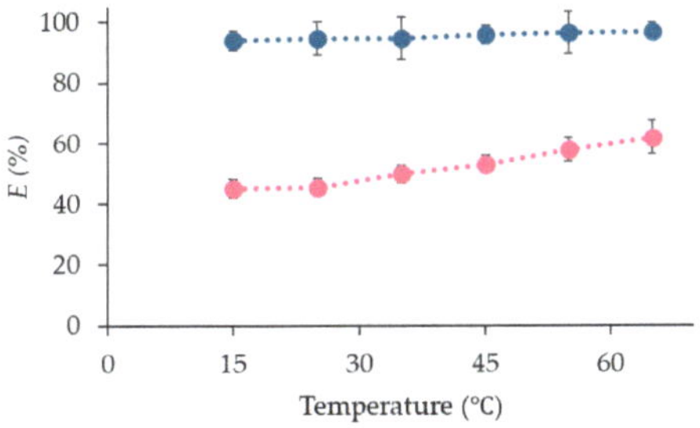

Figure 8. Extraction efficiency of Co(II) from pure water (pink) and from 6 M HCl (blue) at different temperatures.

Temperature does not significantly affect the extraction of Co(II) from HCl. However, when Co(II) is extracted from pure water, the process becomes slightly more favorable at higher temperatures. The fact that E(%) is similar at room temperature and elevated temperatures indicates that the separation can be performed without additional heating, resulting in substantial savings in both energy and cost.

2.3. *Stripping of Co(II)*

After the first cycle of equilibration of the metal-containing IL phase with pure water, up to 80% of stripped Co(II) was obtained. More cycles are needed to completely strip the IL of its Co(II) content using only water (Figure 9 and Table S2). The equilibrium (3) is therefore reached:

$$\overline{2[P_{66614}][CoCl_4]} + \overline{2DecH} \rightleftharpoons Co^{2+} + 4Cl^- + \overline{2[P_{66614}][Dec]} + 2H^+ \quad (3)$$

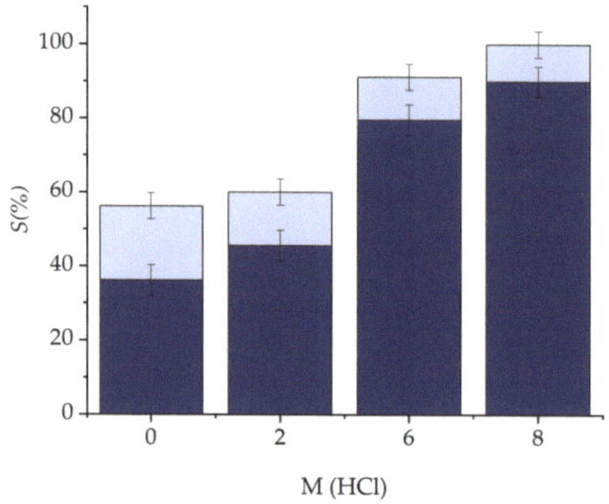

Figure 9. Cumulative stripping (*S*%) of Co(II) from [P_{66614}][Dec] extracted from different HCl feeds (M HCl) utilizing only water. Dark blue in one step, dark blue + light blue after two steps.

Moreover, the 64.4% of Ni(II) was stripped from the IL phase using water after two consecutive cycles from pure water media. The total Co(II) recovery (Equation (7)) is shown in Figure 10.

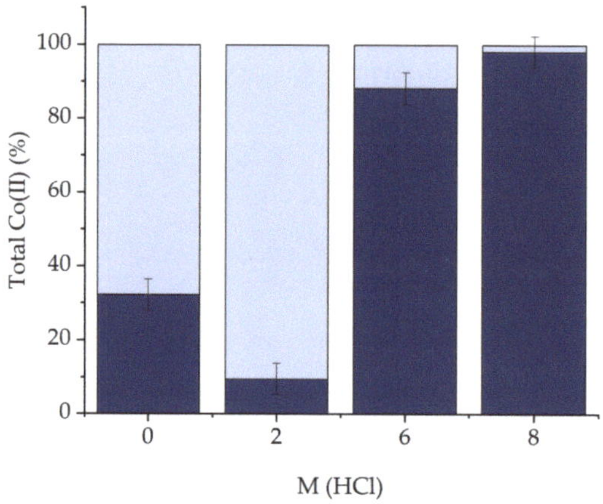

Figure 10. In dark blue, the percentage of recovered Co(II) from 0 to 8 M HCl media. Dark blue + light blue, total Co(II) present in the experiment.

The best conditions for separation of Co(II) from Ni(II) are extraction from 8 M HCl and stripping with water, which was implemented in the membrane separation experiment.

2.4. Membrane Characterization

PIMs were produced by combining PVC and [P_{66614}][Dec] at different weight ratios (20, 50, 70%). Average thickness of the membranes was 0.115 ± 0.02 mm. The resulting PIMs were characterized by means of spectroscopic, mechanical, and thermal properties.

As can be seen in Figure 11, the tensile strength is strongly affected by the composition. The PIM with 20% of [P_{66614}][Dec] shows similar behavior as pure PVC [72], while the membranes with 50% and 70% of [P_{66614}][Dec] display typical stress–strain curves (Figure 11) for flexible materials [73]. The addition of IL [P_{66614}][Dec] to PVC increases elongation at rupture, but decreases the tensile strength of the membrane, which is due to its plasticizing properties [74].

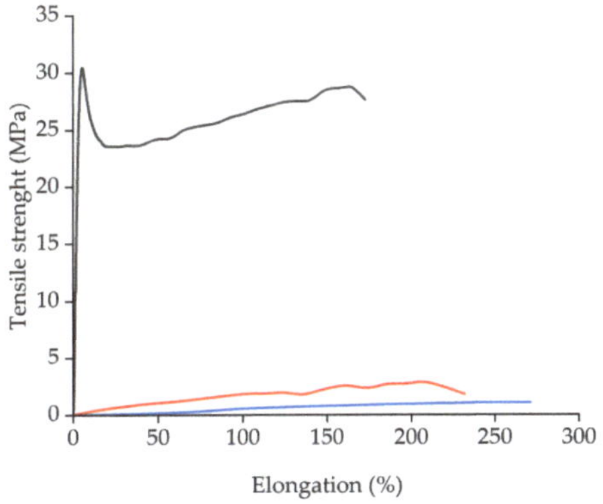

Figure 11. Stress–strain curves of PVC: [P_{66614}][Dec] (80:20) black, PVC: [P_{66614}][Dec] (50:50) red, and PVC: [P_{66614}][Dec] (30:70) blue.

Water-membrane contact angle was measured to assess the effect of the IL on the wettability of the PIM. Good wettability of the membrane is important for successful metal transport [75]. In Table 1 the contact angles are shown for the compositions of the PIMs tested in this work.

Table 1. Contact angle dependence on membrane % weight composition.

PVC (%)	[P_{66614}][Dec] (%)	Contact Angle (θ)
100	0	75.7 ± 0.5
80	20	74.4 ± 1.6
50	50	51.0 ± 2.8
30	70	28.1 ± 5.4

The contact angle of the pure PVC (θ = 75.7°) (Table 1) is reduced by the addition of [P_{66614}][Dec]. Although [P_{66614}][Dec] is hydrophobic, its presence can disrupt the regular hydrophobic domains of pure PVC, leading to a modified surface energy that may enhance water affinity to some extent. This increased chain mobility can lead to a smoother surface, which facilitates better water spreading and results in a lower contact angle [76]. A lower contact angle indicates better wettability, which facilitates the initial wetting of the membrane.

The vibrational spectrum of PVC (Figure 12a) is also deeply modified when the IL is incorporated (Figure 12b). For this characterization only the membrane PVC: [P_{66614}][Dec] (30:70) was considered, as it was the one with the optimal extraction performance (see Section 2.5).

Firstly, the C-H stretching modes at 2920 cm^{-1} become significantly more intense than in the starting polymer, due to the aliphatic tails of the added $[Dec]^-$ anion. New peaks at 1574 and 1728 cm^{-1} (red and orange circles) assigned to the C=O stretching modes of the carboxylate group [77] are present as well. In the used membrane (Figure 12d), the peak at 1574 cm^{-1} disappears, while the peaks at 1640 cm^{-1}r (green circle) and 1728 cm^{-1} increase in intensity. This spectral feature shows that the IL is retained in the membrane after use. Moreover, the peaks' positions in spectrum Figure 12d are diagnostic of the protonation of the carboxylate group [77] which is caused by the prolonged contact with the strongly acidic solution [77]. The latter result is coherent with the proposed equilibrium (2) where the decanoate is protonated when Co(II) is extracted in the IL phase in the PIM. Water is also present in the membrane, as revealed by the broad band centered around 3400 cm^{-1} assigned to the water O-H stretching.

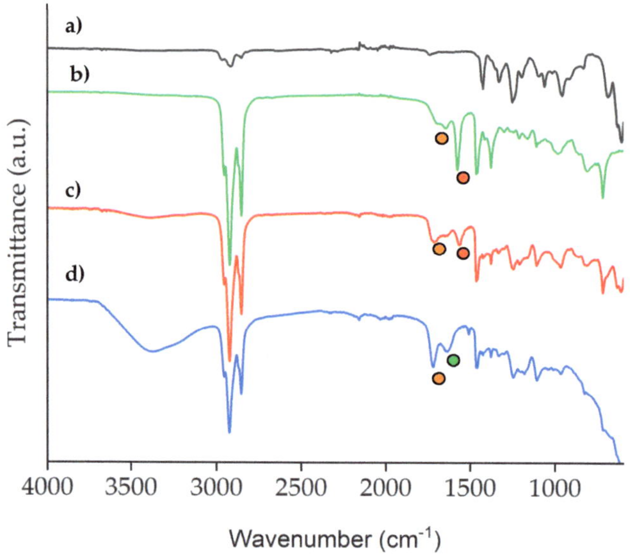

Figure 12. FTIR spectra of (**a**) pure PVC (black); (**b**) pure $[P_{66614}]$[Dec] (green); (**c**) PVC: $[P_{66614}]$[Dec] (30:70) PIM (red); and (**d**) PVC: $[P_{66614}]$[Dec] (30:70) PIM after extraction of Co(II) from 8 M HCl (blue).

The thermal behavior of PIMs was evaluated by differential scanning calorimetry (DSC) which displays a strong dependence upon composition.

In Figure 13, the DSC of pure PVC membrane and PVC: $[P_{66614}]$[Dec] (80:20) presents the glass transition temperature (T_g) at 58 °C. The glass transition becomes increasingly broader in the PIMs with an increased fraction of $[P_{66614}]$[Dec]. Melting peaks appear at −2 °C in PVC: $[P_{66614}]$[Dec] (50:50) (red) and with an increase of the IL fraction shift towards lower temperatures. This feature is clearly related to the included $[P_{66614}]$[Dec] as can be seen in the DSC of the pure liquid which shows three melting peaks at −43 °C, −7 °C, and +4 °C.

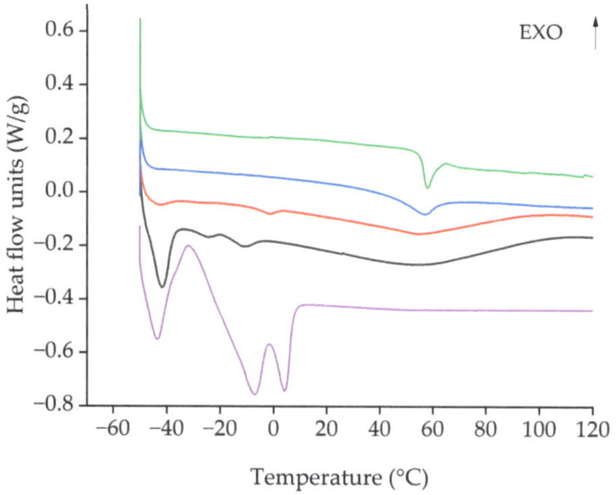

Figure 13. Thermograms of pure PVC (green), PVC: $[P_{66614}]$[Dec] (80:20) (blue), PVC: $[P_{66614}]$[Dec] (50:50) (red), PVC: $[P_{66614}]$[Dec] (30:70) (black), and pure $[P_{66614}]$[Dec] (purple).

The surface morphology of the starting polymer (Figure 14a) also changes upon inclusion of [P_{66614}][Dec] and after use. The initial homogenous surface of PVC is significantly altered by introducing larger granules (around 15 μm) and smaller pore-like structures (around 3 μm) (Figure 14b). These clusters and pores create a rough, heterogeneous surface resulting in a bigger surface area and thus promoting better metal transport. After being in contact with a Co(II)/Ni(II) 8 M HCl solution for 52 h, a roughness in the surface appears (Figure 14c).

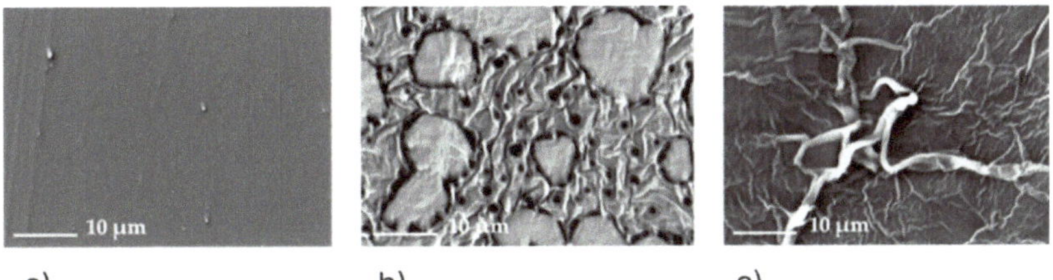

Figure 14. SEM images of (**a**) pure PVC, (**b**) PVC: [P_{66614}][Dec] (30:70) before extraction, and (**c**) PVC: [P_{66614}][Dec] (30:70) after extraction.

2.5. Separation of Co(II) from Ni(II) with PIMs

Co(II) was separated from Ni(II) utilizing a PIM based on 30% PVC and 70% [P_{66614}][Dec] with an experimental setup shown in Figure 15. The membranes with a lower percentage of [P_{66614}][Dec] did not display metal extraction within 48 h while the membrane with higher IL content was too fragile to be usable. A possible explanation of this behavior is that the 30:70 composition allows a sufficiently fast diffusion through the membrane to observe extraction in the typical experimental timeframe. The presence of a "threshold" concentration of the carrier in the membrane to observe transport was previously observed for other systems [46,78]. The working conditions were established based on the best performance obtained in the liquid-liquid extraction experiments (feed containing $[Co]_{aq}$ = 10 mM, $[Ni]_{aq}$ = 10 mM in 8 M HCl, pure water in the stripping phase, T = 25 °C).

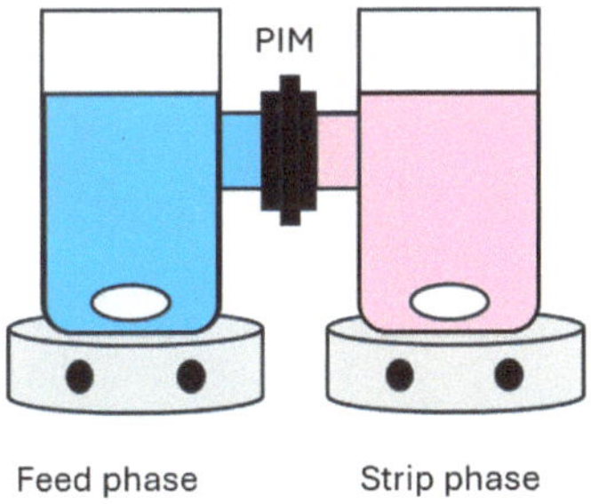

Figure 15. Experimental setup for the separation using the PVC: [P_{66614}][Dec] PIM. The volume of each compartment is 50 mL, contact surface with the membrane 4.90 cm^2, and stirring speed 700 rpm.

The permeation of metal through the membrane consists of three steps: (i) absorption of $[CoCl_4]^{2-}$ into the membrane, (ii) transport through the membrane, and (iii) release of Co(II) from the membrane into the stripping phase (Equation (3)).

In Figure 16a the relative concentration of Co(II) with respect to the initial one in the feed and stripping phases vs. time is plotted. The concentration in the stripping phase increases slowly until ~30 h when an onset is observed. At 50 h, around the 95% of the initial Co(II) is transferred to the stripping phase, while the metal concentration drops below the detection limit in the feed. This implies that ~5% of Co(II) remains incorporated in the membrane. On the other hand, Ni(II) concentration decreases slightly in the feed (~7%), but it is not detected in the stripping phase (Figure 16b).

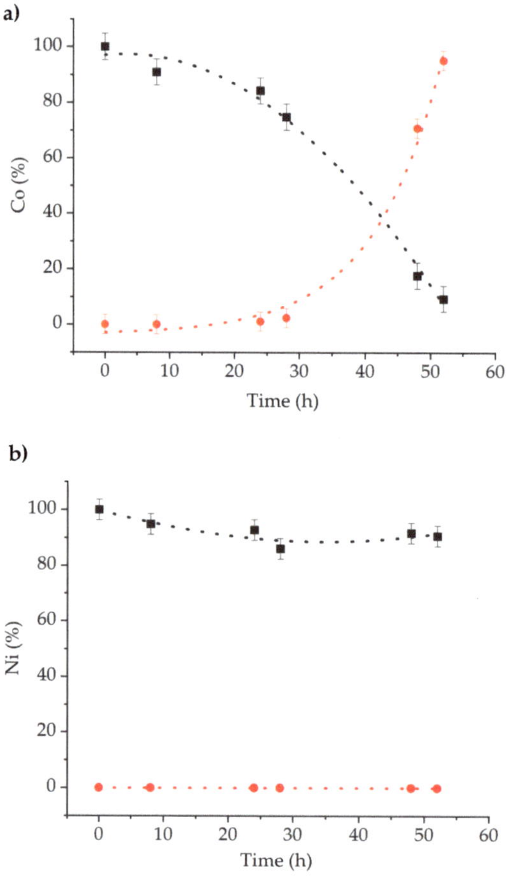

Figure 16. Relative change (%) with respect to initial concentration (10 mM) vs. time of (**a**) Co(II) and (**b**) Ni(II) in the feed (black) and strip (red) phases.

The final pH of the stripping phase was measured and found to be <1.0, indicating that protons are transported through the membrane. This is also supported by the FTIR spectrum of the used membrane (Figure 12). The stripping phase also shows a positive reaction (white precipitate formation) upon the addition of $AgNO_3$, confirming the transfer of Cl^- anions in the aqueous solution.

3. Materials and Methods

3.1. Chemicals

Trihexyl(tetradecyl)phosphonium decanoate ([P_{66614}][Dec]) (>95%) and Trihexyl (tetradecyl)phosphonium chloride ([P_{66614}][Cl]) (>95%) was purchased from IoLiTec (Heilbronn, Germany). $CoCl_2 \cdot 6H_2O$ was purchased from JT Baker (Phillipsburg, NJ, USA), $NiCl_2 \cdot 6H_2O$ were ordered from Sigma-Aldrich (Burlington, MA, USA). NaCl was purchased from Honeywell Fluka. HCl (37% solution in water) was ordered from Sigma-Aldrich. PVC (high molecular weight) was purchased from Sigma-Aldrich. THF was purchased from Sigma-Aldrich. All products were used as received, without any further purification.

3.2. Extraction and Stripping Experiments

Metal extraction experiments were conducted for several aqueous solutions with different HCl or NaCl concentrations containing $CoCl_2$ and $NiCl_2$ (total concentration of each metal = 50 mM). For the extractions, 2.0 mL of the aqueous solution and 2.0 mL of the IL phase were stirred at 1500 rpm for variable times ranging from 1 to 60 min at 25 °C. The IL phase was pre-equilibrated with different concentrations of HCl or NaCl for one hour before use.

The temperature was controlled by immersing the sample tube in a thermostatic bath. The experiments were performed from 15 to 65 °C for 5 min in a thermostatic bath.

The total metal content of the water phases was determined using ICP-OES (Agilent 5800, Palo Alto, CA, USA). Calibration curves were built by analyzing standard solutions in the concentration range for 0–50 mg L^{-1} (Figure S4) and prepared starting from a multi-element standard solution (Merck, Darmstadt, Germany). Argon was used as an internal standard. All the measurements were conducted in triplicate.

The electronic (UV-Vis) spectra of the metal-containing solutions were recorded with a Varian Cary 50 spectrophotometer in a 0.1 and 10 mm quartz cuvette.

The percent extraction (E%) is defined as the amount of metal extracted to the IL phase over the total amount of metal in both phases and is given by the following expression (Equation (4)) [39]:

$$E(\%) = \frac{V_{IL}[M]_{IL}}{V_{aq}[M]_0} \times 100 = \frac{[M]_0 - [M]_{aq}}{[M]_0} \times 100 \quad (4)$$

The volumes of the ionic liquid (V_{IL}) and aqueous phase (V_{aq}) are the volumes of the organic and aqueous phases, which are equal in our experiments. The molar concentrations $[M]_0$, $[M]_{aq}$, and $[M]_{IL}$ are the metal in the initial water phase and in the aqueous and IL phase when the extraction equilibrium is reached.

The D_M (M = Co, Ni) was calculated as follows (Equation (5)) [39]:

$$D_M = \frac{[M]_0 - [M]_{aq}}{[M]_{aq}} \quad (5)$$

Stripping was performed several times, by equilibrating the loaded IL phase with an equal volume of water (2.0 mL) and shaking for 5 min. The aqueous and IL phases were separated for further analysis with ICP-OES. The stripping was evaluated by calculating the S(%), using Equation (6) [38]:

$$S(\%) = \frac{V_{aq,s}[M]_{aq,s}}{V_{IL}\,[M]_{IL}} \times 100 = \frac{[M]_{aq,s}}{[M]_{IL}} \times 100 \quad (6)$$

where $[M]_{IL}$ is the metal concentration in the IL phase after the extraction, $[V]_{IL}$ is the volume of the IL phase, $[V]_{aq,s}$ is the volume of the aqueous phase used for stripping, and $[M]_{aq,s}$ is the metal concentration in the aqueous phase after stripping. After stripping, the Co(II) recovered (R%) was calculated by Equation (7):

$$R\ (\%) = \frac{[Co]_{extracted}}{[Co]_{initial}} \times S(\%) \quad (7)$$

3.3. Membrane Preparation

A set of membranes was prepared by dissolving PVC (0.8, 0.5, 0.3, and 0.2 g) and IL $[P_{66614}]$[Dec] (0.2, 0.5, 0.7, 0.8 g) in 10 mL of THF. The mixture of PVC and IL was stirred on a magnetic stirrer until dissolution was completed. The total mass of each membrane was ~1 g. After dissolving the PVC and IL, the solution was poured into glass Petri plates (Figure 17) and was left to evaporate overnight [79]. Then, membranes were peeled from the Petri dishes and used without further treatments.

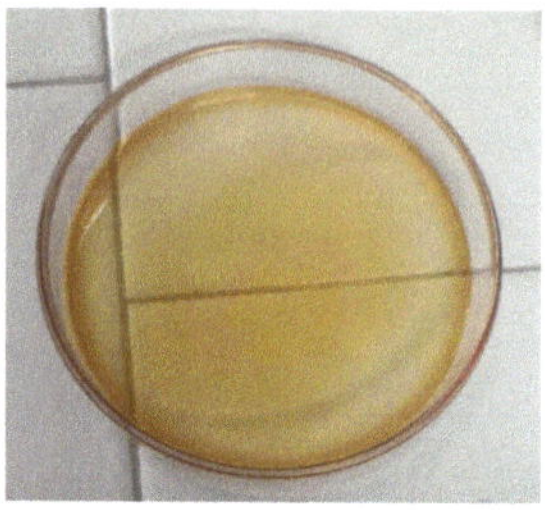

Figure 17. PVC: [P_{66614}][Dec] (30:70) membrane after synthesis.

3.4. *Contact Angle*

The surface contact angle of the resultant PVC membranes was measured by a portable video-based goniometer PGX. Deionized water was slowly dropped onto the surface of the specimens. The angle was measured manually by the three-point method. At least five different locations were measured for each specimen. The indoor temperature was 27 ± 0.5 °C.

3.5. *Elastic Modulus*

Samples were manually cut into 10×60 mm strips and subjected to tensile test using a 34TM-5 dynamometer (Instron LTD., High Wycombe, UK) equipped with a 5 kN loading cell. Samples were pulled until failure at a 10 mm/min rate. Percentage elongation measures the ability of a material to deform under tensile stress before breaking.

3.6. *Microscopy*

A field-emission-gun scanning electron microscope (FE-SEM Jeol JSM7600F Scanning Electron Microscope, JEOL, Tokyo, Japan) was used to observe and characterize the samples. All images were collected at an acceleration voltage of 15 kV, a distance of 15 mm, and at magnifications ranging between 25× and 10,000×. All samples were sputter-coated (Cressington, Watford, UK) with a thin (2–5 nm) layer of gold to improve their electrical conductivity.

3.7. *FTIR*

ATR spectra of pure PVC and PVC: [P_{66614}][Dec] (30:70) membrane before and after extraction were collected using a Fourier transform infrared (FT-IR) spectrometer (Thermo Scientific Nicolet iS-50 FTIR, Monza, Italy) equipped with an ATR module and a deuterated triglycine sulfate (DTGS) detector. Each spectrum was collected using 32 scans and a spectral resolution of 4 cm^{-1}. Wavelength varied from 4000 cm^{-1} to 400 cm^{-1}.

3.8. *DSC*

Samples were manually cut into approximately 3×3 mm squares and weighed to 0.0001 g precision inside 100 µL aluminum pans (Mettler-Toledo, Greifensee, Switzerland). A DSC 3 Stare System differential scanning calorimeter was then used to heat the samples from −50 °C to 120 °C at a 10 °C/min heating rate under continuous nitrogen flow (20 mL/min). Glass transition temperature and peak enthalpies were obtained by elaborating themograms using the STARe software (ver. 16.10, Mettler-Toledo).

3.9. *Extraction with PIMs*

Extractions using PIMs were performed in a setup depicted in Figure 15. The setup was purchased from Tecnovetro s.r.l (Monza, Italy). The volume of the feed and stripping phases were 50 mL each, at room temperature, with a stirring speed of 700 rpm and a membrane contact surface of 4.90 cm^2.

To test the performance of the PVC: [P_{66614}][Dec] (30:70) membrane for the separation of Co(II) from Ni(II), an 8 M HCl solution containing $CoCl_2$ and $NiCl_2$ (metal concentration

10 mM) was prepared and employed as the feed phase. Pure water was used as the stripping phase. The extractions were conducted at room temperature. Feed and stripping phases were periodically sampled, and the metal content was analyzed using ICP-OES.

3.10. Extraction Efficiency in Membrane Separation

The change of the metal concentration in the feed phase was calculated by Equation (8), while the change of the metal concentration in the stripping phase was calculated by Equation (9):

$$\%\ M_{feed} = 100 - \left(\frac{[M_{start}] - [M_{t,\ feed}]}{[M_{start}]}\right) \times 100\% \tag{8}$$

$$\%\ M_{strip} = 100 - \left(\frac{[M_{start}] - [M_{t,\ strip}]}{[M_{start}]}\right) \times 100\% \tag{9}$$

where $[M_{start}]$ is the initial metal concentration in the feed, $[M_{t,feed}]$ is a concentration of metal in the feed phase after t amount of time, and $[M_{t,strip}]$ is a concentration of metal in the stripping phase after certain (t) amount of time.

4. Conclusions

This work shows the applicability of a carboxylic acid containing IL in the Co/Ni separation both as in liquid-liquid extraction and supported on a polymeric membrane.

The efficiency obtained of the extraction of Ni(II) and Co(II) from concentrated HCl solutions shows distinct performance as chloride ion concentrations vary, which is explained by the formation of different speciation of these two metal ions. When extraction occurs from water and NaCl solutions, Co(II) and Ni(II) are both extracted through the coordination of decanoate anions, and a low selectivity for Co(II) is obtained. When extractions are performed from concentrated HCl solutions, the decanoate anion is protonated and is not able to bind metal ions. In such conditions Co(II) is selectively extracted as tetrachloride species. Notably, the best performance in terms of *E*(%) and selectivity towards Co(II) is obtained when the feed is above 6 M HCl. Stripping was performed by using deionized water, which allowed a recovery close to the 100% of the total Co(II) in the feed solution.

PIMs formulated with PVC and the IL $[P_{66614}]$[Dec] successfully extracted Co(II), when a PVC: Dec ratio of 30:70 was employed. The high selectivity for Co(II) over Ni(II) was comparable to that obtained from liquid-liquid extraction. The use of PIMs reduces the amount of IL required and allows the recovery of Co(II) in a single step. However, the extractions with PIMs in this work require a significantly longer time with respect to liquid-liquid experiments. Even so, the high selectivity obtained with the PVC: Dec (30:70) PIM combined with durability in acidic conditions constitute a starting point for further developments towards practical applications. Several improvements of different aspects of IL-based PIMs have been discussed in a recent review [80]. Another limitation for a scale-up is the high concentration of HCl acid required to achieve a high selectivity, which poses environmental and safety concerns. In this context, the improvement of the process kinetics and the use of less aggressive acids would give a great benefit.

Supplementary Materials: The following supporting information can be downloaded at: https://www.mdpi.com/article/10.3390/molecules29194545/s1, Figure S1. Absorption spectrum of Ni(II) aqueous phase in 0 M HCl (blue), 2 M HCl (orange), 6 M HCl (grey), and 8 M HCl (yellow). Figure S2. Ni(II) in $[P_{66614}]$[Dec] IL phase after extraction from 0 M HCl. Figure S3. *E*(%) of Co(II) in $[P_{66614}]$[Dec] containing variable concentrations of HCl (a) and NaCl (b) $[Co]_{aq}$ = 50 mM. Figure S4. ICP-OES calibration curves for (a) Co(II), (b) Ni(II). Table S1. *D* of Co(II) and Ni(II) after extraction with $[P_{66614}]$[Dec] from HCl and NaCl media. Table S2. Cumulative stripping (S%) of Co(II) from $[P_{66614}]$[Dec] extracted from different HCl feeds (M HCl) utilizing only water.

Author Contributions: Methodology, investigation, formal analysis, data curation, writing—original draft preparation, writing—review and editing, A.K.; formal analysis, data curation, writing—review and editing, M.T.; investigation, J.A.R.G.; conceptualization, methodology, supervision, funding acquisition, writing—review and editing, A.M.; methodology, investigation, supervision, writing—original draft preparation, writing—review and editing, M.S. All authors have read and agreed to the published version of the manuscript.

Funding: This research was funded by the University of Udine, in the framework of the Strategic Plan 2022-25—Interdepartmental Research Project ESPeRT. A.M. and M.S. acknowledge the University of Udine for Research financed with European Union funds–NextGenerationEU—MSCA grants D.M. 737/2021—CUPG25F21003390007. A.M. and A.K. acknowledge the results from the PhD programme on Green topics (Action IV.5, DM 1061/2021, cycle XXXVII) carried out with co-financing from the European Union–ESF REACT-EU, PON Research and Innovation 2014–2020, UniUD. M.T. acknowledges the Italian Ministry for University and research for funding through the PRIN2022 call with the project "Wastezilla" (2022HYH95P).

Data Availability Statement: Data are available within the manuscript and Supplementary Materials. Further inquiries can be directed to the authors.

Conflicts of Interest: The authors declare no conflicts of interest.

References

1. Zhao, Y.; Pohl, O.; Bhatt, A.I.; Collis, G.E.; Mahon, P.J.; Rüther, T.; Hollenkamp, A.F. A Review on Battery Market Trends, Second-Life Reuse, and Recycling. *Sustain. Chem.* **2021**, *2*, 167–205. [CrossRef]
2. Tisserant, A.; Pauliuk, S. Matching Global Cobalt Demand under Different Scenarios for Co-Production and Mining Attractiveness. *J. Econ. Struct.* **2016**, *5*, 4. [CrossRef]
3. Gianvincenzi, M.; Mosconi, E.M.; Marconi, M.; Tola, F. Battery Waste Management in Europe: Black Mass Hazardousness and Recycling Strategies in the Light of an Evolving Competitive Regulation. *Recycling* **2024**, *9*, 13. [CrossRef]
4. Murdock, B.E.; Toghill, K.E.; Tapia-Ruiz, N. A Perspective on the Sustainability of Cathode Materials Used in Lithium-Ion Batteries. *Adv. Energy Mater.* **2021**, *11*, 2102028. [CrossRef]
5. Leal Filho, W.; Kotter, R.; Özuyar, P.G.; Abubakar, I.R.; Eustachio, J.H.P.P.; Matandirotya, N.R. Understanding Rare Earth Elements as Critical Raw Materials. *Sustainability* **2023**, *15*, 1919. [CrossRef]
6. Cheng, A.L.; Fuchs, E.R.H.; Karplus, V.J.; Michalek, J.J. Electric Vehicle Battery Chemistry Affects Supply Chain Disruption Vulnerabilities. *Nat. Commun.* **2024**, *15*, 2143. [CrossRef]
7. Alvial-Hein, G.; Mahandra, H.; Ghahreman, A. Separation and Recovery of Cobalt and Nickel from End of Life Products via Solvent Extraction Technique: A Review. *J. Clean. Prod.* **2021**, *297*, 126592. [CrossRef]
8. Xie, Y.; Xu, Y.; Yan, L.; Yang, R. Recovery of Nickel, Copper and Cobalt from Low-Grade Ni–Cu Sulfide Tailings. *Hydrometallurgy* **2005**, *80*, 54–58. [CrossRef]
9. Agatzini-Leonardou, S.; Tsakiridis, P.E.; Oustadakis, P.; Karidakis, T.; Katsiapi, A. Hydrometallurgical Process for the Separation and Recovery of Nickel from Sulphate Heap Leach Liquor of Nickeliferrous Laterite Ores. *Miner. Eng.* **2009**, *22*, 1181–1192. [CrossRef]
10. Harper, G.; Sommerville, R.; Kendrick, E.; Driscoll, L.; Slater, P.; Stolkin, R.; Walton, A.; Christensen, P.; Heidrich, O.; Lambert, S.; et al. Recycling Lithium-Ion Batteries from Electric Vehicles. *Nature* **2019**, *575*, 75–86. [CrossRef]
11. Kovačević, A.; Tolazzi, M.; Sanadar, M.; Melchior, A. Hydrometallurgical Recovery of Metals from Spent Lithium-Ion Batteries with Ionic Liquids and Deep Eutectic Solvents. *J. Environ. Chem. Eng.* **2024**, *12*, 113248. [CrossRef]
12. Makuza, B.; Tian, Q.; Guo, X.; Chattopadhyay, K.; Yu, D. Pyrometallurgical Options for Recycling Spent Lithium-Ion Batteries: A Comprehensive Review. *J. Power Sources* **2021**, *491*, 229622. [CrossRef]
13. Preston, J.S. Solvent Extraction of Cobalt(II) and Nickel(II) by a Quaternary Ammonium Thiocyanate. *Sep. Sci. Technol.* **1982**, *17*, 1697–1718. [CrossRef]
14. Liu, Y.; Nam, S.-H.; Lee, M.-S. A Study on the Separation of Co(II), Ni(II), and Mg(II) by Solvent Extraction with Cationic Extractants. *Bull. Korean Chem. Soc.* **2015**, *36*, 2646–2650. [CrossRef]
15. Mubarok, M.Z.; Yunita, F.E.; Mubarok, M.Z.; Yunita, F.E. Solvent Extraction of Nickel and Cobalt from Ammonia-Ammonium Carbonate Solution by Using LIX 84-ICNS. *Int. J. Nonferr. Metall.* **2015**, *4*, 15–27. [CrossRef]
16. Devi, N.B.; Nathsarma, K.C.; Chakravortty, V. Separation and Recovery of Cobalt(II) and Nickel(II) from Sulphate Solutions Using Sodium Salts of D2EHPA, PC 88A and Cyanex 272. *Hydrometallurgy* **1998**, *49*, 47–61. [CrossRef]
17. Fleitlikh, I.Y.; Pashkov, G.L.; Grigorieva, N.A.; Nikiforova, L.K.; Pleshkov, M.A.; Shneerson, Y.M. Cobalt and Nickel Recovery from Sulfate Media Containing Calcium, Manganese, and Magnesium with a Mixture of CYANEX 301 and a Trialkylamine. *Solvent Extr. Ion Exch.* **2011**, *29*, 782–799. [CrossRef]
18. He, M.; Jin, X.; Zhang, X.; Duan, X.; Zhang, P.; Teng, L.; Liu, Q.; Liu, W. Combined Pyro-Hydrometallurgical Technology for Recovering Valuable Metal Elements from Spent Lithium-Ion Batteries: A Review of Recent Developments. *Green Chem.* **2023**, *25*, 6561–6580. [CrossRef]

19. Sukhbaatar, T.; Dourdain, S.; Turgis, R.; Rey, J.; Arrachart, G.; Pellet-Rostaing, S. Ionic Liquids as Diluents in Solvent Extraction: First Evidence of Supramolecular Aggregation of a Couple of Extractant Molecules. *Chem. Commun.* **2015**, *51*, 15960–15963. [CrossRef]
20. Wongsawa, T.; Traiwongsa, N.; Pancharoen, U.; Nootong, K. A Review of the Recovery of Precious Metals Using Ionic Liquid Extractants in Hydrometallurgical Processes. *Hydrometallurgy* **2020**, *198*, 105488. [CrossRef]
21. Billard, I.; Ouadi, A.; Gaillard, C. Liquid-Liquid Extraction of Actinides, Lanthanides, and Fission Products by Use of Ionic Liquids: From Discovery to Understanding. *Anal. Bioanal. Chem.* **2011**, *400*, 1555–1566. [CrossRef] [PubMed]
22. Vasudeva Rao, P.R.; Venkatesan, K.A.; Rout, A.; Srinivasan, T.G.; Nagarajan, K. Potential Applications of Room Temperature Ionic Liquids for Fission Products and Actinide Separation. *Sep. Sci. Technol.* **2012**, *47*, 204–222. [CrossRef]
23. Kolarik, Z. Ionic Liquids: How Far Do They Extend the Potential of Solvent Extraction of f-Elements? *Sep. Sci. Technol.* **2012**, *31*, 24–60. [CrossRef]
24. Busato, M.; Lapi, A.; D'Angelo, P.; Melchior, A. Coordination of the Co^{2+} and Ni^{2+} Ions in $Tf2N^-$ Based Ionic Liquids: A Combined X-ray Absorption and Molecular Dynamics Study. *J. Phys. Chem. B* **2021**, *125*, 6639–6648. [CrossRef]
25. Busato, M.; D'Angelo, P.; Melchior, A. Solvation of Zn^{2+} Ion in 1-Alkyl-3-Methylimidazolium Bis(Trifluoromethylsulfonyl)Imide Ionic Liquids: A Molecular Dynamics and X-ray Absorption Study. *Phys. Chem. Chem. Phys.* **2019**, *21*, 6958–6969. [CrossRef]
26. Melchior, A.; Gaillard, C.; Gràcia Lanas, S.; Tolazzi, M.; Billard, I.; Georg, S.; Sarrasin, L.; Boltoeva, M. Nickel(II) Complexation with Nitrate in Dry [C4mim][Tf2N] Ionic Liquid: A Spectroscopic, Microcalorimetric, and Molecular Dynamics Study. *Inorg. Chem.* **2016**, *55*, 3498–3507. [CrossRef]
27. Flieger, J.; Flieger, M. Ionic Liquids Toxicity-Benefits and Threats. *Int. J. Mol. Sci.* **2020**, *21*, 6267. [CrossRef] [PubMed]
28. Raj, T.; Chandrasekhar, K.; Park, J.; Varjani, S.; Sharma, P.; Kumar, D.; Yoon, J.J.; Pandey, A.; Kim, S.H. Synthesis of Fatty Acid-Based Ammonium Ionic Liquids and Their Application for Extraction of Co(II) and Ni(II) Metals Ions from Aqueous Solution. *Chemosphere* **2022**, *307*, 135787. [CrossRef]
29. Vavina, A.V.; Seitkalieva, M.M.; Strukova, E.N.; Ananikov, V.P. Fatty Acid-Derived Ionic Liquids as Soft and Sustainable Antimicrobial Agents. *J. Mol. Liq.* **2024**, *410*, 125483. [CrossRef]
30. Gusain, R.; Khatri, O.P. Fatty Acid Ionic Liquids as Environmentally Friendly Lubricants for Low Friction and Wear. *RSC Adv.* **2016**, *6*, 3462–3469. [CrossRef]
31. Parmentier, D.; Metz, S.J.; Kroon, M.C. Tetraalkylammonium Oleate and Linoleate Based Ionic Liquids: Promising Extractants for Metal Salts. *Green Chem.* **2013**, *15*, 205–209. [CrossRef]
32. Parmentier, D.; Vander Hoogerstraete, T.; Metz, S.J.; Binnemans, K.; Kroon, M.C. Selective Extraction of Metals from Chloride Solutions with the Tetraoctylphosphonium Oleate Ionic Liquid. *Ind. Eng. Chem. Res.* **2015**, *54*, 5149–5158. [CrossRef]
33. Yang, Q.; Xu, D.; Zhang, J.; Zhu, Y.; Zhang, Z.; Qian, C.; Ren, Q.; Xing, H. Long-Chain Fatty Acid-Based Phosphonium Ionic Liquids with Strong Hydrogen-Bond Basicity and Good Lipophilicity: Synthesis, Characterization, and Application in Extraction. *ACS Sustain. Chem. Eng.* **2015**, *3*, 309–316. [CrossRef]
34. Saadeh, S.M.; Yasseen, Z.; Sharif, F.A.; Abu Shawish, H.M. New Room Temperature Ionic Liquids with Interesting Ecotoxicological and Antimicrobial Properties. *Ecotoxicol. Environ. Saf.* **2009**, *72*, 1805–1809. [CrossRef] [PubMed]
35. Singh, R.; Mahandra, H.; Gupta, B. Optimization of a Solvent Extraction Route for the Recovery of Mo from Petroleum Refinery Spent Catalyst Using Cyphos IL 102. *Solvent Extr. Ion Exch.* **2018**, *36*, 401–419. [CrossRef]
36. Cieszynska, A.; Wisniewski, M. Selective Extraction of Palladium(II) from Hydrochloric Acid Solutions with Phosphonium Extractants. *Sep. Purif. Technol.* **2011**, *80*, 385–389. [CrossRef]
37. Kogelnig, D.; Stojanovic, A.; Jirsa, F.; Körner, W.; Krachler, R.; Keppler, B.K. Transport and Separation of Iron(III) from Nickel(II) with the Ionic Liquid Trihexyl(Tetradecyl)Phosphonium Chloride. *Sep. Purif. Technol.* **2010**, *72*, 56–60. [CrossRef]
38. Vander Hoogerstraete, T.; Binnemans, K. Highly Efficient Separation of Rare Earths from Nickel and Cobalt by Solvent Extraction with the Ionic Liquid Trihexyl(Tetradecyl)Phosphonium Nitrate: A Process Relevant to the Recycling of Rare Earths from Permanent Magnets and Nickel Metal Hydride Batteries. *Green Chem.* **2014**, *16*, 1594–1606. [CrossRef]
39. Vander Hoogerstraete, T.; Wellens, S.; Verachtert, K.; Binnemans, K. Removal of Transition Metals from Rare Earths by Solvent Extraction with an Undiluted Phosphonium Ionic Liquid: Separations Relevant to Rare-Earth Magnet Recycling. *Green Chem.* **2013**, *15*, 919–927. [CrossRef]
40. Ilyas, S.; Srivastava, R.R.; Kim, H. Selective Separation of Cobalt versus Nickel by Split-Phosphinate Complexation Using a Phosphonium-Based Ionic Liquid. *Environ. Chem. Lett.* **2023**, *21*, 673–680. [CrossRef]
41. Satyawirawan, S.A.; Cattrall, R.W.; Kolev, S.D.; Almeida, M.I.G.S. Improving Co(II) Separation from Ni(II) by Solvent Extraction Using Phosphonium-Based Ionic Liquids. *J. Mol. Liq.* **2023**, *380*, 121764. [CrossRef]
42. Mušović, J.; Tekić, D.; Marić, S.; Jocić, A.; Stanković, D.; Dimitrijević, A. Sustainable Recovery of Cobalt and Lithium from Lithium-Ion Battery Cathode Material by Combining Sulfate Leachates and Aqueous Biphasic Systems Based on Tetrabutylphosphonium-Ionic Liquids. *Sep. Purif. Technol.* **2024**, *348*, 127707. [CrossRef]
43. Eyupoglu, V.; Unal, A. The Extraction and the Removal of Cd(II) Using Polymer Inclusion Membrane Containing Symmetric Room Temperature Ionic Liquid as Ion Carrier. *J. Environ. Chem. Eng.* **2023**, *11*, 110570. [CrossRef]
44. Hernández-Fernández, A.; Iniesta-López, E.; Ginestá-Anzola, A.; Garrido, Y.; Pérez de los Ríos, A.; Quesada-Medina, J.; Hernández-Fernández, F.J. Polymeric Inclusion Membranes Based on Ionic Liquids for Selective Separation of Metal Ions. *Membranes* **2023**, *13*, 795. [CrossRef] [PubMed]

45. Safarpour, M.; Safikhani, A.; Vatanpour, V. Polyvinyl Chloride-Based Membranes: A Review on Fabrication Techniques, Applications and Future Perspectives. *Sep. Purif. Technol.* **2021**, *279*, 119678. [CrossRef]
46. Almeida, M.I.G.S.; Cattrall, R.W.; Kolev, S.D. Recent Trends in Extraction and Transport of Metal Ions Using Polymer Inclusion Membranes (PIMs). *J. Membr. Sci.* **2012**, *415–416*, 9–23. [CrossRef]
47. Hernández-Fernández, F.J.; de los Ríos, A.P.; Mateo-Ramírez, F.; Juarez, M.D.; Lozano-Blanco, L.J.; Godínez, C. New Application of Polymer Inclusion Membrane Based on Ionic Liquids as Proton Exchange Membrane in Microbial Fuel Cell. *Sep. Purif. Technol.* **2016**, *160*, 51–58. [CrossRef]
48. Xu, L.; Zeng, X.; He, Q.; Deng, T.; Zhang, C.; Zhang, W. Stable Ionic Liquid-Based Polymer Inclusion Membranes for Lithium and Magnesium Separation. *Sep. Purif. Technol.* **2022**, *288*, 120626. [CrossRef]
49. Baczyńska, M.; Waszak, M.; Nowicki, M.; Prządka, D.; Borysiak, S.; Regel-Rosocka, M. Characterization of Polymer Inclusion Membranes (PIMs) Containing Phosphonium Ionic Liquids as Zn(II) Carriers. *Ind. Eng. Chem. Res.* **2018**, *57*, 5070–5082. [CrossRef]
50. Santos Klienchen Dalari, B.L.; Lisboa Giroletti, C.; Malaret, F.J.; Skoronski, E.; Hallett, J.P.; Matias, W.G.; Puerari, R.C.; Nagel-Hassemer, M.E. Application of a Phosphonium-Based Ionic Liquid for Reactive Textile Dye Removal: Extraction Study and Toxicological Evaluation. *J. Environ. Manag.* **2022**, *304*, 114322. [CrossRef]
51. Skoronski, E.; Fernandes, M.; Malaret, F.J.; Hallett, J.P. Use of Phosphonium Ionic Liquids for Highly Efficient Extraction of Phenolic Compounds from Water. *Sep. Purif. Technol.* **2020**, *248*, 117069. [CrossRef]
52. Marták, J.; Liptaj, T.; Schlosser, Š. Extraction of Butyric Acid by Phosphonium Decanoate Ionic Liquid. *J. Chem. Eng. Data* **2019**, *64*, 2973–2984. [CrossRef]
53. Blaga, A.C.; Dragoi, E.N.; Tucaliuc, A.; Kloetzer, L.; Cascaval, D. Folic Acid Ionic-Liquids-Based Separation: Extraction and Modelling. *Molecules* **2023**, *28*, 3339. [CrossRef] [PubMed]
54. Alizadeh, S.; Abdollahy, M.; Khodadadi Darban, A.; Mohseni, M. Theoretical and Experimental Comparison of Rare Earths Extraction by [P6,6,6,1,4][Decanoate] Bifunctional Ionic Liquid and D2EHPA Acidic Extractant. *Min. Eng.* **2022**, *180*, 107473. [CrossRef]
55. Xuan, W.; de Souza Braga, A.; Korbel, C.; Chagnes, A. New Insights in the Leaching Kinetics of Cathodic Materials in Acidic Chloride Media for Lithium-Ion Battery Recycling. *Hydrometallurgy* **2021**, *204*, 105705. [CrossRef]
56. Wellens, S.; Thijs, B.; Binnemans, K. An Environmentally Friendlier Approach to Hydrometallurgy: Highly Selective Separation of Cobalt from Nickel by Solvent Extraction with Undiluted Phosphonium Ionic Liquids. *Green Chem.* **2012**, *14*, 1657–1665. [CrossRef]
57. Dhiman, S.; Gupta, B. Partition Studies on Cobalt and Recycling of Valuable Metals from Waste Li-Ion Batteries via Solvent Extraction and Chemical Precipitation. *J. Clean. Prod.* **2019**, *225*, 820–832. [CrossRef]
58. Zhang, C.; Hu, B.; Zhao, S.; Liao, Z.; Wang, M. Separation of Co(II) and Ni(II) from Hydrochloric Acid Leach Liquor by Solvent Extraction and Crystallization. *J. Sustain. Metall.* **2022**, *8*, 91–101. [CrossRef]
59. Hitchcock, P.B.; Seddon, K.R.; Welton, T. Hydrogen-Bond Acceptor Abilities of Tetrachlorometalate(II) Complexes in Ionic Liquids. *J. Chem. Soc. Dalton Trans.* **1993**, 2639–2643. [CrossRef]
60. Bowlas, C.J.; Bruce, D.W.; Seddon, K.R. Liquid-Crystalline Ionic Liquids. *Chem. Commun.* **1996**, 1625–1626. [CrossRef]
61. Skibsted, L.H.; Bjerrum, J. Studies on Cobalt (II) Halide Complex Formation. II. Cobalt (II) Chloride Complexes in 10 M Perchloric Acid Solution. *Acta Chem. Scand. A* **1978**, *32*, 429–434. [CrossRef]
62. Liu, W.; Borg, S.J.; Testemale, D.; Etschmann, B.; Hazemann, J.-L.; Brugger, J. Speciation and Thermodynamic Properties for Cobalt Chloride Complexes in Hydrothermal Fluids at 35–440 °C and 600 Bar: An in-Situ XAS Study. *Geochim. Cosmochim. Acta* **2011**, *75*, 1227–1248. [CrossRef]
63. Bjerrum, J.; Halonin, A.S.; Skibsated, L.H. Studies on Cobalt(II) Halide Complex Formation. I. A Spectrophotometric Study of the Chloro Cobalt(II) Complexes in Strong Aqueous Chloride Solutions. *Acta Chem. Scand. A* **1975**, *29*, 326–332. [CrossRef]
64. Pan, P.; Susak, N.J. Co(II)-Chloride and -Bromide Complexes in Aqueous Solutions up to 5 *m* Na*X* and 90 °C: Spectrophotometric Study and Geological Implications. *Geochim. Cosmochim. Acta* **1989**, *53*, 327–341. [CrossRef]
65. Uchikoshi, M. Determination of the Distribution of Cobalt-Chloro Complexes in Hydrochloric Acid Solutions at 298 K. *J. Solut. Chem.* **2018**, *47*, 2021–2038. [CrossRef]
66. Uchikoshi, M.; Shinoda, K. Determination of Structures of Cobalt(II)-Chloro Complexes in Hydrochloric Acid Solutions by X-ray Absorption Spectroscopy at 298 K. *Struct. Chem.* **2019**, *30*, 945–954. [CrossRef]
67. Lee, M.-S.; Nam, S.-H. Chemical Equilibria of Nickel Chloride in HCl Solution at 25 °C. *Bull. Korean Chem. Soc.* **2009**, *30*, 2203–2207. [CrossRef]
68. Rybka, P.; Regel-Rosocka, M. Nickel(II) and Cobalt(II) Extraction from Chloride Solutions with Quaternary Phosphonium Salts. *Sep. Sci. Technol.* **2012**, *47*, 1296–1302. [CrossRef]
69. Chaverra, D.E.; Restrepo-Baena, O.J.; Ruiz, M.C. Cobalt Extraction from Sulfate/Chloride Media with Trioctyl(Alkyl)Phosphonium Chloride Ionic Liquids. *ACS Omega* **2020**, *5*, 5643–5650. [CrossRef]
70. Lommelen, R.; Vander Hoogerstraete, T.; Onghena, B.; Billard, I.; Binnemans, K. Model for Metal Extraction from Chloride Media with Basic Extractants: A Coordination Chemistry Approach. *Inorg. Chem.* **2019**, *58*, 12289–12301. [CrossRef]
71. Lin, B.; McCormick, A.V.; Davis, H.T.; Strey, R. Solubility of Sodium Soaps in Aqueous Salt Solutions. *J. Colloid Interface Sci.* **2005**, *291*, 543–549. [CrossRef] [PubMed]

72. Zhu, H.; Yang, J.; Wu, M.; Wu, Q.; Liu, J.; Zhang, J. Biobased Plasticizers from Tartaric Acid: Synthesis and Effect of Alkyl Chain Length on the Properties of Poly(Vinyl Chloride. *ACS Omega* **2021**, *6*, 13161–13169. [CrossRef]
73. Yang, J.-X.; Long, Y.-Y.; Pan, L.; Men, Y.-F.; Li, Y.-S. Spontaneously Healable Thermoplastic Elastomers Achieved through One-Pot Living Ring-Opening Metathesis Copolymerization of Well-Designed Bulky Monomers. *ACS Appl. Mater. Interfaces* **2016**, *8*, 12445–12455. [CrossRef] [PubMed]
74. Rahman, M.; Brazel, C.S. Ionic Liquids: New Generation Stable Plasticizers for Poly(Vinyl Chloride). *Polym. Degrad. Stab.* **2006**, *91*, 3371–3382. [CrossRef]
75. Keskin, B.; Yuksekdag, A.; Zeytuncu, B.; Koyuncu, I. Development of Polymer Inclusion Membranes for Palladium Recovery: Effect of Base Polymer, Carriers, and Plasticizers on Structure and Performance. *J. Water Process Eng.* **2023**, *52*, 103576. [CrossRef]
76. Shah, B.L.; Shertukde, V.V. Effect of Plasticizers on Mechanical, Electrical, Permanence, and Thermal Properties of Poly(Vinyl Chloride). *J. Appl. Polym. Sci.* **2003**, *90*, 3278–3284. [CrossRef]
77. Max, J.-J.; Chapados, C. Infrared Spectroscopy of Aqueous Carboxylic Acids: Comparison between Different Acids and Their Salts. *J. Phys. Chem. A* **2004**, *108*, 3324–3337. [CrossRef]
78. Fontàs, C.; Tayeb, R.; Dhahbi, M.; Gaudichet, E.; Thominette, F.; Roy, P.; Steenkeste, K.; Fontaine-Aupart, M.-P.; Tingry, S.; Tronel-Peyroz, E.; et al. Polymer Inclusion Membranes: The Concept of Fixed Sites Membrane Revised. *J. Membr. Sci.* **2007**, *290*, 62–72. [CrossRef]
79. Witt, K.; Radzymińska-Lenarcik, E. Characterization of PVC-Based Polymer Inclusion Membranes with Phosphonium Ionic Liquids. *J. Therm. Anal. Calorim.* **2019**, *138*, 4437–4443. [CrossRef]
80. Zhao, S.; Samadi, A.; Wang, Z.; Pringle, J.M.; Zhang, Y.; Kolev, S.D. Ionic Liquid-Based Polymer Inclusion Membranes for Metal Ions Extraction and Recovery: Fundamentals, Considerations, and Prospects. *Chem. Eng. J.* **2024**, *481*, 148792. [CrossRef]

molecules

MDPI

Article

Non-Targeted Nuclear Magnetic Resonance Analysis for Food Authenticity: A Comparative Study on Tomato Samples

Biagia Musio [1,*], Rosa Ragone [1], Stefano Todisco [1], Antonino Rizzuti [1], Egidio Iorio [2], Mattea Chirico [2], Maria Elena Pisanu [2], Nadia Meloni [3], Piero Mastrorilli [1,4] and Vito Gallo [1,4]

1 Department of Civil, Environmental, Land, Building Engineering and Chemistry (DICATECh), Polytechnic University of Bari, Via Orabona, 4, I-70125 Bari, Italy; rosa.ragone@poliba.it (R.R.); stefano.todisco@poliba.it (S.T.); antonino.rizzuti@poliba.it (A.R.); piero.mastrorilli@poliba.it (P.M.); vito.gallo@poliba.it (V.G.)

2 Istituto Superiore di Sanità, Core Facilities Istituto Superiore Di Sanità, Viale Regina Elena, 299, I-00161 Roma, Italy; egidio.iorio@iss.it (E.I.); mattea.chirico@iss.it (M.C.); mariaelena.pisanu@iss.it (M.E.P.)

3 Agenzia Regionale Protezione Ambientale Lazio, Dipartimento Prevenzione e Laboratorio Integrato, Servizio Coordinamento delle Attività di Laboratorio, Unità Laboratorio Chimico di Latina, Via Mario Siciliano, 1, I-04100 Latina, Italy; nadia.meloni@arpalazio.it

4 Innovative Solutions S.r.l., Spin-Off Company of the Polytechnic University of Bari, Zona H 150/B, I-70015 Noci, Italy

* Correspondence: biagia.musio@poliba.it; Tel.: +39-0805963569

Abstract: Non-targeted NMR is widely accepted as a powerful and robust analytical tool for food control. Nevertheless, standardized procedures based on validated methods are still needed when a non-targeted approach is adopted. Interlaboratory comparisons carried out in recent years have demonstrated the statistical equivalence of spectra generated by different instruments when the sample was prepared by the same operator. The present study focused on assessing the reproducibility of NMR spectra of the same matrix when different operators performed individually both the sample preparation and the measurements using their spectrometer. For this purpose, two independent laboratories prepared 63 tomato samples according to a previously optimized procedure and recorded the corresponding 1D ^{1}H NMR spectra. A classification model was built using the spectroscopic fingerprint data delivered by the two laboratories to assess the geographical origin of the tomato samples. The performance of the optimized statistical model was satisfactory, with a 97.62% correct sample classification rate. The results of this work support the suitability of NMR techniques in food control routines even when samples are prepared by different operators by using their equipment in independent laboratories.

Keywords: metabolomic analysis; NMR; geographical origin; method validation; fingerprint; inter-laboratory comparison; food control; traceability

check for updates

Citation: Musio, B.; Ragone, R.; Todisco, S.; Rizzuti, A.; Iorio, E.; Chirico, M.; Pisanu, M.E.; Meloni, N.; Mastrorilli, P.; Gallo, V. Non-Targeted Nuclear Magnetic Resonance Analysis for Food Authenticity: A Comparative Study on Tomato Samples. *Molecules* **2024**, *29*, 4441. https://doi.org/10.3390/molecules29184441

Academic Editors: Giuseppina Raffaini and Fabio Ganazzoli

Received: 8 August 2024
Revised: 13 September 2024
Accepted: 15 September 2024
Published: 19 September 2024

1. Introduction

In the last decades, applications of metabolomics based on NMR spectroscopy for food control, in terms of quality, safety, and authenticity, have extraordinarily increased [1–9], and many attempts have been made to include NMR protocols in the list of the official routine methods [10–12]. Due to the chemical complexity that generally characterizes food matrices, the non-targeted approach (combined with multivariate statistical analysis) finds many applications in studies on the variety, geographical origin, possible frauds, production, and industrial processing of foodstuffs [13–17]. The non-targeted approach allows getting a large amount of information on the wide range of metabolites (fingerprinting) or a set of selected metabolites (profiling, often referred to as the semi-targeted approach) contained in a complex mixture [16,18–21].

In this context, metabolomic analysis based on ^{1}H NMR spectroscopy presents multiple advantages: it is non-destructive, intrinsically quantitative, not time-consuming, cost-effective, and particularly robust [22].

Specifically, the robustness of ^{1}H NMR spectroscopy is based on the ability to generate comparable spectra for the same set of samples using differently configured instruments. The results of some recent interlaboratory studies demonstrated that the statistical equivalence of NMR spectra can be reached when the FIDs, generated by differently configured spectrometers upon applying optimized acquisition parameters, are opportunely processed. Indeed, inter-laboratory variance can be significantly decreased when the spectra are processed by a single operator compared to multi-operator processing regardless of the software used [23,24]. Furthermore, it has been demonstrated the crucial importance of the method adopted to reduce the raw spectral data to the numerical matrix subsequently employed for the development of a classification model [25–28].

However, these studies did not account for the variability strictly related to sample preparation. To the best of our knowledge, few works report on comparative studies in which each participating laboratory executed the entire analytical protocol from sample management to NMR acquisition. Deborde et al. focused on the standardization of plant extract preparation, setup of NMR instruments (400, 500, and 600 MHz), verification of sample spectra quality, and spectra processing steps. Specifically, the quality of the produced spectra was based on the coefficient of variation in the full width at half maximum (FWHM) and the signal-to-noise ratio (S/N) of two selected peaks (finding values comprised between 5 and 10% depending on the size of the sample set and the spectrometer field). The global variance of the spectra was verified through the score distance in the PCA scores plot along the components PC1 and PC2 [29].

Herein, further steps have been made to demonstrate the robustness and the applicability of NMR data to generate comparable spectra even when the samples are prepared and analyzed independently by two different laboratories using their equipment and following established protocols. First, the protocols for the sample preparation and NMR measurement were optimized based on statistical quality parameters. Next, the statistical equivalence of the pool of spectra produced by the two laboratories was assessed by applying a multivariate data analysis. Ultimately, a classification model was built and validated to discriminate between tomato samples cultivated in two different Italian regions, namely Lazio and Sicily. Details on the optimization of the sample preparation protocol, along with statistical considerations to assess the comparability of the generated spectra and the reliability of the constructed classification model, will be discussed throughout the manuscript.

2. Results and Discussion

2.1. Optimization of Sample Preparation Protocol

Three different protocols for the sample preparation were tested to evaluate both the extraction capability and the sample stability over the analysis time.

A detailed description of the three protocols is reported in Sections 4.1.1–4.1.3, starting from mechanically squeezed tomatoes (P1) [30], followed by lyophilized tomatoes (P2) [31–34], and homogenized tomatoes (P3) [35]. The choice of the most suitable sample preparation protocol was based on two experimental evaluations, namely the extraction capability and the repeatability of the NMR measurements. The extraction capability was verified through the analysis of the metabolic composition of the aqueous extracts obtained upon application of the three different protocols. Spectroscopic investigations suggested that a higher number of metabolites, such as amino acids and carbohydrates, could be extracted from P3 (See Figure S1 in Supplementary Material). Additionally, the precision and repeatability of the three analytical protocols, including sample preparation and 1D ^{1}H NOESY (Nuclear Overhauser Effect Spectroscopy) measurement, were evaluated. For this purpose, ten NMR samples were prepared for each protocol using the same batch of tomatoes. A well-defined signal in the 1D ^{1}H NOESY spectrum at 1.32 ppm was selected, and the area under such a peak was calculated in the ten spectra. The signal selection was based on its satisfactory resolution and the observed stability of the corresponding metabolite over time. In the absence of changes in the NMR spectra, as in the present case, the calculation of the relative standard deviation of a single signal has been demonstrated as a valid parameter to evaluate the repeatability of NMR measurements [23]. The obtained integral values were subjected to descriptive statistics. As shown in Table 1, the lowest value of %RSD was found when P3 was applied for the sample preparation (%RSD = 1.32), suggesting that integral values calculated for the ten prepared samples were more tightly clustered around the mean compared to the cases P1 and P2. Based on the extracting capability and the measurement reliability, P3 was selected as the most suitable sample preparation protocol for this study and, therefore, was followed by the two laboratories for the subsequent NMR measurements.

Table 1. Results of the descriptive statistics applied on the integral values of the signal at 1.32 ppm as contained in ten 1D ^{1}H NOESY spectra recorded for ten analytical samples of the same tomato when the three protocols (P1–P3) were applied.

Statistic Parameter	P1	P2	P3
Median	0.202	0.142	0.303
Mean (μ)	0.200	0.142	0.304
Standard deviation (σ)	0.005	0.003	0.004
%RSD [a]	2.68	1.83	1.32

[a] Relative Standard Deviation percentage calculated as $\mu/\sigma \times 100$.

2.2. *Metabolic Profile of Tomatoes Aqueous Extracts Following P3*

The main classes of water-soluble metabolites were identified by comparing the 1D ^{1}H NOESY spectra of the aqueous extracts from homogenized tomatoes (Figure 1) with those of reference compounds.

The main classes of metabolites detected in the 1D ^{1}H NOESY spectra of the samples under investigation are in agreement with the data reported in the literature [36,37]. They include organic acids as acetic, malic, and citric acids (**7**, **10**, and **11** in Figure 1); carbohydrates as glucose, fructose, and galacturonate (**14**, **16**, **17**, and **18** in Figure 1); amino acids as isoleucine, leucine, valine, threonine, alanine, GABA, glutamine, aspartic acid, tyrosine, and phenylalanine (**1**, **2**, **3**, **5**, **6**, **8**, **9**, **12**, **21**, and **22** in Figure 1); alcohols as ethanol and methanol (**4** and **15** in Figure 1); nucleosides as adenosine and uridine (**19** and **20** in Figure 1); quaternary ammonium compounds as choline and trigonelline (**13** and **23** in Figure 1). The complete list of metabolites contained in the aqueous extracts of tomato as identified via 1D ^{1}H NOESY measurements is reported in Table S1 in Supplementary Material. Characterization was based on literature data and comparison with reference compounds. Among the attributed signals, those at 6.88 and 7.60 ppm were addressed (Figure 1, compound **9**). Based on the comparison with the reference solution, such signals were assigned to the hydrogen atoms of the amide group of glutamine (**9**). Interestingly, such signals are not observed in the NMR spectra reported in the public database when glutamine is dissolved in water or deuterated water at pH = 7 [38]. Conversely, under our conditions (pH = 4.2), the two broad resonances were observed both in the tomato extracts under investigation and a reference solution of pure glutamine. ^{1}H-^{15}N HMQC experiment performed on a reference solution of pure glutamine revealed that the two signals belong to hydrogen atoms bound to the same nitrogen atom at 112 ppm (see Figure S2 in Supplementary Material). Based on the ^{15}N chemical shift value reported in the literature, such nitrogen can be attributed to the amide functional group [39]. In addition, an exchange process between these two hydrogen atoms was observed performing a 2D ^{1}H NOESY-EXSY experiment (see Figure S3 in Supplementary Material). The exchange with water, if any, could not be detected due to suppression of the water signal during the acquisition of the NMR measurement. Moreover, a NOE contact was observed between the signal at 7.60 ppm and the signal at 2.45 ppm (-CγH2-), suggesting a *syn* relation between these hydrogen atoms. Based on these findings, it can be argued that the rate of the rotation around the C-N in the amide moiety is slowed down under our conditions (pH = 4.2), likely due to a stabilization of the iminol form in the tautomeric equilibrium of the amide. The same considerations were made for the aqueous extracts of tomatoes based on the information contained in the 2D ^{1}H NOESY-EXSY experiment (see Figure S4 in Supplementary Material).

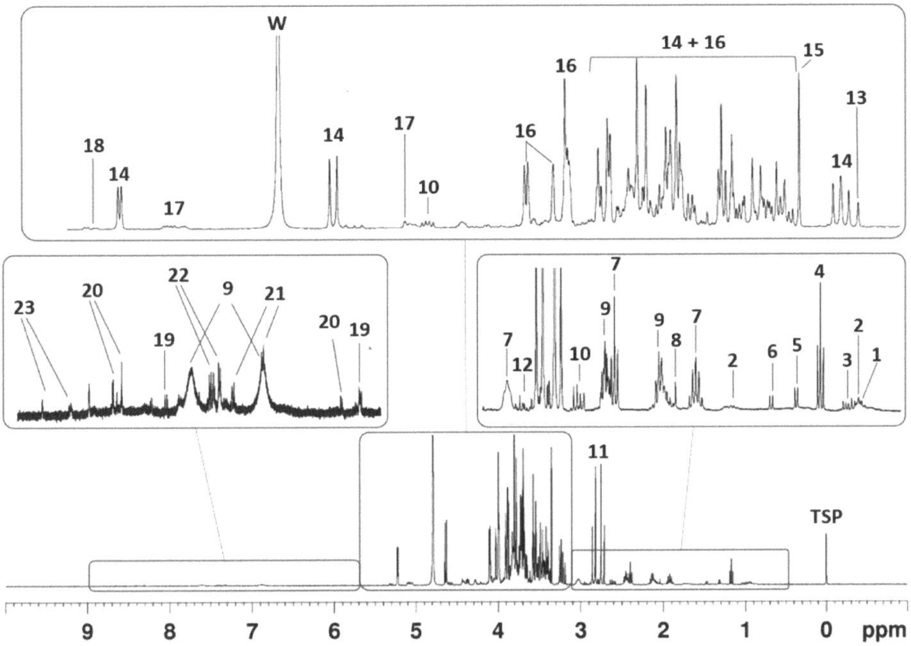

Figure 1. A typical 1D ^{1}H NOESY spectrum of an aqueous extract of a tomato sample (400 MHz). The main classes of metabolites identified via comparison with reference compounds are indicated by increasing numbering. The full chemical shift assignment is reported in Table 1. "W" refers to the residual water signal. The chemical shift scale is referenced to the TSP-d_4 singlet at 0 ppm.

2.3. Statistical Analysis

The numerical matrix obtained from the data treatment described in Section 4.3 was imported into SIMCA 17.0.2 software. A statistical investigation was carried out to assess the comparability of the spectra produced by the two laboratories (Lab1 and Lab2) when they independently prepared the tomato samples according to a well-defined protocol through their equipment. A PCA was performed on the spectral data after a Pareto scaling, which resulted in the most suitable one, to evaluate the sample distribution of the whole dataset containing the spectra recorded by both Lab1 and Lab2. As illustrated in the scores plot (Figure 2a), no significant distance was observed between the group of spectra produced by Lab1 (yellow diamond) and the group of spectra delivered by Lab2 (red triangle). To confirm such a hypothesis, once PCA was applied, the DModX scores plot (Figure 2b) was investigated, assessing that all the spectra produced by the two laboratories were located within the 2-fold DCrit value (2×1.189).

To further confirm the similarity among the spectra produced for the same samples by the two laboratories, a cluster analysis was performed by adopting Euclidean as the Distance Measure and Ward as the Clustering Algorithm. As illustrated in the hierarchical clustering dendrogram (see Figure S5 in Supplementary Material), generally, the spectra produced by the two laboratories for the same sample clustered very closely. Moreover, a pair-wise correlation was attempted, selecting samples as a dimension, Kendall rank correlation as a distance measure, and a correlation cutoff equal to 0.05. The values of correlation coefficients were generally higher than 0.50 both for the replicates produced by Lab1 for the same sample and for the spectra produced by both the laboratories for the same sample (see Figure S6 and Table S2 in Supplementary Material for further details). The evidence obtained from these statistical investigations suggested a satisfactory comparability of the recorded spectra both intra-laboratory (short distance among the replicates produced by Lab1) and inter-laboratory (short distance among the spectra produced by the two laboratories for the same sample).

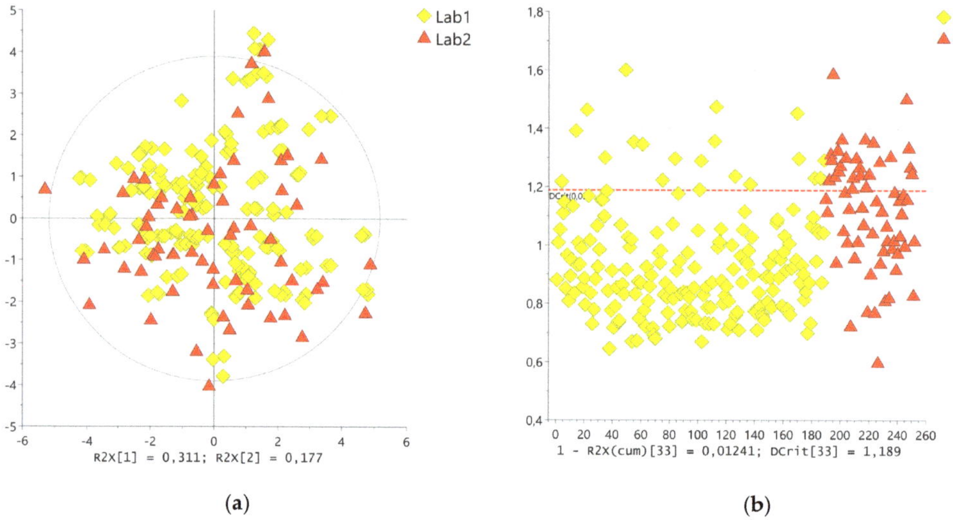

Figure 2. (**a**) PC1/PC2 scores plot related to PCA and (**b**) DModX plots using a dataset composed of all the spectra registered by Lab1 and Lab2. The observations are indicated as yellow diamonds and red triangles for spectra produced by Lab1 and Lab2, respectively.

Once the comparability among the 1D ^{1}H NOESY spectra produced by the two laboratories was demonstrated, the resulting dataset was exploited to build an optimized classification model to assess the geographical origin of the tomato samples. For this purpose, OPLS-DA was adopted as a supervised statistical approach to discriminate between two groups of samples cultivated and collected from Sicily (26 samples) and Lazio (37 samples), respectively. As summarized in Table 2, different combinations of training and validation sets were adopted to verify possible effects on the reliability and prediction capability of the resulting classification models (M1–M9). In all cases, the ratio of samples according to the belonging class, namely Sicily (SI) and Lazio (LA), was kept uniform within the training and the validation sets (ratio SI/LA $\approx$ 1.4).

In the first three cases, two sets of spectra produced by the two laboratories were used to train and validate the models. In the very first case (M1), the training set was composed of 126 out of 189 spectra produced by Lab1 (considering all the replicates) and 42 out of 63 spectra produced by Lab2, randomly extracted from the available spectra (ratio 3:1). The same ratio of 3:1 was maintained for the validation, being formed of 63 spectra from Lab1 and 21 ones from Lab2. Next, to evaluate the effect of the replicates on the overall performance of the classification model, the three replicates produced by Lab1 for each sample were merged based both on the average and median values to train and validate M2 and M3, respectively. Specifically, the merged spectra were used as a training set and validation set in a ratio of 2:1 in M2 as average spectra (Lab1 avg) and in M3 as median spectra (Lab1 med). Ultimately, to verify the interchangeability of the spectra regardless of the producing operator/equipment, four further models, M4–M9, were built and evaluated. In the case of M4, all the spectra produced by Lab1 (189) were used as a training set, while all the spectra recorded by Lab2 (63) were employed to test the model. The average spectrum and the median one were used to train M5 and M6, respectively. In these cases, the spectra produced by Lab2 were employed to validate the models. Lastly, a model was trained by using the 63 spectra recorded by Lab2. Such a model was validated against three different sets composed of the spectra produced by Lab1. Specifically, all spectra, including the replicates, were used in M7; the average spectra were employed in M8 and the median spectra in M9.

Table 2. Summary of the composition of the training set and validation set used to build the OPLS-DA models (M1–M9).

Model	Training Set	Validation Set
M1	Lab1 = 126 Lab2 = 42 Tot. = 168	Lab1 = 63 Lab2 = 21 Tot. = 84
M2	Lab1 avg = 42 Lab2 = 42 Tot. = 84	Lab1 avg = 21 Lab2 = 21 Tot. = 42
M3	Lab1 med = 42 Lab2 = 42 Tot. = 84	Lab1 med = 21 Lab2 = 21 Tot. = 42
M4	Lab1 = 189	Lab2 = 63
M5	Lab1 avg = 63	Lab2 = 63
M6	Lab1 med = 63	Lab2 = 63
M7	Lab2 = 63	Lab1 = 189
M8	Lab2 = 63	Lab1 avg = 63
M9	Lab2 = 63	Lab1 med = 63

Table 3 summarizes the main quality parameters of the nine classification models (M1–M9). The number of predictive (P) and orthogonal components (O) and the total explained variance both in the X and Y matrices were evaluated to assess the main features of the developed model.

Table 3. Summary of quality parameters of OPLS-DA models (M1–M9).

Model	No [a]	R^2X (cum) [b]	R^2Y (cum) [c]	Q^2 (cum) [d]	Q^2 Intercept	R^2 Intercept	F-Value [e]	*p*-Value [f]	Correct Prediction
M1	1P + 8O	0.850	0.767	0.619	−0.444	0.254	13.4641	4.9424×10^{-23}	97.62%
M2	1P + 6O	0.811	0.741	0.505	−0.630	0.365	5.0329	2.3550×10^{-6}	90.48%
M3	1P + 6O	0.810	0.748	0.521	−0.645	0.371	5.3575	9.2400×10^{-7}	92.86%
M4	1P + 8O	0.861	0.802	0.718	−0.351	0.193	24.0347	1.4347×10^{-37}	87.30%
M5	1P + 2O	0.608	0.567	0.419	−0.357	0.215	6.7444	2.0513×10^{-5}	80.95%
M6	1P + 2O	0.606	0.555	0.399	−0.361	0.223	8.9320	1.4372×10^{-13}	80.95%
M7									85.19%
M8	1P + 2O	0.565	0.505	0.308	−0.363	0.242	4.1578	1.5945×10^{-3}	85.71%
M9									85.71%

[a] No indicates the number of predictive (P) and orthogonal (O) components. [b] R^2X (cum) represents the total (predictive and orthogonal) explained variance in model samples (X). [c] R^2Y (cum) represents the cumulative explained variation in the Y matrix. [d] Q^2 (cum) describes the predictive ability of the model based on sevenfold cross-validation. [e] F-value was obtained from the F-test based on the ratio MS Regression/MS Residual (where MS stays for Mean Squares). [f] *p*-value indicates the probability level where a model with this F-value may be the result of just chance. For a significant model, the *p*-value should be lower than 0.05.

M1 and M4 resulted in the most stable and reliable models, being characterized by the highest values of R^2Y (cum) and Q^2 (cum) values, i.e., R^2Y (cum) = 0.767 and Q^2 (cum) = 0.619 for M1; R^2Y (cum) = 0.802 and Q^2 (cum) = 0.718 for M4. The models M2 and M3 showed equally satisfactory values of R^2Y (cum) and Q^2 (cum) values, being around 0.741–0.748 and 0.505–0.521, respectively. Conversely, the quality of the remaining models (M5–M9) was not satisfactory, with R^2Y (cum) and Q^2 (cum) values of 0.505–0.567 and 0.308–0.419, respectively.

The statistical significance of the models was evaluated by computing the p values upon application of analysis of variance (CV-ANOVA) in the cross-validated residuals of the Y-variables. The lowest p-values were obtained for M1 ($p = 4.9424 \times 10^{-23}$) and M4 ($p = 1.4347 \times 10^{-37}$), confirming the highest reliability of these two models.

Permutation tests were performed to check the degree of overfit for the OPLS-DA (number of permutations = 200), whereas the Q^2 intercept value < 0.05 and R^2 intercept value < 0.40 were assumed as indicative of a valid model. As described in Table 3, the computed Q^2 and R^2 intercepts suggested that all the built models can be considered valid and correctly fitted (see Figure S7 in Supplementary Material for further details).

Once the models were fitted on the training sets and the reliability was assessed, the models were used to predict the responses for the observations in the validation set (see Figure S8 in Supplementary Material for further details). The models M1–M3 fitted on a mixture of samples produced by the two laboratories were able to achieve a high correct prediction of the observations in the validation set (90.48–97.62%). In all the other cases (M4–M9), the prediction capability was lower, with a percentage of correct predictions in the range of 80.95–87.30%.

The Receiver Operating Characteristic (ROC) curves were investigated to evaluate the difference in the performance of M1 and M4, which have resulted in the most promising models according to the quality parameters illustrated in Table 3 and the results of CV-ANOVA. The values of Area Under the Curve (AUC) were computed both for M1 (Figure 3a) and M4 (Figure 3b), finding a higher value for the first model (0.996471) compared to the latter (0.974012).

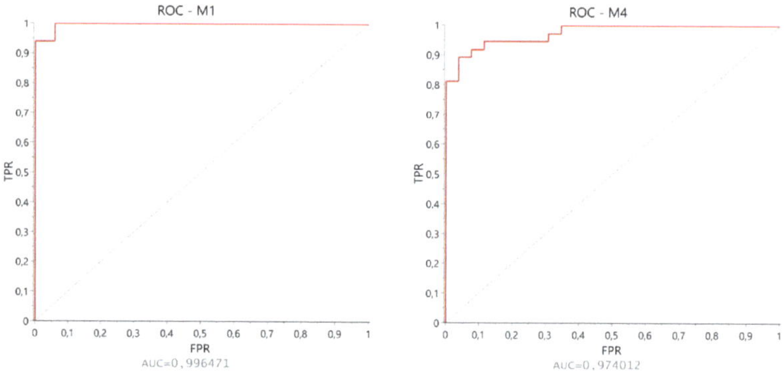

(a) (b)

Figure 3. ROC curves for models (**a**) M1 and (**b**) M4.

3. Discussion

The results of the present study represent a step forward and an integration of the previous ones reporting on the aspects affecting the proficiency of inter-laboratory comparisons dealing with the analysis of food matrices through NMR-based metabolomics. The evaluation of the statistical equivalence of NMR spectra produced by different facilities has been the object of many inter-laboratory comparisons, both for the quantification of well-defined metabolites [40–43] and for screening purposes towards the assessment of food authenticity and traceability [23,44,45]. The present work aimed at establishing the comparability of the 1D ^{1}H NOESY spectra produced by two different laboratories during the analysis of food samples (tomatoes) and the applicability of such spectroscopic data for the construction of an opportune classification model able to discriminate, as a case study, between tomato samples cultivated in two Italian regions, i.e., Lazio and Sicily.

The preparation protocol was deeply investigated in a way to achieve a good compromise in terms of extraction capability, which translates into the amount of metabolites extracted from tomatoes, and satisfactory measurement repeatability. For this purpose, three different preparation protocols were investigated. Following an in-depth analysis of the 1D ^{1}H NOESY spectra, the aqueous extract of homogenized tomato was found to be the most informative in terms of the number of extracted metabolites compared to that obtained from tomato juice or lyophilized tomato. In addition, sample preparation starting from homogenized tomatoes allowed for more repeatable measurements, considering the relative standard deviation (%RSD) computed for the integral of well-defined signals in spectra of ten replicates of the same tomato batch. The optimized protocols for the sample preparation and NMR measurement were performed by two different laboratories utilizing their facilities. An in-depth statistical investigation was carried out to establish the comparability of the produced spectra for the same sample. Specifically, the distance among the spectra was studied by analyzing the distance of the samples within a PCA model (DModX), the distance among the samples according to hierarchical clustering, and the values of the correlation coefficients among the samples. Based on the results of these investigations, the spectra produced by the two laboratories showed a reciprocal very short distance, confirming a satisfactory statistical equivalence among them. The pool of spectra was then used for the construction of the OPLS-DA model to discriminate the tomato samples cultivated in Lazio from those cultivated in Sicily. Different combinations of training and validation sets were investigated, aiming at obtaining a reliable and valid classification model. The best results were observed when a combination of spectra produced by the two laboratories was used to train the model (M1). In this case, the OPLS-DA model resulted as highly reliable and fitted in terms of quality parameters and validation tests. Importantly, this model was found to be highly predictive with a correct prediction rate of around 97% when a mixture of 84 samples produced by both laboratories and unknown to the algorithm was used to query the model (Table 4, M1). Lower performance was observed when the model was trained using all the spectra produced by a single laboratory, and the model was validated using the spectra delivered by the second laboratory (Table 4, M4, and M7). Merging replicates in the form of average (Table 4, M2, M5, and M8) or median (Table 4, M3, M6, and M9) spectra resulted in a slight loss of information with a consequent deterioration in the predictive ability of the model.

The non-targeted approach utilized in this study offers several practical advantages for the food industry. Firstly, its ability to detect a wide range of compounds without prior knowledge allows for a more comprehensive monitoring of food products. This holistic view can enhance the detection of food fraud, ensuring that food products meet regulatory standards and consumer expectations. Secondly, the efficiency of the non-targeted approach in processing large datasets and identifying unique chemical fingerprints could be valuable for establishing traceability systems that are more robust and less dependent on predefined markers. This adaptability is particularly important in a globalized food market, where supply chains are complex and the types of fraud or contamination can vary significantly.

By integrating non-targeted approaches into standard traceability practices, the food industry can develop more resilient and adaptive systems that better respond to emerging challenges and risks, thereby safeguarding public health and maintaining market integrity.

The results described in this work are very encouraging, considering the possibility of building a model trained by a pool of spectra produced by independent laboratories around the world analyzing samples prepared according to a well-established protocol through their facilities. Such data collection may serve for other spectra whose authenticity is unknown to be queried for classification purposes.

Table 4. The Misclassification table shows the proportion of correctly classified observations in the prediction set for the OPLS-DA models (M1–M9). Correctly classified observations are indicated in green. Misclassified observations are indicated in pink.

Model	Class	Prediction Set	Predicted as SI	Predicted as LA	Correct Prediction %	Fisher's Prob.
M1	SI	34	32	2	97.62	3.6×10^{-21}
	LA	50	0	50		
M2	SI	19	16	3	90.48	8.8×10^{-8}
	LA	23	1	22		
M3	SI	19	16	3	92.86	5.8×10^{-9}
	LA	23	0	23		
M4	SI	26	20	6	87.3	3×10^{-9}
	LA	37	2	35		
M5	SI	26	15	11	80.95	7.9×10^{-7}
	LA	37	1	36		
M6	SI	26	15	11	80.95	7.9×10^{-7}
	LA	37	1	36		
M7	SI	78	60	18	85.19	1.5×10^{-22}
	LA	111	10	101		
M8	SI	26	20	6	85.71	2.0×10^{-8}
	LA	37	3	34		
M9	SI	26	20	6	85.71	2.0×10^{-8}
	LA	37	3	34		

4. Materials and Methods

4.1. Materials

3-(Trimethylsilyl)-2,2,3,3-tetradeutero-propionic acid sodium salt (TSP-d_4, CAS N. 24493-21-8, 99%D, Armar Chemicals, Döttingen, Switzerland), hydrochloric acid (HCl, 37%w, CAS N. 7647-01-0; ≥99.5%, Sigma-Aldrich, Milan, Italy), sodium oxalate ($Na_2C_2O_4$, CAS N. 62-76-0; ≥99.5%, Sigma-Aldrich, Milan, Italy), sodium azide (NaN_3, CAS N. 26628-22-8; ≥99.5%, Sigma-Aldrich, Milan, Italy), and deuterium oxide (D_2O, CAS. N. 7789-20-0, 99.86%D, Eurisotop, Saclay, France) were used for sample preparation. Methanol-d_4 (CD_3OD, CAS. N. 811-98-3, 99.80%D, Eurisotop, Saclay, France) was used for temperature calibration. Whatman syringe membrane filters (PTFE, pore size 0.2 μm, diam. 47 mm) were provided by Sigma-Aldrich. NMR tubes (Wilmad WG-1000-7) were provided by ATS Life Sciences Wilmad, Vineland, NJ, United States. A total number of 63 tomato samples were provided by ARPA-Lazio, Rome, Italy. The samples were collected from two different Italian geographical regions (n. 26 samples from Sicily and n. 37 samples from Lazio). All samples were collected according to official recommendations for sampling (Regulations (CE) no. 834/2007, no. 889/2008, no. 1235/2008, and following modifications) [46,47] and processed (homogenized) according to Regulations (CE) no. 401/2006, no. 178/2010, and following modifications [48,49].

The preparation protocol was optimized on tomatoes cv Centus F1—ISI 25765 provided by "Azienda Agricola Tulipa S.r.l.", Stornarella (FG, Italy). Tomatoes were stored at −20 °C until analysis. The following three procedures were tested for the sample preparation: manual squeezing (P1), lyophilization (P2), and homogeneization (P3). For all three procedures, the same buffer solution of sodium oxalate [$(HC_2O_4)^-/(C_2O_4)^{2-}$ 0.11 M, pH 4.2] containing NaN_3 as a bacteriostatic agent was used for the extraction. The buffer was prepared according to the following recipe: $Na_2C_2O_4$ (37 g) was dissolved in distilled water (800 mL) at room temperature. HCl 37%w (about 6.9 mL) was added dropwise, adjusting the pH to a value of 4.2. Next, NaN_3 (170 mg/L) was added. Finally, water was added to the solution to reach a final volume of 1 L.

4.1.1. Method P1 [30]

Tomatoes were defrosted for 60 min at room temperature. Samples were mechanically squeezed and centrifuged for 10 min at 4000× *g*. An aliquot of supernatant (318 μL) was mixed with sodium oxalate buffer (222 μL) and TSP-d_4/D_2O (60 μL). The resulting solution was transferred into an NMR tube.

4.1.2. Method P2 [50]

Tomatoes were freeze-dried at −50 °C and 0.045 atm for 24 h in a lyophilizer (Martin-Christ GmbH, Model Alpha 1-4 LSC, Osterode am Harz, Germany), then they were ground manually employing a mortar and a pestle. The obtained powder was sieved (through a metallic sifter, pore size of 0.5 mm) and stored at room temperature under vacuum in a plastic bag protected from light until analysis. A quantity of 200 mg of sample was weighed and dissolved in 1.8 mL of buffer. The solution was sonicated for 10 min at 40 kHz, vortexed for 5 min at 2500 rpm, and centrifuged for 10 min at 4000× *g*. A volume of 540 μL of supernatant was transferred into an NMR tube and added to 60 μL of TSP-d_4/D_2O solution. The resulting solution was transferred into an NMR tube.

4.1.3. Method P3 [29]

Tomatoes were homogenized and stored at −20 °C. Before analysis, samples were thawed for 60 min at room temperature. An aliquot of 4.0 g of sample was dissolved in 1.0 mL of buffer and vortexed for 5 min at 2500 rpm. The solution was subjected to a thermic treatment for 10 min at 80 °C in a thermostatic bath, followed by a centrifugation step for 10 min at 4000× *g*. The supernatant was filtered off using a syringe filter (PTFE, porosity = 0.2 μm, diameter 47 mm). An aliquot of the filtrate (540 μL) was mixed with TSP/D_2O (60 μL), and the resulting solution was transferred into an NMR tube.

4.2. NMR Measurements

NMR experiments were conducted at 298.1 ± 0.1 K. Before NMR acquisition, the temperature was calibrated using a tube containing pure methanol-d_4 (CD_3OD, 99.80%D) [51].

Lab1 used a Bruker Avance 400 spectrometer equipped with a 5 mm inverse broadband (BBI) probe, an autosampler, and an automatic system for tuning and shimming, using TOPSPIN 3.0 software for acquisition (Bruker BioSpin GmbH, Rheinstetten, Germany). Lab2 used an NMR spectrometer Bruker Avance 400 equipped with a 5 mm inverse broadband (BBI) probe and a manual system for tuning and shimming, using the XWIN-NMR 3.5 operative system for acquisition.

The following acquisition parameters were optimized and adopted to record the 1D ^{1}H NOESY measurements: pulse program = noesygppr1d; size of fid (TD) = 128 K data points; spectral width (SW) = 20 ppm; transmitter offset = 4.70 ppm; dummy scans (ds) = 4; number of scans (ns) = 64; acquisition time = 8.12 s; mixing time (d8) = 0.01 s; recycle delay (d1) = 30 s. Before the analysis, each laboratory performed a calibration of the 90° pulse on the sample solution.

The 1D ^{1}H NOESY FIDs (252) produced by the two different laboratories (189 FIDs by Lab1 and 63 by Lab2) were processed by a single operator using the software MestReNova 11.0 (Mestrelab Research SL, Santiago de Compostela, Spain). The FIDs were zero-filled with 128 K number of points before undergoing a Fourier transformation by applying an exponential multiplication function with a line broadening of 0.1 Hz. The spectrum phase was manually corrected, while the baseline was subjected to an automatic correction. The TSP-d_4 singlet signal was set at δ = 0.00 ppm and used as a chemical shift reference.

4.3. Data Preprocessing and Chemometrics

The raw data (FIDs) derived from the 1D ^{1}H NOESY measurements were processed by a single operator using MestReNova and segmented into regular-sized (0.04 ppm) intervals (buckets) in the range of [10.50, 0.50] ppm. The underlying area of each bucket was calculated and normalized to the total intensity. The areas of the buckets in the region

[5.13, 4.69] ppm, corresponding to the residual water signal, were set to 0. The data were stored as a table with one sample per row and one variable (bucket) per column. The data matrices were imported into the software SIMCA 17.0.2 (Umetrics, Umea, Sweden) or MetaboAnalyst 5.0. The NMR spectra constituted the observations, while the buckets constituted the x-variables. Buckets were centered and subjected to Pareto scaling (each x_j-variable was scaled to $1/\text{sqrt}(\text{sd}_j)$, where sd_j is the standard deviation of the x_j-variable computed around the mean) to avoid noise inflation. An unsupervised method, the Principal Component Analysis (PCA), was applied to obtain an overview of all available data. Then, a supervised approach, the Orthogonal Partial Least Squares Discriminant Analysis (OPLS-DA), was performed to build a model for the classification of tomato samples according to the geographical origin, Lazio (LA) vs. Sicily (SI). The evaluation of the quality of OPLS-DA models was based on the parameters R^2 (goodness-of-fit) and Q^2 (goodness-of-prediction in 7-fold cross-validation). Permutation tests were performed to assess the performance of the OPLS-DA models.

Supplementary Materials: The following supporting information can be downloaded at: https://www.mdpi.com/article/10.3390/molecules29184441/s1, Figure S1: 1D ^{1}H NOESY spectra of aqueous extracts of squeezed tomato (P1), lyophilized tomato (P2), and homogenized tomato (P3); Table S1: List of metabolites contained in the aqueous extracts of tomato and identified via 1D ^{1}H NOESY measurements; Figure S2: A portion of the ^{1}H-^{15}N HMQC of a reference solution of glutamine at pH 4.2; Figure S3: ^{1}H-NOESY/EXSY spectrum of a reference solution of glutamine at pH 4.2; Figure S4: ^{1}H-NOESY/EXSY spectrum of aqueous extracts of tomato; Figure S5: Hierarchical clustering dendrogram; Figure S6: Correlation heatmap; Table S2: Correlation table; Figure S7: Results of the permutation tests; Figure S8: Prediction scores plot (P1/O1) of OPLS-DA models (a) M1, (b) M2, (c) M3, (d) M4, (e) M5, (f) M6, (g) M7, (h) M8, and (i) M9.

Author Contributions: Conceptualization, B.M. and V.G.; methodology, B.M. and R.R.; software, R.R.; validation, B.M., R.R. and S.T.; formal analysis, S.T., A.R., E.I., M.C. and M.E.P.; investigation, S.T. and N.M.; resources, N.M., V.G. and P.M.; data curation, R.R.; writing—original draft preparation, B.M. and R.R.; writing—review and editing, B.M., R.R., S.T., A.R., P.M. and V.G.; visualization, S.T.; supervision, B.M. and V.G.; project administration, V.G. and P.M.; funding acquisition, V.G. All authors have read and agreed to the published version of the manuscript.

Funding: This research was funded by Istituto Poligrafico Zecca dello Stato (IPZS), research agreement CUP: D91I18000970005.

Institutional Review Board Statement: Not applicable.

Informed Consent Statement: Not applicable.

Data Availability Statement: The original contributions presented in the study are included in the article/Supplementary Material, further inquiries can be directed to the corresponding author.

Acknowledgments: Mirco Leoni from ARPA Lazio is gratefully acknowledged for supplying the authentic tomato samples utilized in this study. We are also grateful to Francesco Lo Greco from ARPA Puglia for his contribution to optimizing the sample preparation protocol described in Section 4.1.2.

Conflicts of Interest: Author Vito Gallo was employed by the company Spin-Off Company of the Polytechnic University of Bar. The remaining authors declare that the research was conducted in the absence of any commercial or financial relationships that could be construed as a potential conflict of interest.

References

1. Hatzakis, E. Nuclear Magnetic Resonance (NMR) Spectroscopy in Food Science: A Comprehensive Review. *Compr. Rev. Food Sci. Food Saf.* **2019**, *18*, 189–220. [CrossRef] [PubMed]
2. Abreu, A.C.; Fernández, I. NMR Metabolomics Applied on the Discrimination of Variables Influencing Tomato (Solanum lycopersicum). *Molecules* **2020**, *25*, 3738. [CrossRef] [PubMed]
3. Tahir, H.E.; Arslan, M.; Komla Mahunu, G.; Adam Mariod, A.B.H.; Hashim, S.; Xiaobo, Z.; Jiyong, S.; El-Seedi, H.R.; Musa, T.H. The use of analytical techniques coupled with chemometrics for tracing the geographical origin of oils: A systematic review (2013–2020). *Food Chem.* **2022**, *366*, 130633. [CrossRef] [PubMed]

4. Rifna, E.J.; Pandiselvam, R.; Kothakota, A.; Subba Rao, K.V.; Dwivedi, M.; Kumar, M.; Thirumdas, R.; Ramesh, S.V. Advanced process analytical tools for identification of adulterants in edible oils—A review. *Food Chem.* **2022**, *369*, 130898. [CrossRef]
5. Zhao, J.; Wang, M.; Saroja, S.G.; Khan, I.A. NMR technique and methodology in botanical health product analysis and quality control. *J. Pharm. Biomed. Anal.* **2022**, *207*, 114376. [CrossRef]
6. Suh, J.H. Critical review: Metabolomics in dairy science—Evaluation of milk and milk product quality. *Food Res. Int.* **2022**, *154*, 110984. [CrossRef]
7. Dimitrakopoulou, M.E.; Vantarakis, A. Does Traceability Lead to Food Authentication? A Systematic Review from A European Perspective. *Food Rev. Int.* **2021**, *39*, 537–559. [CrossRef]
8. Colnago, L.A.; Wiesman, Z.; Pages, G.; Musse, M.; Monaretto, T.; Windt, C.W.; Rondeau-Mouro, C. Low field, time domain NMR in the agriculture and agrifood sectors: An overview of applications in plants, foods and biofuels. *J. Magn. Reson.* **2021**, *323*, 106899. [CrossRef] [PubMed]
9. Laghi, L.; Picone, G.; Capozzi, F. Nuclear magnetic resonance for foodomics beyond food analysis. *TrAC—Trends Anal. Chem.* **2014**, *59*, 93–102. [CrossRef]
10. Solovyev, P.A.; Fauhl-Hassek, C.; Riedl, J.; Esslinger, S.; Bontempo, L.; Camin, F. NMR spectroscopy in wine authentication: An official control perspective. *Compr. Rev. Food Sci. Food Saf.* **2021**, *20*, 2040–2062. [CrossRef]
11. Palacios-Jordan, H.; Jané-Brunet, A.; Jané-Brunet, E.; Puiggròs, F.; Canela, N.; Rodríguez, M.A. Considerations on the Analysis of E-900 Food Additive: An NMR Perspective. *Foods* **2022**, *11*, 297. [CrossRef] [PubMed]
12. Ehlers, M.; Horn, B.; Raeke, J.; Fauhl-Hassek, C.; Hermann, A.; Brockmeyer, J.; Riedl, J. Towards harmonization of non-targeted 1H NMR spectroscopy-based wine authentication: Instrument comparison. *Food Control* **2022**, *132*, 108508. [CrossRef]
13. Weljie, A.M.; Newton, J.; Mercier, P.; Carlson, E.; Slupsky, C.M. Targeted pofiling: Quantitative analysis of1H NMR metabolomics data. *Anal. Chem.* **2006**, *78*, 4430–4442. [CrossRef] [PubMed]
14. Mounet, F.; Lemaire-Chamley, M.; Maucourt, M.; Cabasson, C.; Giraudel, J.L.; Deborde, C.; Lessire, R.; Gallusci, P.; Bertrand, A.; Gaudillère, M.; et al. Quantitative metabolic profiles of tomato flesh and seeds during fruit development: Complementary analysis with ANN and PCA. *Metabolomics* **2007**, *3*, 273–288. [CrossRef]
15. Corsaro, C.; Mallamace, D.; Vasi, S.; Ferrantelli, V.; Dugo, G.; Cicero, N. 1H HR-MAS NMR Spectroscopy and the Metabolite Determination of Typical Foods in Mediterranean Diet. *J. Anal. Methods Chem.* **2015**, *2015*, 175696. [CrossRef]
16. Sobolev, A.P.; Thomas, F.; Donarski, J.; Ingallina, C.; Circi, S.; Cesare Marincola, F.; Capitani, D.; Mannina, L. Use of NMR applications to tackle future food fraud issues. *Trends Food Sci. Technol.* **2019**, *91*, 347–353. [CrossRef]
17. Bharti, S.K.; Roy, R. Quantitative 1H NMR spectroscopy. *TrAC - Trends Anal. Chem.* **2012**, *35*, 5–26. [CrossRef]
18. Sobolev, A.P.; Mannina, L.; Proietti, N.; Carradori, S.; Daglia, M.; Giusti, A.M.; Antiochia, R.; Capitani, D. Untargeted NMR-based methodology in the study of fruit metabolites. *Molecules* **2015**, *20*, 4088–4108. [CrossRef]
19. Fiorino, G.M.; Garino, C.; Arlorio, M.; Logrieco, A.F.; Losito, I.; Monaci, L. Overview on Untargeted Methods to Combat Food Frauds: A Focus on Fishery Products. *J. Food Qual.* **2018**, *2018*, 1581746. [CrossRef]
20. Calò, F.; Girelli, C.R.; Wang, S.C.; Fanizzi, F.P. Geographical Origin Assessment of Extra Virgin Olive Oil via NMR and MS Combined with Chemometrics as Analytical Approaches. *Foods* **2022**, *11*, 113. [CrossRef]
21. Oms-Oliu, G.; Hertog, M.L.A.T.M.; Van de Poel, B.; Ampofo-Asiama, J.; Geeraerd, A.H.; Nicolai, B.M. Metabolic characterization of tomato fruit during preharvest development, ripening, and postharvest shelf-life. *Postharvest Biol. Technol.* **2011**, *62*, 7–16. [CrossRef]
22. Riswanto, F.D.O.; Windarsih, A.; Lukitaningsih, E.; Rafi, M.; Fadzilah, N.A.; Rohman, A. Metabolite Fingerprinting Based on1 H-NMR Spectroscopy and Liquid Chromatography for the Authentication of Herbal Products. *Molecules* **2022**, *27*, 1198. [CrossRef] [PubMed]
23. Gallo, V.; Ragone, R.; Musio, B.; Todisco, S.; Rizzuti, A.; Mastrorilli, P.; Pontrelli, S.; Intini, N.; Scapicchio, P.; Triggiani, M.; et al. A Contribution to the Harmonization of Non-targeted NMR Methods for Data-Driven Food Authenticity Assessment. *Food Anal. Methods* **2020**, *13*, 530–541. [CrossRef]
24. Zailer, E.; Holzgrabe, U.; Diehl, B.W.K. Interlaboratory Comparison Test as an Evaluation of Applicability of an Alternative Edible Oil Analysis by 1H NMR Spectroscopy. *J. AOAC Int.* **2017**, *100*, 1819–1830. [CrossRef] [PubMed]
25. Sousa, S.A.A.; Magalhães, A.; Ferreira, M.M.C. Optimized bucketing for NMR spectra: Three case studies. *Chemom. Intell. Lab. Syst.* **2013**, *122*, 93–102. [CrossRef]
26. Karaman, I. Preprocessing and pretreatment of metabolomics data for statistical analysis. In *Advances in Experimental Medicine and Biology*; Springer New York LLC: New York, NY, USA, 2017; Volume 965, pp. 145–161.
27. Mulder, F.A.A.; Tenori, L.; Licari, C.; Luchinat, C. Practical considerations for rapid and quantitative NMR-based metabolomics. *J. Magn. Reson.* **2023**, *352*, 107462. [CrossRef]
28. Ragone, R.; Todisco, S.; Triggiani, M.; Pontrelli, S.; Latronico, M.; Mastrorilli, P.; Intini, N.; Ferroni, C.; Musio, B.; Gallo, V. Development of a food class-discrimination system by non-targeted NMR analyses using different magnetic field strengths. *Food Chem.* **2020**, *332*, 127339. [CrossRef]
29. Deborde, C.; Fontaine, J.X.; Jacob, D.; Botana, A.; Nicaise, V.; Richard-Forget, F.; Lecomte, S.; Decourtil, C.; Hamade, K.; Mesnard, F.; et al. Optimizing 1D 1H-NMR profiling of plant samples for high throughput analysis: Extract preparation, standardization, automation and spectra processing. *Metabolomics* **2019**, *15*, 28. [CrossRef]

30. Musio, B.; Ragone, R.; Todisco, S.; Rizzuti, A.; Latronico, M.; Mastrorilli, P.; Pontrelli, S.; Intini, N.; Scapicchio, P.; Triggiani, M.; et al. A community-built calibration system: The case study of quantification of metabolites in grape juice by qNMR spectroscopy. *Talanta* **2020**, *214*, 120855. [CrossRef]
31. Le Gall, G.; Colquhoun, I.J.; Davis, A.L.; Collins, G.J.; Verhoeyen, M.E. Metabolite profiling of tomato (Lycopersicon esculentum) using 1H NMR spectroscopy as a tool to detect potential unintended effects following a genetic modification. *J. Agric. Food Chem.* **2003**, *51*, 2447–2456. [CrossRef]
32. Zhang, G.; Abdulla, W. On honey authentication and adulterant detection techniques. *Food Control* **2022**, *138*, 108992. [CrossRef]
33. ElNaker, N.A.; Daou, M.; Ochsenkühn, M.A.; Amin, S.A.; Yousef, A.F.; Yousef, L.F. A metabolomics approach to evaluate the effect of lyophilization versus oven drying on the chemical composition of plant extracts. *Sci. Rep.* **2021**, *11*, 22679. [CrossRef]
34. Beteinakis, S.; Papachristodoulou, A.; Mikros, E.; Halabalaki, M. From sample preparation to NMR-based metabolic profiling in food commodities: The case of table olives. *Phytochem. Anal.* **2022**, *33*, 83–93. [CrossRef] [PubMed]
35. Kim, H.K.; Choi, Y.H.; Verpoorte, R. NMR-based metabolomic analysis of plants. *Nat. Protoc.* **2010**, *5*, 536–549. [CrossRef]
36. Chamley, M.L.; Mounet, F.; Deborde, C.; Maucourt, M.; Jacob, D.; Moing, A. NMR-based tissular and developmental metabolomics of tomato fruit. *Metabolites* **2019**, *9*, 93. [CrossRef]
37. Hohmann, M.; Christoph, N.; Wachter, H.; Holzgrabe, U. 1H NMR profiling as an approach to differentiate conventionally and organically grown tomatoes. *J. Agric. Food Chem.* **2014**, *62*, 8530–8540. [CrossRef] [PubMed]
38. Human Metabolome Database: 1H NMR Spectrum (1D, 500 MHz, H_2O, Experimental) (HMDB0000641). Available online: https://hmdb.ca/spectra/nmr_one_d/1452 (accessed on 13 September 2024).
39. Tjandra, N.; Bax, A. Solution NMR Measurement of Amide Proton Chemical Shift Anisotropy in 15N-Enriched Proteins. Correlation with Hydrogen Bond Length§. *J. Am. Chem. Soc.* **1997**, *119*, 8076–8082. [CrossRef]
40. Bauer, M.; Bertario, A.; Boccardi, G.; Fontaine, X.; Rao, R.; Verrier, D. Reproducibility of 1H-NMR integrals: A collaborative study. *J. Pharm. Biomed. Anal.* **1998**, *17*, 419–425. [CrossRef]
41. Chen, Z.; Lian, X.; Zhou, M.; Zhang, X.; Wang, C. Quantitation of L-cystine in Food Supplements and Additives Using 1H qNMR: Method Development and Application. *Foods* **2023**, *12*, 2421. [CrossRef]
42. Okaru, A.O.; Scharinger, A.; Rajcic de Rezende, T.; Teipel, J.; Kuballa, T.; Walch, S.G.; Lachenmeier, D.W. Validation of a Quantitative Proton Nuclear Magnetic Resonance Spectroscopic Screening Method for Coffee Quality and Authenticity (NMR Coffee Screener). *Foods* **2020**, *9*, 47. [CrossRef]
43. Bourafai-Aziez, A.; Jacob, D.; Charpentier, G.; Cassin, E.; Rousselot, G.; Moing, A.; Deborde, C. Development, Validation, and Use of 1H-NMR Spectroscopy for Evaluating the Quality of Acerola-Based Food Supplements and Quantifying Ascorbic Acid. *Molecules* **2022**, *27*, 5614. [CrossRef] [PubMed]
44. Piccinonna, S.; Ragone, R.; Stocchero, M.; Del Coco, L.; De Pascali, S.A.; Schena, F.P.; Fanizzi, F.P. Robustness of NMR-based metabolomics to generate comparable data sets for olive oil cultivar classification. An inter-laboratory study on Apulian olive oils. *Food Chem.* **2016**, *199*, 675–683. [CrossRef] [PubMed]
45. Ward, J.L.; Baker, J.M.; Miller, S.J.; Deborde, C.; Maucourt, M.; Biais, B.; Rolin, D.; Moing, A.; Moco, S.; Vervoort, J.; et al. An inter-laboratory comparison demonstrates that [1H]-NMR metabolite fingerprinting is a robust technique for collaborative plant metabolomic data collection. *Metabolomics* **2010**, *6*, 263–273. [CrossRef] [PubMed]
46. Commission Regulation (EU)-889/2008-EUR-Lex. Available online: https://eur-lex.europa.eu/legal-content/IT/TXT/?uri=CELEX:32008R0889 (accessed on 16 September 2024).
47. Commission Regulation (EU)-1235/2008-EUR-Lex. Available online: https://eur-lex.europa.eu/legal-content/EN/ALL/?uri=CELEX:32008R1235 (accessed on 16 September 2024).
48. Commission Regulation (EU)-178/2010-EUR-Lex. Available online: https://eur-lex.europa.eu/legal-content/EN/ALL/?uri=CELEX:32010R0178 (accessed on 16 September 2024).
49. Commission Regulation (EU)-401/2006-EUR-Lex. Available online: https://eur-lex.europa.eu/legal-content/EN/TXT/?uri=CELEX:32006R0401 (accessed on 16 September 2024).
50. Jlilat, A.; Ragone, R.; Gualano, S.; Santoro, F.; Gallo, V.; Varvaro, L.; Mastrorilli, P.; Saponari, M.; Nigro, F.; D'Onghia, A.M. A non-targeted metabolomics study on Xylella fastidiosa infected olive plants grown under controlled conditions. *Sci. Rep.* **2021**, *11*, 1070. [CrossRef]
51. Chemistry, C. Related compounds. *J. Med. Pharm. Chem.* **2001**, *2*, 1941–1944.

molecules
MDPI

Article

Cellulose Nanocrystal-Based Emulsion of Thyme Essential Oil: Preparation and Characterisation as Sustainable Crop Protection Tool

Francesca Baldassarre [1,2,*], Daniele Schiavi [3], Veronica Di Lorenzo [3], Francesca Biondo [1], Viviana Vergaro [1,2], Gianpiero Colangelo [4], Giorgio Mariano Balestra [3] and Giuseppe Ciccarella [1,2,*]

1 Department of Biological and Environmental Sciences, UdR INSTM of Lecce University of Salento, Via Monteroni, 73100 Lecce, Italy; francesca.biondo@unisalento.it (F.B.); viviana.vergaro@unisalento.it (V.V.)
2 Institute of Nanotechnology, CNR NANOTEC, Consiglio Nazionale delle Ricerche, Via Monteroni, 73100 Lecce, Italy
3 Department of Agriculture and Forest Sciences (DAFNE), University of Tuscia, Via S. Camillo de Lellis, snc, 01100 Viterbo, Italy; schiavi@unitus.it (D.S.); veronica.dilorenzo@unitus.it (V.D.L.); balestra@unitus.it (G.M.B.)
4 Department of Engineering for Innovation, University of Salento, Via Monteroni, 73100 Lecce, Italy; gianpiero.colangelo@unisalento.it
* Correspondence: francesca.baldassarre@unisalento.it (F.B.); giuseppe.ciccarella@unisalento.it (G.C.); Tel.: +39-0832-299469 (F.B.); +39-0832-319810 (G.C.)

Abstract: Essential oil-based pesticides, which contain antimicrobial and antioxidant molecules, have potential for use in sustainable agriculture. However, these compounds have limitations such as volatility, poor water solubility, and phytotoxicity. Nanoencapsulation, through processes like micro- and nanoemulsions, can enhance the stability and bioactivity of essential oils. In this study, thyme essential oil from supercritical carbon dioxide extraction was selected as a sustainable antimicrobial tool and nanoencapsulated in an oil-in-water emulsion system. The investigated protocol provided high-speed homogenisation in the presence of cellulose nanocrystals as stabilisers and calcium chloride as an ionic crosslinking agent. Thyme essential oil was characterised via GC-MS and UV-vis analysis, indicating rich content in phenols. The cellulose nanocrystal/essential oil ratio and calcium chloride concentration were varied to tune the nanoemulsions' physical–chemical stability, which was investigated via UV-vis, direct observation, dynamic light scattering, and Turbiscan analysis. Transmission electron microscopy confirmed the nanosized droplet formation. The nanoemulsion resulting from the addition of crosslinked nanocrystals was very stable over time at room temperature. It was evaluated for the first time on *Pseudomonas savastanoi pv. savastanoi*, the causal agent of olive knot disease. In vitro tests showed a synergistic effect of the formulation components, and in vivo tests on olive seedlings demonstrated reduced bacterial colonies without any phytotoxic effect. These findings suggest that crosslinked cellulose nanocrystal emulsions can enhance the stability and bioactivity of thyme essential oil, providing a new tool for crop protection.

Keywords: cellulose nanocrystals; thyme essential oil; nanoemulsions; phenols; biopesticides; olive knot disease

Citation: Baldassarre, F.; Schiavi, D.; Di Lorenzo, V.; Biondo, F.; Vergaro, V.; Colangelo, G.; Balestra, G.M.; Ciccarella, G. Cellulose Nanocrystal-Based Emulsion of Thyme Essential Oil: Preparation and Characterisation as Sustainable Crop Protection Tool. *Molecules* **2023**, *28*, 7884. https://doi.org/10.3390/molecules28237884

Academic Editors: Giuseppina Raffaini and Fabio Ganazzoli

Received: 9 November 2023
Revised: 29 November 2023
Accepted: 29 November 2023
Published: 30 November 2023

1. Introduction

The massive use of synthetic antimicrobial agrochemicals in agrifood raises several concerns about environmental and toxicological pollution [1,2]. The synthetic pesticide market is in decline, while biopesticides, which have been estimated to conspicuously grow by 2025, could offer an innovative way to achieve greater sustainability in agricultural practices, even matching the growing preference of consumers for natural and safer products [3–5]. In this context, essential oils (EOs) represent a valid and ecofriendly alternative to chemicals and actual biopesticides [6,7]. These plant extracts are rich in aromatic secondary metabolites with antimicrobial effects and plant defence mechanisms against several pathogenic organisms. Phenolic compounds such as carvacrol, thymol, coumarins, limonene, eugenol, and menthol possess antibacterial, antifungal, antiviral, antimycotic, antiparasitic, insecticidal, antioxidant, and antiseptic properties. Therefore, the use of EOs and their constituents ranges from medicine to agriculture as biopesticides, and use in food preservatives and additives in food packaging materials [8]. EOs are ecofriendly products because of their volatility, which allows for their removal from the environment. However, this volatility is a limit to their bioactivity, which is also compromised by decomposition under light and oxygen exposure during application or storage.

The application of nanotechnology leads to important innovations in products, including EO formulations, refining their physicochemical properties and functions [9–12]. EOs need to be encapsulated in emulsion form to be dispersible in water and to improve stability and bioavailability. Colloidal stability is also required to avoid gravity-related problems such as creaming or sedimentation. Nanoemulsions (NEs) offer improved wettability, improved diffusion capacity, and superior mechanical/chemical stability through the formation of nanometric droplets. These properties also reduce volatilisation and degradation of active ingredients, increasing target site penetration and bioactivity [13]. NE formulations are crucial for the water dispersion of lipophilic and/or poorly water-soluble compounds such as EOs, pesticides, or foodstuffs [14–16]. The following Scheme 1 presents the potential features of EO NEs for agricultural application.

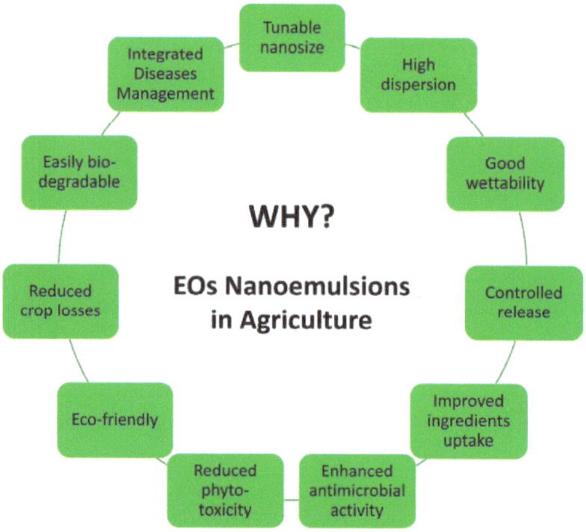

Scheme 1. Benefits of using essential oils nanoemulsions in agriculture.

These systems are generally composed of a water and an oil phase with the presence of surfactants, amphiphilic molecules which provide a decrease in the interfacial tension between the two immiscible phases. NEs differ from microemulsions (MEs) not only due to the formation of nanosized droplets, ranging from 20 to 200 nm, but also due to their kinetic and long-term stability due to their high- and low-energy methods of preparation. Furthermore, NEs require a lower quantity of surfactants than MEs, reducing potential toxicological problems [17]. The use of surfactants and emulsifiers minimises or prevents the occurrence of Ostwald ripening, prevents coalescence, and improves the antimicrobial activity of EOs [18]. Emulsifiers are a subcategory of surfactants which prevent oil droplet aggregation, increasing colloidal stability. Food-grade synthetic and natural emulsifiers are being used in NE formulations, such as polyoxyethylene sorbitan, phospholipids like lecithin, proteins, polysaccharides (gum arabic and pectin), and saponins [19–21]. NE stabilisation can also be carried out via solid particle addition, referred to as the Pickering method. Organic and inorganic particles retard oil evaporation and avoid colloid coalescence, improving essential oil NEs' antimicrobial activity for cosmetic, pharmaceutic, and agrifood applications [22]. Several spherical, rod-like, and plate-like particles can be used to obtain Pickering emulsions. Spherical inorganic particles, such as titanium oxides, alumina, and silica, offer good stability but present environmental problems [23,24]. Protein nanoparticles, soy, gelatin, and other polysaccharide nanoparticles as well as polysaccharide/protein complex nanoparticles have been studied [25].

Cellulose nanoparticles are great stabilisers compared with other types of particles due to their biocompatibility, biodegradability, thermomechanical behaviour, and costs. Cellulose nanocrystals (CNCs), cellulose nanofibers (CNFs), and microfibrillated cellulose (MFC) have been used in NEs and MEs, in both native and modified forms [26–28]. Furthermore, CNCs are very interesting additives due to the better control of their morphology and chemical changes, and for the reproducibility of their emulsion formation. The hydroxyl groups on the surface of the CNCs give this nanomaterial an amphiphilic characteristic that is useful for stabilising oil–water emulsions. Indeed, the negative charge of the CNCs favours the colloidal stabilisation of NE nanoparticles [29]. CNCs display interesting biological properties when it comes to microorganism interactions, which have been recently explored to develop crop protection tools, together with other natural active ingredients, such as chitosan, starch, and gallic acid [30,31]. Furthermore, several works have reported on the smart combination of CNCs as biostabilisers and EOs as green pesticides [32,33]. CNCs-stabilised emulsions of clove, oregano, and thyme white essential oils showed enhanced antimicrobial activity against food-related microorganisms and larvae, stronger than that of pure EOs [29,33,34]. In addition, the encapsulation of thymol and eugenol EOs has been effectively achieved with a new emulsification method using an unmodified cellulose shell, achieving high antimould activity, which is useful for ecological pre- and postharvest pathogen control [35]. Thymol, the primary phenolic component of thyme (*Thymus vulgaris*) essential oil, displays rapid activity against gram-negative and gram-positive bacteria compared with other plant metabolites [36,37]. Recently, we found a great inhibition activity towards *Xylella fastidiosa* for thymol, which was improved through the carrier action of $CaCO_3$ nanocrystals [38,39].

In this work, thyme EO (Th-EO) from an ecofriendly extraction process was characterised with GC-MS and UV-vis analysis and used for the first time as a crop protection tool against *Pseudomonas savastanoi pv. Savastanoi* (Psav). This gram-negative bacterium causes olive knot disease, and its management depends on agronomic practices and preventive chemical treatments, including with copper salts [40]. Copper-based agrochemicals can accumulate in the soil and cause harm to plants, nontarget organisms, and humans [41]. The European Commission has strict regulations on the use of such chemicals, prompting the need for alternative options. Despite some progress, olive knot disease continues to be a threat to olive crops in the Mediterranean region. Therefore, it is important to explore alternative management methods [42–45].

In detail, NEs were prepared by exploiting the stabilisation action of CNCs and using $CaCl_2$ as an ionic crosslinking agent, resulting in the obtainment of CNCs@Th-EO NEs. Stability was investigated through a visual method, dynamic light scattering, and Turbiscan analysis. Nanodroplet morphology was observed using transmission electronic microscopy. Samples were characterised using UV-vis spectrometry to obtain absorption spectra and total phenolic content. Stability studies confirmed a long-term physical–chemical stability after 30 days of storage at room temperature (RT). Three in vitro tests showed a great inhibition action of Th-EO towards Psav that was improved with NE application. This action was confirmed via in vivo testing, which provided a reduction in epiphytic survival in infected olive plants after 7–14 days post-inoculum (dpi), without phytotoxic effects. Our data demonstrate that Th-EO is a valid biopesticide and its bioactivity is improved by emulsification in the presence of CNCs and $CaCl_2$, thanks to the formation of a very stable nanodroplet suspension.

2. Results and Discussion

2.1. Chemical Composition of Thyme Essential Oil

Th-EO from Licofarma s.r.l. company was extracted from *Thymus vulgaris* L. using a supercritical CO_2 extraction process. The yield of Th-EO was over 2% (*w*/*w*) and its density was 0.95 g/mL. The obtained pure oil was stored at RT until utilisation for chemical composition and further studies. Th-EO was light yellow in colour and had a characteristic, sharp odour. Extraction methods, as well as geographical location, plant species, harvest time, and climate, can influence the quality and composition of EO [46].

We first quantified the total phenol content (TPC) with the Folin–Ciocalteu colorimetric method (Section 3.4.2), detecting a TPC of 219 ± 19 µg GAE/mg Th-EO. The phenolic content of plant extracts significantly affects their antioxidant and antimicrobial activities [8,47]. Phenols and phenolic acid are bioactive phytochemicals consisting of a single substituted phenolic ring, and their antimicrobial activity is due to the position and number of hydroxyl groups. Toxicological mechanisms consist of membrane disruption, cell wall complexation, adhesin binding, and enzyme inactivation [48].

GC-MS analysis was exploited to identify the main compounds of EO. The most abundant compound in our Th-EO was *o*-cymene, followed by thymol. Other compounds were present in undetectable traces. The chemical composition obtained using GC-MS is shown in Table 1 with the chemical formulas of the identified compounds.

Table 1. Chemical composition of selected *Thymus vulgaris* L. EO, extracted with supercritical CO_2.

Peak	Retention Time	Area %	Identified Compound	Formula	MW
1	10.783	76.65	*o*-Cymene	$C_{10}H_{14}$	134
2	22.864	23.35	Thymol	$C_{10}H_{14}O$	150

Our results are partially in accordance with those found by other authors. Thyme EO is generally composed of *p*-cymene, linalool, thymol, and carvacrol. These last compounds are responsible for antimicrobial activity [49]. Some variations have also been found for thyme white essential oil, which is mainly composed of thymol and *p*-cymene [50].

Thymol (2-isopropyl-5-methylphenol) is the main monoterpene phenol found in extracts from plants of the *Lamiaceae* family, such as *Thymus*, *Thymbra*, and *Origanum*, but it is also present in other species. It is a very interesting substance with many potential applications in different fields, from pharmaceutical use to foodstuffs, for which it is registered by the European Commission as a safe flavouring. Nevertheless, there are many works assessing its antibacterial and antifungal activity towards a broad spectrum of pathogens [36].

2.2. Physical–Chemical Properties of Nanoemulsions

2.2.1. Preparation of CNCs@Th-EO NEs and Oil Entrapment Efficiency

The potential of EOs as biopesticides is related to nanoencapsulation strategies. In this context, the delivery of active ingredients used as pesticides via NEs is central, as shown in the recent literature [7].

We formulated oil in water (O/W) NEs using Tween 80 as a surfactant, ethanol as a cosurfactant to increase the solubilisation of active ingredients, and CNCs as stabilisation agents, just as described in the Materials and Methods Section 3.3. Tween 80 and Tween 20 are the most used surfactants for EO emulsions because they are effective for the achievement of colloidal stability. Furthermore, nonionic surfactants are usually applicated in agriculture for their nontoxicity, for their ecocompatibility, and because they are not affected by pH and ionic strength [16,51,52].

The oil/surfactant ratio (*v*:*v*) was maintained at 2:1, just as described in the Materials and Methods Section 3.3; instead, two Th-EO:CNCs ratios (*w*:*w*) were investigated to obtain NEs with different oil content (% *v*/*v*). CNCs were added as solid particles to form steric protection at the O/W interface with the aim of long-term stability, which is widely discussed in subsequent paragraphs. Furthermore, $CaCl_2$ was investigated as an ionic crosslinker. The aim was to enhance the emulsification action of CNCs by establishing salt bridges inside the cellulose network, as has been experimented for different polysaccharide-based systems [53–55]. Ca^{2+} ions intercalate between cellulose nanocrystals, forming electrostatic interactions with the negatively charged carboxyl groups (–COO^-) of nanocellulose chains. Formulations with and without the salt were prepared to evaluate the chemical composition and stability of CNCs@Th-EO NEs. The following Scheme 2 presents the flowchart of the investigated procedures and methodologies.

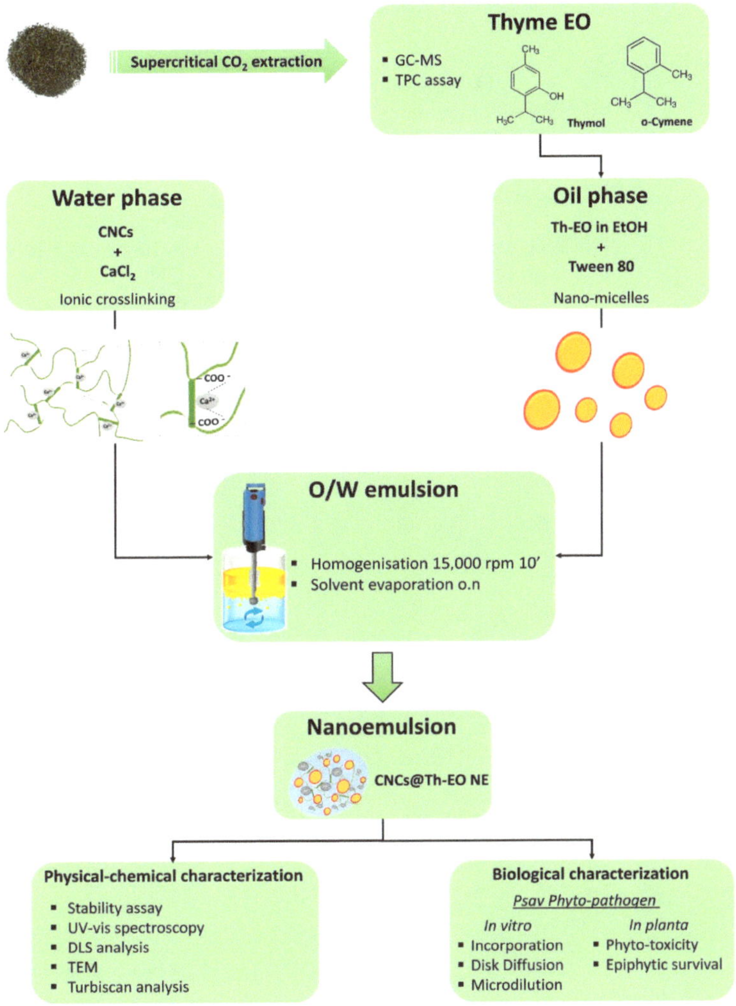

Scheme 2. Flowchart of the process studied for the CNCs@Th-EO NE production and methodologies for their characterisation.

Table 2 presents the formulated NEs, indicating their initial composition, their oil entrapment efficiency according to UV-vis measurements, and their TPC data after preparation.

Table 2. Nanoemulsion formulations with Th-EO encapsulation data after solvent evaporation (300 rpm, overnight at room temperature under fume hood).

Sample	Oil Content (% *v*/*v*)	$CaCl_2$ (3 mM)	Oil Entrapment Efficiency % *	TPC (μg GAE/mg Th-EO) ¥
CNCs@Th-EO NE_1	10	Yes	100	236 ± 12
CNCs@Th-EO NE_2	10	No	100	226 ± 3
CNCs@Th-EO NE_3	1.5	Yes	100	218 ± 31
CNCs@Th-EO NE_4	1.5	No	100	226 ± 14

* Data obtained from UV-vis measurements and Equation (1). ¥ TPC assay at the same EO concentration of 20 μg/mL.

All samples after preparation appeared homogeneously white in colour, with no visible free oil or creaming, showing the successful emulsification of Th-EO. The oil entrapment was 100%, as indicated by both the oil retention percentage data and the TPC assay. The NE TPC data are close to those of free oil at the same Th-EO concentration (see previous paragraph).

The oil entrapment efficiency data indicated that emulsion formulation (initial oil content and $CaCl_2$ addition) did not influence the Th-EO loading capacity. It can be assumed that the stabilising action of CNCs is effective enough to trap any amount of oil introduced, regardless of the EO concentration and crosslinking step. This finding is in line with previous works about cellulose-based emulsions of EOs; at low cellulose particle concentrations, the EO type (different polarity) mainly influenced the emulsion process [32].

Furthermore, the UV spectra of free Th-EO and NE showed no changes in absorption peak wavelengths after encapsulation, suggesting there were no structural modifications of phytochemicals following the emulsification process (see Figure 1).

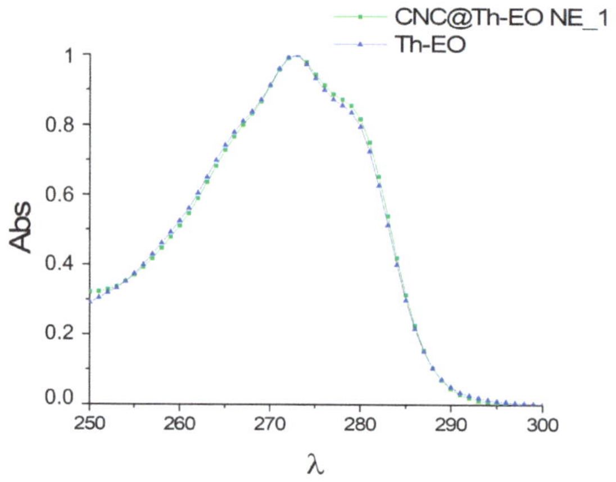

Figure 1. UV spectra of Th-EO before and after encapsulation in CNCs@Th-EO NE_1 formulation.

2.2.2. Nanoemulsion Stability

Oil entrapment efficiency provides a qualitative assessment of the performance of a given encapsulation process, while the emulsion stability indexes relate to the ability of a given emulsifier/oil system to contrast the spontaneous phase separation.

The four formulations were assessed daily through visual observation after solvent evaporation (time 0) and during the two weeks after preparation (at 1, 7, and 14 days). The solvent evaporation was conducted via continuous stirring (300 rpm) overnight at room temperature under the fume hood. The NEs were stored at RT and at 4 °C. The gravitational stability was verified via centrifugation of sample aliquots as described in the Materials and Methods section. Stability indexes were calculated following Equations (2) and (3). Oil retention was also analysed after 30 days by quantifying Th-EO in the remaining emulsion volume through UV absorption using Equation (1).

First of all, surfactant addition is necessary to better solubilise EOs. NEs without Tween 80 showed complete phase separation for both oil concentrations (10 and 1.5% *v*/*v*). The incorporation of almost 5% of surfactant is generally reported for efficient nanoemulsion production due to its influence on oil droplet aggregation. Several studies have investigated surfactant flexibility and ability to tune the hydrophilic–lipophilic balance (HLB), including the synergistic effect from a mixture of nonionic surfactants [16,56]. In our work, Tween 80 was used in combination with CNCs, ensuring a loading efficiency of 100% Th-EO (see Table 2). In terms of emulsion formation and stability, a drastic creaming phenomenon was observed, reaching an SI % of 10 already after 1 day without CNCs. The role of the $CaCl_2$ crosslinker and the influence of the EO concentration were then studied. The following Table 3 presents the stability parameters of CNCs@Th-EO NEs (see Table 2) stored at RT in the dark.

Table 3. Stability towards shear (ES) values and stability index (SI) values at days 0, 7, and 14, and oil retention percentage after 30 days of storage. These parameters refer to the four formulations of CNCs@Th-EO NE (see Table 2).

	CNCs@Th-EO NE_1 *	CNCs@Th-EO NE_2 *	CNCs@Th-EO NE_3 *	CNCs@Th-EO NE_4 *
ES %	100	80	100	100
SI % 0 d	100	100	100	100
SI % 1 d	100	85	100	90
SI % 7 d	100	85	100	90
SI % 14 d	100	85	100	90
Oil retention % 30 d ¥	100	50	100	100

* Stored at RT in the dark. ¥ Data obtained from UV-vis measurements and Equation (1).

All NEs after solvent evaporation (time 0 d) remained homogeneous for the first 24 h, as indicated by the SI percentages. Stability towards centrifugation shear indicated a loss of stability for the 10% *v*/*v* oil sample, without a crosslinker (CNCs@Th-EO NE_2). Moreover, no considerable changes were observed for the other emulsions following centrifugation. A minor phase separation was observed for samples without $CaCl_2$ after the first day of storage; SI percentages were 85% and 90%, respectively, for CNCs@Th-EO NE_2 and CNCs@Th-EO NE_4 (10% *v*/*v* and 1.5% *v*/*v* oil samples). In these samples, we observed a clear cream layer which remained unchanged over time, as indicated by the measured SI percentages (two weeks after preparation). In addition, the CNCs@Th-EO NE_2 sample showed a significant loss of oil retention (50%) in the remaining emulsion layer, as determined using oil quantification. The UV-vis spectra of the oil in the cream and emulsion layers of the CNCs@Th-EO NE_2 formulation are shown in Supplementary Figure S1, which illustrates the reduction in EO retention. We observed a small decrease in emulsion volume for CNCs@Th-EO NE_2 after storage, so the loss of oil retention is not due to evaporation of the unstabilised EO but is related to the phase separation caused by the creaming phenomenon. The oil retention data were also confirmed via TPC quantification. No differences were detected or measured for NEs stored at 4 °C, demonstrating that storage temperature does not affect the produced Th-EO formulations, as shown in Supplementary Table S1.

The stability data suggested that the stabilising effect of CNCs was strong and fundamental; the ES and SI percentages were high for all samples and remained stable for 14 days. However, the best results were obtained with $CaCl_2$, which enhanced the ability of CNCs to form stable emulsions due to the strong electrostatic network. The crosslinked network provided inhibition of coalescence and creaming phenomena with maximum oil entrainment, regardless of the initial EO content. This efficient EO coverage easily led to emulsion stability over time and after centrifugation, resulting in uniform droplet distribution, as confirmed via subsequent analysis. This mechanism is necessary to prevent destabilisation, as demonstrated for EO emulsions based on CNCs and CNFs [57].

Increasing the oil concentration in a formulation could affect the resulting nanoemulsion's stability [58]. Despite the increase in oil content, our CNCs@Th-EO NE_1 formulation (10% *v*/*v* concentration of Th-EO) showed excellent physicochemical stability. No differences were found between CNCs@Th-EO NE_1 and CNCs@Th-EO NE_3, which have different oil contents but the same concentrations of CNCs and $CaCl_2$ (1.5% *w*/*v* and 3 mM, respectively), suggesting that the increase in CNCs concentration is not necessary exploiting the ionic crosslinking of Ca^{2+}. Mikulcová et al. demonstrated an improvement in the stability of EO emulsions by increasing the amount of cellulose, particularly for MFC, which provided a stronger three-dimensional fibril–droplet network than that formed by CNCs [32]. An effect of oil type, viscosity, and polarity has also been suggested [57]. Shin et al. observed a floating creamy layer for the samples with lower content of CNCs (as mg CNCs/mL of oil) that was not sufficient for the efficient EO droplets covering [50]. We suggest a synergistic action among crosslinked CNCs in the aqueous phase and the Th-EO/Tween 80 mixture of the oil fraction, which achieved oil droplet covering and coalescence blocking.

Nanoemulsion instability can result from particle aggregation or dissolution due to the Ostwald ripening phenomenon which usually occurs on the first days after the preparation and is dependent on the oil phase fraction in the NE system [16]. Therefore, dynamic light scattering (DLS) analysis was applied to determine the size and ζ-potential of NE droplets and their colloidal stability over time, in terms of polydispersity index (PdI) and average hydrodynamic diameter (Z-average diameter). We again analysed the contribution of the oil fraction in the presence of CNCs and with and without crosslinking.

2.2.3. Nanodroplet Size and Colloidal Stability over Time

Size and ζ-potential of droplets are important parameters impacting the NEs' colloidal stability over time. Furthermore, the PdI gives information about sample uniformity that is crucial to detect potential coalescence and/or flocculation phenomena. These data were recorded using DLS analysis, a common technique for determining the size distribution of nanocolloid suspensions. These measurements require dilution of the samples to avoid multiple scattering due to aggregation as a result of electrostatic interactions. Therefore, this light scattering assay is also suitable for determining the stability of NEs after dilution, which can affect emulsion performance [59].

Figure 2 reports the DLS plots, Z-average diameters, and PdI versus ageing time (days) for all the produced NEs.

First, the four NEs showed a PdI below 0.4 and remained below 0.4 after storage, suggesting monodisperse oil droplet formation and good formulation homogeneity, consistent with agricultural applications [16]. The addition of $CaCl_2$ improved colloidal stability just as observed in previous studies (paragraph 2.2.2). The formulations with $CaCl_2$ (CNCs@Th-EO NE_1 and CNCs@Th-EO NE_3) showed no changes in DLS parameters over time, contrary to the others (CNCs@Th-EO NE_2 and CNCs@Th-EO NE_4). In particular, the CNCs@Th-EO NE_2 sample (10% *v*/*v* oil without $CaCl_2$) showed a doubling of the Z-average diameter with a slight reduction in PdI after 7–14 days, indicating that a first coalescence phenomenon had already occurred after 7 days without flocculation or sedimentation. This behaviour is in line with what is suggested by the NE observation (creaming phenomenon) and the stability values in Table 3. Furthermore, the formulations with the lowest oil content (CNCs@Th-EO NE_3 and CNCs@Th-EO NE_4) formed smaller nanodroplets than the 10% *v*/*v* concentrated samples. This can be explained by the increased interfacial area of the droplets due to the higher oil concentration. As the number of CNCs was the same for all formulations, there was less cellulose available to stabilise the interfacial area. Consequently, an increase in EO concentration would result in less extensive coverage of the droplets' surface by the available CNCs, leading to an increase in droplet volume with a consequent increase in Z-average diameter that reduces the total interfacial area. Huaping Yu et al. reported that the size of the clove oil droplets produced via homogenisation depended on the contribution of the stabiliser when a low number of CNCs was used [34]. These data are in line with our outcomes for the last NEs. The same trend was observed for cellulose-based EO MEs [33,35]. Finally, we can deduce that the crosslinking by Ca^{2+} compensates for the inefficient coverage of the droplet surface due to excess oil, thus increasing the stability of NEs without increasing the CNCs amount.

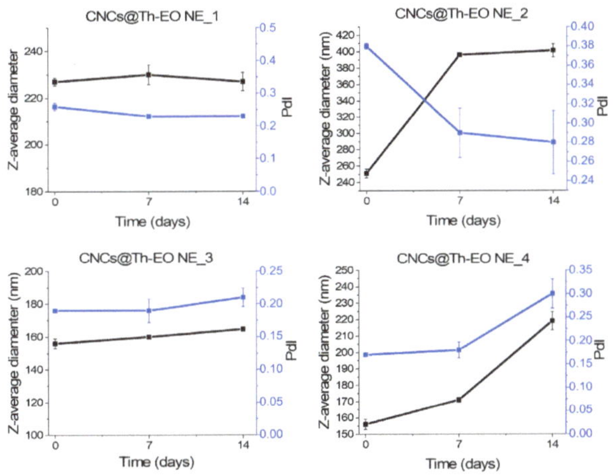

Figure 2. Z-average diameter (-■- black line) and PdI (-■- blue line) versus time (days) of the four formulated NEs measured via DLS at 0.1 mg/mL in distilled ultrapure water.

Concerning the ζ-potential parameter, any variations were recorded between samples and over time. We recorded ζ-potential values in the range of −25–−27 mV for all NEs, which remained unchanged after storage. Since Tween 80 is a nonionic surfactant, the negative ζ-potential is expected to be contributed by CNCs, which showed a ζ-potential of -36.7 ± 3 mV at 0.1 mg/mL in ultrapure water. A value of −25 mV provided a strong enough electrostatic repulsion to prevent droplet aggregation, stabilising the NEs. The increase in the ζ-potential values of NEs suggests structural changes in oil nanoparticles that may be related to instability problems, as indicated by the increase in droplet size with ageing time [60]. This destabilisation process related to NEs is known as Ostwald ripening, and it also involves a diffusive transfer of the EO from smaller to larger droplets [61]. For this reason, it is important to cover and stabilise nanodroplets with polymers or nanoparticles. In our experiments, the ζ-potential did not change over time, which is in line with the recorded slight variations in the Z-average diameter. Supplementary Table S2 presents the DLS parameters of the CNCs@Th-EO NE_1 sample over time. This formulation showed excellent dilution stability; the nanoparticle size and ζ-potential remained constant even after a 1/1000 dilution (necessary to perform appropriate DLS measurements). These data are consistent with the absence of observed phase separation, as discussed in the previous section. The Z-average diameter remained around 230 nm, suggesting that the high-energy homogenisation method resulted in the spontaneous formation of CNCs-stabilised nanoscale droplets, as indicated by the recorded colloidal stability (see ζ-potential and PdI parameters). CNCs nanodimensions ensure a robust coating of OE micelles that promotes emulsification by blocking the Ostwald's maturation mechanism [62]. An alternative way to kinetically improve EO emulsion stability is the exploitation of lipids [63]. Spherical cellulose nanocrystals produced Pickering emulsions, recording a decrease in microdroplet size and an increase in emulsion ratio as the CNC concentration increased [29]. Therefore, the morphology of the particles is also critical in producing stable emulsions and determining the size of the droplets.

Our data demonstrated that the addition of the crosslinker improves the emulsification potential of CNCs by producing a uniform distribution of emulsion nanodroplets even at the highest Th-EO concentration of 10% v/v. Therefore, the CNCs@Th-EO NE_1 formulation (10% v/v of Th-EO with $CaCl_2$) was selected for the following characterisations thanks to its high Th-EO concentration and retention over time and its good kinetic stability.

2.2.4. CNCs and NEs Droplet Morphology

CNCs nanodimensions in 6% w/v aqueous gel from CelluloseLab were confirmed via SEM analysis. Supplementary Figure S2 presents a representative SEM image of CNCs in which we can observe the nanoneedle morphology as indicated by the product data sheet.

The morphology of CNCs@Th-EO NE_1 was characterised via TEM. First, TEM analysis revealed the formation of nanomicelles of 23.8 ± 4 nm deriving from surfactant molecule interaction with Th-EO (see Supplementary Figure S3). Supplementary Figure S3A,B show the presence of CNCs, such as a network in which nanomicelles were immersed. Figure 3 presents two representative TEM images of CNCs@Th-EO NE_1 nanodroplets.

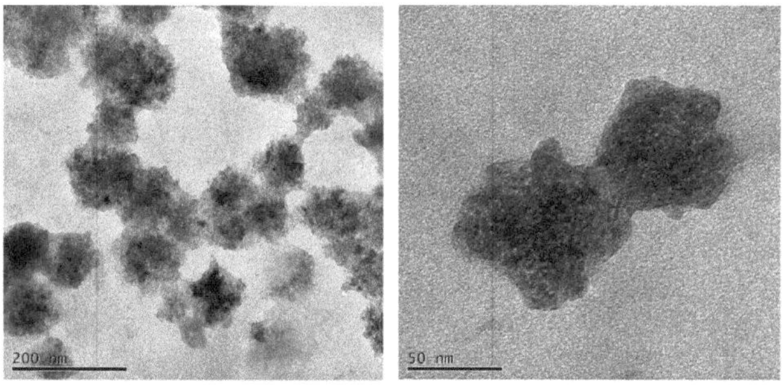

Figure 3. TEM images of nanodroplets of CNCs@Th-EO NE_1 formulation at different magnifications.

We observed spherical and homogeneous droplets in which we could visualise the single micelles. The nanodimensions of the emulsion were also confirmed in agreement with the measured hydrodynamic diameters reported in Supplementary Table S2. TEM images displayed droplets with a diameter of 109.4 ± 18 nm; hydrodynamic diameter (~230 nm) is bigger than effective colloidal diameter because of water molecule presence.

Our observation is in line with the literature on pesticide nanoemulsions, which occur in spherical shapes or with core shell-like structures due to a few clusters of nanomicelles, formed during preparation [16]. The small droplet size could be attributed to the effective adsorption of crosslinked CNCs on oil micelles as well as to the downsizing effect of the homogenisation process, as previously indicated by DLS data [34].

The observed droplet aggregation is due to rearrangement of particles when dried on a copper grid for TEM analysis. The advantages of NEs over MEs are their smaller drop sizes, which provide a formulation with increased wettability, spreadability, and bioavailability. However, NEs performance in agriculture such as in other applications, could be affected by long-term instability [64]. This characteristic was evaluated using Turbiscan analysis.

2.2.5. Long-Term Stability of Nanoemulsion with Turbiscan LabExpert

The higher encapsulation performance in the CNCs@Th-EO NE_1 formulation may be contributed by the excellent emulsifying properties of CNCs following the ionic crosslinking of Ca^{2+}. Optical observation as well as DLS analysis demonstrated the physical–chemical stability of this NE. Emulsions stabilised by solid colloidal nanoparticles, referred to as Pickering emulsions, were generally characterised by long-term stability [32]; we verified this issue via Turbiscan LabExpert analysis during the first 24 h after NE preparation (following o.n. solvent evaporation) and after 30 days of storage at RT. These measurements were effectuated on native samples without any dilution. The instrument software (Turbiscan Easy Soft) calculates the TSI value (see Equation (4)) that is used to predict dispersion stability [65]; the smaller TSI value corresponds to a more stable system. In this study, TSI variation over 24 h of analysis was monitored, comparing the CNCs@Th-EO NE_1 immediately after preparation and after 30 days. TSI plots are presented in Figure 4.

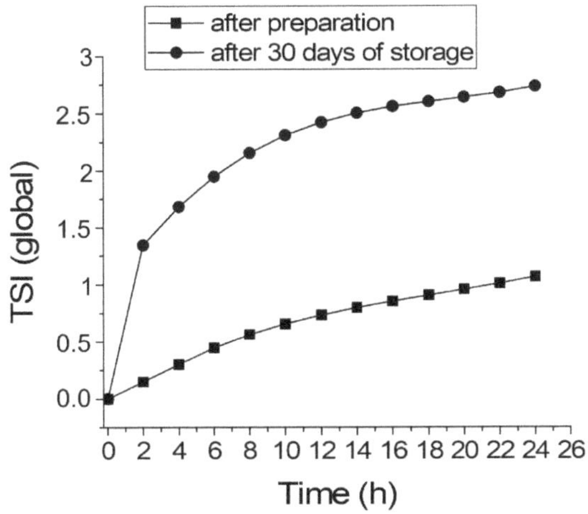

Figure 4. TSI values over 24 h of analysis with Turbiscan LabExpert on CNCs@Th-EO NE_1 formulation without dilution, after preparation (following solvent evaporation), and after 30 days of storage.

The instrument software indicated that TSI values below 0.5 correspond to a not significant chance condition, TSI values in the range 0.5–1 correspond to an early stage of destabilisation, and TSI values in the range 1–3 correspond to a destabilisation phase; values above 3 indicate great destabilisation of the system. The first three phases are not visible to the naked eye. Therefore, we observed that the CNCs@Th-EO NE_1 formulation reached an early destabilisation stage after 24 h, remaining in the destabilisation phase (TSI below 3) after 30 days of storage. These data are consistent with the stability index values in Table 3. We observed no visible change in this formulation, which remained homogeneous and without sedimentation, flocculation, or creaming processes, as just described in Section 2.2.2. These qualitative observations were confirmed via Turbiscan LabExpert analysis, which showed no ripples in the Δ backscattering (BS) plot, as reported in Supplementary Figure S4.

2.3. Biological Properties of Th-EO and CNCs@Th-EO NE

The antimicrobial properties of Th-EO are well known, and research has led to a better understanding of the mechanisms responsible for its behaviour. The phenolic components of the essential oil appear to play an important role in its antimicrobial activity, particularly against bacteria, as other studies have shown. Membrane disruptions followed by depolarisation, altered ion exchange, and cytoplasmic leakage are the most likely hypotheses, although multisite action cannot be excluded [66]. Indeed, thymol as itself, which was one the main constituents of the Th-EO used in this work, was positively used to inhibit *R. solanacearum* and several *Xanthomonas* species, the causal agents of bacterial wilt and leaf spot in many crops [36]. A great growth inhibition activity of this compound has been demonstrated in *X. fastidiosa* cells and has been greatly enhanced by nanoencapsulation and smart delivery [39]. Even cymene was positively assayed for its antimicrobial properties on several microorganisms, including nematodes, fungi, and food-borne bacteria, in both its natural forms (para and ortho) [67,68]. To our knowledge, this is the first report on the antimicrobial activity of an o-cymene-based product on phytopathogenic bacteria.

Our Th-EO antimicrobial activity was first tested on Psav via incorporation in agarised KB. The colony count revealed a complete growth inhibition comparable to that of copper sulphate at the field dose when the essential oil was used at a concentration higher than 1% v/v. Even at lower concentrations (0.5% v/v), a remarkable inhibition (85%) was achieved (see Figure 5).

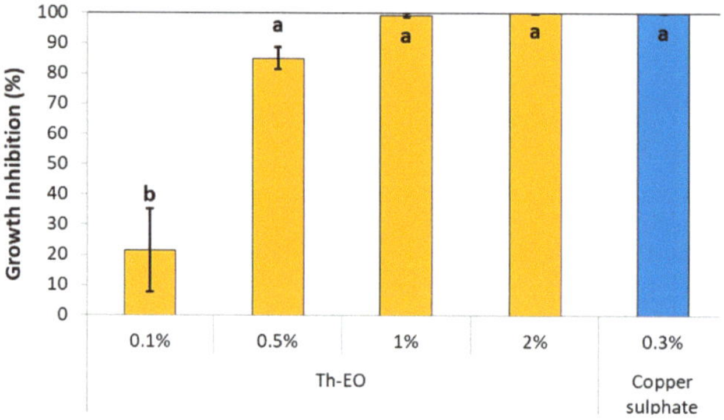

Figure 5. Antimicrobial properties of Th-EO on Psav when incorporated in agarised media. Data are represented as the mean and SD; different letters (a, b) show significantly different values after one-way ANOVA followed by Tukey's HSD post hoc test were performed.

In terms of biocompatibility, no adverse effects were observed on the leaf development of olive plants treated with Th-EO and the CNCs used in this work (see Table 4). As a matter of fact, NBI, which was calculated using the ratio of chlorophyll and flavanol contents in leaves, gives a reliable indication of the health status of the plants: this index considers plants to be in good shape when most of the absorbed nitrogen is used for primary metabolic functions, such as chlorophyll synthesis, while plants could be subjected to abiotic or biotic stress when secondary metabolic products demand more nitrogen, lowering the NBI values [69,70].

Table 4. Biological parameters observed over time on olive seedlings treated with thyme essential oil, CNCs, and water. Means and SDs are reported after one-way ANOVA was performed (ns indicated not statistically significant).

Treatment	Parameter	1 dpt	7 dpt	14 dpt
Th-EO 0.5% v/v	Chlorophylls (DU)	52 ± 2 ns	50.9 ± 2 ns	53.5 ± 2 ns
	Flavonols (DU)	2.0 ± 0.1 ns	1.9 ± 0.1 ns	2.0 ± 0.2 ns
	NBI	26.0 ± 1 ns	26.8 ± 1.6 ns	27.0 ± 1.4 ns
	Leaf area (cm^2)	-	-	5.1 ± 0.6 ns
CNCs 0.5% v/v	Chlorophylls (DU)	54.7 ± 2 ns	50.7 ± 3 ns	50.3 ± 2.0 ns
	Flavonols (DU)	2.0 ± 0.2 ns	1.9 ± 0.2 ns	1.9 ± 0.3 ns
	NBI	27.4 ± 2 ns	25.7 ± 1.5 ns	27.4 ± 2 ns
	Leaf area (cm^2)	-	-	5.3 ± 1 ns
Water	Chlorophylls (DU)	51.9 ± 2 ns	57.2 ± 3 ns	56.3 ± 3 ns
	Flavonols (DU)	1.9 ± 0.3 ns	1.9 ± 0.2 ns	2.0 ± 0.2 ns
	NBI	28.3 ± 1.5 ns	29.8 ± 2 ns	29.0 ± 3 ns
	Leaf area (cm^2)	-	-	5.1 ± 0.7 ns

Several studies have already pointed out the absence of toxicity for plants treated with CNCs, confirming our results, but when it comes to essential oils, the outcomes can be more unpredictable, since many factors are involved in the biological activity of EOs, such as temperature, humidity, and concentration [71]. However, this experiment highlighted the possibility of using an effective antibacterial amount (0.5% *v*/*v*) of Th-EOs without damaging the olive plants' basal growth functions, such as leaf development and nitrogen metabolism.

Given the interesting preliminary results about the biological activity of Th-EO on Psav and olive plants, we moved towards the characterisation of the antimicrobial activity of the nanoemulsion. CNCs@Th-EO NE_1 was picked from among the proposed formulations due to its good stability over time, lack of sedimentation and flocculation, and high retention of Th-EO, as previously stated. We first compared the antimicrobial activity of the selected NE with that of Th-EO alone using a simple disc diffusion test. Interestingly, when the NE was used at the same concentration as the EO, a wider inhibition halo around the disc could be appreciated, as can be observed in the plot in Figure 6.

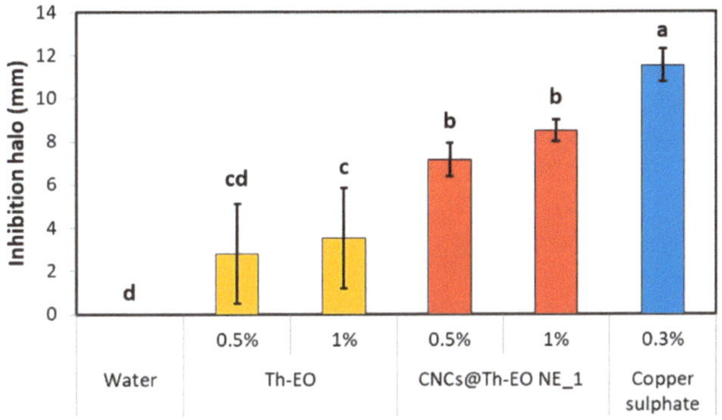

Figure 6. Inhibition halos produced by Th-EO and CNCs@Th-EO NE_1 in the disc diffusion test. Data are represented as the mean and SD; different letters (a, b, c, d) show significantly different values after one-way ANOVA followed by Tukey's HSD post hoc test were performed.

This could be explained by considering the encapsulated form of EO instead of the free form, which could have resulted in less volatilisation or dispersion of the oil [72]. The advantages of encapsulating EO with nanomaterials have already been reported by several authors, who pointed out an increased stability and an increase in antimicrobial activity [73,74]. Furthermore, the synergistic effect of these molecules was explored and confirmed by Abbasi et al. (2023), who proposed a Th-EO and carboxymethylcellulose coating for postharvest applications [75].

Since there was a need for a quantitative determination of CNCs@Th-EO NE_1's inhibition activity, we tested it on Psav through a microdilution method. The count of developed colonies after it was exposed to increasing concentrations of the NE in a growth-promoting broth revealed the capability of the compound to fully inhibit the bacteria starting from doses higher than 0.05% *v*/*v*, while lower doses of 0.1% *v*/*v* of NE could inhibit the bacterial growth by 90%, still in a comparable way to the inhibition displayed by copper at the field dose (see Figure 7).

As CNCs have been shown to have unique antimicrobial mechanisms on phytopathogenic bacteria, such as inhibition of swimming motility and biofilm production, as well as induction of cell flocculation in liquid media, we hypothesised a synergistic effect of nanocrystals and Th-EO [71]. The presence of CNCs in the formulation could have resulted in the bacterial cell being more exposed to the drug, preventing it from moving freely in the medium and adhering to surfaces, and of course preventing the EO from settling or separating from the liquid phase.

This behaviour was confirmed in the artificially inoculated plants, where the epiphytic survival of Psav was monitored for 14 days (see Figure 8).

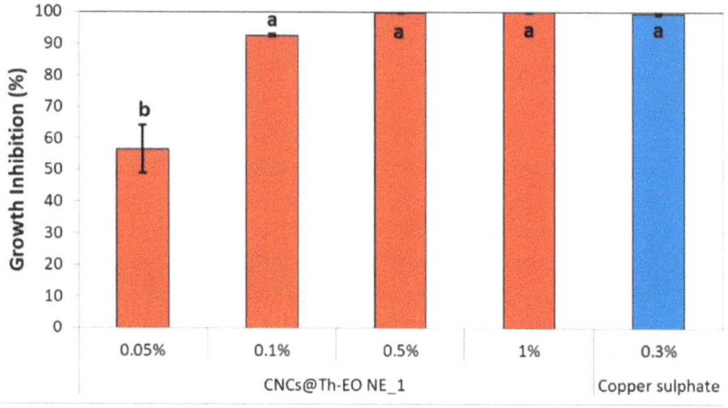

Figure 7. Growth inhibition percentages displayed by increasing doses of CNCs@Th-EO NE_1 on Psav using a microdilution assay. Data are represented as the mean and SD; different letters (a, b) show significantly different values after one-way ANOVA followed by Tukey's HSD post hoc test were performed.

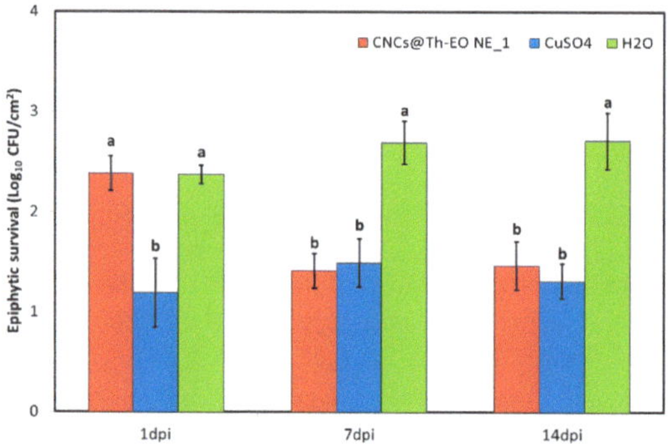

Figure 8. Epiphytic survival of Psav inoculated on olive seedlings after being treated with 0.5% *v*/*v* CNCs@Th-EO NE_1, 0.3% *w*/*v* copper sulphate, and water. Data are represented as the mean and SD; different letters (a, b) show significantly different values after one-way ANOVA followed by Tukey's HSD post hoc test were performed.

At 1 dpi, only copper showed an appreciable effect in lowering the Psav epiphytic population (1.21 CFU/cm^2), while the NE showed similar values to the negative control treatment (2.38 and 2.37 CFU/cm^2, respectively). This could be explained considering the great capability of the formulation to retain the encapsulated active ingredients, preventing it from being available as soon as it comes into contact with the bacterial cells. On the contrary, a few days after the application, the inhibition activity of the EO could be appreciated. Indeed, the re-isolation of the bacteria from the leaves highlighted the capability of the compound to reduce up to one log unit (1.41 CFU/cm^2) the bacteria survival in a comparable way to that of copper sulphate after seven days from inoculation (1.48 CFU/cm^2). The same trend was recorded at 14 dpi, since the recovered colonies from NE- and $CuSO_4$-treated plants were statistically similar (1.46 and 1.31 CFU/cm^2, respectively). Lowering the capability of phytopathogenic bacteria to survive outside the host is a valid strategy to decrease the risk of infections, since the epiphytic phase represents an important source of inoculum [76]. As a matter of fact, Psav preventive control methods heavily revolve around the use of protectants, such as cupric salts and biocontrol agents, and the observance of good agronomic practices to avoid the opening of artificial wounds which could promote the pathogen's ingress, especially considering the bacteria's ability to persist on the host over the seasons [77]. For these reasons, further studies are planned to better assess the capability of the NE to maintain its antimicrobial properties over time, especially in field conditions, where environmental components, such as light, temperature, air humidity, and precipitations play a fundamental role in the kinetics of agrochemicals. Given the collected data, we believe the proposed nanoencapsulation method could provide an effective way to deliver volatile and instable compounds such as essential oils, while maintaining, if not boosting, their biological properties.

3. Materials and Methods

3.1. Materials

CNCs were purchased from CelluloseLab (212-2 Garland Court, Enterprise Bldg., Fredericton, NB, Canada, E3B 5A3), in 6% *w*/*v* aqueous gel. Licofarma s.r.l. (Via Lecce 90/92, Galatina (LE), Italy; https://www.licofarma.com/, accessed on 17 May 2019) provided thyme essential oil (Th-EO) via supercritical CO_2 extraction. The oil was stored at room temperature and used without any purification. All chemicals and organic solvents were of the highest purity commercially available from Sigma-Aldrich (Milano, Italy). The bacterial strain of *Pseudomonas savastanoi pv. savastanoi* (Psav) PvBa206 was maintained and periodically subcultured on King's B (KB) medium Petri dishes incubated at 27 °C for 48 h [78]. One-year-old olive tree seedlings of the cultivar Leccino that were propagated by cuttings, 50 cm high, and single-stemmed were used in this work. Seedlings were propagated by cuttings, 50 cm high, and single-stemmed. Olive tree seedlings were grown in a glasshouse at 25 ± 2 °C during the day and 16 ± 2 °C during the night with a relative air humidity of 65%.

3.2. Identification of EO Constituents via Gas Chromatography/Mass Spectrometry

Chemical analysis of Th-EO was performed via gas chromatography/mass spectrometry (GC-MS), using the Agilent Technologies, 7820A GC system with HP-5MS column (5% phenyl-methyl-polysiloxane; 30 m × 0.25 mm i.d., 0.2 μm film thickness). Helium was used as carrier gas at a flow rate of 1 mL/min with ionisation voltage of 70 eV. The injection volume of EO was 1 μL in hexane. The injector was maintained at 250 °C. The oven temperature was maintained at 40 °C for 1 min followed by an increment of 3 °C/min, and finally held at 250 °C. Mass range scanned was 40–160 amu. The peaks of the mass spectra obtained for the compounds were compared with those from the NIST Mass Spectrometry Data Center.

3.3. Preparation of CNCs-Stabilised Th-EO Nanoemulsions

CNCs@Th-EO NEs were prepared by mixing the oil phase, Th-EO and surfactant Tween 80 in ethanol, and the water phase, CNCs in distilled water with and without 3 mM of $CaCl_2$. The ratio Th-EO:Tween 80 (*v*:*v*) was maintained 2:1. We investigated two Th-EO:CNCs ratios, 1:1 and 6:1 (*w*:*w*), to prepare NEs with two Th-EO concentrations (1.5 and 10 % *v*/*v*). The oil/ethanol ratio was always 1:1 (*v*:*v*). First, CNCs suspension was mixed with 3 mM of $CaCl_2$ (or only water in the experiments without $CaCl_2$) with continuous stirring at 500 rpm for 5 min. Then the oil phase was gradually added to the water phase with continuous stirring, and then the mixture was emulsified using an Ultra-Turrax blender model IKA T25 (IKA Werke, Staufen, Germany) at 15,000 rpm for 10 min. NEs were agitated at 300 rpm o.n. at RT under the fume hood for ethanol evaporation. Solvent removal was easily verified by quantifying the volume reduction. The obtained samples were stored at RT and 4 °C for further characterisations. The Table 5 presents the contained components of the prepared NEs.

Table 5. Components and their concentrations that were used for the NE preparation.

Sample	Th-EO:CNCs (*w*:*w*)	Oil Concentration (% *v*/*v*)	Th-EO:Tween 80 (*v*:*v*)	Th-EO:EtOH (*v*:*v*)	$CaCl_2$
CNCs@Th-EO NE_1	6:1	10	2:1	1:1	3 mM
CNCs@Th-EO NE_2	6:1	10	2:1	1:1	0
CNCs@Th-EO NE_3	1:1	1.5	2:1	1:1	3 mM
CNCs@Th-EO NE_4	1:1	1.5	2:1	1:1	0

3.4. *Characterisations*

3.4.1. UV–Vis Spectroscopy and Oil Retention

The readings for UV–vis spectra of Th-EO and resulting NEs were recorded in the range of 250–350 nm using a Varian-Cary 500 spectrophotometer. The unknown concentration was obtained with reference to a standard curve using Th-EO standard solutions in ethanol at known concentrations in the range of 50–0.1 mg/mL, and the line was fitted using Origin software (OriginPro 2016 64bit) (Abs values at λ_{max} = 273 nm were multiplied by dilution factor).

Oil retention over storage time was evaluated via EO quantification, which was performed using spectrophotometric analysis to record UV-Vis absorption spectra at 273 nm, and referring to the standard curve. Oil retention percentage was calculated according to the following equation:

$$\text{Oil retention } \% = \frac{\text{amount of EO quantified in NE}}{\text{amount of EO added to NE}} \times 100 \quad (1)$$

3.4.2. Total Phenolic Content

Total phenolic content was estimated spectrophotometrically according to the Folin–Ciocalteu colorimetric method. The reaction mixture was prepared by mixing 50 μL of EO or NEs (20 μg/mL of oil), 50 μL of 10% Folin–Ciocalteu's reagent dissolved in 750 μL of distilled water, and 500 μL of 7% $NaHCO_3$. The samples were incubated at RT for 90 min in the dark. The absorbance was determined at λ_{max} = 740 nm. It was calibrated against gallic acid standards (concentration range: 20–1 μg/mL) and the results were expressed as μg gallic acid equivalents (GAE)/mg EO. Data presented are average values of three measurements for each sample.

3.4.3. Stability Study

Emulsion storage stability was evaluated: visual transitions from steady state to creaming and coalescence for a period of 15 days were noted in graduated tubes. Nanoemulsion stability (%) was measured in duplicates at 0, 1, 7, and 14 days. The emulsion stability index (SI) was expressed as the formed emulsion layer volume (V_{emuls}) relative to the total sample volume (V_{total}). The SI was calculated using the following equation:

$$\text{SI } \% = \frac{V_{emuls}}{V_{total}} \times 100 \quad (2)$$

Stability towards shear was evaluated using centrifugation methodology. Samples were centrifuged at 10,000 rpm for 5 min at 20 °C in graduated tubes. The centrifugation resulted in an oily phase at the top, an emulsion phase in the middle, and an aqueous phase at the bottom. Emulsion stability (ES) was determined using the following equation:

$$\text{ES } \% = \frac{\text{remaining emulsion volume}}{\text{initial emulsion volume}} \times 100 \quad (3)$$

3.4.4. Droplet Size and Colloidal Stability

Sample dilution was performed to study stability against phase separation based on particle size distribution, polydispersity index, and ζ-potential measurements through DLS.

CNCs@Th-EO NEs were analysed with a Nano ZS90 (Malvern Instruments, Cambridge, UK) instrument. Preliminary DLS tests indicated the optimum sample concentration of 0.1 mg/mL. The potential analysis of particles was carried out via laser Doppler velocimetry (LDV). Measurements were performed at RT, in filtered distilled water (0.45 µm), at the refractive index of cellulose (1.469). The ζ-potential values are reported as the mean of 5 measurements; each of them was derived from 10 different runs to establish measurement repeatability. Particle size distribution data are reported as the mean of 3 measurements, each of them derived from 15 different runs to establish measurement repeatability.

3.4.5. CNCs and NEs Morphological Analysis

CNCs were observed with scanning electronic microscopy (SEM). A drop of the sample was placed on silicon support and dried at room temperature and then was viewed under a SEM MERLIN ZEISS, with an FEG source, at an accelerating voltage of 20 kV, using short exposure time (a few tens of seconds).

The droplet morphology of CNCs@Th-EO NE was analysed with transmission electron microscopy (TEM). A drop of NE (10 µL) was placed on a standard carbon-coated 200-mesh copper grid and left at RT o.n. The TEM micrographs were acquired by analysing the grid under a JEOL JEM 1400Plus microscope with LaB6 source at an accelerating voltage of 80 kV.

3.4.6. Stability Measurement of the Nanoemulsion Using Turbiscan LabExpert

Nanoemulsion stability was estimated using Turbiscan LabExpert, after preparation and after 30 days of storage at room temperature in the dark. This instrument has two synchronous detectors and a near-infrared light source (λ = 880 nm). The transmission detector receives the light flux transmitted (T) through the sample; the backscattering detector captures the backscattered light (BS). The reading head acquires transmissions and backscattering data either at a chosen position on the sample cell or every 40 µm, while moving along the 55 mm cell height. The recorded backscattering intensity of radiation is proportional to particle concentration. An important factor obtained with the Turbiscan instrument is related to the Turbiscan stability index (TSI). It monitors the destabilisation kinetics versus ageing time. It sums all the variations detected in the sample (size and/or concentration) at a given ageing time. The higher the TSI is, the worse the stability of the sample is. These stability index results have been used to compare the stability of many samples. The formula related to the TSI is reported in Equation (4):

$$\mathrm{TSI} = \sqrt{\frac{\sum_{i=1}^{n}(x_i - x_{BS})^2}{n-1}} \tag{4}$$

where x_i is the mean backscattering for every minute of measurement, x_{BS} is the mean x_i, and n is the number of scans [79,80].

Nanoemulsions without dilution were placed in a sample bottle (20 mL) and were scanned every 10 min for 24 h at 27 °C. After the internal changes were monitored, the TSI was calculated to evaluate NE stability with Turbiscan Easy Soft and provide a unique parameter.

3.5. Biological Study

3.5.1. Preliminary Biological Activity of Th-EO and CNCs

Extracted Th-EO was evaluated for its antimicrobial properties on Psav by incorporating it in agarised media [81]. Briefly, an aliquot of Th-EO was added to KB medium to reach the desired concentrations (0.1, 0.5, 1, 2% *v*/*v*). Then, 100 µL of a 10^3 CFU/mL suspension made from a fresh Psav culture was uniformly streaked onto the plates. After an incubation of 48 h at 27 °C, developed colonies were counted and the growth inhibition (expressed as percentage) was calculated as follows:

$$\text{Growth Inhibition } \% = \frac{\text{Negative control Colonies} - \text{Treatment Colonies}}{\text{Negative control Colonies}} \times 100 \quad (5)$$

KB alone and KB amended with 0.3% *w*/*v* copper sulphate pentahydrate were used as negative and positive controls, respectively [43]. Each thesis consisted of three replicates. The experiment was repeated twice.

Effects of Th-EO and CNCs were studied on olive plants to preventively assess the phytotoxicity of the NEs. Olive plants (10 per thesis) were spray-treated with a 0.5% *v*/*v* suspension of Th-EO and a 0.5% *v*/*v* suspension of CNCs until runoff. At 1, 7, and 14 days post-treatment (dpt), 8 measurements per plant were taken using a leaf clipper (Dualex 4 Scientific, FORCE-A, Orsay Cedex, France) to quantify the chlorophyll and the flavonol contents, expressed as Dualex unities (DUs). The nitrogen balance index (NBI) was calculated as the ratio of the two values [82]. At 14 dpt, two leaves per plant were harvested and their area was measured using the software ImageJ (version 1.51j8) (NIH, Bethesda, MD, USA) (accessed on Windows 10) (Microsoft, Redmond, WA, USA) [83]. Water was used as control. The experiment was repeated twice.

3.5.2. Antimicrobial Properties of Th-EO Nanoemulsion

The highest-performing NEs in terms of kinetic stability and Th-EO content were tested on Psav to quantify its antimicrobial activity. First, a disc diffusion test was designed to assess the differences between Th-EO alone and incorporated in CNCs in terms of the inhibition halo [84]. Sterile paper discs were placed on KB plates previously inoculated with 100 µL of a 10^6 CFU/mL Psav suspension, then 10 µL of different suspensions (0.5, 1% *v*/*v*) was pipetted on the discs. After 48 h of incubation at 27 °C, the inhibition halo was measured. Water and copper were used as controls as previously mentioned. Each thesis consisted of five replicates.

Afterwards, the inhibition of the selected NE was deeply investigated using a microdilution test: 20 µL of a 10^4 CFU/mL Psav suspension was added to 80 µL of Luria–Bertani broth previously amended with the substances to reach the final concentrations of 0.05, 0.1, 0.5, and 1% *v*/*v*. After 24 h of incubation at 27 °C under continuous orbital shacking, several decimal dilutions were obtained and 100 µL from each was plated on KB. After 48 h of incubation at 27 °C, developed colonies were counted [85]. The growth inhibition percentage was calculated as described in Equation (5). Each thesis consisted of three replicates.

The antimicrobial properties of the proposed NE were eventually tested on olive plants, via observing the effects of the nanomaterials on the epiphytic survival of the bacterium. Plants were treated as reported before, then they were spray-inoculated after 24 h with a 10^6 CFU/mL Psav suspension, they were bagged, and the air humidity of the growth chamber was raised to 80%. At 1, 7, and 14 dpi (days post-inoculation), 10 leaves per thesis (1 leaf per plant) were collected and washed in PBS (phosphate-buffered saline) using a homogeniser (Stomacher 400 Circulator, Seward Ltd., Worthing, UK) set at 150 rpm for 4 min. Several dilutions were plated on KB agar plates, which were incubated at 27 °C for 48 h. The number of developed colonies was counted and divided by the total area of the harvested leaves to obtain the final value of Log_{10} CFU/cm^2 [31]. In each test, water and copper were used as controls. The experiments were repeated twice.

4. Conclusions

The urge to find sustainable agrochemicals as alternatives to traditional pesticides has led to the exploration of innovative antimicrobial compounds. Nanoencapsulation could represent a suitable way to enhance the biological properties of natural active ingredients, which often present limitations to final field application due to volatility, phytotoxicity, and poor miscibility. In this context, essential oils represent a valid and ecofriendly alternative to chemicals and actual biopesticides.

We produced an o/w nanoemulsion of thyme essential oil derived from supercritical CO_2 extraction and composed of *o*-cymene and thymol, which are well-known bioactive phytochemicals. Nanoemulsion preparation was studied, exploiting the stabilisation action of CNCs and varying initial concentrations of EOs and an ionic crosslinker. The presence of CNCs in the aqueous phase of the formulations was associated with great encapsulation efficiency and stability of Th-EO, even with a high oil content. However, the best physical–chemical stability over time at room temperature was obtained in the presence of a crosslinked cellulose network, which was able to maintain 100% oil retention and a constant hydrodynamic diameter of nanodroplets. These features were demonstrated via a stability study, EO quantification assays, and DLS parameter monitoring. The nanodimensions of the produced formulation were confirmed using TEM morphological analysis. UV-vis spectroscopy and a TPC assay suggested that the bioactives of Th-EO were not altered after encapsulation and remained stably entrapped for 30 days, as confirmed via Turbiscan LabExpert analysis.

Many essential oils, despite the numerous reports on their antimicrobial and antioxidant properties, have rarely found an effective delivery method based on sustainable molecules, such as organic polymers. In this work, we have demonstrated for the first time that is possible to formulate thyme essential oil with cellulose nanocrystals crosslinked by calcium ions to obtain a very stable nanoemulsion which showed greater inhibition against the causal agent of olive knot disease than free oil under the same conditions. This interesting bioactivity was demonstrated using different biological assays, both in vitro and *in planta*, highlighting the high antimicrobial activity of our nanoemulsion without displaying any phytotoxic effect. We firmly believe that this approach could be further deepened to investigate different bioactive molecules as well as different pathosystems.

Supplementary Materials: The following supplementary information can be downloaded at https://www.mdpi.com/article/10.3390/molecules28237884/s1: Figure S1: UV-vis spectra of Th-EO in cream layer and remaining emulsion volume of CNCs@Th-EO NE_2 formulation after 30 days of storage at room temperature; Table S1: TPC data of nanoemulsions after storage at room temperature and at 4 °C; Table S2: DLS parameters of CNCs@Th-EO NE_1 formulation over time; Figure S2: SEM image of used CNCs; Figure S3: TEM images of Th-EO/surfactant micelles in CNCs@Th-EO NE_1 formulation at different magnifications; B is a zoomed image of A and D is a zoomed image of C; Figure S4: Δ backscattering % versus height (mm) plot of CNCs@Th-EO NE_1 formulation at T 0 and T 30 days, following Turbiscan Lab Tower scanning every 2 h for 24 h.

Author Contributions: Conceptualisation, F.B. (Francesca Baldassarre) and D.S.; methodology, F.B. (Francesca Baldassarre), D.S., V.D.L. and F.B. (Francesca Biondo); validation, F.B. (Francesca Baldassarre) and D.S.; formal analysis, F.B. (Francesca Baldassarre) and D.S.; investigation, V.D.L., F.B. (Francesca Biondo), G.C. (Gianpiero Colangelo), F.B. (Francesca Baldassarre) and D.S.; resources, G.C. (Gianpiero Colangelo), G.M.B. and G.C. (Giuseppe Ciccarella); data curation, F.B. (Francesca Baldassarre) and D.S.; writing—original draft preparation, F.B. (Francesca Baldassarre); writing—review and editing, F.B. (Francesca Baldassarre), D.S. and V.V.; visualisation, F.B. (Francesca Baldassarre); supervision, F.B. (Francesca Baldassarre), G.M.B. and G.C. (Giuseppe Ciccarella); project administration, G.C. (Giuseppe Ciccarella); funding acquisition, G.M.B. and G.C. (Giuseppe Ciccarella). All authors have read and agreed to the published version of the manuscript.

Funding: This research was funded by the Ministero Dell'istruzione, Dell'universita' e Della Ricerca, Project NanotEcnologie chiMiche green per la protEzione Sostenibile delle plante (NEMESI) ARS01_01002 CUP: F36C18000180005, Regione Puglia, Project Research for Innovation (REFIN), "Sintesi di un Sistema Teranostico a Base di Nano-Cellulosa per la Detection e la Cura Dei Tumori" (code: 0B988883) and by Ministry of University and Research (MUR) initiative "Departments of Excellence" (Law 232/2016) DAFNE Project 2023-27 "Digital, Intelligent, Green and Sustainable (acronym: D.I.Ver.So)".

Institutional Review Board Statement: Olive tree seedlings were used in this study. The olive tree seedlings of the cultivar Leccino were provided by the nursery Azienda Agricola Vivai Piante Fortunato p.a. Luca located in *Sammichele di Bari*, Italy and used as stated before.

Informed Consent Statement: Not applicable.

Data Availability Statement: All data are available in the publication.

Acknowledgments: We thank Leonardo Rescio of Licofarma s.r.l. for the supply of the thyme essential oil derived from supercritical CO_2 extraction which was used in our experimentation. We thank Bernardetta Anna Tenuzzo of the Department of Biological and Environmental Sciences of the University of Salento for technical support to the project activities.

Conflicts of Interest: The authors declare no conflict of interest.

References

1. Van Maele-Fabry, G.; Gamet-Payrastre, L.; Lison, D. Residential exposure to pesticides as risk factor for childhood and young adult brain tumors: A systematic review and meta-analysis. *Environ. Int.* **2017**, *106*, 69–90. [CrossRef] [PubMed]
2. Hazra, D.; Purkait, A. Role of Pesticide Formulations for Sustainable Crop Protection and Environment Management: A Review. *J. Pharmacogn. Phytochem.* **2019**, *8*, 686–693.
3. Thakore, Y. The biopesticide market for global agricultural use. *Ind. Biotechnol.* **2006**, *2*, 194–208. [CrossRef]
4. Isman, M.B. A renaissance for botanical insecticides? *Pest Manag. Sci.* **2015**, *71*, 1587–1590. [CrossRef] [PubMed]
5. Mattos, B.D.; Tardy, B.L.; Magalhães, W.L.; Rojas, O.J. Controlled release for crop and wood protection: Recent progress toward sustainable and safe nanostructured biocidal systems. *J. Control. Release* **2017**, *262*, 139–150. [CrossRef] [PubMed]
6. Menossi, M.; Ollier, R.P.; Casalongué, A.C.; Alvarez, A.V. Essential oil-loaded bio-nanomaterials for sustainable agricultural applications. *J. Chem. Technol. Biotechnol.* **2021**, *96*, 2109–2122. [CrossRef]
7. Pavoni, L.; Pavela, R.; Cespi, M.; Bonacucina, G.; Maggi, F.; Zeni, V.; Canale, A.; Lucchi, A.; Bruschi, F.; Benelli, G. Green Micro- and Nanoemulsions for Managing Parasites, Vectors and Pests. *Nanomaterials* **2019**, *9*, 1285. [CrossRef]
8. Vasile, C.; Sivertsvik, M.; Miteluţ, A.C.; Brebu, M.A.; Stoleru, E.; Rosnes, J.T.; Tănase, E.E.; Khan, W.; Pamfil, D.; Cornea, C.P.; et al. Comparative Analysis of the Composition and Active Property Evaluation of Certain Essential Oils to Assess their Potential Applications in Active Food Packaging. *Materials* **2017**, *10*, 45. [CrossRef]
9. Kumar, S.; Nehra, M.; Dilbaghi, N.; Marrazza, G.; Hassan, A.A.; Kim, K.-H. Nano-based smart pesticide formulations: Emerging opportunities for agriculture. *J. Control. Release* **2019**, *294*, 131–153. [CrossRef]
10. Biondo, F.; Baldassarre, F.; Vergaro, V.; Ciccarella, G. Chapter 3—Controlled Biocide Release from Smart Delivery Systems: Materials Engineering to Tune Release Rate, Biointeractions, and Responsiveness. In *Micro and Nano Technologies*; Balestra, G.M., Fortunati, E., Eds.; Elsevier: Amsterdam, The Netherlands, 2021; pp. 31–147. ISBN 978-0-12-823394-8.
11. Baldassarre, F.; Tatulli, G.; Vergaro, V.; Mariano, S.; Scala, V.; Nobile, C.; Pucci, N.; Dini, L.; Loreti, S.; Ciccarella, G. Sonication-Assisted Production of Fosetyl-Al Nanocrystals: Investigation of Human Toxicity and In Vitro Antibacterial Efficacy against Xylella fastidiosa. *Nanomaterials* **2020**, *10*, 1174. [CrossRef]
12. Bettini, S.; Pagano, R.; Valli, L.; Giancane, G. Drastic nickel ion removal from aqueous solution by curcumin-capped Ag nanoparticles. *Nanoscale* **2014**, *6*, 10113–10117. [CrossRef] [PubMed]
13. Pavoni, L.; Perinelli, D.R.; Bonacucina, G.; Cespi, M.; Palmieri, G.F. An Overview of Micro- and Nanoemulsions as Vehicles for Essential Oils: Formulation, Preparation and Stability. *Nanomaterials* **2020**, *10*, 135. [CrossRef] [PubMed]
14. Ali, E.O.M.; Shakil, N.A.; Rana, V.S.; Sarkar, D.J.; Majumder, S.; Kaushik, P.; Singh, B.B.; Kumar, J. Antifungal activity of nano emulsions of neem and citronella oils against phytopathogenic fungi, Rhizoctonia solani and Sclerotium rolfsii. *Ind. Crop. Prod.* **2017**, *108*, 379–387. [CrossRef]
15. Jiang, H.; Zhong, S.; Schwarz, P.; Chen, B.; Rao, J. Chemical composition of essential oils from leaf and bud of clove and their impact on the antifungal and mycotoxin inhibitory activities of clove oil-in-water nanoemulsions. *Ind. Crop. Prod.* **2022**, *187*, 115479. [CrossRef]
16. Mustafa, I.F.; Hussein, M.Z. Synthesis and Technology of Nanoemulsion-Based Pesticide Formulation. *Nanomaterials* **2020**, *10*, 1608. [CrossRef] [PubMed]
17. Kale, S.N.; Deore, S.L. Emulsion Micro Emulsion and Nano Emulsion: A Review. *Syst. Rev. Pharm.* **2016**, *8*, 39–47. [CrossRef]
18. Jang, Y.; Park, J.; Song, H.Y.; Choi, S.J. Ostwald Ripening Rate of Orange Oil Emulsions: Effects of Molecular Structure of Emulsifiers and Their Oil Composition. *J. Food Sci.* **2019**, *84*, 440–447. [CrossRef]
19. Dammak, I.; Sobral, P.J.D.A.; Aquino, A.; das Neves, M.A.; Conte-Junior, C.A. Nanoemulsions: Using emulsifiers from natural sources replacing synthetic ones—A review. *Compr. Rev. Food Sci. Food Saf.* **2020**, *19*, 2721–2746. [CrossRef]
20. Bai, L.; Huan, S.; Gu, J.; McClements, D.J. Fabrication of oil-in-water nanoemulsions by dual-channel microfluidization using natural emulsifiers: Saponins, phospholipids, proteins, and polysaccharides. *Food Hydrocoll.* **2016**, *61*, 703–711. [CrossRef]
21. Hu, Q.; Gerhard, H.; Upadhyaya, I.; Venkitanarayanan, K.; Luo, Y. Antimicrobial eugenol nanoemulsion prepared by gum arabic and lecithin and evaluation of drying technologies. *Int. J. Biol. Macromol.* **2016**, *87*, 130–140. [CrossRef]
22. Jamali, S.N.; Assadpour, E.; Feng, J.; Jafari, S.M. Natural antimicrobial-loaded nanoemulsions for the control of food spoilage/pathogenic microorganisms. *Adv. Colloid Interface Sci.* **2021**, *295*, 102504. [CrossRef]
23. Xu, M.; Zhang, W.; Pei, X.; Jiang, J.; Cui, Z.; Binks, B.P. CO_2/N_2 triggered switchable Pickering emulsions stabilized by alumina nanoparticles in combination with a conventional anionic surfactant. *RSC Adv.* **2017**, *7*, 29742–29751. [CrossRef]
24. Demina, P.A.; Grigoriev, D.O.; Kuz'micheva, G.M.; Bukreeva, T.V. Preparation of pickering-emulsion-based capsules with shells composed of titanium dioxide nanoparticles and polyelectrolyte layers. *Colloid J.* **2017**, *79*, 198–203. [CrossRef]

25. Rayner, M.; Marku, D.; Eriksson, M.; Sjöö, M.; Dejmek, P.; Wahlgren, M. Biomass-based particles for the formulation of Pickering type emulsions in food and topical applications. *Colloids Surf. A Physicochem. Eng. Asp.* **2014**, *458*, 48–62. [CrossRef]
26. Yadykova, A.Y.; Ilyin, S.O. Nanocellulose-stabilized bitumen emulsions as a base for preparation of nanocomposite asphalt binders. *Carbohydr. Polym.* **2023**, *313*, 120896. [CrossRef]
27. Korábková, E.; Kašpárková, V.; Vašíček, O.; Víchová, Z.; Káčerová, S.; Valášková, K.; Urbánková, L.; Vícha, J.; Münster, L.; Skopalová, K.; et al. Pickering emulsions as an effective route for the preparation of bioactive composites: A study of nanocellulose/polyaniline particles with immunomodulatory effect. *Carbohydr. Polym.* **2024**, *323*, 121429. [CrossRef] [PubMed]
28. Guo, X.; Wang, X.; Wei, Y.; Liu, P.; Deng, X.; Lei, Y.; Zhang, J. Preparation and properties of films loaded with cellulose nanocrystals stabilized Thymus vulgaris essential oil Pickering emulsion based on modified tapioca starch/polyvinyl alcohol. *Food Chem.* **2024**, *435*, 137597. [CrossRef]
29. Dong, H.; Ding, Q.; Jiang, Y.; Li, X.; Han, W. Pickering emulsions stabilized by spherical cellulose nanocrystals. *Carbohydr. Polym.* **2021**, *265*, 118101. [CrossRef]
30. Francesconi, S.; Ronchetti, R.; Camaioni, E.; Giovagnoli, S.; Sestili, F.; Palombieri, S.; Balestra, G.M. Boosting Immunity and Management against Wheat *Fusarium* Diseases by a Sustainable, Circular Nanostructured Delivery Platform. *Plants* **2023**, *12*, 1223. [CrossRef]
31. Schiavi, D.; Balbi, R.; Giovagnoli, S.; Camaioni, E.; Botticella, E.; Sestili, F.; Balestra, G.M. A Green Nanostructured Pesticide to Control Tomato Bacterial Speck Disease. *Nanomaterials* **2021**, *11*, 1852. [CrossRef]
32. Mikulcová, V.; Bordes, R.; Kašpárková, V. On the preparation and antibacterial activity of emulsions stabilized with nanocellulose particles. *Food Hydrocoll.* **2016**, *61*, 780–792. [CrossRef]
33. Zhou, Y.; Sun, S.; Bei, W.; Zahi, M.R.; Yuan, Q.; Liang, H. Preparation and antimicrobial activity of oregano essential oil Pickering emulsion stabilized by cellulose nanocrystals. *Int. J. Biol. Macromol.* **2018**, *112*, 7–13. [CrossRef]
34. Yu, H.; Huang, G.; Ma, Y.; Liu, Y.; Huang, X.; Zheng, Q.; Yue, P.; Yang, M. Cellulose nanocrystals based clove oil Pickering emulsion for enhanced antibacterial activity. *Int. J. Biol. Macromol.* **2021**, *170*, 24–32. [CrossRef]
35. Shlosman, K.; Rein, D.M.; Shemesh, R.; Koifman, N.; Caspi, A.; Cohen, Y. Encapsulation of Thymol and Eugenol Essential Oils Using Unmodified Cellulose: Preparation and Characterization. *Polymers* **2022**, *15*, 95. [CrossRef]
36. Marchese, A.; Orhan, I.E.; Daglia, M.; Barbieri, R.; Di Lorenzo, A.; Gortzi, O.; Izadi, M.; Nabavi, S.M. Antibacterial and antifungal activities of thymol: A brief review of the literature. *Food Chem.* **2016**, *210*, 402–414. [CrossRef]
37. Li, J.; Chang, J.W.; Saenger, M.; Deering, A. Thymol nanoemulsions formed via spontaneous emulsification: Physical and antimicrobial properties. *Food Chem.* **2017**, *232*, 191–197. [CrossRef]
38. Baldassarre, F.; De Stradis, A.; Altamura, G.; Vergaro, V.; Citti, C.; Cannazza, G.; Capodilupo, A.L.; Dini, L.; Ciccarella, G. Application of calcium carbonate nanocarriers for controlled release of phytodrugs against *Xylella fastidiosa* pathogen. *Pure Appl. Chem.* **2020**, *92*, 429–444. [CrossRef]
39. Baldassarre, F.; Schiavi, D.; Ciarroni, S.; Tagliavento, V.; De Stradis, A.; Vergaro, V.; Suranna, G.P.; Balestra, G.M.; Ciccarella, G. Thymol-Nanoparticles as Effective Biocides against the Quarantine Pathogen *Xylella fastidiosa*. *Nanomaterials* **2023**, *13*, 1285. [CrossRef] [PubMed]
40. Gardan, L.; Bollet, C.; Abu Ghorrah, M.; Grimont, F.; Grimont, P.A.D. DNA Relatedness among the Pathovar Strains of Pseudomonas syringae subsp. savastanoi Janse (1982) and Proposal of *Pseudomonas savastanoi* sp. nov. *Int. J. Syst. Evol. Microbiol.* **1992**, *42*, 606–612. [CrossRef]
41. Lamichhane, J.R.; Osdaghi, E.; Behlau, F.; Köhl, J.; Jones, J.B.; Aubertot, J.-N. Thirteen decades of antimicrobial copper compounds applied in agriculture. A review. *Agron. Sustain. Dev.* **2018**, *38*, 28. [CrossRef]
42. Saito, H.; Yamashita, Y.; Sakata, N.; Ishiga, T.; Shiraishi, N.; Usuki, G.; Nguyen, V.T.; Yamamura, E.; Ishiga, Y. Covering Soybean Leaves with Cellulose Nanofiber Changes Leaf Surface Hydrophobicity and Confers Resistance Against *Phakopsora pachyrhizi*. *Front. Plant Sci.* **2021**, *12*, 726565. [CrossRef]
43. Schiavi, D.; Francesconi, S.; Taddei, A.R.; Fortunati, E.; Balestra, G.M. Exploring cellulose nanocrystals obtained from olive tree wastes as sustainable crop protection tool against bacterial diseases. *Sci. Rep.* **2022**, *12*, 6149. [CrossRef]
44. Pannucci, E.; Caracciolo, R.; Romani, A.; Cacciola, F.; Dugo, P.; Bernini, R.; Varvaro, L.; Santi, L. An hydroxytyrosol enriched extract from olive mill wastewaters exerts antioxidant activity and antimicrobial activity on *Pseudomonas savastanoi* pv. savastanoi and Agrobacterium tumefaciens. *Nat. Prod. Res.* **2019**, *35*, 2677–2684. [CrossRef]
45. Sisto, A.; Morea, M.; Baruzzi, F.; Palumbo, G. Differentiation of *Pseudomonas syringae* subsp. Savastonoi Strains Isolated from Various Host Plants by Restriction Fragment Lengh Polymorphism. *Phytopathol. Mediterr.* **2002**, *41*, 63–71.
46. Kim, J.-E.; Lee, J.-E.; Huh, M.-J.; Lee, S.-C.; Seo, S.-M.; Kwon, J.H.; Park, I.-K. Fumigant Antifungal Activity via Reactive Oxygen Species of *Thymus vulgaris* and *Satureja hortensis* Essential Oils and Constituents against *Raffaelea quercus-mongolicae* and *Rhizoctonia solani*. *Biomolecules* **2019**, *9*, 561. [CrossRef]
47. Brahmi, F.; Abdenour, A.; Bruno, M.; Silvia, P.; Alessandra, P.; Danilo, F.; Drifa, Y.-G.; Fahmi, E.M.; Khodir, M.; Mohamed, C. Chemical composition and in vitro antimicrobial, insecticidal and antioxidant activities of the essential oils of *Mentha pulegium* L. and *Mentha rotundifolia* (L.) Huds growing in Algeria. *Ind. Crops Prod.* **2016**, *88*, 96–105. [CrossRef]
48. Cowan, M.M. Plant Products as Antimicrobial Agents. *Clin. Microbiol. Rev.* **1999**, *12*, 564–582. [CrossRef]

49. Bozin, B.; Mimica-Dukic, N.; Simin, N.; Anackov, G. Characterization of the Volatile Composition of Essential Oils of Some Lamiaceae Spices and the Antimicrobial and Antioxidant Activities of the Entire Oils. *J. Agric. Food Chem.* **2006**, *54*, 1822–1828. [CrossRef]
50. Shin, J.; Na, K.; Shin, S.; Seo, S.-M.; Youn, H.J.; Park, I.-K.; Hyun, J. Biological Activity of Thyme White Essential Oil Stabilized by Cellulose Nanocrystals. *Biomolecules* **2019**, *9*, 799. [CrossRef] [PubMed]
51. Balasubramani, S.; Rajendhiran, T.; Moola, A.K.; Diana, R.K.B. Development of nanoemulsion from Vitex negundo L. essential oil and their efficacy of antioxidant, antimicrobial and larvicidal activities (*Aedes aegypti* L.). *Environ. Sci. Pollut. Res.* **2017**, *24*, 15125–15133. [CrossRef] [PubMed]
52. Ghosh, V.; Mukherjee, A.; Chandrasekaran, N. Eugenol-loaded antimicrobial nanoemulsion preserves fruit juice against, microbial spoilage. *Colloids Surf. B Biointerfaces* **2014**, *114*, 392–397. [CrossRef] [PubMed]
53. Lu, H.; Li, X.; Tian, T.; Yang, H.; Quan, G.; Zhang, Y.; Huang, H. The pH-responsiveness carrier of sanxan gel beads crosslinked with $CaCl_2$ to control drug release. *Int. J. Biol. Macromol.* **2023**, *250*, 126298. [CrossRef] [PubMed]
54. Qu, R.-J.; Wang, Y.; Li, D.; Wang, L.-J. Rheological behavior of nanocellulose gels at various calcium chloride concentrations. *Carbohydr. Polym.* **2021**, *274*, 118660. [CrossRef] [PubMed]
55. Doustdar, F.; Olad, A.; Ghorbani, M. Effect of glutaraldehyde and calcium chloride as different crosslinking agents on the characteristics of chitosan/cellulose nanocrystals scaffold. *Int. J. Biol. Macromol.* **2022**, *208*, 912–924. [CrossRef]
56. Du, Z.; Wang, C.; Tai, X.; Wang, G.; Liu, X. Optimization and Characterization of Biocompatible Oil-in-Water Nanoemulsion for Pesticide Delivery. *ACS Sustain. Chem. Eng.* **2016**, *4*, 983–991. [CrossRef]
57. Souza, A.G.; Ferreira, R.R.; Paula, L.C.; Setz, L.F.; Rosa, D.S. The effect of essential oil chemical structures on Pickering emulsion stabilized with cellulose nanofibrils. *J. Mol. Liq.* **2020**, *320*, 114458. [CrossRef]
58. Heydari, M.; Amirjani, A.; Bagheri, M.; Sharifian, I.; Sabahi, Q. Eco-friendly pesticide based on peppermint oil nanoemulsion: Preparation, physicochemical properties, and its aphicidal activity against cotton aphid. *Environ. Sci. Pollut. Res.* **2020**, *27*, 6667–6679. [CrossRef]
59. Feng, J.; Zhang, Q.; Liu, Q.; Zhu, Z.; McClements, D.J.; Jafari, S.M. Chapter 12—Application of Nanoemulsions in Formulation of Pesticides. In *Nanoemulsions*; Jafari, S.M., McClements, D.J., Eds.; Academic Press: Cambridge, MA, USA, 2018; pp. 379–413. ISBN 978-0-12-811838-2.
60. Chen, H.; Zhong, Q. Physical and antimicrobial properties of self-emulsified nanoemulsions containing three synergistic essential oils. *Int. J. Food Microbiol.* **2022**, *365*, 109557. [CrossRef]
61. Trujillo-Cayado, A.L.; Santos, J.; Calero, N.; Alfaro-Rodríguez, M.; Muñoz, J. Strategies for reducing Ostwald ripening phenomenon in nanoemulsions based on thyme essential oil. *J. Sci. Food Agric.* **2020**, *100*, 1671–1677. [CrossRef]
62. Razavi, M.S.; Golmohammadi, A.; Nematollahzadeh, A.; Fiori, F.; Rovera, C.; Farris, S. Preparation of cinnamon essential oil emulsion by bacterial cellulose nanocrystals and fish gelatin. *Food Hydrocoll.* **2020**, *109*, 106111. [CrossRef]
63. Zhang, Y.; Zhong, Q. Physical and antimicrobial properties of neutral nanoemulsions self-assembled from alkaline thyme oil and sodium caseinate mixtures. *Int. J. Biol. Macromol.* **2020**, *148*, 1046–1052. [CrossRef]
64. Díaz-Blancas, V.; Medina, D.I.; Padilla-Ortega, E.; Bortolini-Zavala, R.; Olvera-Romero, M.; Luna-Bárcenas, G. Nanoemulsion Formulations of Fungicide Tebuconazole for Agricultural Applications. *Molecules* **2016**, *21*, 1271. [CrossRef]
65. Huang, K.; Liu, R.; Zhang, Y.; Guan, X. Characteristics of two cedarwood essential oil emulsions and their antioxidant and antibacterial activities. *Food Chem.* **2021**, *346*, 128970. [CrossRef]
66. Schiavi, D.; Francesconi, S.; Bischetti, G.; Giovanale, G.; Fortunati, E.; Balestra, G.M. Antibacterial activity of coumarin as an innovative organic control strategy for *Xanthomonas euvesicatoria* pv. *euvesicatoria*. *J. Plant Dis. Prot.* **2021**, *129*, 181–187. [CrossRef]
67. Marchese, A.; Arciola, C.R.; Barbieri, R.; Silva, A.S.; Nabavi, S.M.; Sokeng, A.J.T.; Izadi, M.; Jafari, N.J.; Suntar, I.; Daglia, M.; et al. Update on Monoterpenes as Antimicrobial Agents: A Particular Focus on p-Cymene. *Materials* **2017**, *10*, 947. [CrossRef]
68. Laquale, S.; Avato, P.; Argentieri, M.P.; Bellardi, M.G.; D'addabbo, T. Nematotoxic activity of essential oils from Monarda species. *J. Pest Sci.* **2018**, *91*, 1115–1125. [CrossRef]
69. Ben Abdallah, F.; Philippe, W.; Goffart, J.P. Comparison of optical indicators for potato crop nitrogen status assessment including novel approaches based on leaf fluorescence and flavonoid content. *J. Plant Nutr.* **2018**, *41*, 2705–2728. [CrossRef]
70. Bracke, J.; Elsen, A.; Adriaenssens, S.; Schoeters, L.; Vandendriessche, H.; Labeke, M.-C. Application of Proximal Optical Sensors to Fine-Tune Nitrogen Fertilization: Opportunities for Woody Ornamentals. *Agronomy* **2019**, *9*, 408. [CrossRef]
71. Schiavi, D.; Taddei, A.R.; Balestra, G.M. Investigating Cellulose Nanocrystals' Biocompatibility and Their Effects on *Pseudomonas syringae* pv. *tomato Epiphytic Survival for Sustainable Crop Protection. Horticulturae* **2023**, *9*, 525. [CrossRef]
72. Pirzada, T.; de Farias, B.V.; Mathew, R.; Guenther, R.H.; Byrd, M.V.; Sit, T.L.; Pal, L.; Opperman, C.H.; Khan, S.A. Recent advances in biodegradable matrices for active ingredient release in crop protection: Towards attaining sustainability in agriculture. *Curr. Opin. Colloid Interface Sci.* **2020**, *48*, 121–136. [CrossRef]
73. Vettraino, A.M.; Zikeli, F.; Mugnozza, G.S.; Vinciguerra, V.; Tabet, D.; Romagnoli, M. Lignin nanoparticles containing essential oils for controlling *Phytophthora cactorum* diseases. *For. Pathol.* **2022**, *52*, e12739. [CrossRef]
74. Rajkumar, V.; Gunasekaran, C.; Paul, C.A.; Dharmaraj, J. Development of encapsulated peppermint essential oil in chitosan nanoparticles: Characterization and biological efficacy against stored-grain pest control. *Pestic. Biochem. Physiol.* **2020**, *170*, 104679. [CrossRef]

75. Abbasi, M.; Dastjerdi, A.M.; Seyahooei, M.A.; Shamili, M.; Madani, B. Postharvest control of green and blue molds on Mexican lime fruit caused by *Penicillium* species using *Thymus vulgaris* essential oil and carboxy methyl cellulose. *J. Plant Dis. Prot.* **2023**, *130*, 1017–1026. [CrossRef]
76. Doan, H.K.; Ngassam, V.N.; Gilmore, S.F.; Tecon, R.; Parikh, A.N.; Leveau, J.H.J. Topography-Driven Shape, Spread, and Retention of Leaf Surface Water Impacts Microbial Dispersion and Activity in the Phyllosphere. *Phytobiomes J.* **2020**, *4*, 268–280. [CrossRef]
77. Lamichhane, J.R.; Varvaro, L. Epiphytic *Pseudomonas savastanoi* pv. *savastanoi can infect and cause olive knot disease on Olea europaea subsp. cuspidata. Australas. Plant Pathol.* **2013**, *42*, 219–225. [CrossRef]
78. King, E.O.; Ward, M.K.; Raney, D.E. Two simple media for the determination of pyocianine and fluorescein. *J. Lab. Clin. Med.* **1954**, *44*, 301–307.
79. Wiśniewska, M. Influences of polyacrylic acid adsorption and temperature on the alumina suspension stability. *Powder Technol.* **2010**, *198*, 258–266. [CrossRef]
80. Kang, W.; Xu, B.; Wang, Y.; Li, Y.; Shan, X.; An, F.; Liu, J. Stability mechanism of W/O crude oil emulsion stabilized by polymer and surfactant. *Colloids Surf. A Physicochem. Eng. Asp.* **2011**, *384*, 555–560. [CrossRef]
81. Wiegand, I.; Hilpert, K.; Hancock, R.E.W. Agar and broth dilution methods to determine the minimal inhibitory concentration (MIC) of antimicrobial substances. *Nat. Protoc.* **2008**, *3*, 163–175. [CrossRef]
82. Cerovic, Z.G.; Masdoumier, G.; Ben Ghozlen, N.; Latouche, G. A new optical leaf-clip meter for simultaneous non-destructive assessment of leaf chlorophyll and epidermal flavonoids. *Physiol. Plant.* **2012**, *146*, 251–260. [CrossRef]
83. Easlon, H.M.; Bloom, A.J. Easy Leaf Area: Automated digital image analysis for rapid and accurate measurement of leaf area. *Appl. Plant Sci.* **2014**, *2*, 1400033. [CrossRef]
84. Balouiri, M.; Sadiki, M.; Ibnsouda, S.K. Methods for in vitro evaluating antimicrobial activity: A review. *J. Pharm. Anal.* **2016**, *6*, 71–79. [CrossRef]
85. Valgas, C.; De Souza, S.M.; Smânia, E.F.A.; Smânia, A., Jr. Screening methods to determine antibacterial activity of natural products. *Braz. J. Microbiol.* **2007**, *38*, 369–380. [CrossRef]

molecules

MDPI

Article

Low-Hydrophilic HKUST−1/Polymer Extrudates for the PSA Separation of CO_2/CH_4

Muhamad Tahriri Rozaini [1,2], Denys I. Grekov [2], Mohamad Azmi Bustam [1,*] and Pascaline Pré [2,*]

1 Centre of Research in Ionic Liquids, CORIL, Chemical Engineering Department, Universiti Teknologi Petronas, Bandar Seri Iskandar 32610, Perak, Malaysia; muhamad_21000026@utp.edu.my or muhamad-tahriri.bin-rozaini@imt-atlantique.fr

2 GEnie des Procédés Environnement-Agroalimentaire (GEPEA) UMR-CNRS 6144, Department of Energy Systems and Environment, IMT Atlantique, 44300 Nantes, France; denys.grekov@imt-atlantique.fr

* Correspondence: azmibustam@utp.edu.my (M.A.B.); pascaline.pre@imt-atlantique.fr (P.P.)

Abstract: HKUST−1 is an MOF adsorbent industrially produced in powder form and thus requires a post-shaping process for use as an adsorbent in fixed-bed separation processes. HKUST−1 is also sensitive to moisture, which degrades its crystalline structure. In this work, HKUST−1, in the form of crystalline powder, was extruded into pellets using a hydrophobic polymeric binder to improve its moisture stability. Thermoplastic polyurethane (TPU) was used for that purpose. The subsequent HKUST−1/TPU extrudate was then compared to HKUST−1/PLA extrudates synthesized with more hydrophilic polymer: polylactic acid (PLA), as the binder. The characterization of the composites was determined via XRD, TGA, SEM-EDS, and an N_2 adsorption isotherm analysis. Meanwhile, the gas-separation performances of HKUST−1/TPU were investigated and compared with HKUST−1/PLA from measurements of CO_2 and CH_4 isotherms at three different temperatures, up to 10 bars. Lastly, the moisture stability of the composite materials was investigated via an aging analysis during storage under humid conditions. It is shown that HKUST−1's crystalline structure was preserved in the HKUST−1/TPU extrudates. The composites also exhibited good thermal stability under 523 K, whilst their textural properties were not significantly modified compared with the pristine HKUST−1. Furthermore, both extrudates exhibited larger CO_2 and CH_4 adsorption capacities in comparison to the pristine HKUST−1. After three months of storage under atmospheric humid conditions, CO_2 adsorption capacities were reduced to only 10% for HKUST−1/TPU, whereas reductions of about 25% and 54% were observed for HKUST−1/PLA and the pristine HKUST−1, respectively. This study demonstrates the interest in shaping MOF powders by extrusion using a hydrophobic thermoplastic binder to operate adsorbents with enhanced moisture stability in gas-separation columns.

Keywords: shaping; HKUST−1; MOF-polymer composite; extrusion; hydrophobic

Citation: Rozaini, M.T.; Grekov, D.I.; Bustam, M.A.; Pré, P. Low-Hydrophilic HKUST−1/Polymer Extrudates for the PSA Separation of CO_2/CH_4. *Molecules* **2024**, *29*, 2069. https://doi.org/10.3390/molecules29092069

Academic Editors: Fabio Ganazzoli and Giuseppina Raffaini

Received: 28 March 2024
Revised: 24 April 2024
Accepted: 25 April 2024
Published: 30 April 2024

1. Introduction

Biogas production has been increasing in recent years thanks to the implementation of multiple renewable energy policies motivated by economic and environmental benefits. From 2010 to 2019, it was estimated that global biogas production increased from 65 GW to 120 GW, of which 70% originated from Europe [1]. According to the International Energy Agency (IEA), global biogas demand is expected to reach up to 872 TWh in 2040 [2], leading to a huge potential market for this type of renewable energy. Biogas is produced from the anaerobic digestion of various organic wastes, such as sewage sludge, agricultural and crop residues, and animal dung, as well as industrial organic wastes and wastewater. Biogas consists of three main components: methane (45–70%), carbon dioxide (24–40%), and nitrogen (1–17%) [3]. Other gases that are present in biogas composition are water vapor, oxygen, hydrogen sulfide, ammonia, carbon monoxide, and traces of halogenated hydrocarbons, siloxanes, and toluene [4]. Biogas can be burned directly on-site to produce heat and electricity. However, biogas energy density is low compared to natural gas (NG) since it contains a large fraction of carbon dioxide in addition to other secondary contaminants. Therefore, biogas needs to be purified to produce biomethane, having a composition matching the specifications for injections into gas grids.

Biogas upgrading can be achieved via numerous technologies, such as water/physical/chemical scrubbing, cryogenic separation, membrane separation, pressure swing adsorption (PSA), and vacuum pressure swing adsorption (VPSA) [5,6]. In the context of this study, we are interested in the removal of CO_2 from biogas via PSA, avoiding the use of a vacuum in the desorption step that would then be replaced with desorption in atmospheric pressure. Because vacuum desorption is mainly responsible for the high energy costs of VPSA processes, better energy performances by PSA separation are foreseen. The choice of adsorbent is one of the key factors in designing such a process.

Thermodynamic and kinetic properties of the adsorbent determine the bed working capacities and the separation performances of the whole unit in terms of methane productivity, purity, and rate of recovery. Good resistance to attrition, thermal stability over long lifetimes, and hydrophobicity are also essential to make a suitable adsorbent for such a separation. Amongst the conventional adsorbents applied for biogas upgrading in VPSA processes are zeolites and carbon molecular sieves (CMS) [7].

Recently, metal–organic frameworks (MOFs) have been gaining attention for their potential application in gas separation owing to their inherent properties, such as high specific surface area, large porosity, and tunable pore size [8,9]. In the literature, MOFs have been extensively studied for their capability to separate CO_2 from CH_4 [10–12]. Amongst the materials investigated, HKUST−1 has been identified as a good candidate for CO_2/CH_4 separation because of its good CO_2/CH_4 selectivity [13,14]. The CO_2 capture performance of HKUST−1 at low pressure is influenced by the affinity of open-metal sites with CO_2, whereas at high pressure, it is governed by the surface area of HKUST−1 [15]. Figure 1 shows the literature comparison of CO_2 and CH_4 adsorption capacities of HKUST−1 with other MOFs, as well as conventional adsorbents, at 298 K for the pressure conditions of one bar and five bars, respectively [16–29]. It can be seen that CO_2 is preferably adsorbed than CH_4 for HKUST−1 at both pressure conditions. On the one hand, the CO_2 adsorption capacity of HKUST−1 at both pressure conditions is better than other MOFs, such as PCN-68 and MIL-101 (Cr), as well as the conventional adsorbent CMS. On the other hand, the MOF-74 adsorbent family exhibits larger CO_2 adsorption capacities than HKUST−1 under both pressure conditions. Similarly, at one bar, the CO_2 adsorption capacity of zeolite 13X surpasses that of HKUST−1, though this trend is reversed at a higher pressure of five bars. Nevertheless, HKUST−1 is one of the few MOFs that are commercially available [30], making the procurement of large-scale amounts of material with consistent quality easier. However, one of the main drawbacks of using HKUST−1 as an adsorbent for CO_2 capture from biogas is its sensitivity towards moisture, which may still be present at low concentrations in the biogas feed, even after the drying step. It is difficult to provide the exact value of leftover moisture in the biogas prior to the upgrading process, as this value may vary depending on dehumidification methods (e.g., condensation and absorption), though interested readers may refer to a notable study by Golmakani et al. [31], which summarizes the range of water dew point reduction in biogas according to different dehumidification processes. Nevertheless, the crystalline structure of HKUST is degraded when exposed to humidity, and this consequently leads to a drastic reduction in its CO_2 adsorption capacities [32,33].

HKUST−1 could be synthesized via different synthesis routes, such as solvothermal, microwave, sonochemical, and mechanochemical synthesis [34–42]. HKUST−1 synthesized through these methods is usually obtained in a powder form of millimetric size, which is not convenient for use in adsorption columns because the packing of fine powder causes restrictions in the flow of gas, thus resulting in large pressure losses across the column [43]. To overcome this issue, fine crystalline adsorbent powder needs to be shaped into larger size particle forms, such as granules, tablets, or monoliths.

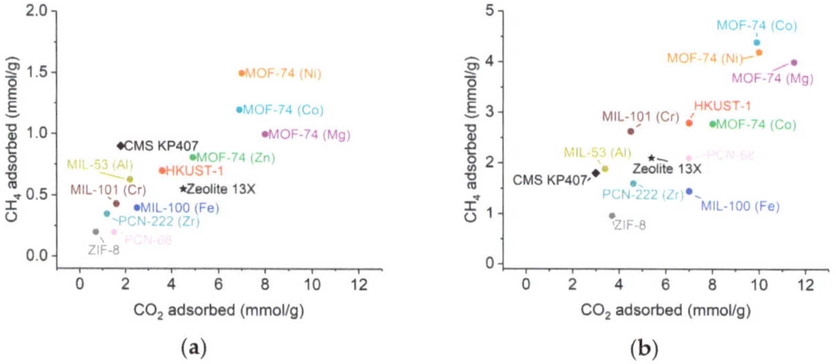

Figure 1. (**a**). CO_2 and CH_4 adsorption capacities comparison for different MOFs at 298 K and 1 bar. (**b**) CO_2 and CH_4 adsorption capacities comparison for different MOFs at 298 K and 5 bars.

MOF shaping can be performed either with or without the use of a binding agent [43]. The usage of a binding agent in the shaping process may significantly modify the MOF's intrinsic properties. In particular, it can help promote the macrostructure's mechanical strength of the adsorbent particle and improve its chemical and thermal stability while still maintaining its intrinsic porosity and adsorption properties. For example, in a study by Cousin-Saint Remi et al. [44], ZIF-8 was shaped by a simple extrusion–crushing–sieving (ECS) approach using different binder recipes, i.e., cellulose–acetate (CA), polyvinylchloride (PVC), polyvinylformal (PVF), polyetherimide (PEI), and polystyrene (PS). The ZIF-8 composites were synthesized using 15 wt% of each binder, and it was revealed that their ethanol adsorption capacities were similar to those of the pristine ZIF-8. Furthermore, this study demonstrated that by increasing the binding agent mass fraction from 7 wt% to 30 wt%, the mechanical stability of the ZIF-8 composites was improved, and the composite made up of a PVDF binder displayed the most robust structure. In addition, it was pointed out that the composite moisture stability was dependent on the binding agent employed and that the use of PVDF as a binder yielded the most stable composite when exposed to humid conditions.

In another notable study by Hastürk et al. [45], MIL-160 (Al) and MIL-101 (Cr) were shaped via the freeze–casting method (extrusion-based method) using different hydrophilic polymeric binders, i.e., polyacrylic acid (PAA), sodium polyacrylate (PAANa), polyethylene glycol (PEG), polyvinyl alcohol (PVA) and polyvinyl pyrrolidone (PVP). This study demonstrated that the usage of a hydrophilic binder enhances the water uptake capacity of the MOFs. Both MIL-160 (Al)/MIL-101 (Cr)@polymer composites displayed an increase in water uptake capacities in the low-pressure region in comparison to the respective pristine materials.

Similarly, in our previous work [46], a pristine HKUST−1 was shaped by simple extrusion using thermoplastic polylactic acid (PLA) as the binding agent. It was shown that the HKUST−1's crystalline structure, morphology, and textural properties, as well as CO_2/CH_4 adsorption capacities, were preserved in the synthesized HKUST−1/PLA composite when compared to the pristine HKUST−1. However, the moisture stability was not significantly improved in comparison to the pristine HKUST−1 [47,48]. It is, therefore, interesting to discover whether the replacement of PLA with another less-hydrophilic thermoplastic polymer as a binding agent could improve the adsorbent moisture stability.

The main objective of this research is to assess the effect of using a low-hydrophilic polymeric binder in the shaping extrusion process on the properties of an HKUST−1 adsorbent composite. For that purpose, thermoplastic polyurethane (TPU) was selected as a polymeric binding agent in order to compare the properties of HKUST−1/TPU and HKUST−1/PLA composites. Thermoplastic polyurethane (TPU) is an elastomeric polymer with a molecular configuration consisting of hard-segment and soft-segment blocks that provide properties such as high ductility, toughness, durability, flexibility, biocompatibility, and biostability [49]. The rigidity and hardness of TPU originate from the hard segment, whereas the flexibility and elastomeric properties originate from the soft segment. TPU is more hydrophobic than PLA, as demonstrated in several other studies [50,51].

To verify the successful shaping of HKUST−1 with TPU, structural and textural properties, as well as CO_2 and CH_4 adsorption equilibrium data for HKUST−1/TPU, were measured and subsequently compared with pristine HKUST−1 and HKUST−1/PLA composites synthesized from the same extrusion process as reported in [46]; however, we used thermoplastic polylactic acid (PLA) as the binding agent. The hydrophilicity of the two polymers was quantified in this study by conducting surface wettability tests (Figure S1). The effect of methanol washing on the textural properties and adsorption capacities of HKUST−1 powder was assessed to interpret differences observed between the composites and pristine HKUST−1. Finally, the stability of the samples under humid conditions was analyzed to assess the impact of the polymer's hydrophobicity on the moisture stability of the composites.

2. Results and Discussion

2.1. Sample Characterization

The structural analysis of the samples was investigated through an XRD analysis. Figure 2 illustrates XRD peaks observed for HKUST−1/TPU, HKUST−1/PLA, pristine HKUST−1, TPU, and PLA. Pure TPU exhibited a characteristic broad peak around 20° due to the diffraction from the (110) planes of the TPU soft segments [52,53], whereas pure PLA exhibited a strong peak at 16.8° due to diffraction from (110) and/or (200) planes [54]. Additionally, pristine HKUST−1 exhibited characteristic peaks at 6.7°, 9.5°, 11.6°, and 13.4°, which can be attributed to the (200), (220), (222), and (400) crystal planes of HKUST−1 [46].

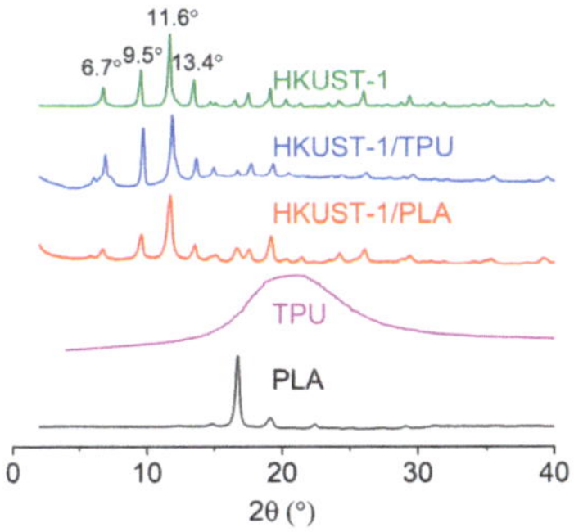

Figure 2. XRD of TPU, PLA, pristine HKUST−1 and its composites.

The XRD pattern for HKUST−1/TPU closely resembled the one for HKUST−1/PLA, where peaks associated with pristine HKUST−1 were clearly present in both composites, whereas peaks associated with pure TPU or PLA were indistinguishable in the HKUST−1/TPU and HKUST−1/PLA samples due to their low loading in the composites. Nevertheless, the XRD analysis confirms the presence of HKUST−1 particles in both composites after the shaping process.

Scanning electron microscopy (SEM) imaging was used to characterize the surface morphology of the adsorbent materials. Figure 3 compares the morphology observed between HKUST−1/TPU, HKUST−1/PLA, and the pristine HKUST−1. Most of the pristine HKUST−1 particles exhibited an octahedron shape, though there were also large particles of an irregular shape. Morphologies of the surface of HKUST−1/TPU and HKUST−1/PLA show that the particles of HKUST−1 were not totally encapsulated by the polymeric binder after shaping. Furthermore, it can be observed that particles in the HKUST−1/TPU composite were held together by fibrous TPU polymers, whereas particles in the HKUST−1/PLA composite were surrounded by amorphous PLA. It is likely that the formation of the fiber grid observed in HKUST−1/TPU occurred during the synthesis process of the composite, as typical commercial filaments of TPU and PLA exhibited a smooth and dense surface (Figure 4). The obtained SEM imaging of both composites demonstrates that the shaping process, using a 10% mass of either one of the polymeric binders, yielded a composite in which HKUST−1 particles remained accessible for gas adsorption.

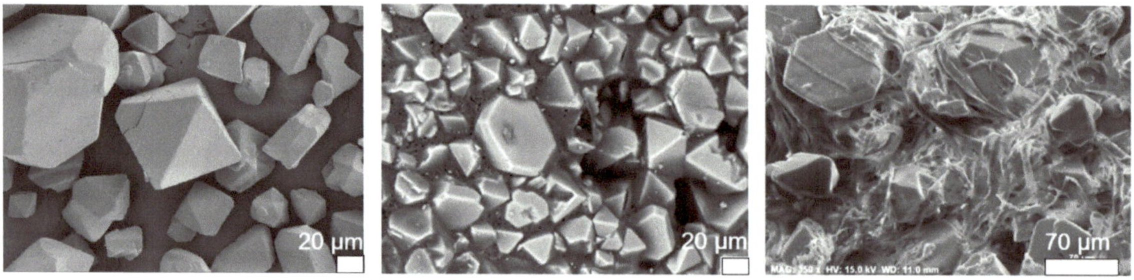

(a) (b) (c)

Figure 3. SEM image of (**a**) pristine HKUST−1. (**b**) HKUST−1/PLA. Reproduced from [46]. (**c**) HKUST−1/TPU.

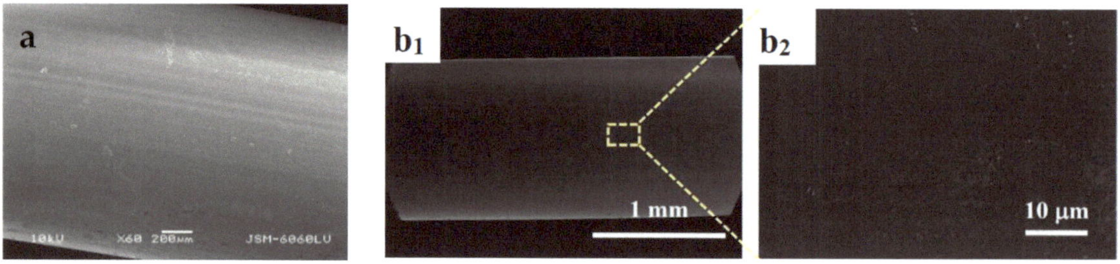

Figure 4. (**a**) SEM image of neat PLA filament. Image reproduced from [55]. (**b$_1$**,**b$_2$**) SEM image of neat TPU filament at different magnification. Images reproduced with permission from [56].

The EDS spectra of HKUST−1/TPU and HKUST−1/PLA are presented in Figures 5a and 5b, respectively. Qualitatively, the peaks corresponding to the expected main elements in the composites are evident, namely, C, O, and Cu. C and O elements were present in both HKUST−1 and the polymeric binder, whereas the Cu element was only present in the pristine HKUST−1. It should be noted that the difference in an element's relative content in HKUST−1/TPU and HKUST−1/PLA was not exploited as the samples that were used for the analysis were not flat, which rendered the quantitative analysis of EDS unreliable. Nevertheless, the presence of element peaks in the composite was similar to the EDS spectra of the pristine HKUST−1 powder reported in other studies [57,58], which is indicative of the preservation of the HKUST−1 crystals in both composites.

Figure 6 displays elemental mapping for HKUST−1/TPU and HKUST−1/PLA. The mapping reveals a uniform distribution of C (represented by blue color) and O (represented by green color) elements over the surface of the composites because these elements were present in both the MOF and binder. However, the Cu element (represented by red color) had a more heterogeneous distribution as this element was only present in HKUST−1. By combining the mapping of the Cu and C elements together, we could observe that there was a clear separation between the Cu element in HKUST−1 and the C element in the polymeric binder of both composites. This separation, clearly observed from the elemental mapping, is a good indication that no degradation reaction occurred between HKUST−1 and the polymeric binders (TPU or PLA) during shaping. It should be noted here that there is a grayish section in the elemental mapping that corresponds to the area where the EDS analysis was unable to detect the elements due to shadowing.

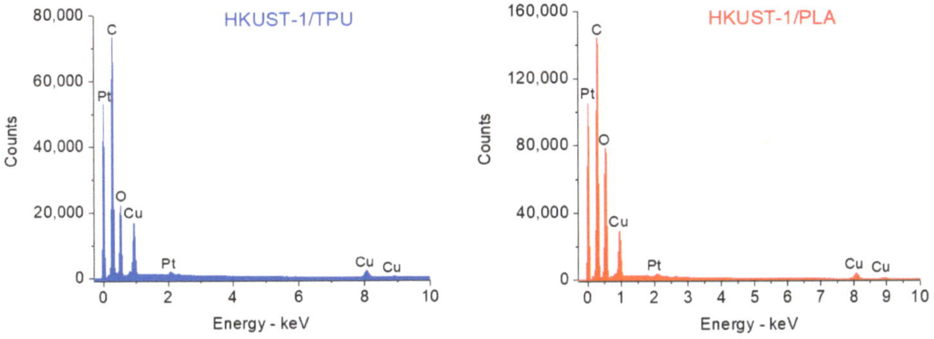

(**a**) (**b**)

Figure 5. (**a**) EDS spectra for HKUST−1/TPU. (**b**) EDS spectra for HKUST−1/PLA.

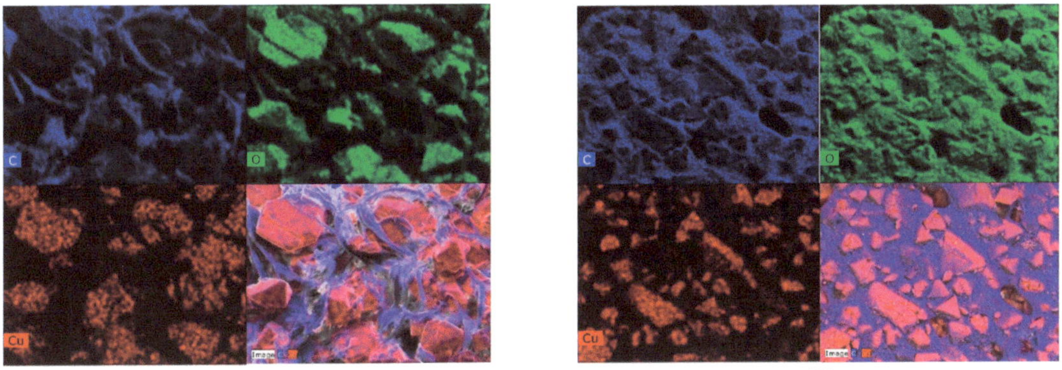

(**a**) (**b**)

Figure 6. (**a**) EDS mapping for HKUST−1/TPU. (**b**) EDS mapping for HKUST−1/PLA.

Nitrogen physisorption isotherms are shown in Figure 7 on both linear and logarithmic scales. All isotherms featured a type I shape relevant to highly microporous solids [59]. The N_2 adsorption capacities of HKUST−1/TPU and HKUST−1/PLA were slightly larger than the pristine HKUST−1's, which signifies that the pristine HKUST−1 particles in both composites remained accessible to gas adsorption, as shown by SEM imaging. In addition to that, it can be seen that nitrogen filling in the lowest pressure range ($P/P_0 < 10^{-4}$) was different for both composites when compared to the pristine HKUST−1 powder. This indicates some changes related to the accessibility of the primary adsorption sites located in the microporous domain after shaping. Furthermore, the N_2 adsorption isotherm of pure TPU and pure PLA (Figure S2, Supporting Information) reveals that both polymeric binders absorbed a very negligible amount of N_2 in comparison to pristine HKUST−1 and its composites, which signifies that both TPU and PLA did not contribute to the slightly larger N_2 adsorption capacity denoted for the two composites. Meanwhile, when pristine HKUST−1 was washed with methanol, an increase in the N_2 adsorption capacity could be observed. Therefore, the increase in the N_2 adsorption capacity for both composites could be explained by the effect of "washing" with methanol during the shaping process.

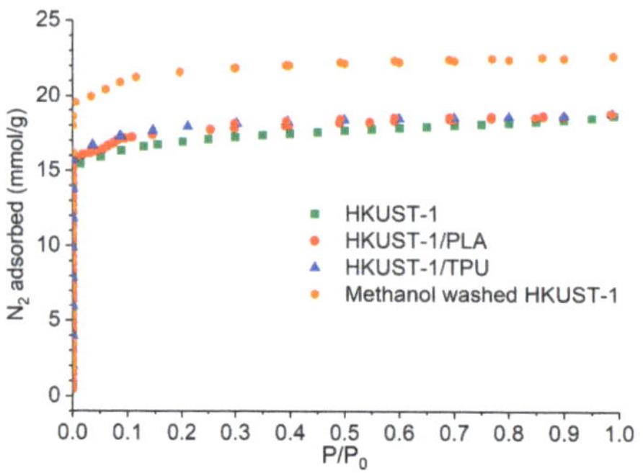

(a)

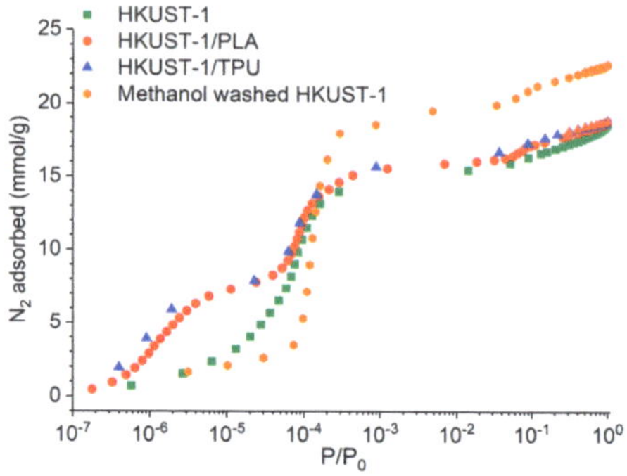

(b)

Figure 7. N_2 adsorption isotherm plot for HKUST−1/TPU, HKUST−1/PLA, pristine HKUST−1 and methanol-washed HKUST−1 in (**a**) linear scale and in (**b**) log scale. Data for HKUST−1/PLA and HKUST−1 was taken from previous work [46].

Table 1 lists the BET surface area and the pore volume data derived from 77K-N_2 isotherms for HKUST−1/TPU, HKUST−1/PLA, pristine HKUST−1, and methanol-washed HKUST−1. As expected, the micropore volumes of both HKUST−1/TPU and HKUST−1/PLA were slightly higher than pristine HKUST−1's, matching the changes observed in the low-pressure region of the N_2 isotherms. The computed BET surface areas of HKUST−1/TPU and HKUST−1/PLA appeared a bit larger than that of pristine HKUST−1. Once again, these trends could be explained by the "washing" of the composites with methanol, as methanol-washed HKUST−1 recorded an increase in the BET surface area and pore volume in comparison to the pristine HKUST−1. Additionally, when pristine HKUST−1 was washed with either DMF or chloroform, an increase in the BET surface area and/or pore volume could also be observed (Figure S3 and Table S2, Supporting Information), which may have resulted from residual reagents present in the pores washed away by the solvents.

Table 1. BET Surface area, pore volume of HKUST−1, methanol-washed HKUST−1, HKUST−1/TPU and HKUST−1/PLA. Data for HKUST−1 and HKUST−1/PLA was taken from previous work [46].

Sample	S_{BET} (m^2/g)	Micropore Volume (cm^3/g)	Total Pore Volume (cm^3/g)
HKUST−1	1500	0.46	0.65
HKUST−1/TPU	1557	0.50	0.65
HKUST−1/PLA	1528	0.54	0.65
Methanol-washed HKUST−1	1956	0.60	0.79

2.2. Thermal and Mechanical Stability

The TGA profiles for pristine HKUST−1 and its composites, as well as for the neat PLA and TPU, are shown in Figure 8. The pristine HKUST−1 was thermally stable up to 593 K, whereas PLA started to degrade at 613 K. Meanwhile, the thermal degradation behavior of TPU can be divided into two stages; the first stage of decomposition occurred between 553 K and 613 K, while the second stage occurred between 663 K and 733 K. The reason for the two-stage degradation was related to the decomposition behavior of urethane bonds in the hard segments and polyol groups in the soft segments of the TPU polymer [60,61].

The thermal degradation of HKUST−1/TPU and HKUST−1/PLA proceeded in two steps; a first mass loss occurred between 350 K–410 K, which consisted of a 3% and 5% weight loss for HKUST−1/TPU and HKUST−1/PLA, respectively, which was associated with the loss of leftover solvent molecules (chloroform, DMF or methanol) that remained trapped inside the pores; the second mass loss started around 560 K and 590 K for HKUST−1/TPU and HKUST−1/PLA, respectively, which can be attributed to the start of the framework and polymeric binder degradation. Interestingly, the mass loss due to trapped solvent molecules is significantly less for HKUST−1/TPU in comparison to HKUST−1/PLA, which could be due to the fibrous nature of TPU in the composite, as seen in the SEM imaging, limiting the entrapment of the solvent after the shaping process. Furthermore, the decomposition behavior of both the hard and soft segments of TPU was no longer distinguishable in the HKUST−1/TPU composite. It could be observed that both the HKUST−1/TPU and HKUST−1/PLA composites displayed a lower degradation temperature than pristine HKUST−1 and their respective pure polymeric binders. This could be attributed to the presence of metal from MOFs in the composite that may have acted as a catalyst for polymer degradation, as concluded in several other studies [54,62,63].

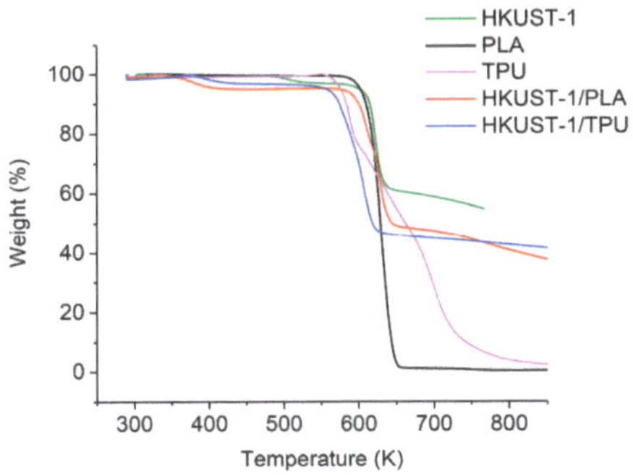

Figure 8. TGA profile for TPU, PLA, pristine HKUST−1 and its composites. Data for HKUST−1 and PLA was taken from previous work [46].

The attrition values of the samples were investigated to determine their mechanical stabilities. An adsorbent with a high attrition value could lead to problems when operating the gas-separation unit, such as bed clogging or an increase in pressure drops inside the adsorption column. Table 2 compares the attrition values measured for HKUST−1/TPU and HKUST−1/PLA with commercial adsorbents and MOF extrudates from other studies. These values were determined using the same attrition test standard according to the D4058-96 ASTM norm [64]. The attrition value of HKUST−1/TPU was only slightly lower in comparison to the one of HKUST−1/PLA, but both samples possessed comparable mechanical stability compared with other commercial adsorbents, as reported in [65]. This shows that TPU and PLA, used at a low loading rate as binding agents, are suitable for making HKUST−1 adsorbent composites with good mechanical resistance to attrition. To improve the mechanical stability of HKUST−1 composites, it could be possible to increase the concentration of the binder, but there is a risk of decreasing the gas-separation performance of the composites because of pore blockages, as observed for the HKUST−1/PLA produced at a 20 wt% binder loading (Figure S4).

Table 2. Attrition percentage of HKUST−1/TPU, HKUST−1/PLA, conventional adsorbent and MOF extrudates.

Sample	Attrition Loss (% wt)	Reference
HKUST−1/TPU	0.4	This study
HKUST−1/PLA	0.5	[46]
Zeolite 3A	≤0.2	[65]
Zeolite 4A	≤0.2	
Zeolite 5A	≤0.2	
Zeolite 13X	≤0.2	
AC-Norit RZN_1	0.2	[66]
UiO-66 extrudate	1.4	

2.3. CO_2 and CH_4 Adsorption Measurements

Methane and carbon dioxide adsorption isotherms (expressed as mmol/g of the adsorbent), which were measured at 298 K for HKUST−1/TPU, HKUST−1/PLA, and pristine HKUST−1, are presented in Figure 9. In a pressure range of less than one bar, both CO_2 and CH_4 adsorption capacities were similar for all the samples and appeared to be linear with the equilibrium pressure. In a pressure range between 1 and 10 bars, the shape of the CO_2 isotherms for all the samples was no longer linear with the equilibrium pressure. The CO_2 adsorption capacities tended to reach a plateau, which was, however, not observable in the tested equilibrium pressure conditions. The CH_4 adsorption isotherms of all the materials in that same pressure range remained, however, almost linear with the equilibrium pressure.

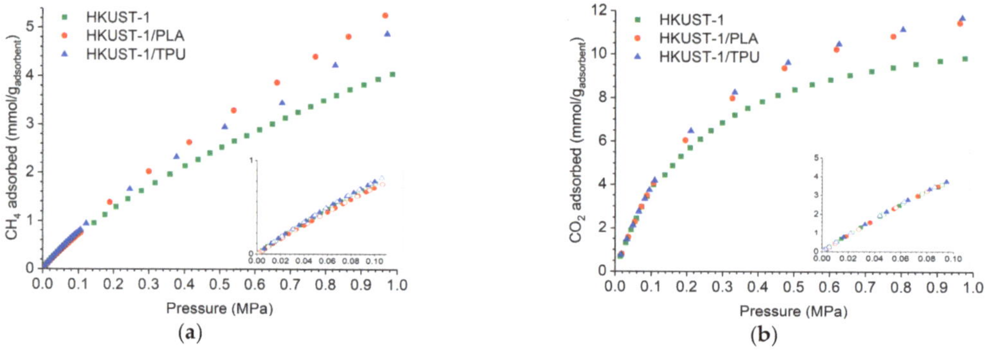

Figure 9. Gravimetric adsorption isotherms of (**a**) CH_4 and (**b**) CO_2 on HKUST−1 and its composites at 298 K. The inset displays the adsorption isotherm at equilibrium pressure up to 1 bar. Data for HKUST−1 and HKUST−1/PLA was taken from previous work [46].

The CO_2 and CH_4 adsorption capacities of the HKUST−1/TPU composite were similar to HKUST−1/PLA and pristine HKUST−1 at equilibrium pressures of less than one bar. However, as the equilibrium pressure increased, both composites exhibited larger CO_2 and CH_4 adsorption capacities than the pristine HKUST−1, which may be attributed to their larger BET surface areas and micropore volumes. The CO_2 adsorption isotherm of HKUST−1/TPU closely resembled that of HKUST−1/PLA, which suggests that TPU as a binding agent does not have a different effect from PLA on CO_2 adsorption capacities. Similarly, the CH_4 adsorption capacities of HKUST−1/TPU were comparable to those of HKUST−1/PLA in the upper range of the equilibrium pressure.

Previous N_2 adsorption isotherm measurements reveal that both composites exhibited higher BET surface areas and pore volumes than the pristine HKUST−1, which may be explained by the washing effect with methanol. Therefore, it is interesting to compare the adsorption performances of the active HKUST−1 particles present in both composites with both pristine and methanol-washed HKUST−1 powders, as displayed in Figure 10. From the normalized CO_2 adsorption capacities, it is shown that at 298 K, HKUST−1 particles in both composites had nearly equal adsorption capacities. In addition, the embedded particles exhibited higher CO_2 adsorption capacities than the pristine HKUST−1 but slightly lower capacities (by around 10%) than the methanol-washed HKUST−1 powder. This could be attributed to partial pore blockage by the thermoplastic binder.

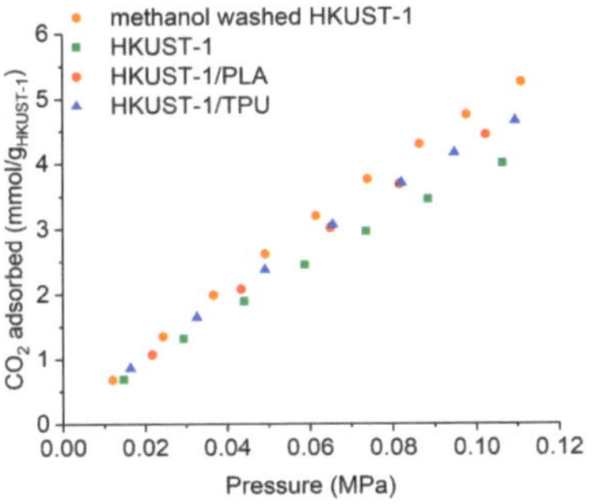

Figure 10. Normalized CO_2 adsorption isotherms compared for pristine HKUST−1, methanol-washed HKUST−1, HKUST−1/PLA and HKUST−1/TPU.

2.4. *Effect of Temperature on Adsorption Isotherms*

Figure 11 shows the CO_2 and CH_4 adsorption isotherms of all the materials measured at 273 K, 298 K, and 303 K. Unsurprisingly, it can be observed that an increase in temperature resulted in a decrease in both CO_2 and CH_4 adsorption capacities. Furthermore, both composites had comparable CO_2 and CH_4 adsorption capacities at any given temperature.

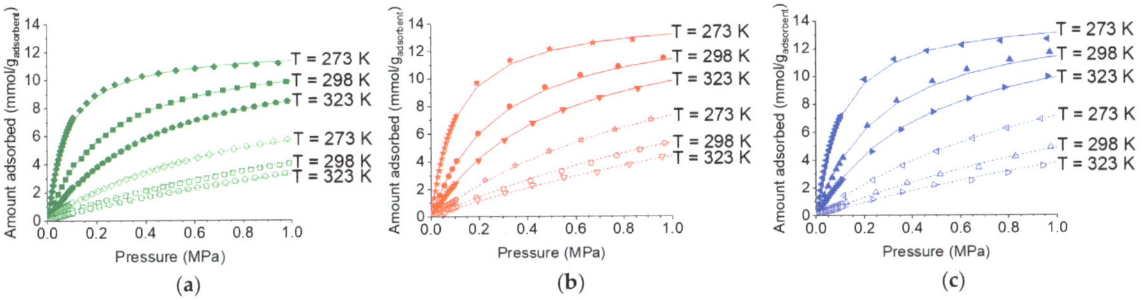

Figure 11. Gravimetric adsorption isotherms of CH_4 and CO_2 at different temperatures for (**a**) pristine HKUST−1, (**b**) HKUST−1/PLA, and (**c**) HKUST−1/TPU. Continuous line represents dual-site Langmuir modeling, whereas filled and unfilled symbols represent CO_2 and CH_4 adsorption, respectively. Isotherm data for pristine HKUST−1 and HKUST−1/PLA were taken from previous work [46].

2.5. *Temperature Dependent Isotherm Modeling and Isosteric Heat of Adsorption*

The determination of the isosteric heat of adsorption Q_{ST} requires a linear regression of the equilibrium data. Thus, to ensure the accuracy of the calculation, an appropriate thermodynamic model was chosen, ensuring good fitting with the experimental isotherm data in the whole temperature range. The dual-site Langmuir model was applied in this study to describe the pure component isotherm data of all the materials, taking into account the influence of temperature, according to the following equations:

$$q_{eq,i} = q_{s1,i} \cdot \frac{K_{1,i} \cdot P_i}{1+(K_{1,i} \cdot P_i)} + q_{s2,i} \cdot \frac{K_{2,i} \cdot P_i}{1+(K_{2,i} \cdot P_i)}$$
$$K_{1,i} = k_{a1,i} e^{k_{a2,i} \cdot \left(\frac{1}{T} - \frac{1}{T_{ref}}\right)} \quad (1)$$
$$K_{2,i} = k_{b1,i} e^{k_{b2,i} \cdot \left(\frac{1}{T} - \frac{1}{T_{ref}}\right)}$$

$q_{s1,i}$ and $q_{s2,i}$ were the saturation capacities of component i in the gas mixture on site 1 and site 2, respectively; $K_{1,I}$ and $K_{2,i}$ were the equilibrium constants of component i in the gas mixture on site 1 and site 2; $k_{a1,i}$ and $k_{b1,i}$ were the pre-exponential constants for the temperature dependence of $K_{1,i}$ and $K_{2,i}$, respectively; $k_{a2,i}$ and $k_{b2,i}$ were the exponential terms for the temperature dependence of $K_{1,i}$ and $K_{2,i}$, respectively; P_i was the pressure of gas component i in equilibrium with the adsorbed phase; $q_{eq,i}$ was the amount adsorbed of component i at equilibrium; T_{ref} was the reference temperature. The goodness of fitting was quantified considering the determination coefficient values R^2, as presented in Table S1 (Supporting Information).

The application of the dual-site Langmuir model to describe the experimental CO_2 adsorption isotherms up to 10 bars reveals that the monolayer saturation capacity of adsorption site 1, q_{s1}, was higher than the monolayer saturation capacity of adsorption site 2, q_{s2}, for all the samples. It is likely that q_{s1} corresponds to the saturation of the polarized adsorption sites located near the open-metal sites of HKUST−1, whereas qs_2 describes the monolayer saturation capacity over sites near the ligand, as proposed in [13,67]. In the case of CH_4, the values of q_{s1} derived from the dual-site Langmuir model were found superior to q_{s2} for all the samples. However, according to the literature [13,68], the preferential adsorption sites of CH_4 on HKUST−1 were located in the octahedral cages of the ligand, whereas adsorption close to the metal sites was less favored due to their lesser accessibility. Therefore, q_{s1} most likely represents the monolayer CH_4 saturation capacity near the ligand, whereas q_{s2} describes the adsorption capacity of CH_4 for the sites near the open-metal sites of the HKUST−1 crystalline structure.

Once the fitting of the isotherm data with the dual-site Langmuir model was established, the value of Q_{ST} could be determined from the linear regression of the equilibrium data. Figure 12 presents the CO_2/CH_4 isosteric heats of adsorption calculated from the Clausius–Clapeyron equation at different loadings of the adsorbed gas for pristine HKUST−1, HKUST−1/TPU, and HKUST−1/PLA. It could be observed that the CO_2 and CH_4 heats of adsorption were constant for all the samples as the loading of the adsorbed gas increased. Both HKUST/TPU and HKUST−1/PLA possessed lower CO_2 adsorption heat than pristine HKUST−1. It could be proposed that the presence of TPU in the composite lessened the interaction intensity between the CO_2 molecules and adsorption sites on HKUST−1. Interestingly, the HKUST−1/PLA composite exhibited a slightly lower CH_4 adsorption heat compared to pristine HKUST−1, whereas HKUST−1/TPU and pristine HKUST−1 showed similar CH_4 adsorption heats. This would mean that the presence of TPU in the adsorbent composite did not influence the interactions between CH_4 and adsorption sites of HKUST−1, contrary to CO_2.

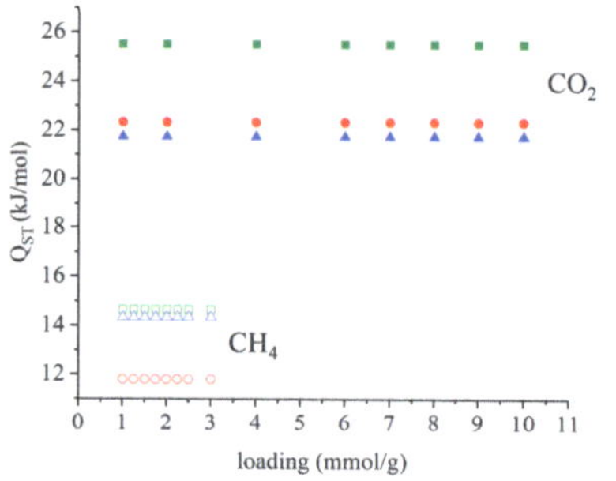

Figure 12. CO_2/CH_4 isosteric heats of adsorption for HKUST−1/TPU (blue triangle), HKUST−1/PLA (red circle) and pristine HKUST−1 (green square). Data for pristine HKUST−1 and HKUST−1/PLA were taken from previous work [46].

2.6. Prediction of CO_2/CH_4 Co-Adsorption Isotherm and IAST Selectivites

By using the dual-site Langmuir isotherm model for the fitting of CO_2 and CH_4 equilibrium data, the co-adsorption isotherms of an equimolar mixture of CO_2/CH_4, representative as an average to the composition of an inlet biogas stream [4], were predicted using IAST for all the materials. Figure 13 describes the predicted co-adsorption isotherms of HKUST−1/TPU, HKUST−1/PLA, and pristine HKUST−1 at 298 K, up to 10 bars. Both HKUST−1/TPU and HKUST−1/PLA composites were predicted to have larger CO_2 and CH_4 co-adsorption capacities compared with pristine HKUST−1. Furthermore, for all the materials, CO_2 was more preferably adsorbed than CH_4 in these conditions.

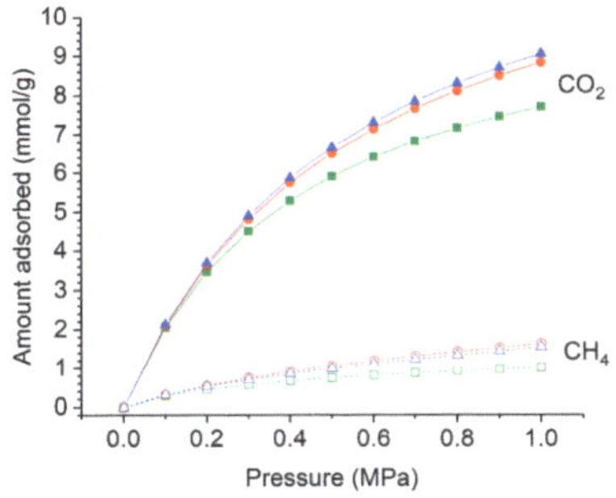

Figure 13. IAST-predicted co-adsorption isotherms for equimolar CO_2/CH_4 mixtures on HKUST−1 (green square), HKUST−1/PLA (red circle) and HKUST−1/TPU (blue triangle) at 298 K as a function of total bulk pressure. Data for pristine HKUST−1 and HKUST−1/PLA were taken from previous study [46].

The adsorbent working capacity is one of the key characteristics in designing a PSA process. The working capacity is defined as the difference between the adsorbed quantities determined under equilibrium at the operating adsorption and purging pressures, respectively. Assuming a PSA process of biogas upgrading, where the adsorption pressure and purging pressure are 10 bars and 1 bar, respectively, the predicted CO_2 and CH_4 working capacities between HKUST−1/TPU and HKUST−1/TPU are very similar to each other. This suggests that the usage of either one or the other composite will result in similar gas-separation performances.

All the samples exhibited a better affinity towards CO_2 than CH_4. For all the materials, the ratio of equilibrium capacities of pure components was around 2. The prediction of co-adsorption isotherms via IAST allowed for the determination of the equilibrium selectivities of an equimolar binary mixture. Figure 14 presents the CO_2/CH_4 co-adsorption selectivities as a function of the equilibrium pressure at 298 K for HKUST−1/TPU, HKUST−1/PLA, and the pristine HKUST−1, respectively. It could be observed that CO_2 was more preferentially adsorbed than CH_4 for all the materials. Additionally, pristine HKUST−1 had the highest selectivity value in the whole equilibrium pressure range, followed by HKUST−1/TPU and HKUST−1/PLA. Furthermore, as the equilibrium pressure was greater than 3 bars, the selectivities of HKUST−1/TPU and HKUST−1/PLA were noticeably diminished, even if the variations remained small, whereas the selectivity of the pristine HKUST−1 did not vary significantly. This could be explained by the larger CH_4 adsorption capacities of the composites, which lowered the separation selectivity despite their larger CO_2 adsorption capacities. When comparing both the composites, HKUST−1/TPU was shown to be slightly more selective towards CO_2 than HKUST−1/PLA, as the former had a slightly lower CH_4 adsorption capacity than the latter.

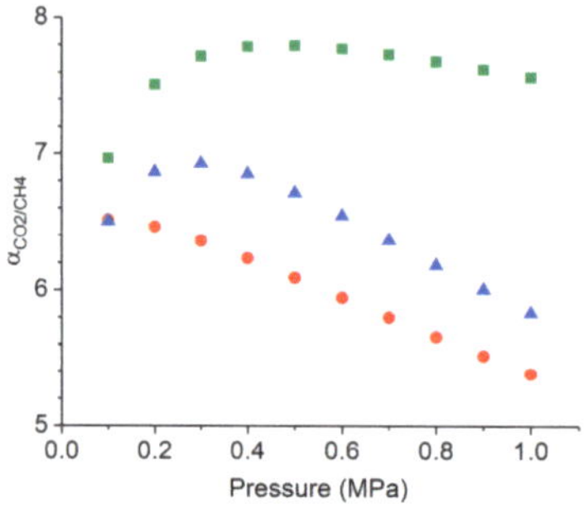

Figure 14. IAST-predicted selectivities for equimolar CO_2/CH_4 mixtures on pristine HKUST−1 (green square), HKUST−1/PLA (red circle) and HKUST−1/TPU (blue triangle) at 298 K as a function of total bulk pressure. Data for pristine HKUST−1 and HKUST−1/PLA were taken from previous study [46].

2.7. Aging along Exposure in Humid Conditions

A water contact angle analysis was conducted on both polymers (Figure S1) to determine their surface wettability and, thus, the hydrophobicity of the material. The average water contact angles for TPU and PLA are presented in Table 3. Based on the water contact angle value of each polymer, it can be concluded that TPU was more hydrophobic than PLA. Therefore, the presence of TPU as a binding agent instead of PLA could contribute to the improvement of the moisture stability of the HKUST−1 composite, which would corroborate the findings of other studies [69–71].

Table 3. Average value of water contact angle onto the surface of TPU and PLA.

Polymer	Average Contact Angle (°)
PLA	66.9
TPU	90.3

HKUST−1 is known as a MOF that is sensitive to water as the open-metal sites of HKUST−1 have a high affinity with water molecules, which results in the formation of Cu-O bonds and thus leads to the disintegration of the HKUST−1 framework [72,73]. Figure 15 displays the H_2O adsorption isotherm for HKUST−1/TPU, HKUST−1/PLA, and pristine HKUST−1 at 298 K. As expected, the pristine HKUST−1 was able to adsorb a larger quantity of water than the extruded composites when the relative humidity (RH) increased. Furthermore, the accessible pores of the pristine HKUST−1 sample started to be completely filled with water at $P/P_0 \approx 0.17$. Meanwhile, the presence of either TPU or PLA in the composite had an effect on lowering the quantity of the adsorbed water molecules as the relative pressure increased. It is possible that the polymeric binder partially hindered the access of the water molecules to certain open-metal sites in HKUST−1. Interestingly, it can be noticed that the accessible pores in HKUST−1/PLA started to be filled with water at a similar relative pressure as pristine HKUST−1, while this was not true in HKUST−1/TPU as the accessible pores only started to be filled at $P/P_0 \approx 0.27$, which could be a result of the hydrophobic nature of TPU reducing the interaction intensity of the MOF open-metal sites with the water.

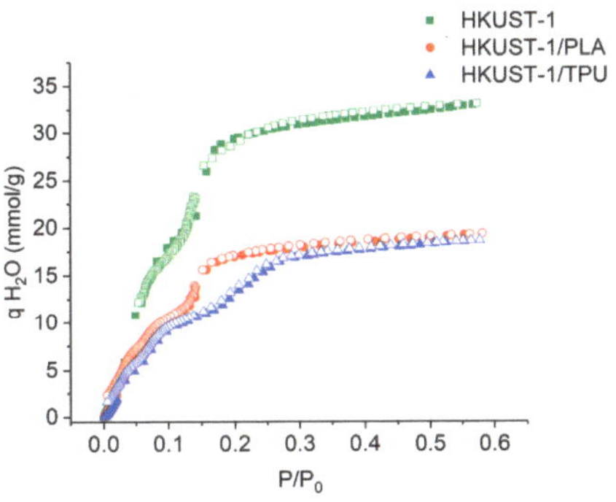

Figure 15. H_2O adsorption isotherm plot for HKUST−1/TPU, HKUST−1/PLA and pristine HKUST−1 at 298 K.

The composite and pristine samples were stored inside a humid environment (RH = 40 ± 5%) for a duration of 3 months, and the samples were re-characterized during this period to investigate the aging of the materials. The value of air RH was sufficiently high to ensure that the pores of all the samples could be filled with humid air based on the previous H_2O isotherm plot for HKUST−1 and its composites. Figure 16 presents the variation in the BET surface areas as well as those of the CO_2 adsorption capacities at one bar and 298 K for HKUST−1/TPU, HKUST−1/PLA, and the pristine HKUST−1 after 3 months of storage in a humid environment. As expected, pristine HKUST−1 showed degradation of both the BET surface and CO_2 adsorption capacities after 3 months of storage in a humid environment. Meanwhile, HKUST−1/PLA had a similar degradation pattern as the pristine HKUST−1 during the first month of storage, but the degradation seemed to stabilize after 1 month. Interestingly, HKUST−1/TPU exhibited less sensitivity to degradation under humid exposure than HKUST−1/PLA during the first month, which, moreover, seemed to be halted after 1 month of storage. We hypothesized that since TPU is more hydrophobic than PLA, it would contribute to a slower degradation of HKUST−1 in the composite. Additionally, both polymeric binders may have hindered some access to the MOF open-metal sites, which are the preferential adsorption sites for water molecules, which could also explain the stabilization of the degradation for both composites after 1 month of storage.

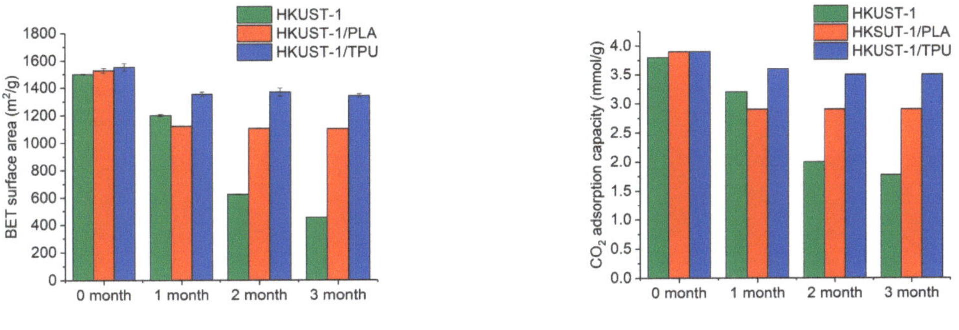

Figure 16. Variation of (**a**) BET surface area and (**b**) CO_2 adsorption capacity of pristine HKUST−1, HKUST−1/PLA and HKUST−1/TPU extrudates stored in humid conditions for 3 months.

3. Materials and Methods

3.1. Materials

HKUST−1 (also known as Cu-BTC) is a MOF also commercially known as Basolite@C300, a trademark of BASF (Beaumont, TX USA) SE. This material, denoted as the pristine HKUST−1, was supplied in powder form by Sigma Aldrich (Saint Louis, MO, USA). Its specific surface area, as specified by the supplier, is in the range of 1500–2100 m^2/g, and its bulk density is 0.35 g/cm^3. In addition, the particles of Basolite@C300 have an average size of 15.96 μm. Apart from that, another sample denoted as methanol-washed HHKUST−1 was also prepared by treating/washing the pristine HKUST−1 with methanol. TPU filament (Python Flex) was purchased from FormFutura (Amsterdam, The Netherlands). The melting temperature of the TPU is in the range of 493 K–523 K, according to the supplier.

3.2. Synthesis of HKUST−1/TPU Composite

Prior to synthesis, pristine HKUST−1 powder and TPU, as received, were degassed under a vacuum at 473 K and 383 K, respectively.

The shaping extrusion process applied to produce HKUST−1/TPU was the same as the one employed to produce the HKUST−1/PLA composite and is described in detail in [46]. Briefly, 0.1 g of TPU was dissolved inside 1 mL of solvent (DMF) using an ultrasonic bath at 328 K for the duration of 1 h. Once TPU was dissolved, 0.9 g of pristine HKUST−1 powder was gradually added to the solution, and further sonification was performed for 30 min to obtain a homogenous mixture that contained 10 wt% binder content. The HKUST−1/TPU suspension was then inserted into a 5 mL DB syringe, followed by its extrusion. Next, the extruded HKUST−1/TPU was briefly washed with methanol to promote an exchange with DMF. Methanol, in having a lower boiling point than DMF, promoted a thorough drying of the HKUST−1/TPU composite. The drying step was performed overnight at 383 K and under vacuum to remove the leftover solvent molecules (DMF or methanol). The dried HKUST−1/TPU composite was then cut using scissors into small cylinders of about 1–2 mm in length. Figure 17 illustrates the synthesis process of HKUST−1/TPU.

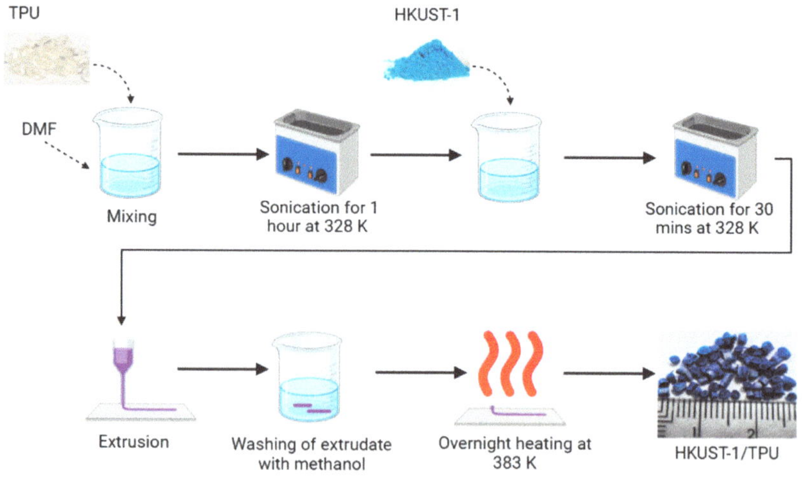

Figure 17. Schematic figure of the shaping process of HKUST−1/TPU composite shaping. Dashed line arrow signifies addition of material inside a recipient whereas continuous line arrow signifies the order of the synthesis step.

3.3. Scanning Electron Microscopy

A JEOL (Peabody, MA, USA) JSM 7600F high-resolution scanning electron microscope was used to collect images of the samples using a 15 kV electron beam, and it was equipped with both backscattered electron (BSE) and secondary electron (SE) detectors. The material samples were deposited on double-sided carbon tape and metalized with Pt. BSE imaging was used to carry out an energy-dispersive X-ray spectroscopy (EDS) element mapping of the samples.

3.4. Powder X-ray Diffraction (XRD)

A Bruker D8 Advance (Billerica, MA, USA) diffractometer equipped with a copper anode (λ = 1.5406 Å) was used to collect XRD patterns. Data were collected in the 2θ range from 5 to 50°, with a step of 0.02° and a scan speed of 1°/min.

3.5. Thermogravimetric Analysis

Thermogravimetric analysis (TGA) measurements were performed using a Setaram (Caluire, France) SETSYS Evolution thermogravimetric analyzer. A total of 5 mg of samples was heated in platinum crucibles from an ambient temperature of up to 1000 K under 20 mL/L of dry N_2 flow at a heating rate of 10 °C/min. The blank was subtracted to correct the TG signal. Prior to analysis, both HKUST−1 composite sample were kept in a desiccator for a prolonged time, more than 1 month, and heated at 383 K overnight under vacuum.

3.6. Characterization of Textural Properties

The material-specific surface area was determined using 77 K-N_2 adsorption isotherm data, assuming the BET theory. The total porous volume was determined from experimental N_2 sorption data at P/P_0 = 0.98. The micropore volume was derived by applying the t-plot model to the N_2 adsorption isotherms.

The N_2 adsorption equilibrium data were obtained using a 3 Flex manometric adsorption analyzer from Micromeritics (Norcross, GA, USA). The instrument was equipped with pressure transducers, allowing measurements in the domain of relative pressure (P/P_0) ranging between 10^{-7} and 1, with a 0.15% precision of the absolute pressure reading. The selected pressure range for the BET surface area calculation was chosen in the domain of $10^{-7} \leq P/P_0 \leq 10^{-2}$ to respect the four consistency criteria of the BET equation, as suggested by Rouquerol et al. [74]. Prior to isotherm measurement, the sample was degassed at 383 K under vacuum for at least 72 h. The void volume of the cell containing the sample was evaluated from helium expansion measured at an ambient temperature and at 77 K.

3.7. Attrition Test

The mechanical stability of the samples was characterized through the attrition test according to the standard D4058-96 ASTM norm. Briefly, 0.2 g mass of material was introduced into a glass vial and was rolled at a frequency of 60 revolutions per minute (rpm) for 30 min. Afterward, the sample was passed through a 500 μm sieve to recover fine particles. The attrition percentage was calculated as follows.

$$\text{Attrition } (\%) = \frac{\text{initial mass} - \text{recovered mass above 500 } \mu\text{m}}{\text{initial mass}} \times 100 \quad (2)$$

3.8. CO_2 and CH_4 Adsorption Isotherms

CO_2 and CH_4 adsorption isotherms were measured using two manometric pieces of equipment. The isotherm data in the pressure range from 1 to 10 bars were collected using the Pressure-Composition Thermodynamics (PCT)-Pro (manometric equipment from SETARAM, Caluire, France). In the low-pressure range, less than 1 bar, the isotherm data were obtained with the 3 Flex apparatus from Micromeritics. In both the low- and high-pressure ranges, adsorption isotherms data were collected at three temperatures: 273 K, 298 K, and 323 K. Prior to each measurement, the samples were degassed under a dynamic vacuum at 383 K for 12 h, and the sample holder dead volume was measured from helium expansion.

3.9. Isosteric Heat of Adsorption

The heat of the adsorption of the components of a gas mixture is a key thermodynamic variable for the design of practical gas-separation processes such as pressure swing and thermal swing adsorption [75,76]. Knowledge of the heat of adsorption helps to determine the extent of adsorbent temperature changes within the adsorbent bed during the adsorption and regeneration processes, which ultimately govern the gas-separation performance. Apart from that, it also allows for the quantification of the adsorbent–adsorbate interaction intensity. The isosteric heats of the adsorption were derived from the application of the Clausius–Clapeyron equation:

$$\ln\frac{P_2}{P_1} = \frac{Q_{ST}}{R} \times \left(\frac{1}{T_1} - \frac{1}{T_2}\right) \quad (3)$$

where Q_{ST} was the isosteric heat of adsorption, T was the temperature, and R was the universal gas constant with a value of 8.314 J/mol K. The values of Q_{ST} were determined for different gas loadings, regressing the isotherm data measured at three different temperatures.

3.10. Ideal Adsorption Solution Theory (IAST)

The Ideal Adsorption Solution Theory, developed by Myers and Prausnitz [77], is a thermodynamic model enabling the prediction of co-adsorption isotherms of gas mixtures. The theory assumes that the gas-adsorbed phase system is analogous to a vapor-liquid equilibrium state following Raoult's law [78]. It relies on three major assumptions: (i) the change in the thermodynamic properties of the adsorbent when gas molecules adsorb is negligible compared to the change in those for the adsorbate; (ii) each adsorbed species has access to the same area of the adsorbent surface; (iii) the Gibbs definition applies to the adsorbed phase [77]. IAST provides a solid theoretical foundation for predicting multi-component adsorption isotherms from single-component adsorption isotherms. IAST has been found to reliably predict the co-adsorption isotherms and selectivities of CO_2/CH_4 mixtures in MOF adsorbents [20,79].

The computational process of the IAST model is described in detail elsewhere [77,80,81]. In this work, IAST isotherm calculation was performed with the aid of the IAST++ program to assess the separation performance of binary equimolar CO_2/CH_4 mixtures at 298 K [81]. Based on the prediction of the IAST co-adsorption isotherms, the equilibrium selectivity of the adsorbent samples $\alpha_{i/j}$ could be determined in the whole range of tested pressure and temperature:

$$\alpha_{i/j} = \frac{x_{i,}/y_i}{x_{j,}/y_j} \quad (4)$$

where x_i and x_j were the molar fraction of components i and j in the adsorbed phase; and y_i and y_j were the molar fractions of components i and j in the gas phase.

3.11. Water Contact Angle

The water contact angle over the polymer binding agents was measured using the sessile droplet method. Prior to analysis, a flat film of the TPU or PLA sample was prepared using the solvent casting technique. Briefly, 1 g of TPU or PLA was dissolved in DMF or chloroform, respectively. The dissolved polymer was then cast into a glass Petri dish and heated at 383 K overnight to remove the solvent and obtain thermoplastic film samples. Once a flat film sample of thermoplastic was obtained, a distilled water droplet was deposited from a syringe on the surface of the sample. An image of the water droplet was immediately taken by a high-speed digital microscope camera (Amscope (Irvine, CA, USA) MU1000), and the contact angle, θ, between the droplet and the surface of the samples was determined using the ImageJ software (version 1.53t) [82]. The water contact angle can be used as an indicator of surface wettability: when $\theta < 90°$, the sample is considered hydrophilic; when $90° < \theta < 120°$, the sample is hydrophobic; and when $\theta > 120°$, the sample is super-hydrophobic. Each test was repeated five times, and the reported results were the average of these five measurements.

3.12. Water Adsorption Isotherms and Material Aging under Humid Atmosphere

The measurement of H_2O adsorption isotherms was performed using the manometric equipment, a 3 Flex apparatus from Micromeritics. Water adsorption isotherm data were collected at 298 K from 0 to 2.1 kPa. Prior to each measurement, the material samples were degassed under a dynamic vacuum at 393 K for 12 h, and the sample holder dead volume was measured from helium expansion.

Material aging and stability to moisture were assessed during storage under atmospheric humid conditions by leaving the adsorbent samples inside a room at a controlled temperature of 25 ± 5 °C and at a relative humidity (RH) of 40 ± 5% for a duration of 3 months. The properties of the stored samples were then re-characterized via measurements of the N_2 adsorption isotherms at 77 K and CO_2 adsorption isotherms up to 1 bar at 298 K.

4. Conclusions

In this work, hydrophobic TPU was used as a binding agent for the shaping of HKUST−1 powder using an extrusion process. The resulting composite was characterized, and its properties were compared with those of synthesized HKUST−1/PLA, obtained after the same shaping process using PLA as a more hydrophilic polymeric binder. The characterization confirms the successful shaping of HKUST−1 powder using TPU as a binder. The HKUST−1/TPU composite exhibited comparable textural properties, thermal stability, and mechanical stability to the HKUST−1/PLA composite. HKUST−1/TPU demonstrated comparable equilibrium adsorption capacities and IAST selectivities as HKUST−1/PLA for CO_2/CH_4 separation. The adsorption capacities of both composites were shown to be larger than the HKUST−1 pristine powder. Such an improvement was attributed to the methanol washing effect applied during the composite preparation before their drying. Methanol-washed HKUST−1 powder was characterized by the largest adsorption capacities when compared with pristine powder and both the PLA and TPU composites. Additionally, HKUST−1/TPU had a higher heat of adsorption for CO_2 than for CH_4, and these data are not dependent on the amount of gas adsorbed. Finally, as TPU was more hydrophobic than PLA, the use of that polymer as a binding agent contributed to a decrease in the degradation rate of the adsorbent after storage in a humid environment for several months. On the whole, this study demonstrates the feasibility of using TPU as a polymeric binder for the shaping of commercial HKUST−1 powder. The extrusion process results in the production of an adsorbent well-suited to be used in an industrial gas-separation process thanks to its good adsorption performance, mechanical and thermal properties, and stability after a long period of storage in a humid atmosphere.

Supplementary Materials: The following supporting information can be downloaded at https://www.mdpi.com/article/10.3390/molecules29092069/s1, Figure S1: Image of water drop onto the surface of PLA and TPU; Figure S2: N_2 adsorption isotherm plot for TPU and PLA; Figure S3: N_2 adsorption isotherms on HKUST−1 and solvent-washed HKUST−1; Figure S4: Normalize CO_2 adsorption isotherm plot for pristine HKUST−1, methanol-washed HKUST−1 and HKUST−1/PLA composites with different binder fraction; Table S1: Fitting Parameters of the dual-site Langmuir Isotherm Model for the CO_2 and CH_4 pure isotherms on HKUST−1, HKUST−1/PLA and HKUST−1/TPU; Table S2: BET Surface area, pore volume of HKUST−1 and the respective solvent-washed HKUST−1.

Author Contributions: Conceptualization, D.I.G., P.P. and M.A.B.; data curation, M.T.R.; formal analysis, M.T.R.; funding acquisition, M.A.B. and P.P.; investigation, M.T.R., D.I.G., P.P. and M.A.B.; methodology, M.T.R., D.I.G., P.P. and M.A.B.; project administration, D.I.G., P.P. and M.A.B.; resources, M.A.B. and P.P.; software, D.I.G. and P.P.; supervision, D.I.G., P.P. and M.A.B.; writing—original draft, M.T.R.; writing—review and editing, D.I.G. and P.P. All authors have read and agreed to the published version of the manuscript.

Funding: This research was funded by Yayasan Universiti Teknologi PETRONAS (YUTP)-PRG 2022 grant number 015PBC-014, Yayasan Universiti Teknologi PETRONAS (YUTP)-FRG 2021 grant number 015LC0-364 and IMT Atlantique, providing half a PhD scholarship.

Institutional Review Board Statement: Not applicable.

Informed Consent Statement: Not applicable.

Data Availability Statement: The original contributions presented in the study are included in the article/Supplementary Material; further inquiries can be directed to the corresponding author/s.

Acknowledgments: The authors thank the Centre of Research in Ionic Liquids, CORIL, Department of Chemical Engineering, Universiti Teknologi PETRONAS, and the Department of Energy Systems and Environment (GEPEA laboratory), IMT Atlantique, for their support in this collaborative work.

Conflicts of Interest: The authors declare no conflicts of interest.

References

1. Pavičić, J.; Mavar, K.N.; Brkić, V.; Simon, K. Biogas and Biomethane Production and Usage: Technology Development, Advantages and Challenges in Europe. *Energies* **2022**, *15*, 2940. [CrossRef]
2. IEA. Outlook for Biogas and Biomethane: Prospects for Organic Growth. 2020. Available online: https://www.iea.org/reports/outlook-for-biogas-and-biomethane-prospects-for-organic-growth (accessed on 3 January 2024).
3. Khan, I.U.; Othman, M.H.D.; Hashim, H.; Matsuura, T.; Ismail, A.F.; Rezaei-DashtArzhandi, M.; Azelee, I.W. Biogas as a renewable energy fuel—A review of biogas upgrading, utilisation and storage. *Energy Convers. Manag.* **2017**, *150*, 277–294. [CrossRef]
4. Bharathiraja, B.; Sudharsana, T.; Jayamuthunagai, J.; Praveenkumar, R.; Chozhavendhan, S.; Iyyappan, J. Biogas production—A review on composition, fuel properties, feed stock and principles of anaerobic digestion. *Renew. Sustain. Energy Rev.* **2018**, *90*, 570–582. [CrossRef]
5. Aghel, B.; Behaein, S.; Wongwises, S.; Shadloo, M.S. A review of recent progress in biogas upgrading: With emphasis on carbon capture. *Biomass Bioenergy* **2022**, *160*, 106422. [CrossRef]
6. Ahmed, S.F.; Mofijur, M.; Tarannum, K.; Chowdhury, A.T.; Rafa, N.; Nuzhat, S.; Kumar, P.S.; Vo, D.-V.N.; Lichtfouse, E.; Mahlia, T.M.I. Biogas upgrading, economy and utilization: A review. *Environ. Chem. Lett.* **2021**, *19*, 4137–4164. [CrossRef]
7. Shah, G.; Ahmad, E.; Pant, K.; Vijay, V. Comprehending the contemporary state of art in biogas enrichment and CO_2 capture technologies via swing adsorption. *Int. J. Hydrogen Energy* **2021**, *46*, 6588–6612. [CrossRef]
8. Jiao, L.; Seow, J.Y.R.; Skinner, W.S.; Wang, Z.U.; Jiang, H.-L. Metal–organic frameworks: Structures and functional applications. *Mater. Today* **2019**, *27*, 43–68. [CrossRef]
9. Ghazvini, M.F.; Vahedi, M.; Nobar, S.N.; Sabouri, F. Investigation of the MOF adsorbents and the gas adsorptive separation mechanisms. *J. Environ. Chem. Eng.* **2021**, *9*, 104790. [CrossRef]
10. Ullah, S.; Bustam, M.A.; Assiri, M.A.; Al-Sehemi, A.G.; Gonfa, G.; Mukhtar, A.; Kareem, F.A.A.; Ayoub, M.; Saqib, S.; Mellon, N.B. Synthesis and characterization of mesoporous MOF UMCM-1 for CO_2/CH_4 adsorption; an experimental, isotherm modeling and thermodynamic study. *Microporous Mesoporous Mater.* **2020**, *294*, 109844. [CrossRef]
11. Salehi, S.; Anbia, M.; Razavi, F. Improving CO_2/CH_4 and CO_2/N_2 adsorptive selectivity of cu-BTC and MOF-derived nanoporous carbon by modification with nitrogen-containing groups. *Environ. Prog. Sustain.* **2020**, *39*, 13302. [CrossRef]
12. Li, C.-N.; Wang, S.-M.; Tao, Z.-P.; Liu, L.; Xu, W.-G.; Gu, X.-J.; Han, Z.-B. Green Synthesis of MOF-801 (Zr/Ce/Hf) for CO_2/N_2 and CO_2/CH_4 Separation. *Inorg. Chem.* **2023**, *62*, 7853–7860. [CrossRef]
13. Teo, H.W.B.; Chakraborty, A.; Kayal, S. Evaluation of CH_4 and CO_2 adsorption on HKUST−1 and MIL-101 (Cr) MOFs employing Monte Carlo simulation and comparison with experimental data. *Appl. Therm. Eng.* **2017**, *110*, 891–900. [CrossRef]
14. Asadi, T.; Ehsani, M.R.; Ribeiro, A.M.; Loureiro, J.M.; Rodrigues, A.E. CO_2/CH_4 Separation by Adsorption using Nanoporous Metal organic Framework Copper-Benzene-1, 3, 5-tricarboxylate Tablet. *Chem. Eng. Technol.* **2017**, *36*, 1231–1239. [CrossRef]
15. Chong, K.C.; Lai, S.O.; Mah, S.K.; Thiam, H.S.; Chong, W.C.; Shuit, S.H.; Lee, S.S.; Chong, W.E. A Review of HKUST−1 Metal-Organic Frameworks in Gas Adsorption. *Conf. Ser. Earth Environ. Sci.* **2023**, *1135*, 012030. [CrossRef]
16. Yu, D.; Yazaydin, A.O.; Lane, J.R.; Dietzel, P.D.C.; Snurr, R.Q. A combined experimental and quantum chemical study of CO_2 adsorption in the metal–organic framework CPO-27 with different metals. *Chem. Sci.* **2013**, *4*, 3544–3556. [CrossRef]
17. Millward, A.R.; Yaghi, O.M. Metal−organic frameworks with exceptionally high capacity for storage of carbon dioxide at room temperature. *J. Am. Chem. Soc.* **2005**, *127*, 17998–17999. [CrossRef]
18. Wu, H.; Zhou, W.; Yildirim, T. High-capacity methane storage in metal−organic frameworks M2 (dhtp): The important role of open metal sites. *J. Am. Chem. Soc.* **2009**, *131*, 4995–5000. [CrossRef] [PubMed]
19. Ye, S.; Jiang, X.; Ruan, L.-W.; Liu, B.; Wang, Y.-M.; Zhu, J.-F.; Qiu, L.-G. Post-combustion CO_2 capture with the HKUST−1 and MIL-101 (Cr) metal–organic frameworks: Adsorption, separation and regeneration investigations. *Microporous Mesoporous Mater.* **2013**, *179*, 191–197. [CrossRef]

20. Hamon, L.; Jolimaître, E.; Pirngruber, G.D. CO_2 and CH_4 separation by adsorption using Cu-BTC metal−organic framework. *Ind. Eng. Chem. Res* **2010**, *49*, 7497–7503. [CrossRef]
21. Xian, S.; Peng, J.; Zhang, Z.; Xia, Q.; Wang, H.; Li, Z. Highly enhanced and weakened adsorption properties of two MOFs by water vapor for separation of CO_2/CH_4 and CO_2/N_2 binary mixtures. *Chem. Eng. J.* **2015**, *270*, 385–392. [CrossRef]
22. Chanut, N.; Wiersum, A.D.; Lee, U.-H.; Hwang, Y.K.; Ragon, F.; Chevreau, H.; Bourrelly, S.; Kuchta, B.; Chang, J.-S.; Serre, C.; et al. Observing the effects of shaping on gas adsorption in metal-organic frameworks. *Eur. J. Inorg. Chem.* **2016**, *27*, 4416–4423. [CrossRef]
23. Bourrelly, S.; Llewellyn, P.L.; Serre, C.; Millange, F.; Loiseau, T.; Férey, G. Different adsorption behaviors of methane and carbon dioxide in the isotypic nanoporous metal terephthalates MIL-53 and MIL-47. *J. Am. Chem. Soc* **2005**, *127*, 13519–13521. [CrossRef] [PubMed]
24. Kayal, S.; Chakraborty, A. Activated carbon (type Maxsorb-III) and MIL-101 (Cr) metal organic framework based composite adsorbent for higher CH_4 storage and CO_2 capture. *Chem. Eng. J.* **2018**, *334*, 780–788. [CrossRef]
25. Yuan, D.; Zhao, D.; Sun, D.; Zhou, H.-C. An isoreticular series of metal–organic frameworks with dendritic hexacarboxylate ligands and exceptionally high gas-uptake capacity. *Angew. Chem.* **2010**, *122*, 5485–5489. [CrossRef]
26. Lv, D.; Shi, R.; Chen, Y.; Chen, Y.; Wu, H.; Zhou, X.; Xi, H.; Li, Z.; Xia, Q. Selective adsorptive separation of CO_2/CH_4 and CO_2/N_2 by a water resistant zirconium–porphyrin metal–organic framework. *Ind. Eng. Chem. Res.* **2018**, *57*, 12215–12224. [CrossRef]
27. Awadallah-F, A.; Hillman, F.; Al-Muhtaseb, S.A.; Jeong, H.K. Adsorption equilibrium and kinetics of nitrogen, methane and carbon dioxide gases onto ZIF-8, Cu10%/ZIF-8, and Cu30%/ZIF-8. Ind. *Eng. Chem. Res.* **2019**, *58*, 6653–6661. [CrossRef]
28. Rocha, L.A.; Andreassen, K.A.; Grande, C.A. Separation of CO_2/CH_4 using carbon molecular sieve (CMS) at low and high pressure. *Chem. Eng. Sci.* **2017**, *164*, 148–157. [CrossRef]
29. Cavenati, S.; Grande, C.A.; Rodrigues, A.E. Adsorption equilibrium of methane, carbon dioxide, and nitrogen on zeolite 13X at high pressures. *J. Chem. Eng. Data* **2004**, *49*, 1095–1101. [CrossRef]
30. Ren, J.; Dyosiba, X.; Musyoka, N.M.; Langmi, H.W.; Mathe, M.; Liao, S. Review on the current practices and efforts towards pilot-scale production of metal-organic frameworks (MOFs). *Coord. Chem. Rev.* **2017**, *352*, 187–219. [CrossRef]
31. Golmakani, A.; Nabavi, S.A.; Wadi, B.; Manovic, V. Advances, challenges, and perspectives of biogas cleaning, upgrading, and utilisation. *Fuel* **2022**, *317*, 123085. [CrossRef]
32. Álvarez, J.R.; Sánchez-González, E.; Pérez, E.; Schneider-Revueltas, E.; Martínez, A.; Tejeda-Cruz, A.; Islas-Jácome, A.; González-Zamora, E.; Ibarra, I.A. Structure stability of HKUST−1 towards water and ethanol and their effect on its CO_2 capture properties. *Dalton Trans.* **2017**, *46*, 9192–9200. [CrossRef]
33. Al-Janabi, N.; Hill, P.; Torrente-Murciano, L.; Garforth, A.; Gorgojo, P.; Siperstein, F.; Fan, X. Mapping the Cu-BTC metal–organic framework (HKUST−1) stability envelope in the presence of water vapour for CO_2 adsorption from flue gases. *Chem. Eng. J.* **2015**, *281*, 669–677. [CrossRef]
34. Ediati, R.; Dewi, S.K.; Hasan, M.R.; Kahardina, M.; Murwani, I.K.; Nadjib, M. Mesoporous HKUST−1 synthesized using solvothermal method. *Rasayan J. Chem.* **2019**, *12*, 1653–1659. [CrossRef]
35. Morales, E.M.C.; Méndez-Rojas, M.A.; Torres-Martínez, L.M.; Garay-Rodríguez, L.F.; López, I.; Uflyand, I.E.; Kharisov, B.I. Ultrafast synthesis of HKUST−1 nanoparticles by solvothermal method: Properties and possible applications. *Polyhedron* **2021**, *210*, 115517. [CrossRef]
36. Nobar, S.N. Cu-BTC synthesis, characterization and preparation for adsorption studies. *Mater. Chem. Phys.* **2018**, *213*, 343–351. [CrossRef]
37. Guo, L.; Du, J.; Li, C.; He, G.; Xiao, Y. Facile synthesis of hierarchical micro-mesoporous HKUST−1 by a mixed-linker defect strategy for enhanced adsorptive removal of benzothiophene from fuel. *Fuel* **2021**, *300*, 120955. [CrossRef]
38. Armstrong, M.; Sirous, P.; Shan, B.; Wang, R.; Zhong, C.; Liu, J.; Mu, B. Prolonged HKUST−1 functionality under extreme hydrothermal conditions by electrospinning polystyrene fibers as a new coating method. *Microporous Mesoporous Mater.* **2018**, *270*, 34–39. [CrossRef]
39. Vehrenberg, J.; Vepsäläinen, M.; Macedo, D.S.; Rubio-Martinez, M.; Webster, N.A.S.; Wessling, M. Steady-state electrochemical synthesis of HKUST−1 with polarity reversal. *Microporous Mesoporous Mater.* **2020**, *303*, 110218. [CrossRef]
40. Vepsäläinen, M.; Macedo, D.S.; Gong, H.; Rubio-Martinez, M.; Bayatsarmadi, B.; He, B. Electrosynthesis of HKUST−1 with flow-reactor post-processing. *Appl. Sci.* **2021**, *11*, 3340. [CrossRef]
41. Liu, P.; Zhao, T.; Cai, K.; Chen, P.; Liu, F.; Tao, D.-J. Rapid mechanochemical construction of HKUST−1 with enhancing water stability by hybrid ligands assembly strategy for efficient adsorption of SF6. *Chem. Eng. J.* **2022**, *437*, 135364. [CrossRef]
42. Stolar, T.; Batzdorf, L.; Lukin, S.; Žilić, D.; Motillo, C.; Friščić, T.; Emmerling, F.; Halasz, I.; Užarević, K. In situ monitoring of the mechanosynthesis of the archetypal metal–organic framework HKUST−1: Effect of liquid additives on the milling reactivity. *Inorg. Chem.* **2017**, *56*, 6599–6608. [CrossRef]
43. Ntouros, V.; Kousis, I.; Pisello, A.L.; Assimakopoulos, M.N. Binding Materials for MOF Monolith Shaping Processes: A Review towards Real Life Application. *Energies* **2022**, *15*, 1489. [CrossRef]
44. Cousin-Saint-Remi, J.; Finoulst, A.-L.; Jabbour, C.; Baron, G.V.; Denayer, J.F.M. Selection of binder recipes for the formulation of MOFs into resistant pellets for molecular separations by fixed-bed adsorption. *Microporous Mesoporous Mater.* **2020**, *304*, 109322. [CrossRef]

45. Hastürk, E.; Höfert, S.-P.; Topalli, B.; Schlüsener, C.; Janiak, C. Shaping of MOFs via freeze-casting method with hydrophilic polymers and their effect on textural properties. *Microporous Mesoporous Mater.* **2020**, *295*, 109907. [CrossRef]
46. Rozaini, M.T.; Grekov, D.I.; Bustam, M.A.; Pré, P. Shaping of HKUST−1 via Extrusion for the Separation of CO_2/CH_4 in Biogas. *Separations* **2023**, *10*, 487. [CrossRef]
47. Yu, W.; Sun, L.; Li, M.; Li, M.; Lei, W.; Wei, C. FDM 3D printing and properties of PBS/PLA blends. *Polymers* **2023**, *15*, 4305. [CrossRef] [PubMed]
48. Rajakaruna, R.A.; Subeshan, B.; Asmatulu, E. Fabrication of hydrophobic PLA filaments for additive manufacturing. *J. Mater. Sci.* **2022**, *57*, 8987–9001. [CrossRef] [PubMed]
49. Nofar, M.; Mohammadi, M.; Carreau, P.J. Effect of TPU hard segment content on the rheological and mechanical properties of PLA/TPU blends. *J. Appl. Polym. Sci* **2020**, *137*, 49387. [CrossRef]
50. Lis-Bartos, A.; Smieszek, A.; Frańczyk, K.; Marycz, K. Fabrication, characterization, and cytotoxicity of thermoplastic polyurethane/poly (lactic acid) material using human adipose derived mesenchymal stromal stem cells (hASCs). *Polymers* **2018**, *10*, 1073. [CrossRef] [PubMed]
51. Oliaei, E.; Kaffashi, B.; Davoodi, S. Investigation of structure and mechanical properties of toughened poly (l-lactide)/thermoplastic poly (ester urethane) blends. *J. Appl. Polym. Sci.* **2016**, 133. [CrossRef]
52. Muñoz-Chilito, J.; Lara-Ramos, J.A.; Marín, L.; Machuca-Martínez, F.; Correa-Aguirre, J.P.; Hidalgo-Salazar, M.A.; García-Navarro, S.; Roca-Blay, L.; Rodríguez, L.A.; Mosquera-Vargas, E.; et al. Morphological Electrical and Hardness Characterization of Carbon Nanotube-Reinforced Thermoplastic Polyurethane (TPU) Nanocomposite Plates. *Molecules* **2023**, *28*, 3598. [CrossRef] [PubMed]
53. Kumar, S.; Gupta, T.K.; Varadarajan, K.M. Strong, stretchable and ultrasensitive MWCNT/TPU nanocomposites for piezoresistive strain sensing. *Compos. Part B* **2019**, *117*, 107285. [CrossRef]
54. Dai, X.; Cao, Y.; Shi, X.; Wang, X. Non-isothermal crystallization kinetics, thermal degradation behavior and mechanical properties of poly (lactic acid)/MOF composites prepared by melt-blending methods. *RSC Adv.* **2016**, *6*, 71461–71471. [CrossRef]
55. Gregor-Svetec, D.; Leskovšek, M.; Leskovar, B.; Elesini, U.S.; Vrabič-Brodnjak, U. Analysis of PLA composite filaments reinforced with lignin and polymerised-lignin-treated NFC. *Polymers* **2021**, *13*, 2174. [CrossRef]
56. Yang, T.; Hu, J.; Wang, P.; Edeleva, M.; Cardon, L.; Zhang, J. Two-step approach based on fused filament fabrication for high performance graphene/thermoplastic polyurethane composite with segregated structure. *Compos. Part A Appl. Sci. Manuf.* **2023**, *174*, 107719. [CrossRef]
57. Bhoria, N.; Basina, G.; Pokhrel, J.; Reddy, K.S.K.; Anastasiou, S.; Balasubramanian, V.V.; AlWahedi, Y.F.; Karanikolos, G.N. Functionalization effects on HKUST−1 and HKUST−1/graphene oxide hybrid adsorbents for hydrogen sulfide removal. *J. Hazard. Mater.* **2020**, *394*, 122565. [CrossRef] [PubMed]
58. Cortés-Súarez, J.; Celis-Arias, V.; Beltra, H.I.; Tejeda-Cruz, A.; Ibarra, I.A.; Romero-Ibarra, E.; Sánchez-González, E.; Loera-Serna, S. Synthesis and characterization of an SWCNT@ HKUST−1 composite: Enhancing the CO_2 adsorption properties of HKUST−1. *ACS Omega* **2019**, *4*, 5275–5282. [CrossRef] [PubMed]
59. Cychosz, K.A.; Guillet-Nicolas, R.; García-Martínez, J.; Thommes, M. Recent advances in the textural characterization of hierarchically structured nanoporous materials. *Chem. Soc. Rev.* **2017**, *46*, 389–414. [CrossRef]
60. Kanbur, Y.; Tayfun, U. Investigating mechanical, thermal, and flammability properties of thermoplastic polyurethane/carbon nanotube composites. *J. Thermoplast. Compos. Mater.* **2018**, *31*, 1661–1675. [CrossRef]
61. Wu, W.; Huang, W.; Tong, Y.; Huang, J.; Wu, J.; Cao, X.; Zhang, Q.; Yu, B.; Li, R.K.Y. Self-assembled double core-shell structured zeolitic imidazole framework-8 as an effective flame retardant and smoke suppression agent for thermoplastic polyurethane. *Appl. Surf. Sci.* **2023**, *610*, 155540. [CrossRef]
62. Evans, K.A.; Kennedy, Z.C.; Arey, B.W.; Christ, J.F.; Schaef, H.T.; Nune, S.K.; Erikson, R.L. Chemically active, porous 3D-printed thermoplastic composites. *ACS Appl. Mater. Interfaces* **2018**, *10*, 15112–15121. [CrossRef] [PubMed]
63. Zhang, J.; Li, Z.; Qi, X.; Zhang, W.; Wang, D.-Y. Size tailored bimetallic metal-organic framework (MOF) on graphene oxide with sandwich-like structure as functional nano-hybrids for improving fire safety of epoxy. *Compos. Part B* **2020**, *188*, 107881. [CrossRef]
64. *ASTM D4058-96*; Standard Test Method for Attrition and Abrasion of Catalysts and Catalyst Carriers. ASTM International: West Conshohocken, PA, USA, 2020.
65. Shah, B.B.; Kundu, T.; Zhao, D. Mechanical properties of shaped metal-organic frameworks. *Top. Curr. Chem.* **2019**, *377*, 25. [CrossRef] [PubMed]
66. Khabzina, Y.; Dhainaut, J.; Ahlhelm, M.; Richter, H.-J.; Reinsch, H.; Stock, N.; Farrusseng, D. Synthesis and shaping scale-up study of functionalized UiO-66 MOF for ammonia air purification filters. *Ind. Eng. Chem. Res.* **2018**, *57*, 8200–8208. [CrossRef]
67. Supronowicz, B.; Mavrandonakis, A.; Heine, T. Interaction of small gases with the unsaturated metal centers of the HKUST−1 metal organic framework. *J. Phys. Chem. C* **2013**, *117*, 14570–14578. [CrossRef]
68. García-Pérez, E.; Gascón, J.; Morales-Flórez, V.; Castillo, J.M.; Kapteijn, F.; Calero, S. Identification of adsorption sites in Cu-BTC by experimentation and molecular simulation. *Langmuir* **2009**, *25*, 1725–1731. [CrossRef] [PubMed]
69. Chae, Y.S.; Park, S.; Kang, D.W.; Kim, D.W.; Kang, M.; Choi, D.S.; Choe, J.H.; Hong, C.S. Moisture-tolerant diamine-appended metal–organic framework composites for effective indoor CO_2 capture through facile spray coating. *Chem. Eng. J.* **2022**, *433*, 133856. [CrossRef]

70. DeCoste, J.B.; Denny, M.S., Jr.; Peterson, G.W.; Mahle, J.J.; Cohen, S.M. Enhanced aging properties of HKUST−1 in hydrophobic mixed-matrix membranes for ammonia adsorption. *Schem. Sci.* **2016**, *7*, 2711–2716. [CrossRef] [PubMed]
71. Park, J.; Chae, Y.S.; Kang, D.W.; Kang, M.; Choe, J.H.; Kim, S.; Kim, J.Y.; Jeong, Y.W.; Hong, C.S. Shaping of a metal–organic framework–polymer composite and its CO_2 adsorption performances from humid indoor air. *ACS Appl. Mater. Interfaces* **2021**, *13*, 25421–25427. [CrossRef] [PubMed]
72. Xue, W.; Zhang, Z.; Huang, H.; Zhong, C.; Mei, D. Theoretical insights into the initial hydrolytic breakdown of HKUST−1. *J. Phys. Chem. C* **2019**, *124*, 1991–2001. [CrossRef]
73. Todaro, M.; Alessi, A.; Sciortino, L.; Agnello, S.; Cannas, M.; Gelardi, F.M.; Buscarino, G. Investigation by Raman Spectroscopy of the Decomposition Process of HKUST−1 upon Exposure to Air. *J. Spectrosc.* **2016**, *2016*, 8074297. [CrossRef]
74. Rouquerol, J.; Rouquerol, F.; Llewellyn, P.; Maurin, G.; Sing, K. *Adsorption by Powders and Porous Solids: Principles, Methodology and Applications*; Academic Press: Cambridge, MA, USA, 2013.
75. Sircar, S.; Mohr, R.; Ristic, C.; Rao, M.B. Isosteric heat of adsorption: Theory and experiment. *J. Phys. Chem. B* **1999**, *103*, 6539–6546. [CrossRef] [PubMed]
76. Tian, Y.; Wu, J. Differential heat of adsorption and isosteres. *Langmuir* **2017**, *33*, 996–1003. [CrossRef] [PubMed]
77. Myers, A.L.; Prausnitz, J.M. Thermodynamics of mixed-gas adsorption. *AIChE J.* **1965**, *11*, 121–127. [CrossRef]
78. Walton, K.S.; Sholl, D.S. Predicting multicomponent adsorption: 50 years of the ideal adsorbed solution theory. *AIChE J.* **2015**, *61*, 2757–2762. [CrossRef]
79. Heymans, N.; SVaesen; De Weireld, G. A complete procedure for acidic gas separation by adsorption on MIL-53 (Al). *Microporous Mesoporous Mater.* **2012**, *154*, 93–99. [CrossRef]
80. Simon, C.M.; Smit, B.; Haranczyk, M. pyIAST: Ideal adsorbed solution theory (IAST) Python package. *Comput. Phys. Commun.* **2016**, *200*, 364–380. [CrossRef]
81. Lee, S.; Lee, J.H.; Kim, J. User-friendly graphical user interface software for ideal adsorbed solution theory calculations. *Korean J. Chem. Eng.* **2018**, *35*, 214–221. [CrossRef]
82. Rasband, W.S. "ImageJ". U.S. National Institutes of Health, Bethesda, Maryland. Available online: https://imagej.nih.gov/ij/ (accessed on 8 February 2023).

molecules

MDPI

Article

Assessing the Limit of CO_2 Storage in Seawater as Bicarbonate-Enriched Solutions

Selene Varliero [1], Samira Jamali Alamooti [1], Francesco Pietro Campo [2,3], Giovanni Cappello [2], Stefano Cappello [2], Stefano Caserini [4], Federico Comazzi [1,2], Piero Macchi [1,*] and Guido Raos [1,*]

[1] Department of Chemistry, Materials and Chemical Engineering "Giulio Natta", Politecnico di Milano, Via Luigi Mancinelli 7, 20131 Milano, Italy
[2] Limenet®, Via Giovanni Amendola 4-6, 23900 Lecco, Italy
[3] Department of Civil and Environmental Engineering, Politecnico di Milano, Piazza Leonardo Da Vinci 32, 20133 Milano, Italy
[4] Department of Engineering and Architecture, Università di Parma, Parco Area delle Scienze 59, 43124 Parma, Italy
* Correspondence: piero.macchi@polimi.it (P.M.); guido.raos@polimi.it (G.R.)

Abstract: The dissolution of CO_2 in seawater in the form of bicarbonate ions is an attractive alternative to storage in geological formations, on the condition that the storage is stable over long periods and does not harm the marine environment. In this work, we focus on the long-term chemical stability of CO_2 absorbed in seawater as bicarbonate by monitoring the physico-chemical properties of the solutions (pH, dissolved inorganic carbon and alkalinity) in six different sets of experiments on both natural and artificial seawater lasting up to three months. The bicarbonate treatment of natural seawater consists of mixing it with pre-equilibrated solutions obtained from the reaction of CO_2 and $Ca(OH)_2$, with the same pH as natural seawater. This was achieved with a pilot plant working with tons of seawater, while small-scale laboratory experiments were carried out by adding sodium bicarbonate to artificial seawater solutions. If the increase in the overall carbon concentration in the final mixture does not exceed a critical threshold (about 1000–1500 μmol/L), the resulting bicarbonate-rich solutions are found to be stable for over three months.

Keywords: CO_2 storage; climate change mitigation; marine chemistry; solution equilibria; carbonate system

Citation: Varliero, S.; Jamali Alamooti, S.; Campo, F.P.; Cappello, G.; Cappello, S.; Caserini, S.; Comazzi, F.; Macchi, P.; Raos, G. Assessing the Limit of CO_2 Storage in Seawater as Bicarbonate-Enriched Solutions. *Molecules* **2024**, *29*, 4069. https://doi.org/10.3390/molecules29174069

Academic Editor: Antonin Chapoy

Received: 23 July 2024
Revised: 23 August 2024
Accepted: 26 August 2024
Published: 28 August 2024

1. Introduction

The permanent storage of carbon dioxide (CO_2) is vital in virtually all mitigation scenarios compatible with ambitious climate targets. CO_2 storage could be used both for the CO_2 captured from the flue gas of industrial processes and for the CO_2 sequestered from the atmosphere through artificial processes [1].

The most developed approach for storing CO_2 is geological storage, namely the injection of CO_2 into geological formations, e.g., in deep saline aquifers [2]. Because the pace and scaling of geological CO_2 storage deployment have fallen short of expectations, and considering that this approach is unfeasible in many geographical areas [3–5], there is increasing interest in alternative solutions that could provide permanent storage of large quantities of CO_2.

Many authors have proposed and studied the storage of carbon dioxide in seawater [6–10], which already contains 98% of the overall CO_2 in the combined ocean-atmosphere system [11]. The large majority of this (86.5%, on average) is actually in the form of bicarbonate ions (HCO_3^-) [11]. Marine storage of CO_2 in the form of bicarbonate ions has the potential to last for geologic times, on the order of 10,000 years [12–14]. Rau and Caldeira [6,15] proposed a method called Accelerated Weathering of Limestone (AWL), consisting of the reaction of CO_2 from power plants' exhaust gas with seawater and calcium carbonate minerals ($CaCO_3$), namely calcite or aragonite, with a final discharge into the ocean of an ionic solution rich in bicarbonates. The overall "weathering" reaction may be summarized as follows:

$$CaCO_3(s) + CO_2(g) + H_2O(l) \rightarrow Ca^{2+}(aq) + 2HCO_3^-(aq) \quad (1)$$

This method has progressed from the laboratory level [16] to a feasibility case study [17], to a pilot-scale reactor [18], and to modeling of local impacts on seawater carbonate chemistry [19]. An improvement of this method, named buffered accelerated weathering of limestone (BAWL), has been proposed by Caserini et al. [9]. With this approach, CO_2 is used in stoichiometric excess with respect to the carbonate minerals, but calcium hydroxide [$Ca(OH)_2$, also known as slaked lime, SL] is added in the final stages of the process to produce a buffered ionic solution at the same pH as seawater. De Marco et al. [20] investigated mass and energy balances and the costs of applying BAWL to the capture and storage of CO_2 from the flue gas of an existing industrial source, and concluded that the process is technically feasible and economically viable.

One intrinsic shortcoming of the AWL and BAWL is the slow rate of the reaction between aqueous CO_2 and limestone. As a consequence, big plants treating large amounts of seawater would be necessary for marine storage of CO_2. The process implemented by Limenet® company [21] is an evolution of BAWL that attempts to overcome this problem by the direct combination of CO_2 with $Ca(OH)_2$, to induce the overall reaction:

$$2CO_2(aq) + Ca(OH)_2(s) + H_2O(l) \rightarrow Ca^{2+}(aq) + 2HCO_3^-(aq) \quad (2)$$

The reaction is carried out in specially designed reactors, where CO_2 is first dissolved in seawater, and then $Ca(OH)_2$ is added to give a bicarbonate-enriched solution with a pH equal to that of natural seawater. As an additional benefit, the solution has high alkalinity, thus increasing the buffering capacity of seawater against acidification [22]. For this reason, these technologies are classified as Ocean Alkalinity Enhancement (OAE) processes. The SL employed in reaction (2) is typically produced by calcination of limestone, an energy-intensive process that produces one mol of CO_2 per mol of $CaCO_3$. Any additional CO_2 emissions can be avoided by using renewable energies for the calcination and by sequestering the CO_2 with one-half of the produced $Ca(OH)_2$. Therefore, ideally this process enables the net sequestration of one mol of CO_2 per mol of $CaCO_3$. Several recent scientific studies address the possible beneficial or harmful consequences of OAE implementations on marine biota [23,24], and the future efficiency of its large-scale implementation [25,26].

The fundamental question that inspired this research is whether the increased amount of bicarbonate in seawater remains stable over time and, therefore, fulfills the requirements for permanent storage. The aim is also to identify the optimal relative amounts of seawater, CO_2, and $Ca(OH)_2$ that avoid CO_2 degassing as well as abiotic or biotic precipitation of carbonate minerals. These are two of the strongest pitfalls of such approaches, as carbonate precipitation would lead to the re-emission of CO_2 into the atmosphere by a reaction that is essentially the reverse of (1):

$$Ca^{2+}(aq) + 2HCO_3^-(aq) \rightarrow CaCO_3(s) + CO_2(g) + H_2O(l). \quad (3)$$

These questions were prompted, among other things, by analogous studies of the stability of seawater treated by ocean liming (OL) operations [7,8,12]. OL consists of the direct dispersion of $Ca(OH)_2$ on the surface of seawater to induce additional absorption of atmospheric CO_2 [12]. Those studies demonstrated that, apart from causing potentially harmful spikes in seawater pH, such OAE operations may also be ineffective because they can trigger unwanted side reactions like (3). While classical ocean liming is an unequilibrated process, the injection of a bicarbonate solution has the inherent advantage of leaving the seawater pH unaltered. In fact, the dissolution of calcium hydroxide occurs in a closed system and with the exact amount of water needed. Only afterward is the bicarbonate-enriched marine solution released into the sea at the same pH. This pH-equilibrated marine solution implies fewer serendipities and unpredictable behaviors than ocean liming, especially pH spikes and possible precipitation of carbonates. By pH-equilibrated, we indicate a solution with the same pH as natural seawater.

Equilibrium with respect to pH and any other chemical reaction within the aqueous phase does not automatically imply equilibrium with respect to other phases, including the formation or dissolution of minerals and the uptake or release of gaseous atmospheric CO_2 [11]. In this respect, it is important to stress that the ocean surface is heavily supersaturated in carbonate minerals, implying a high risk of precipitation. A sudden and uncontrolled increase in the local concentration of carbonate ions may trigger the nucleation and therefore the precipitation of carbonate minerals. In particular, the aragonite saturation state ranges between 2.7 and 3.7 in the Mediterranean Sea [27]. It is defined and calculated by the following equation:

$$\Omega_{Ar} = \frac{\left[Ca^{2+}\right]\left[CO_3^{2-}\right]}{K_{SP}} \quad (4)$$

where $\left[Ca^{2+}\right]$ and $\left[CO_3^{2-}\right]$ are the molar concentrations of calcium and carbonate ions, while K_{SP} is the stoichiometric solubility product of aragonite in seawater [27]. The aragonite saturation state is considered a useful indicator of the risk of precipitation [7,28,29], even though it is more soluble than calcite, as precipitation of the latter is inhibited by the high concentration of magnesium in seawater [30].

This work aims to assess the storage efficiency of CO_2, converted into bicarbonate ions, in seawater. In particular, it is important to quantify the limit of bicarbonate additions without causing side effects such as the precipitation of carbonate minerals (e.g., aragonite or calcite) that may occur several days or even weeks after treatment. With this in mind, we have tested the stability of seawater solutions containing an enhanced concentration of bicarbonate ions in two distinct sets of experiments:

(a) Natural seawater treated with the Limenet® process at a site located in the harbor of La Spezia (Italy) and subsequently transferred to our laboratory at the Politecnico di Milano for long-term monitoring;
(b) Artificial seawater prepared and treated in the laboratory with controlled additions of sodium bicarbonate.

Furthermore, we have evaluated the durability of CO_2 stored in the form of dissolved bicarbonates through measurements of pH, Dissolved Inorganic Carbon (DIC), and Total Alkalinity (TA).

Within the scope of our study, it is important to stress that DIC approximately coincides with the sum of C contained in HCO_3^- and CO_3^{2-} because the smaller contribution of CO_2 can be ignored in seawater, and no other inorganic C is present. On the other hand, TA is approximately the sum of the quantities of HCO_3^- and 2 times CO_3^{2-}. Both indicators are therefore useful for monitoring the C content in seawater. Our observations have been correlated with the calculated saturation states (Ω) of calcite and aragonite [Equation (4)]. We monitored these parameters over long periods, ranging from a few days up to three months, allowing us to assess the stability of the treated solutions.

2. Results

Table 1 summarizes the series of experiments we conducted to test the stability of bicarbonate-enriched seawater solutions. The first column contains labels used throughout the manuscript to indicate a series of samples and experimental conditions. These can be classified according to the following variables (see Section 4 for more details):

(1) Mode: Carbon was added to the solutions either in a single step or by multiple additions over a period of several days.
(2) Seawater: We used either natural seawater (collected from the Mediterranean Sea at La Spezia) or artificial seawater (prepared from purified water and inorganic salts).

(3) Environment: We measured the evolution of the treated solutions either in an open atmosphere or in closed cabinets with a fixed volume of enclosed air (ca. 300 L). We call the experiments as "mixed" where we temporarily opened the cabinet to perform the addition of sodium bicarbonate.
(4) Treatment: The alkalinization of seawater was obtained either with a concentrated solution of sodium bicarbonate or through the Limenet® process. The latter implies the formation of calcium bicarbonate from the neutralization of carbon dioxide and calcium hydroxide, as described in the Introduction and in Section 4. These treatments are indicated in the table as $NaHCO_3$ and $Ca(HCO_3)_2$, respectively.
(5) $Max\Delta_{DIC}$: The largest theoretical amount of added carbon (in μmol/L) for a series of experiments. It is a theoretical value because it represents the expected increase in DIC, assuming ideal addition without degassing or precipitation.
(6) Initial DIC: In the experiments with natural seawater, the measured initial DIC was 2370 μmol/L for SN1/SN2 and 2470 μmol/L for MN. In the experiments with artificial seawater (MA and SA), the initial DIC was set to 2000 μmol/L [31] or to 2800 μmol/L, obtained from the dissolution of $NaHCO_3$.
(7) Duration: This refers to the longest duration of a set of experiments. Measurements were carried out in the laboratory for up to 90 days.

Table 1. Series of seawater samples and experiments. Each row represents a set of experiments conducted with different DIC additions.

Code	Mode	Seawater	Environment	Treatment	$Max\Delta_{DIC}$ (μmol/L)	Initial DIC (μmol/L)	Duration (Days)
SN1	Single	Natural	Open	$Ca(HCO_3)_2$	7510	2370	90
SN2	Single	Natural	Open	$Ca(HCO_3)_2$	5650	2370	90
SA	Single	Artificial	Closed	$NaHCO_3$	800	2000	3
MAM	Multiple	Artificial	Mixed	$NaHCO_3$	3200	2000	24
MAC	Multiple	Artificial	Closed	$NaHCO_3$	400	2800	16
MN	Multiple	Natural	Closed	$NaHCO_3$	1000	2470	52

In Figure 1, we report results from the experiments of types SN1 and SN2, which are characterized by different values of $Max\Delta_{DIC}$. The measurements lasted up to 90 days, which is one of the longest periods ever reported in the literature for this type of study. The numbers next to each code (e.g., 70 in "SN1-70") indicate the theoretical added DIC, in μmol/L. We measured the pH, DIC, and TA with variable frequency. We also report the results of concomitant control experiments on untreated natural seawater (SW) used as a reference. The average starting pH of the SW samples we analyzed is ca. 8.1, close to the values reported in the literature for the Mediterranean [27]. We point out that the solutions monitored in SN1 and SN2 experiments were static, as we did not continuously stir or vibrate them to mimic the natural motion of the ocean surface. Some stirring was nonetheless applied almost daily, at least in the initial phases of the experiments, as part of the sampling operations.

A few minutes after the initial dissolution ("day 0"), all the samples share the same pH as SW, apart from the two solutions with the highest Δ_{DIC} (7510 μmol/L for SN1 and 5650 μmol/L for SN2), which have a lower pH. This is probably caused by partial precipitation of carbonate minerals occurring in the initial stages of the treatment, before the first pH measurement. Nonetheless, even in these two solutions, the pH increases until day 18, when the gap with the other solutions is greatly reduced, even though it remains below that of SW. The pH of the solutions with an added DIC below 270 μmol/L does not show a systematic trend compared to SW, although the differences with respect to SW are always below 0.04, well within the precision limits of the measurements. This behavior indicates that pH is not significantly affected by low DIC additions. For solutions with carbon addition between 360 and 1500 μmol/L, the pH is consistently higher than in SW, proportional to the theoretical concentration. Note that a small increase in pH is expected to be beneficial for the marine environment, considering that the oceans have already undergone significant acidification (the average pH has decreased from 8.11 in 1985 to 8.05 in 2021) due to the enhanced absorption of CO_2 from the atmosphere [32], and that a surface ocean pH as low as recent times is uncommon in the last two million years [33].

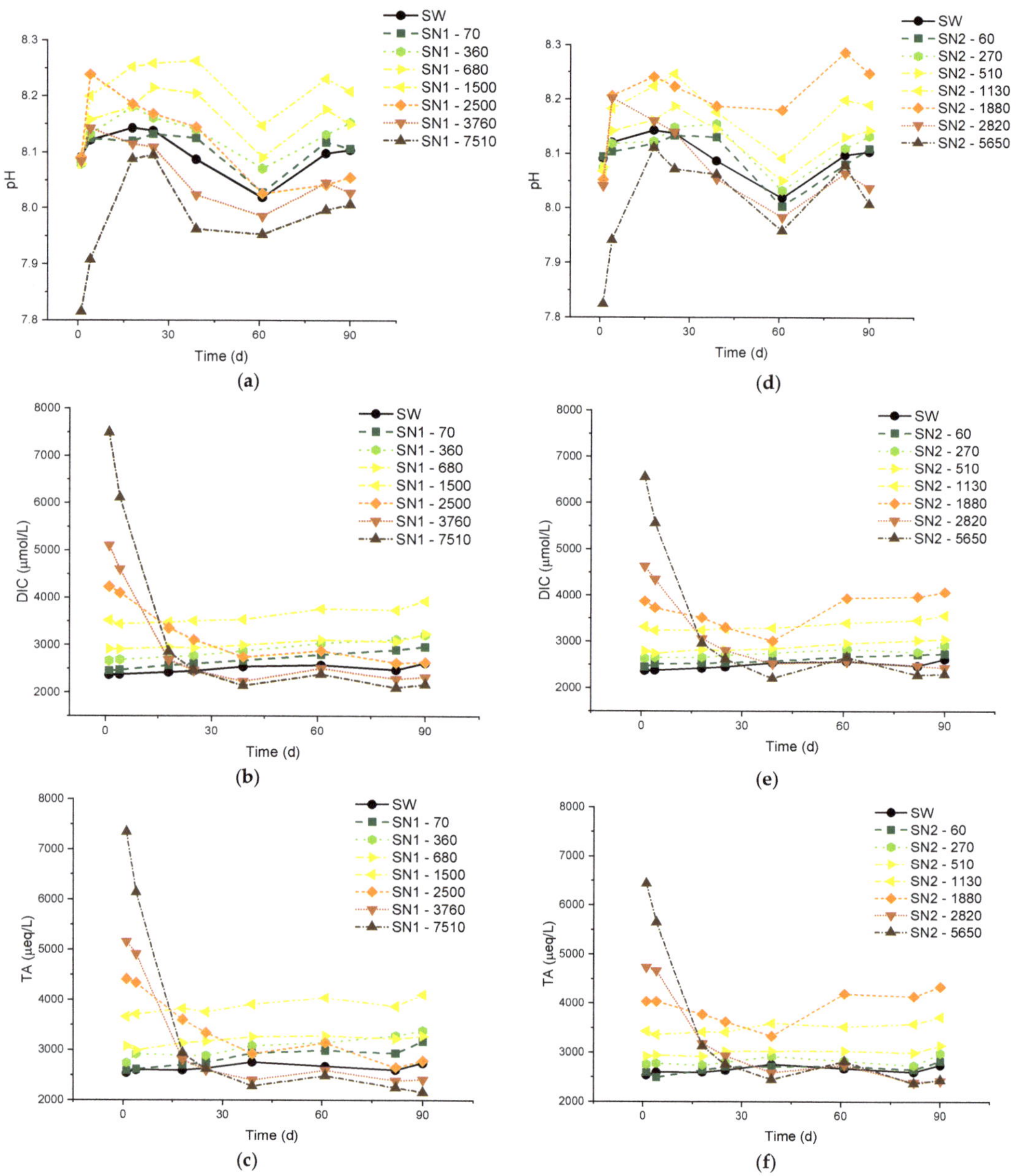

Figure 1. Measured pH, alkalinity, and DIC values over 90 days. Graphs (**a**–**c**) refer to SN1, and graphs (**d**–**f**) refer to SN2.

The rest of Figure 1 reports results for the DIC [panels (b) and (e)] and the TA [panels (c) and (f)]. The measurements of these quantities started on "day 1", immediately after the arrival of the seawater samples at our laboratory. The overall behavior of these quantities is consistent with our pH measurements. In both the SN1 and SN2 series of experiments, the two solutions treated with the largest additions show a decrease in DIC and TA to levels lower than in SW within approximately 30 days. Note that, for most of the samples, the measurements of DIC indicate values already lower than the sum of the initial DIC and the theoretical Δ_{DIC} (see again Table 1). This suggests the occurrence of some precipitation and degassing for high DIC additions, which will be taken into account in the formulation of the process efficiency, below. On the other hand, untreated SW and the solutions with Δ_{DIC} equal to 1500 μmol/L or lower show a slight increase in TA and DIC for the entire duration of the monitoring.

The precipitation of carbonates from the most concentrated solutions is not surprising, considering the natural supersaturation of seawater [27]. The saturation states Ω of all solutions under examination can be computed from the measured pH, TA, and DIC values [11], and they show some variation. We should consider that the samples were not stored in a temperature-controlled ambient; therefore, the Ω of untreated natural seawater also fluctuated during the control period: the initial Ω was 6.45 and 4.20 for calcite and aragonite, respectively, and the two quantities varied in the ranges 5.15–8.84 (calcite) and 3.34–5.69 (aragonite) without the occurrence of precipitation (Tables A1 and A2 in Appendix A). Of course, analogous oscillations also affected the treated solutions. Therefore, for each measurement, we focus on the saturation of the treated solutions (Ω_i) relative to the saturation of the control SW measured on the same day (Ω_{SW}), using the ratio:

$$r\Omega = \Omega_i/\Omega_{SW}. \tag{5}$$

Calcite and aragonite share the same rΩ because the solubility products disappear from the denominators when computing Equation (5).

The results are reported in Figure 2. The samples with carbon additions of 5650 μmol/L and 2820 μmol/L are those with the largest rΩ on day 1, which rapidly decreases due to observed massive precipitation. The samples with carbon additions of 1500 μmol/L (for the SN1 experiments) and 1130 μmol/L (for the SN2 experiments) have the largest stable rΩ values, respectively equal to 1.94 and 1.68 (average values). So, according to the present study, these rΩ's could be considered safe threshold values, below which precipitation of carbonate minerals does not occur in our samples.

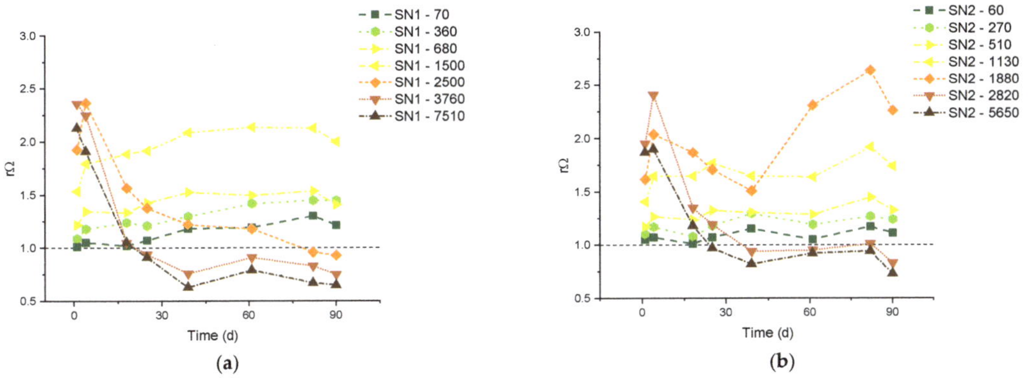

Figure 2. Relative supersaturation rΩ of aragonite and calcite in the SN1 (**a**) and SN2 (**b**) experiments.

Figure 3 reports results from the SA experiments on artificial seawater with a single addition of alkalinity in the form of $NaHCO_3$ powder. Additional data are contained in

Table A3 in Appendix A. We tested carbon concentrations of 2000, 2400, and 2800 μmol/L. Each experiment was repeated twice. Considering the value of 2000 μmol/L as a baseline close to untreated natural seawater (see again Table 1), these experiments are labeled as Δ_{DIC} = 0, 400, and 800, respectively. The SA experiments were monitored in a sealed cabinet, which also allowed for the measurement of CO_2 concentration in the atmosphere. The variation of CO_2 over time should reflect degassing from the solution.

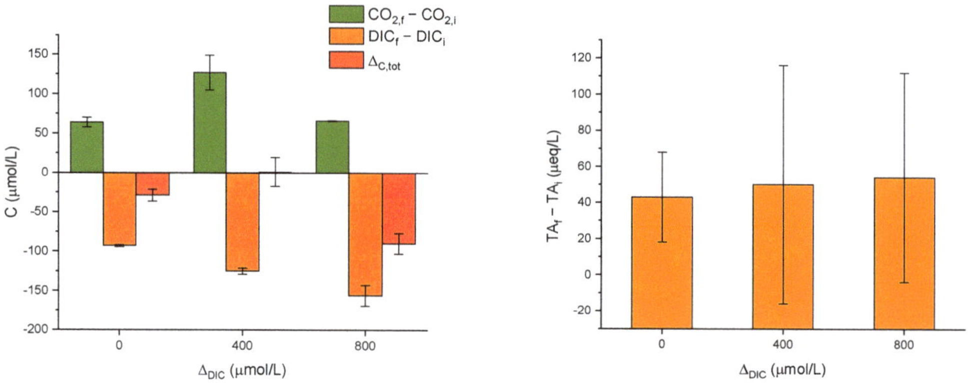

Figure 3. Results of the SA experiments; the error bars refer to individual measurements.

The pH stabilizes in all the SA experiments, from 7.93 to 8.03. Instead, the TA shows sizeable fluctuations, which are largely due to the technical difficulty of these measurements. As shown in Figure 3, in all three additions, the DIC measured just after the dosage decreases at the end of the experiment to about 100–150 μmol/L, depending on the dosage (values reported as DIC_f-DIC_i). This gap increases with the DIC addition, suggesting degassing of CO_2. This hypothesis is confirmed by the measured increase in atmospheric CO_2 ($CO_{2,f}-CO_{2,i}$), although it is not consistent with the DIC addition. Overall, we can define $\Delta_{C,tot}$ as the sum of DIC_f-DIC_i and $CO_{2,f}-CO_{2,i}$. We see that all the experiments show a loss of carbon which is not present either in solution or in air. The missing carbon is likely due to minor precipitation of carbonates. We were not able to retrieve the expected quantities in the form of powder after filtration, precisely because these were very small.

Another laboratory experiment (MAM in Table 1) was carried out with eight regular additions, starting again from 2000 μmol/L up to a theoretical DIC of 5200 μmol/L (hence, a Δ_{DIC} of 3200 μmol/L).

The results of the MAM experiment are reported in Figure 4. The measured DIC increases, but it is progressively lower than the expected value. It is noteworthy that the last addition did not produce any increase in DIC. The total alkalinity, also shown in Figure 4, reflects the same behavior as DIC, though with a pair of outliers on day 6, possibly due to a calibration pitfall. It should be considered, in fact, that the precision of DIC measurement (repeated 3–4 times for each sampling) is much superior to that of TA (single measurement for each sampling).

Even accounting for the lower precision, the drop in TA (compared to the theoretical value) seems to be delayed with respect to the drop in DIC (see again Figure 4). For example, after the third addition on day 8, the TA still matches the theoretical value, while the DIC does not. This may be ascribed to some CO_2 degassing occurring after the first additions, while the loss of carbon by precipitation (with a concurrent decrease in DIC and TA) would be triggered only subsequently. Indeed, the formation of a few particles was visually observed at two stages of the MAM experiments:

(1) A few days after the third injection of $NaHCO_3$ (with a theoretical DIC of 3200 μmol/L), some precipitates floated on the surface of the solution;

(2) At the endpoint of the experiment (theoretical DIC = 5200 µmol/L), a significant number of precipitates stuck on the wall and bottom of the beaker were observed.

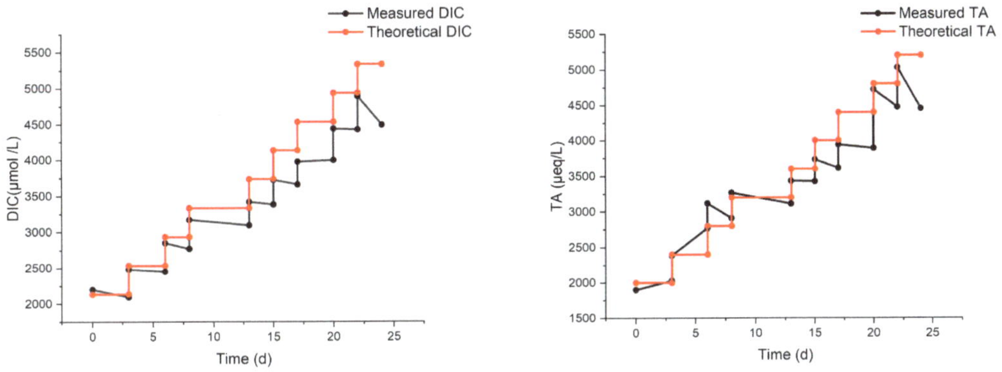

Figure 4. Measured DIC and TA from the MAM experiment on artificial seawater with multiple bi-carbonate dosages over 24 days.

The first episode of precipitation occurred during the longest shift at a fixed concentration, enough to allow precipitation. This is the point where the differences between the measured and the theoretical DIC and TA start to increase significantly. Calculated Ω_{Ar} rises from 0.88 (on day 0) to 6.37 (on day 22) and then drops due to precipitation.

The precipitates from the MAM experiment were collected and analyzed by XRD. The diffraction pattern, shown in Figure 5, has clear signatures of the presence of aragonite. The large bump at low diffraction angles is mainly due to scattering from the sample holder and air, while the second one at higher angles is likely due to an amorphous carbonate phase and small precipitation nuclei [30]. From the diffraction pattern it is not possible to recognize any other crystal form than aragonite (and certainly exclude the presence of calcite), despite the fact that aragonite is more soluble (it has a higher K_{SP}) than calcite. It is well known that kinetic factors may dominate over thermodynamic ones in the precipitation of carbonates from seawater [34].

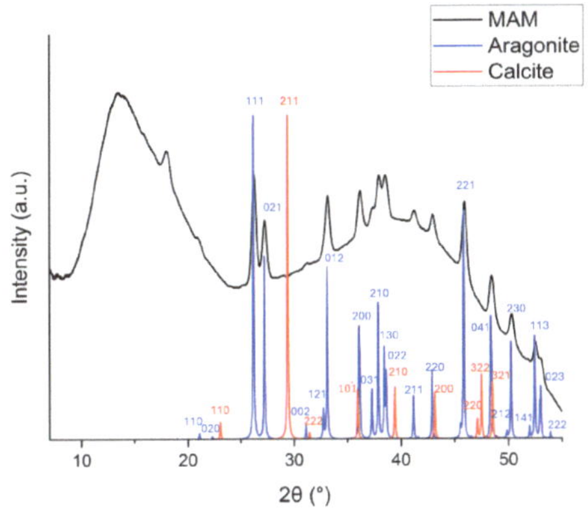

Figure 5. The XRD pattern of the precipitate collected at the end of the MAM experiment (black curve). Simulated diffraction patterns of calcite (red) and aragonite (blue) are also displayed.

Finally, we describe the MAC and MN experiments. They were carried out to compare the response of artificial and natural seawater to alkalinity addition. These experiments lasted 16 and 52 days, respectively, with an $NaHCO_3$ addition one week after the start of the experiments. The final theoretical DIC concentration was chosen in both cases to be greater than or equal to 3200 μmol/L, which triggered the precipitation of aragonite in the MAM experiment (Figure 4). The environment was sealed for the entire duration of these experiments. As shown in Figure 6, continuous decreases in DIC and TA are observed from the start of the MAC experiment, indicating continuous degassing and precipitation, consistent with the measured increase in CO_2 concentration in the surrounding atmosphere (Figure 7). The results from the MN experiment in Figure 8 show a similar trend in DIC, while the measurements of TA are more erratic but stable, which may indicate degassing and, to a lesser extent, some precipitation.

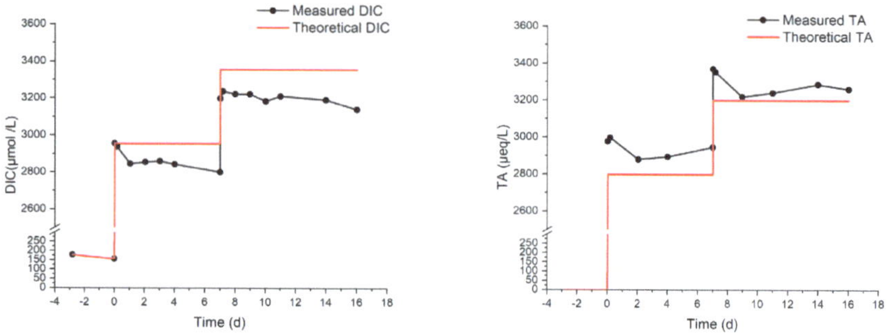

Figure 6. DIC and TA from the MAC experiment in artificial seawater with two-step bicarbonate dosage. Initial TA is assumed to be 0 because it was below the detection limit of the instrument, while for DIC the starting point was measurable by the instrument.

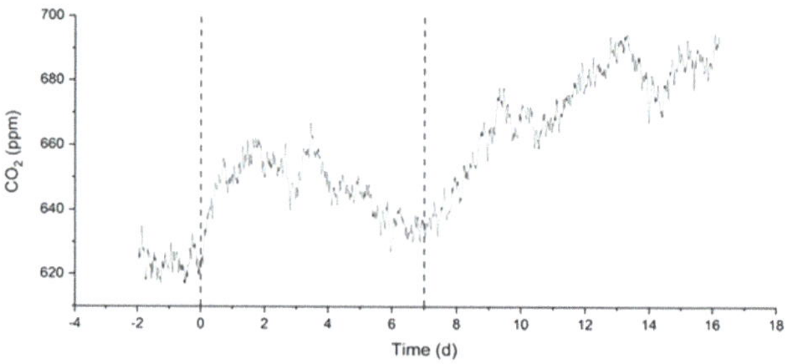

Figure 7. Measured pressure of CO_2 (in atm) from a MAC experiment in artificial seawater with two-step bicarbonate dosage. Dashed lines indicate the additions of $NaHCO_3$ on days 0 and 7.

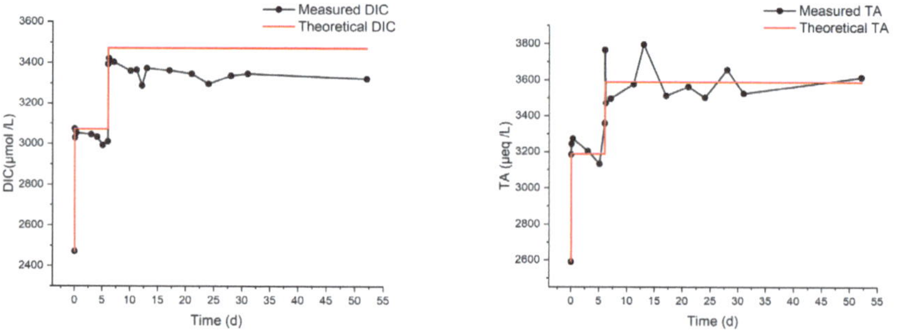

Figure 8. DIC and TA from the MN experiment on natural seawater with two-step bicarbonate dosage.

3. Discussion

The experiments described in the previous section enable us to widen the perspective on the processes for treating seawater with buffered solutions enriched with CO_2. The overall purpose of the experiments was to assess the efficiency of the alkalinity enhancement process (i.e., the fraction of CO_2 actually introduced into seawater, mainly as bicarbonates) and its efficacy (i.e., the stability over time of the solutions, without precipitation of minerals or degassing of CO_2). Here, we concentrate on the discussion of the SN experiments, which are based on the application of the revised BAWL technology implemented by Limenet® on natural seawater.

The hypotheses underlying the BAWL technology that we wanted to test are:

a. By injecting a CO_2 solution pre-equilibrated at the same pH as natural seawater, one induces the least perturbation to the chemical equilibria of the carbonate system and to the natural environment. In particular, the pH should remain constant both after the initial treatment and over longer times;
b. CO_2 remains in the seawater solution mainly in the form of bicarbonate, so that the alkalinity and carbon content should increase, without precipitation of mineral phases or degassing of CO_2;
c. The efficiency is high, meaning that the measured increase of DIC matches the added quantity over a long time.

One major concern for marine sequestration approaches is that seawater is already oversaturated with calcium carbonates. Therefore, any further addition increases the risk of precipitation and degassing. All results indicate that there is indeed an upper limit, above which it is impossible to increase the carbon content of seawater. This affects the CO_2 storage and the method efficiency, i.e., hypotheses (b) and (c). Below the critical concentration, all the previous interrelated hypotheses are simultaneously verified.

The natural seawater solutions treated with the Limenet® process had a stable pH around the natural value of 8.1, up to DIC additions of 1500 μmol/L (Figure 1). Therefore, there are no special concerns about hypothesis (a). Also, the DIC and TA are stable when seawater is treated within this concentration limit, showing an average variation of 3 to 4%, the same as observed for untreated natural seawater. Statistical descriptors of the data are collected in Tables A4 and A5 in Appendix A.

The DIC and TA drop by more than 60% when seawater is treated with the most concentrated solutions (see more details in Tables A4–A6). The decrease in carbon content observed for DIC additions > 1500 μmol/L is probably due to a combination of CO_2 degassing and precipitation of carbonate minerals. Once nucleation triggers the precipitation of carbonates, it can quickly proceed to significantly reduce Ω, in addition or in synergy with degasification.

The critical Ω of aragonite and calcite were recognized as important indicators of the likelihood of precipitation [7,8]. Marion et al. [35] suggested 18.8 and 12.3 for Ω_{Ca} and Ω_{Ar}, respectively. In more specific experiments on OAE, Moras et al. [7] reported aragonite formation at much lower supersaturations and suggested a safe threshold of $\Omega_{Ar} = 5$ to avoid "runaway" precipitation. In our SN1-1500 samples, there is no evidence of precipitation even if the Ω_{Ar} has an average value of 7.7. Such discrepancies among the defined thresholds may originate from several factors. First of all, we point out that the supersaturation states are not measured directly, but they are calculated by geochemical software that may apply different models. Secondly, one should take into account the specific technologies and chemicals used in the OAE operations, as well as the origin of the seawater (location, temperature, salinity, etc.). Finally, there are factors such as the presence of organic matter, pollutants, colloidal particles, and marine organisms that are not taken into account in the evaluation of Ω_{Ar}, but they can certainly affect precipitation reactions [36–38]. For these reasons, we suggest the increase of Ω relative to that of the starting SW [$r\Omega$, see Equation (5)] as a possible indicator for defining a safe OAE application.

Notwithstanding the different approaches to defining the threshold, when the limit is reached, the carbon storage efficiency drops significantly. The efficiency [$\eta(t)$] can be defined as the ratio between the observed increase in the carbon content of seawater and the theoretical one (Δ_{DIC}). Our notation indicates that it is a time-dependent quantity.

Let DIC(t) and $DIC_{SW}(t)$ be the measured values of DIC for a given treatment and for untreated natural seawater, measured in the laboratory at the same time t. These two concentrations change over time, also due to processes that are unrelated to the loss of carbon, such as water evaporation and biological activity (the samples were kept in the lab at room temperature, in open glass bottles).

We obtain the efficiency as the product of two factors. The first (η_0) depends on phenomena occurring during the initial addition of carbon, the second one (η_{St}) during the subsequent stability tests:

$$\eta(t) = \eta_0 \times \eta_{St}(t). \tag{6}$$

These are given by:

$$\eta_0 = \frac{\mathrm{DIC}(0) - \mathrm{DIC_{SW}}(0)}{\Delta_{\mathrm{DIC}}} \tag{7}$$

and:

$$\eta_{St}(t) = \frac{1}{r(t)} \times \frac{\mathrm{DIC}(t) - \mathrm{DIC_{SW}}(t)}{\mathrm{DIC}(0) - \mathrm{DIC_{SW}}(0)} \tag{8}$$

where:

$$r(t) = \frac{\mathrm{DIC_{SW}}(t)}{\mathrm{DIC_{SW}}(0)} \tag{9}$$

The value of η_0 takes into account non-idealities that may occur in the reactor and in the line from the reactor to the delivery point, which reduce the amount of carbon taken up by the seawater solutions before discharge. Our estimates, based on the extrapolation of DIC data measured on day 1 (see Figure 9), lead to $\eta_0 \approx 80\%$ for $\Delta_{DIC} \geq 360$ µmol/L. This value could be increased by optimizing the process parameters. The efficiency of stability includes a correction factor $r(t)$ that takes into account the already mentioned phenomena, which also occur in natural seawater under our laboratory conditions and affect all the DIC values, even though they are unrelated to the loss of carbon.

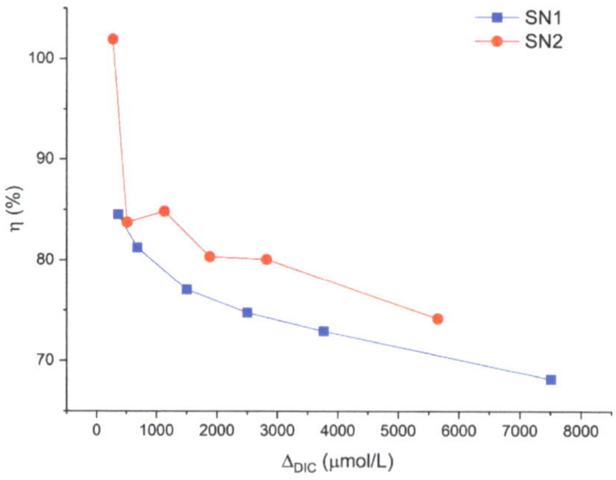

Figure 9. Process efficiency on day 1 as a function of DIC addition (Δ_{DIC}).

Figure 10 shows the η_{St} trends for samples with Δ_{DIC} higher than 270 µmol/L. The data for lower concentrations are not reported here because they are subject to very large errors. All samples with carbon addition between 510 and 1500 µmol/L share a similar trend: an average stability efficiency between 88% and 94% and a standard deviation of 8–9% (except for the 510 µmol/L theoretical DIC addition, for which the standard deviation was 16%). This implies an overall process efficiency of the order of 70%.

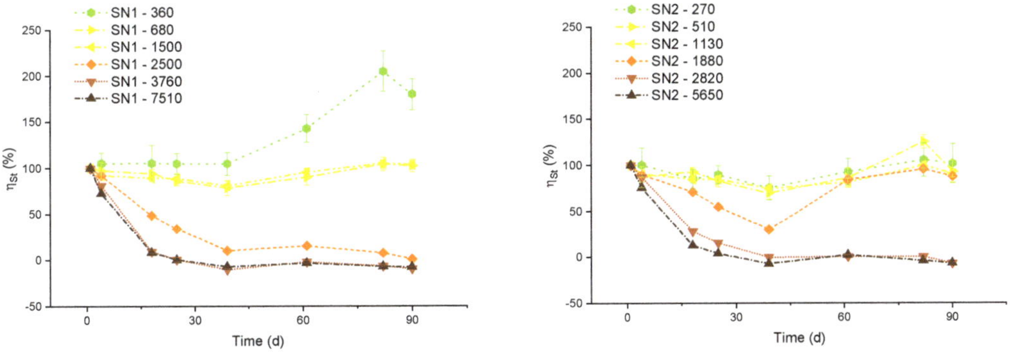

Figure 10. Stability efficiency over time. The efficiency of SN1 (**a**) and SN2 (**b**) samples are represented together. The name of the series represents the μmol/L of carbon theoretically added to the solution (Δ_{DIC}).

The sample with Δ_{DIC} equal to 360 μmol/L shows an efficiency that grows far above the 100% limit. This anomalous behavior is likely due to contamination of the sample after day 39, as it is not observed in all the other samples.

On the other hand, for the samples with Δ_{DIC} higher than 1500 μmol/L, the efficiency drops dramatically within a few days. For the highest concentrations, the efficiency is actually close to zero or even negative. A negative efficiency indicates a final DIC content lower than in untreated seawater. This agrees with the observed decrease of DIC in Figure 1 and the runaway precipitation of carbonate minerals, similar to the discussion by Moras et al. [7], Hartmann et al. [8], and Varliero et al. [39].

A final remark on efficiency is related to CO_2 equilibrium with the atmosphere. Figure 1a,d shows a small increase in pH from day 1 to day 4 for all the samples, including seawater. This is likely due to the equilibration of the solution with the atmosphere by degassing. The importance of degassing is also highlighted by the experiments with small Δ_{DIC} in artificial seawater (SA and MAC, see Figures 3, 6 and 7). In those experiments, atmospheric CO_2 increased without precipitation. Indeed, the pH of artificial seawater is generally lower than that of natural seawater, so it is understandable that degassing is more prominent.

4. Materials and Methods

4.1. Natural Seawater

Natural seawater has been used for two experimental configurations: single and multiple alkalinity dosages. Seawater has been sampled on two different occasions. Sampling for the SN1 and SN2 experiments occurred in September and October 2022 in La Spezia (Liguria, Italy) at the CSSN (Naval Support and Experimentation Center; coordinates: 44.095863, 9.862471). The MN experiment used water collected in February 2024 in La Spezia Bay (44.1013006, 9.8280323), and was stored in glass or polycarbonate Nalgene containers.

4.2. Artificial Seawater

Artificial seawater was prepared by dissolving NaCl, Na_2SO_4, KCl, $MgCl_2{\cdot}6H_2O$, and $CaCl_2$ salts in purified water, with the relative abundances proposed by Roy et al. [40] reported in Table 2. It was then stored in polycarbonate Nalgene tanks. All salts were Labkem (located in Barcelona, Spain) products, purchased from Labbox, and used without further purification.

Table 2. Concentration of salts in artificial seawater [40]. Amount expressed as grams in each liter of distilled water added.

Salts	Concentration (g/L)
NaCl	25.14
Na_2SO_4	4.18
KCl	0.79
$MgCl_2 \cdot 6H_2O$	11.19
$CaCl_2$	1.20

4.3. *Treatment with Ca(HCO$_3$)$_2$*

Figure 11 shows a schematic block diagram of the Limenet® system as implemented in La Spezia. Using a draft pump, about 25 L/s of seawater was collected at a depth of 2 m. After about 10 s, a gaseous stream of 100% CO_2 was injected. After about 180 s, a slurry of $Ca(OH)_2$ was dosed into the acidic stream of seawater and CO_2 to reach the same pH as fresh seawater (i.e., about pH 8.1). The slurry was composed of 30 parts seawater and 1 part $Ca(OH)_2$ by weight. The proportion of CO_2 and seawater was controlled by a flux valve, while the amount of $Ca(OH)_2$ was verified by weighing the hydroxide consumed. Table 3 summarizes the proportion of seawater, CO_2, and $Ca(OH)_2$.

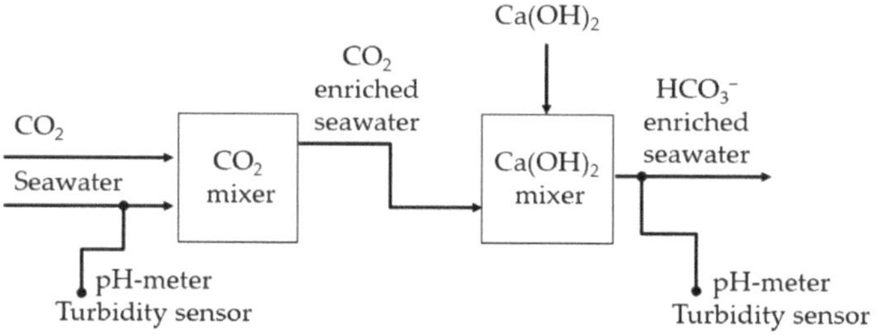

Figure 11. Scheme of the Limenet® process applied to produce a high alkaline solution with natural seawater, and the sensors used to control the system.

Table 3. Seawater and calcium hydroxide used to produce samples SN1 and SN2.

	SN1	SN2
Seawater (m^3)	3000	4000
$Ca(OH)_2$ (ton)	0.874	0.874
CO_2 (ton)	1.000	1.000

pHSense 5–381 and TurbSense SN—TSIR—9667 probes were used to monitor pH and turbidity in the system. CO_2 was provided by AirLiquide, while $Ca(OH)_2$ powder was supplied by Unicalce.

The bicarbonate-enriched seawater exiting the plant was mixed with natural seawater to recreate different dilution ratios. Three sets of samples were produced: SN1 with a ratio of 3000 m^3/ton between seawater and CO_2; SN2 and SN3 with a ratio of 4000 m^3/ton (see Table A6 for SN3). The bicarbonate-enriched solutions collected were diluted with fresh seawater, using variable proportions, namely 1:0, 1:1, 1:4, 1:10, 1:20, and 1:100 mass ratios between the alkaline solution and fresh seawater (see Table 4 for the corresponding Δ_{DIC}).

After preparation, the containers were capped and transported on the same day to the laboratory of the Department of Chemistry, Politecnico di Milano, without any thermostatic storage device or other conditioning.

DIC and TA analysis was carried out within 24 h after collection. It was repeated once a week for one month and then twice a week for the last two months, for a total of 90 days.

Table 4. Conversion from dilution ratios to dissolved inorganic carbon added initially to the solution (Δ_{DIC}).

Dilution Ratio	SN1 Δ_{DIC} (µmol/L)	SN2 Δ_{DIC} (µmol/L)
SW	0	0
1:0	7510	5650
1:1	3760	2820
1:2	2500	1880
1:4	1500	1130
1:10	680	510
1:20	360	270
1:100	70	60

Each sample was stored in two 500-mL borosilicate glass bottles and uncapped to allow them to reach equilibrium with CO_2 under laboratory conditions. On day 1, pH and conductivity measurements were carried out to check the consistency between the two containers. We excluded the measurements on day 53 from Section 2 because the first bottles of each sample were almost empty and therefore more affected by evaporation. In Figure 1, for some solutions (especially SN2–1880), there is a visible gap between day 39 (last measurement from the first bottle) and day 61 (first measurement from the second bottle).

4.4. Treatment with $NaHCO_3$

Experiments SA, MAM, MAC, and MN took place at the Politecnico di Milano. In these experiments, powdered sodium bicarbonate ($NaHCO_3$) was added to 4.5 L of natural seawater.

$NaHCO_3$ was a Labkem product from Labbox, and used without further purification.

In the SA experiments, sodium bicarbonate was added in a single dosage (2.0, 2.4, and 2.8 mmol/L). 2 mmol/L is the value of $NaHCO_3$ suggested by Millero [31] for artificial seawater to mimic the natural seawater pH and alkalinity. These experiments were repeated twice. Furthermore, a control test, without $NaHCO_3$ addition, was conducted.

After $NaHCO_3$ addition, the beaker was confined inside a sealed poly(methyl methacrylate) plexiglass cabinet with a volume of 0.335 m^3 to avoid exchanges of air with the external environment of the laboratory, having an air/water volumetric ratio of 74.3. The windows were opened approximately two hours before the analysis to maintain the concentration of CO_2 similar among different experiments and to allow CO_2 equilibration.

Probes were placed inside the cabinet to continuously measure pH, conductivity, and temperature of the artificial seawater. A CO_2 sensor was used to measure its concentration (in ppm) in the atmosphere inside the cabinet. DIC and alkalinity were analyzed before and immediately after the $NaHCO_3$ addition. At the end of the experiment, i.e., after about 48–72 h, the cabinet was opened, and all measurements were repeated.

The MAM experiments were performed in artificial seawater. Sodium bicarbonate was dosed in multiple stages, opening the cabinet for dosages and samplings. The addition was done step by step over 24 days, from 2000 to 5200 µmol/L.

The MN and MAC experiments were performed with 4 L of solution instead of 4.5 L, thus with an air/water volumetric ratio of 83.35. The cabinet was closed for the entire duration of the experiments, and sample suction and alkalinity injection were done through a 150 mL syringe by piping from the inside to the outside of the cabinet and controlled by a manually driven valve. $NaHCO_3$ was pre-dissolved in a treated solution sampled by the syringe and then re-injected into the solution. To maintain the volume of the solution, treated seawater samples were kept outside the cabinet and added to replace the seawater sampled for measuring the DIC and TA. Before the first injection, the artificial and natural seawater were equilibrated with air inside the closed cabinet for three and one day, respectively. TA, DIC, pH, and conductivity were measured by periodic sampling, and CO_2 concentration in the air was continuously recorded.

For all experiments, temperature was not controlled; the maximum and minimum values recorded during the entire duration of the experiments were about 21 and 16 °C, respectively.

4.5. Measurements

Before the first measurements of a new bottle, each sample was vacuum filtrated with sieves of 2–3 μm cut-off to remove large particles that could affect the subsequent analyses. Moreover, filtration allows for the identification of the precipitates' nature and composition by X-ray diffraction analysis (XRD) using a Rigaku-Synergy-S single-crystal diffractometer. This equipment was necessary given the small amount of precipitate that did not allow a classical powder XRD measurement.

pH and conductivity were measured using electrode sensors from MATTLER TOLEDO Seven excellence. The pH probe was calibrated every two weeks according to the NIST scale; then, the values were corrected on the total scale, as suggested by Badocco et al. [41].

Total alkalinity was measured by automatic titration (Hanna Instruments HI84531). The pH probe was calibrated every two weeks while the pumping system was calibrated every day.

Dissolved inorganic carbon was measured by acidification and non-dispersive infrared absorbance (Analytik Jena multi NC 2100S). The machine calculates DIC concentration as the average of three measurements. If the average has a variation coefficient higher than 2%, a fourth measurement is provided, and one is discarded. We verified the calibration by measuring a 2500 μmol/L standard.

Atmospheric CO_2 was measured using a sensor (ITSENSOR RCO2-W) located inside the cabinet.

4.6. Speciation and Phase Equilibria Simulation

The supersaturation Ω of aragonite has been calculated with the CO2SYS Excel Macro version 2.5 [42], using salinity, temperature, DIC, and pH as input data to characterize the carbonate system. The software was set on the pH total scale, using constants from Mehrbach [43] refit by Dickson and Millero [44] for the carbonate system, Dickson [45] for $KHSO_4$, and Uppström [46] for B_T. Practical salinity was calculated from the measured conductivity [47]. The calculation of Ω in CO2SYS does not consider the variation of Ca^{2+} due to the dissolution of $Ca(OH)_2$ and precipitation of $CaCO_3$, so the value was corrected as suggested by Moras et al. [7].

For the experiments in artificial seawater, a set of simulations was performed to determine the concentrations of $NaHCO_3$. The aim was to ensure that Ω of aragonite did not exceed 5, i.e., the threshold value above which seawater is so oversaturated as to cause the precipitation of carbonates and the consequent release of CO_2 into the atmosphere [8]. These simulations were performed with PHREEQC software version 3.7.0 [48], with the dataset "phreeqc.dat".

5. Conclusions

We have presented a series of experiments on bicarbonate-enriched seawater, including both natural and artificial variants. The aim was to assess the factors affecting the stability and overall efficiency of the storage process, against adverse mechanisms such as CO_2 degassing and precipitation of carbonate minerals [see e.g., Equation (3)].

The experiments on natural seawater presented in this work enable us to conclude that, for carbon additions up to 1500 μmol/L, the carbonate system and the carbon storage efficiency are stable over time. Mixing seawater with calcium bicarbonate solutions prepared with the Limenet® process results in stable preservation of CO_2 for over three months. Notably, the duration of these experiments is almost unprecedented for this kind of study. On the other hand, higher concentrations (with total DIC of ca. 4100 μmol/L, equivalent to a carbon addition of about 1800 μmol/L) may lead to precipitation and loss of efficiency. Experiments on artificial seawater, treated with solid $NaHCO_3$, show precipitation and degassing for an increase in carbon content of ca. 1200 μmol/L, corresponding to a total DIC of 3200 μmol/L.

Considering the uncertainties of our measurements and environmental variance, we may conclude that a safe limit for the increase in carbon content in our seawater samples is about 1000 μmol/L. It is also important to consider that the precipitation observed above this threshold occurs only after several days. In a real-world application in a marine environment, this delay is likely sufficient to achieve significant dilution and avoid this pitfall, even for higher DIC additions.

Supplementary Materials: The following supporting information can be downloaded at: https://www.mdpi.com/article/10.3390/molecules29174069/s1. The Supporting Material containing the data related to this study is available as a zipped Excel File.

Author Contributions: Conceptualization, G.C., S.C. (Stefano Cappello), S.C. (Stefano Caserini), P.M. and G.R.; data curation, F.C., S.J.A. and S.V.; formal analysis, G.R. and S.V.; investigation G.C., S.C. (Stefano Cappello), F.C., S.J.A. and S.V.; methodology, S.J.A., P.M. and S.V.; supervision, P.M. and G.R.; writing—original draft preparation, F.P.C., F.C., S.J.A. and S.V.; writing—review and editing, S.C. (Stefano Caserini), P.M. and G.R. All authors have read and agreed to the published version of the manuscript.

Funding: The experiments: whose results are presented in this paper, are funded partly by Limenet®, partly by a contract of Hyrogas SIA (Latvia) with the Politecnico di Milano. The work of S.J.A. is funded by MUR with a DM117 scholarship.

Institutional Review Board Statement: Not applicable.

Informed Consent Statement: Not applicable.

Data Availability Statement: One Excel file containing the data related to this study is included within the supporting information.

Acknowledgments: The authors thank CSSN—Centro di Supporto e Sperimentazione Navale that host the experimental facility in La Spezia.

Conflicts of Interest: Some authors (Francesco Pietro Campo, Giovanni Cappello, Stefano Cappello, Federico Comazzi) are affiliated with Limenet®, which owns the patent (PCT/IB2022/051464) of the process producing the marine bicarbonate solution analyzed in this study. The remaining authors have no conflicts of interest to declare.

Appendix A

Table A1. Saturation state (Ω) of aragonite for SN1 set of samples over time.

Time (d)	SW	SN1-7510	SN1-3760	SN1-2500	SN1-1500	SN1-680	SN1-360	SN1-70
1	4.21	8.94	9.91	8.11	6.46	5.12	4.60	4.25
4	4.30	8.21	9.67	10.20	7.73	5.82	5.08	4.53
18	4.03	4.25	4.22	6.33	7.61	5.41	5.01	4.10
25	4.20	3.82	3.96	5.80	8.05	6.03	5.09	4.51
39	3.69	2.33	2.81	4.49	7.72	5.65	4.81	4.34
61	3.34	2.65	3.05	3.95	7.14	5.01	4.76	3.99
82	3.69	2.48	3.05	3.53	7.88	5.68	5.37	4.81
90	4.60	2.99	3.44	4.26	9.18	6.50	6.68	5.57

Table A2. Saturation state (Ω) of aragonite for SN2 set of samples over time.

Time (d)	SW	SN2-5650	SN2-2820	SN2-1880	SN2-1130	SN2-510	SN2-270	SN2-60
1	4.21	7.88	8.21	6.83	5.93	4.92	4.61	4.42
4	4.30	8.20	10.39	8.79	7.11	5.45	5.03	4.58
18	4.03	4.75	5.45	7.53	6.64	5.01	4.36	4.07
25	4.20	4.07	4.99	7.17	7.45	5.58	4.97	4.50
39	3.69	3.03	3.46	5.58	6.08	4.84	4.78	4.23
61	3.34	3.09	3.19	7.72	5.48	4.31	3.99	3.50
82	3.69	3.48	3.73	9.76	7.09	5.35	4.69	4.32
90	4.60	3.37	3.80	10.39	8.00	6.12	5.71	5.10

Table A3. Data from SA experiments. Each row refers to a single experiment. Δ_{DIC} is the addition of $NaHCO_3$. pH_f is the final pH. (TA_f-TA_i) and (DIC_f-DIC_i) are the differences between the final values of TA and DIC and those referred to measurements taken just after the addition of bicarbonate. $CO_{2,f}-CO_{2,i}$ indicates the variation of CO_2 in the gas phase, expressed as μmol of gaseous CO_2 per L of solution volume. $\Delta_{C,tot}$ is the total variation of carbon in the system, considering the atmosphere and the solution contribution. Ω_{Ar} is the calculated aragonite saturation state, at the beginning of each experiment, right after the bicarbonate addition.

Δ_{DIC} (μmol/L)	pH_f	TA_f-TA_i (μeq/L)	$CO_{2,f}$--$CO_{2,I}$ (μmol/L)	DIC_f--DIC_i (μmol/L)	$\Delta_{C,tot}$ (μmol/L)	Ω_{Ar}
0	8.03	18	70	−92	−22	2.58
0	7.93	68	57	−94	−37	2.28
400	7.98	116	105	−122	−17	2.96
400	7.96	−16	149	−129	20	2.53
800	8.00	112	66	−169	−103	3.37
800	8.01	−4	66	−143	−77	3.71

Table A4. Average, standard deviation, and averaged percentage variation (AV%) for SN1 of DIC and TA during the three months of sample analysis.

Δ_{DIC}	DIC (μmol/L)	AV%	TA (μmol/L)	AV%
0	2483 ± 87	4%	2661 ± 92	3%
7510	3294 ± 2035	62%	3373 ± 1950	58%
3760	2935 ± 1106	38%	3079 ± 1120	36%
2500	3135 ± 644	21%	3348 ± 652	19%
1500	3633 ± 169	5%	3910 ± 199	5%
680	3036 ± 116	4%	3237 ± 193	6%
360	2915 ± 206	7%	3085 ± 239	8%
70	2705 ± 199	7%	2883 ± 241	8%

Table A5. Average, standard deviation, and averaged percentage variation (AV%) for SN2 of DIC and TA during the three months of sample analysis.

Δ_{DIC}	DIC (μmol/L)	AV%	TA (μmol/L)	AV%
0	2483 ± 87	4%	2661 ± 92	3%
5650	3245 ± 1637	50%	3371 ± 1552	46%
2820	3021 ± 864	29%	3131 ± 928	30%
1880	3576 ± 471	13%	3842 ± 434	11%
1130	3358 ± 109	3%	3547 ± 155	4%
510	2888 ± 108	4%	3030 ± 95	3%
270	2751 ± 97	4%	2844 ± 106	4%
60	2594 ± 99	4%	2694 ± 118	4%

Table A6. Average, standard deviation, and averaged percentage variation (AV%) for SN3 of DIC and TA during the three months of sample analysis.

Δ_{DIC}	DIC (μmol/L)	AV%	TA (μmol/L)	AV%
0	2472 ± 77	3%	2686 ± 102	4%
2820	2645 ± 1003	38%	2789 ± 1081	39%
1130	3417 ± 110	3%	3758 ± 226	6%
510	2904 ± 94	3%	3134 ± 148	5%
270	2773 ± 88	3%	2936 ± 175	6%
60	2556 ± 91	4%	2756 ± 121	4%

References

1. Intergovernmental Panel on Climate Change (IPCC) Technical Summary. *Climate Change 2022—Mitigation of Climate Change: Working Group III Contribution to the Sixth Assessment Report of the Intergovernmental Panel on Climate Change*; Cambridge University Press: Cambridge, UK, 2023; pp. 51–148.
2. Celia, M.A.; Bachu, S.; Nordbotten, J.M.; Bandilla, K.W. Status of CO_2 Storage in Deep Saline Aquifers with Emphasis on Modeling Approaches and Practical Simulations. *Water Resour. Res.* **2015**, *51*, 6846–6892. [CrossRef]
3. Wang, N.; Akimoto, K.; Nemet, G.F. What Went Wrong? Learning from Three Decades of Carbon Capture, Utilization and Sequestration (CCUS) Pilot and Demonstration Projects. *Energy Policy* **2021**, *158*, 112546. [CrossRef]
4. Lane, J.; Greig, C.; Garnett, A. Uncertain Storage Prospects Create a Conundrum for Carbon Capture and Storage Ambitions. *Nat. Clim. Chang.* **2021**, *11*, 925–936. [CrossRef]
5. Global CCS Institute. *Global Status of CCS 2023*; Global CCS Institute: Melbourne, Australia, 2023.
6. Rau, G.H.; Caldeira, K. Enhanced Carbonate Dissolution: A means of sequestering waste CO_2 as ocean bicarbonate. *Energy Convers. Manag.* **1999**, *40*, 1803–1813. [CrossRef]
7. Moras, C.A.; Bach, L.T.; Cyronak, T.; Joannes-Boyau, R.; Schulz, K.G. Ocean Alkalinity Enhancement—Avoiding Runaway CaCO3 Precipitation during Quick and Hydrated Lime Dissolution. *Biogeosciences* **2022**, *19*, 3537–3557. [CrossRef]
8. Hartmann, J.; Suitner, N.; Lim, C.; Schneider, J.; Marín-Samper, L.; Arístegui, J.; Renforth, P.; Taucher, J.; Riebesell, U. Stability of Alkalinity in Ocean Alkalinity Enhancement (OAE) Approaches—Consequences for Durability of CO_2 Storage. *Biogeosciences* **2023**, *20*, 781–802. [CrossRef]
9. Caserini, S.; Cappello, G.; Righi, D.; Raos, G.; Campo, F.; De Marco, S.; Renforth, P.; Varliero, S.; Grosso, M. Buffered Accelerated Weathering of Limestone for Storing CO_2: Chemical Background. *Int. J. Greenh. Gas Control* **2021**, *112*, 103517. [CrossRef]
10. Ringham, M.; Hirtle, N.; Shaw, C.; Lu, X.; Herndon, J.; Carter, B.; Eisaman, M. A Comprehensive Assessment of Electrochemical Ocean Alkalinity Enhancement in Seawater: Kinetics, Efficiency, and Precipitation Thresholds. *EGUsphere* **2024**, preprint. [CrossRef]
11. Zeebe, R.E.; Wolf-Gladrow, D.A. *CO_2 in Seawater: Equilibrium, Kinetics, Isotopes*; Gulf Professional Publishing: Houston, TX, USA, 2001.
12. Renforth, P.; Henderson, G. Assessing Ocean Alkalinity for Carbon Sequestration. *Rev. Geophys.* **2017**, *55*, 636–674. [CrossRef]
13. Middelburg, J.J.; Soetaert, K.; Hagens, M. Ocean Alkalinity, Buffering and Biogeochemical Processes. *Rev. Geophys.* **2020**, *58*, e2019RG000681. [CrossRef]
14. Eisaman, M.D.; Geilert, S.; Renforth, P.; Bastianini, L.; Campbell, J.; Dale, A.W.; Foteinis, S.; Grasse, P.; Hawrot, O.; Löscher, C.R.; et al. Assessing the Technical Aspects of Ocean-Alkalinity-Enhancement Approaches. *State Planet* **2023**, *2-oae2023*, 1–29. [CrossRef]
15. Caldeira, K.; Rau, G.H. Accelerating Carbonate Dissolution to Sequester Carbon Dioxide in the Ocean: Geochemical Implications. *Geophys. Res. Lett.* **2000**, *27*, 225–228. [CrossRef]
16. Rau, G.H. CO_2 Mitigation via Capture and Chemical Conversion in Seawater. *Environ. Sci. Technol.* **2011**, *45*, 1088–1092. [CrossRef] [PubMed]
17. Chou, W.-C.; Gong, G.-C.; Hsieh, P.-S.; Chang, M.-H.; Chen, H.-Y.; Yang, C.-Y.; Syu, R.-W. Potential Impacts of Effluent from Accelerated Weathering of Limestone on Seawater Carbon Chemistry: A Case Study for the Hoping Power Plant in Northeastern Taiwan. *Mar. Chem.* **2015**, *168*, 27–36. [CrossRef]
18. Kirchner, J.S.; Berry, A.; Ohnemüller, F.; Schnetger, B.; Erich, E.; Brumsack, H.-J.; Lettmann, K.A. Reducing CO_2 Emissions of a Coal-Fired Power Plant via Accelerated Weathering of Limestone: Carbon Capture Efficiency and Environmental Safety. *Environ. Sci. Technol.* **2020**, *54*, 4528–4535. [CrossRef]
19. Kirchner, J.S.; Lettmann, K.A.; Schnetger, B.; Wolff, J.-O.; Brumsack, H.-J. Carbon Capture via Accelerated Weathering of Limestone: Modeling Local Impacts on the Carbonate Chemistry of the Southern North Sea. *Int. J. Greenh. Gas Control* **2020**, *92*, 102855. [CrossRef]
20. De Marco, S.; Varliero, S.; Caserini, S.; Cappello, G.; Raos, G.; Campo, F.; Grosso, M. Techno-Economic Evaluation of Buffered Accelerated Weathering of Limestone as a CO_2 Capture and Storage Option. *Mitig. Adapt. Strateg. Glob. Chang.* **2023**, *28*, 17. [CrossRef]
21. Limenet®, United States Patent and Trademark—Office. Apparatus and Method for Accelerated Dissolution of Carbonates with Buffered. European Patent PHPCT/IB2022/051464. WO2022175885, 29 July 2024.
22. Gattuso, J.-P.; Hansson, L. *Acidification: Background and History*; Oxford University Press: Oxford, UK, 2011.
23. Camatti, E.; Valsecchi, S.; Caserini, S.; Barbaccia, E.; Santinelli, C.; Basso, D.; Azzellino, A. Short-Term Impact Assessment of Ocean Liming: A Copepod Exposure Test. *Mar. Pollut. Bull.* **2024**, *198*, 115833. [CrossRef]
24. Fakhraee, M.; Li, Z.; Planavsky, N.J.; Reinhard, C.T. A Biogeochemical Model of Mineral-Based Ocean Alkalinity Enhancement: Impacts on the Biological Pump and Ocean Carbon Uptake. *Environ. Res. Lett.* **2023**, *18*, 044047. [CrossRef]
25. Schwinger, J.; Bourgeois, T.; Rickels, W. On the Emission-Path Dependency of the Efficiency of Ocean Alkalinity Enhancement. *Environ. Res. Lett.* **2024**, *19*, 074067. [CrossRef]
26. Paul, A.J.; Haunost, M.; Goldenberg, S.U.; Hartmann, J.; Sánchez, N.; Schneider, J.; Suitner, N.; Riebesell, U. Ocean Alkalinity Enhancement in an Open Ocean Ecosystem: Biogeochemical Responses and Carbon Storage Durability. *EGUsphere* **2024**, preprint. [CrossRef]

27. Álvarez, M.; Sanleón-Bartolomé, H.; Tanhua, T.; Mintrop, L.; Luchetta, A.; Cantoni, C.; Schroeder, K.; Civitarese, G. The CO_2 System in the Mediterranean Sea: A Basin Wide Perspective. *Ocean. Sci.* **2014**, *10*, 69–92. [CrossRef]
28. Suitner, N.; Faucher, G.; Lim, C.; Schneider, J.; Moras, C.A.; Riebesell, U.; Hartmann, J. Ocean Alkalinity Enhancement Approaches and the Predictability of Runaway Precipitation Processes—Results of an Experimental Study to Determine Critical Alkalinity Ranges for Safe and Sustainable Application Scenarios. *EGUsphere* **2024**, preprint. [CrossRef]
29. Schulz, K.G.; Bach, L.T.; Dickson, A.G. *Seawater Carbonate Chemistry Considerations for Ocean Alkalinity Enhancement Research: Theory, Measurements, and Calculations*; State Planet: SP 2; Copernicus Publications (EGU): Vienna, Austria, 2023; Chapter 2; pp. 1–14. [CrossRef]
30. Zhang, Z.; Xie, Y.; Xu, X.; Pan, H.; Tang, R. Transformation of Amorphous Calcium Carbonate into Aragonite. *J. Cryst. Growth* **2012**, *343*, 62–67. [CrossRef]
31. Millero, F.J. The Marine Inorganic Carbon Cycle. *Chem. Rev.* **2007**, *107*, 308–341. [CrossRef]
32. Available online: https://www.eea.europa.eu/en/analysis/indicators/ocean-acidification#:~:text=Seawater%20pH%20has%20decreased%20from,modifying%20ecosystem%20services%20like%20fisheries (accessed on 22 May 2024).
33. Intergovernmental Panel on Climate Change (IPCC) Technical Summary. *Climate Change 2021—The Physical Science Basis: Working Group I Contribution to the Sixth Assessment Report of the Intergovernmental Panel on Climate Change*; Cambridge University Press: Cambridge, UK, 2023; pp. 35–144.
34. Morse, J.W.; Arvidson, R.S.; Lüttge, A. Calcium Carbonate Formation and Dissolution. *Chem. Rev.* **2007**, *107*, 342–381. [CrossRef]
35. Marion, G.M.; Millero, F.J.; Feistel, R. Precipitation of Solid Phase Calcium Carbonates and Their Effect on Application of Seawater S A-T-P Models. *Ocean. Sci.* **2009**, *5*, 285–291. [CrossRef]
36. Jiang, L.; Feely, R.A.; Carter, B.R.; Greeley, D.J.; Gledhill, D.K.; Arzayus, K.M. Climatological Distribution of Aragonite Saturation State in the Global Oceans. *Glob. Biogeochem. Cycles* **2015**, *29*, 1656–1673. [CrossRef]
37. Zhang, D.; Lin, Q.; Xue, N.; Zhu, P.; Wang, Z.; Wang, W.; Ji, Q.; Dong, L.; Yan, K.; Wu, J.; et al. The Kinetics, Thermodynamics and Mineral Crystallography of $CaCO_3$ Precipitation by Dissolved Organic Matter and Salinity. *Sci. Total Environ.* **2019**, *673*, 546–552. [CrossRef]
38. Cyronak, T.; Schulz, K.G.; Jokiel, P.L. The Omega Myth: What Really Drives Lower Calcification Rates in an Acidifying Ocean. ICES. *J. Mar. Sci.* **2016**, *73*, 558–562. [CrossRef]
39. Varliero, S.; Buono, A.; Caserini, S.; Raos, G.; Macchi, P. Chemical Aspect of Ocean Liming for CO_2 Removal: Dissolution Kinetics of Calcium Hydroxide in Seawater. *ACS Eng. Au* **2024**, *4*, 422–431. [CrossRef]
40. Roy, R.N.; Roy, L.N.; Vogel, K.M.; Porter-Moore, C.; Pearson, T.; Good, C.E.; Millero, F.J.; Campbell, D.M. The Dissociation Constants of Carbonic Acid in Seawater at Salinities 5 to 45 and Temperatures 0 to 45 °C. *Mar. Chem.* **1993**, *44*, 249–267. [CrossRef]
41. Badocco, D.; Pedrini, F.; Pastore, A.; di Marco, V.; Marin, M.G.; Bogialli, S.; Roverso, M.; Pastore, P. Use of a Simple Empirical Model for the Accurate Conversion of the Seawater PH Value Measured with NIST Calibration into Seawater PH Scales. *Talanta* **2021**, *225*, 122051. [CrossRef] [PubMed]
42. Lewis, E.; Wallace, D. *MS Excel Program Developed for CO_2 System Calculations*; ORNL/CDIAC-593 105a (Co2sys_v2.5) [Code]; Carbon Dioxide Information Analysis Center Location: Oak Ridge, TN, USA, 2011.
43. Mehrbach, C.; Culberson, C.H.; Hawley, J.E.; Pytkowicx, R.M. Measurement of the Apparent Dissociation Constants of Carbonic Acid in Seawater at Atmospheric Pressure. *Limnol. Oceanogr.* **1973**, *18*, 897–907. [CrossRef]
44. Dickson, A.G.; Millero, F.J. A Comparison of the Equilibrium Constants for the Dissociation of Carbonic Acid in Seawater Media. Deep Sea Research Part A. *Oceanogr. Res. Pap.* **1987**, *34*, 1733–1743. [CrossRef]
45. Dickson, A.G. Standard Potential of the Reaction: AgCl(s) + 12H2(g) = Ag(s) + HCl(Aq), and the Standard Acidity Constant of the Ion HSO_4^- in Synthetic Sea Water from 273.15 to 318.15 K. *J. Chem. Thermodyn.* **1990**, *22*, 113–127. [CrossRef]
46. Uppström, L.R. The Boron/Chlorinity Ratio of Deep-Sea Water from the Pacific Ocean. *Deep. Sea Res. Oceanogr. Abstr.* **1974**, *21*, 161–162. [CrossRef]
47. Lewis, E.L.; Perkin, R.G. The Practical Salinity Scale 1978: Conversion of Existing Data. Deep Sea Research Part A. *Oceanogr. Res. Pap.* **1981**, *28*, 307–328. [CrossRef]
48. Parkhurst, D.; Appelo, C. Description of Input and Examples for PHREEQC Version 3: A Computer Program for Speciation, Batch-Reaction, One-Dimensional Transport, and Inverse Geochemical Calculations. *US Geol. Surv. Tech. Methods* **2013**, *6*, 497.

molecules

MDPI

Article

Viscosity Flow Curves of Agar and the *Bounded Ripening Growth* Model of the Gelation Onset

Vincenzo Villani

Dipartimento di Scienze, Università della Basilicata, 85100 Potenza, Italy; vincenzo.villani@unibas.it

Abstract: The gelation kinetics of agar aqueous solutions were studied by means of the viscosity flow curves using a coaxial Couette cylinder viscometer. The viscosity curves show an unusual sigmoidal trend or an exponential decay to a viscous steady state. An original theory of gelation kinetics was developed considering the coarsening of increasingly larger and more stable clusters due to Ostwald ripening and the breakup of clusters that were too large due to the instability of rotating large particles induced by the shear rate. The developed *Bounded Ripening Growth* model takes into account the trend of the viscosity curves by means of an autocatalytic process with negative feedback on aggregation according to the logistic kinetic equation, in which the constants $k_1(\gamma)$ and $k_-(\nu)$ are governed by the surface tension and shear rate, respectively. A dimensionless equation based on the difference between the Weber number and the ratio of the inverse kinetic constant to forward constant, accounts for the behavior of the dispersed phase in equilibrium conditions or far from the hydrostatic equilibrium.

Keywords: gelation; gelation onset; hydrogels; Weber number; logistic equation; agar solution; Ostwald ripening; rotating liquid drops

check for updates

Citation: Villani, V. Viscosity Flow Curves of Agar and the *Bounded Ripening Growth* Model of the Gelation Onset. *Molecules* **2024**, *29*, 1293. https://doi.org/10.3390/molecules29061293

Academic Editors: Fabio Ganazzoli, Giuseppina Raffaini and Borislav Angelov

Received: 14 February 2024
Revised: 11 March 2024
Accepted: 12 March 2024
Published: 14 March 2024

1. Introduction

The gelation (or *sol-gel* transition) of polymer solutions is a hot topic of scientific and technological interest [1]. In particular, the preparation of hydrogels is important in the food, cosmetic, pharmaceutical, medical and bioplastics industries; furthermore, it is fundamental in the fabrication of 3D scaffolds for tissue engineering [2–5]. From the rheological point of view there are many open problems, such as the optimization of the formulation, the control of the aggregation kinetics and the crosslinking of the polymer material [6].

The onset of gelation arises from the formation of a transient fluctuating network of particles interacting reversibly through short-range attractive interactions lightly exceeding the thermal energy kT, as in the Baxter sticky sphere model [7]. The average cluster size diverges strongly with time near gelation and, in an experimental system, the position of the gel point is associated with the inflection point on the viscosity flow curve or a substantial increase in the high-frequency storage modulus [8].

In this paper, the gelation onset of agar polymer solutions was studied by determining the viscosity curves as a function of time, $\eta = \eta(t; \nu, c, T)$, using a Couette coaxial cylinder rotational viscometer. The shear rate ν, concentration c, temperature T and rheological history during experiments were varied. The viscometry method has been widely used in the determination of the gelation time from the inflection point on the viscosity flow curve [9].

In general, the coarsening kinetics of dispersed clusters is given by the Ostwald ripening [10] according to the Voorhees equation [11]:

$$4\pi R^2 \frac{dR}{dt} = \mu \cdot J$$

$$J = -D \oint_S \nabla c \cdot dS$$

The equation represents the flow of matter across the surface cluster of radius R according to the first Fick equation, where μ is the molar volume of the aggregate and J is the diffusion flux integral. The equation is valid for both growing or dissolving particles, giving rise to an exponential growth of the aggregate phase at the expense of the smaller particles:

$$R^3 = R_0^3 \cdot \exp(k \cdot t)$$

The concentration B of the dispersed particles is given by the Kelvin equation [12], where B_∞ is the equilibrium concentration of the gel state and γ is the surface tension:

$$B(R) = B_\infty \cdot \exp(\frac{2\gamma \cdot \mu}{kT \cdot R})$$

The evolution of the particle size distribution function $f(t, R)$ is given by the partial differential equation of Alexandrov and Alexandrova [13], where D is the diffusion coefficient of particles:

$$\frac{\partial f(R,t)}{\partial t} + \frac{\partial}{\partial R}(\frac{dR}{dt} \cdot f) = \frac{\partial}{\partial R}(D \cdot f)$$

These theories take into account the asymptotic state of gelation process when larger clusters growth at the expense of smaller ones in an unbounded way.

In this work, an original coarsening model, which we call the *Bounded Ripening Growth* (BRG) of the aggregation of elementary particles at the onset of gelation has been developed, taking into account the surface tension of the dispersed particles (Laplace's equation), the instability of rotating liquid drops (Brown's equation) and the diffusive processes (Fick's first law) in which the larger and more stable particles grow at the expense of the smaller and more unstable particles, which dissolve in the elementary particles and diffuse below the action of the concentration gradient (Ostwald ripening). The dispersion viscosity is a linear function of the volume fraction of the dispersed phase according to the Einstein equation.

A logistic kinetics equation is obtained as a function of the concentration of the dispersed phase, in which the forward constant is controlled by the surface tension and the inverse constant by the applied shear rate.

2. Material and Methods Section

The aqueous solutions of agar (food additive E406) at 1 and 1.5% by weight are prepared at a temperature of 80 °C. Furthermore, the blend agar 1%–hyaluronic acid 0.5% (aqueous solution of sodium hyaluronate 1%) was considered.

The cooling of the samples to the target values of 60, 50, 45 and 40 °C was accomplished by coupling the Couette cell of the viscosimeter (ViscoQC Anton Paar, Anton Paar, Graz, Austria) to a heated and refrigerated circulating bath (Haake DC30, Thermo Haake, Karlsruhe, Germany). Viscosity flow curves of 1 h were collected with a time step of 30 s in the viscosity range of 100 mPa s. The rotational frequency of 60 or 30 rpm (revolutions per minute) was applied.

3. Experimental Section

When the aqueous solutions of agar at 1% or 1.5% are cooled to values of 45 or 50 °C, we observe the onset of the gelation transition, with a higher temperature for the more concentrated solution. At the gelling point, the solution becomes heterogeneous with the formation of dispersed aggregates, which gradually become larger until the formation of the gel phase, corresponding to a connected agarose chains network. The gelation kinetics are monitored via the viscosity flow curves $\eta = \eta(t)$. At the onset temperatures (45 °C for agar at 1% and 50 °C for agar at 1.5%), the curves show the appearance of an unusual sigmoidal trend towards a viscous steady state (Figure 1).

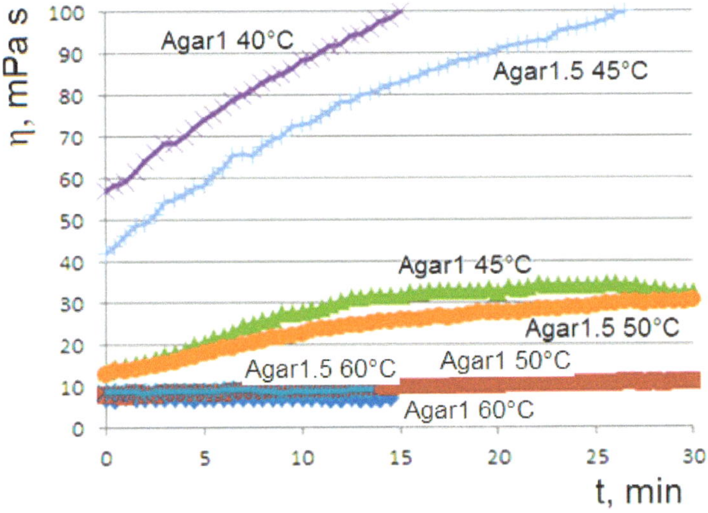

Figure 1. Viscosity flow curves at 60, 50, 45 and 40 °C for the 1% agar solution (*Agar*1 in labels) and at 60, 50 and 45 °C for the 1.5% agar (*Agar*1.5 in labels). The applied rotational speed is 60 rpm.

The dependence of the gelation kinetics on the shear rate was highlighted by the means of the viscosity curves at different rotational speeds; by increasing the shear rate, the achievement of the steady state in the gelation process is favored (Figure 2).

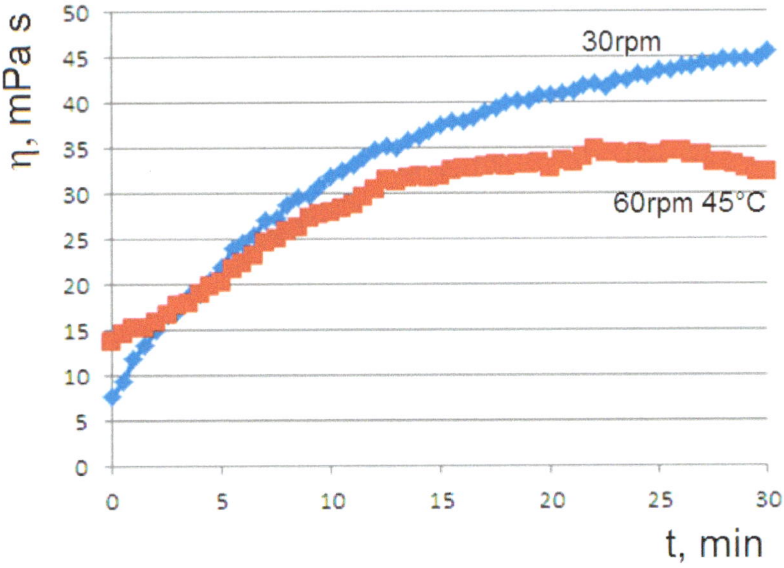

Figure 2. Viscosity flow curves at 45 °C for the 1% agar solution at rotational speeds of 60 (blue line) or 30 rpm (red).

The role played by the shear rate is demonstrated by the viscosity graph obtained after a pause in flow for a sufficiently long time (45 min): the flow–pause–flow experiment. In this first rheological history experiment, when the test resumes after the pause, the viscosity starts from high values due to the formation of the gel state. However, the viscosity rapidly decays, due to the applied shear rate, towards the viscous steady state observed in the initial curve (Figure 3). This behavior is explained later by the proposed model.

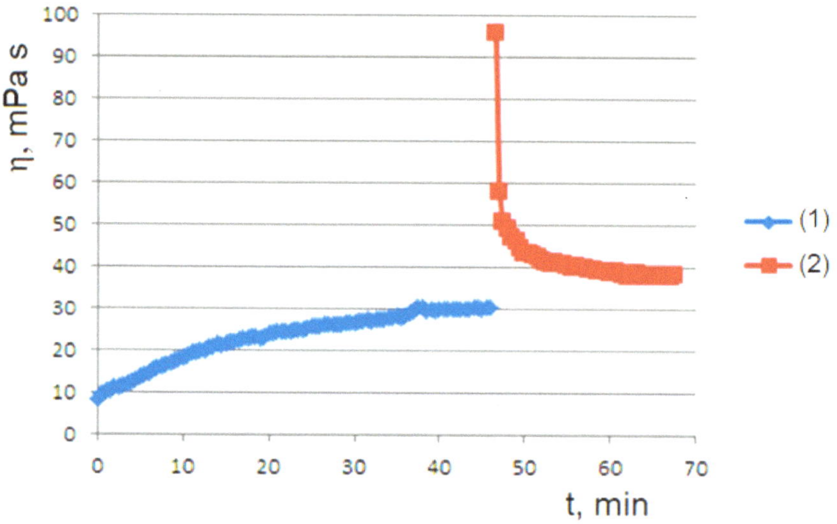

Figure 3. The rheological history experiment of flow–pause–flow: the initial viscosity curve (1) is followed by a 60 min pause and then by a final viscosity curve (2). An agar solution at 1% and a rotational speed of 60 rpm are used.

A second rheological history experiment of gelling–mixing–flow was carried out using a succession of viscometric curves interspersed with the mechanical homogenization of the sample. At 45 °C for the 1% sample (Figure 4), we obtain a series of curves that relax from top to bottom to steady states, highlighting that mechanical stirring has produced an initial concentration of dispersed phase greater than the final concentration $B_0 > B_\infty$ (supersaturated state). On the contrary, at 50 °C for the 1.5% sample (Figure 5), we obtain a series of curves that converge from bottom to top to steady states; this is consistent with an initial concentration of the dispersed phase that is lower than the final concentration $B_0 < B_\infty$ (undersaturated state), which occurs at a higher temperature. Furthermore, in both cases, we observe convergence to progressively higher values of equilibrium concentration B_∞ by iterating the stirring–gelling cycle. In all cases, as we will see, the observed curves are consistent with the *Bounded Ripening Growth* model proposed in this work.

The trend of the viscosity curves is confirmed in two-component hydrogels. Figure 6 shows the curves of the blend agar 1%–hyaluronic acid 0.5% *versus* the agar 1% reference solution at temperatures from 60 to 40 °C. At 45 °C, the sigmoidal curves of the two systems are perfectly overlapped, indicating that the long hyaluronic chains adsorbed on the agarose network do not interfere in the clusters coarsening.

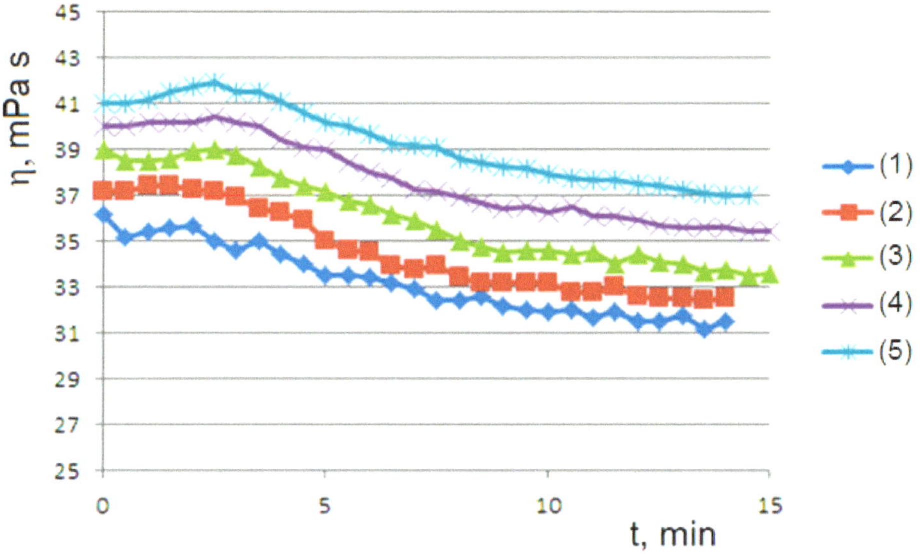

Figure 4. The rheological history experiment of gelling–mixing–flow: a succession of viscosity curves (from (1) to (5)) from the bottom to top at 45 °C with homogenization of the sample at the end of each test. An agar solution at 1% and rotational speed of 60 rpm are used.

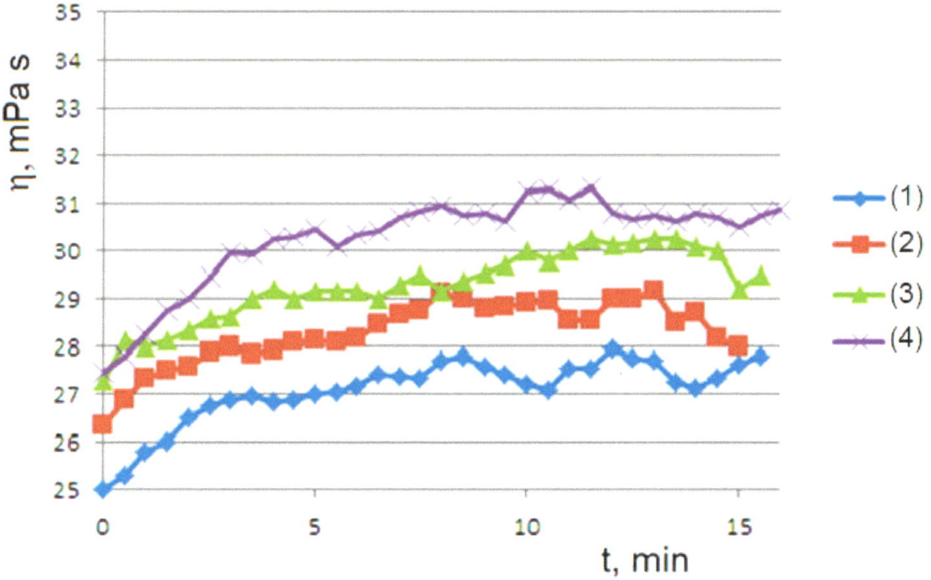

Figure 5. The rheological history experiment of gelling–mixing–flow: a succession of viscosity curves (from (1) to (4)) from the bottom to top at 50 °C with homogenization of the sample at the end of each test. An agar solution at 1% and rotational speed of 60 rpm are used.

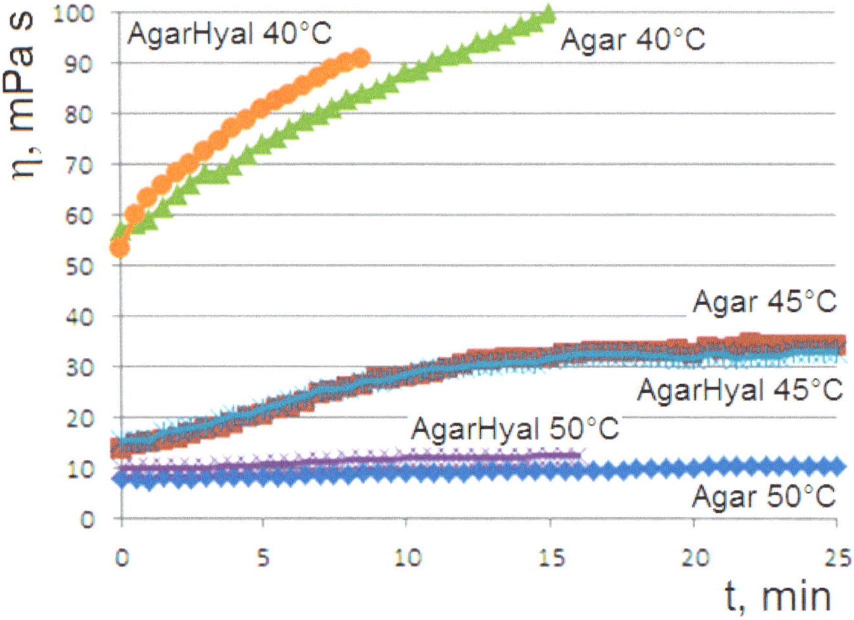

Figure 6. Viscosity curves at 50, 45 and 40 °C (decreasing from the bottom to top) for the blend (agar 1%–hyaluronic acid 0.5% aqueous solution) (*AgarHyal* in the label) *vs* the agar 1% reference solution (*Agar* in the label). The applied rotational speed is 60 rpm.

4. Theoretical Section

4.1. Bounded Ripening Growth Model

The *Bounded Ripening Growth* model of gelation is developed, taking into account the growth of aggregates due to the driving force of surface tension according to Ostwald ripening and the breakup of aggregates via negative shear rate feedback, due to the instability of clusters that are too large. Finally, the viscous steady state given by the formation–destruction equilibrium of the aggregates is reached [14–16].

The agarose macromolecules at a temperature of about 50 °C (depending on the concentration of the aqueous solution) couple (coil-to-helix transition), giving rise to the double helix elementary sol particles A [17]. The double helices have pending chains that allow the formation of increasingly large clusters B, according to exponential coarsening.

Let us consider the proposed *Bounded Ripening Growth* model. In the first step of gelation, the minimization of the surface free energy of the system prevails, which favors the growth of the clusters. For simplicity, we assume Laplace's law for spherical particles dispersed in the continuous medium (1), where Δp is the Laplace pressure across the particle surface:

$$\Delta p = \frac{2 \cdot \gamma}{R}$$

The *Ostwald ripening* mechanism is the basis of the increase in the size of the dispersed particles (2) (Figure 7).

The smaller *sol* aggregates tend to spontaneously dissolve (the feedforward effect) due to the high Laplace pressure and low surface tension, freeing the elementary particles; therefore, the free particles spread in the aqueous medium towards the larger clusters and down the concentration gradient in accordance with Fick's first Law; finally, their adsorption reduces the interfacial energy of the system.

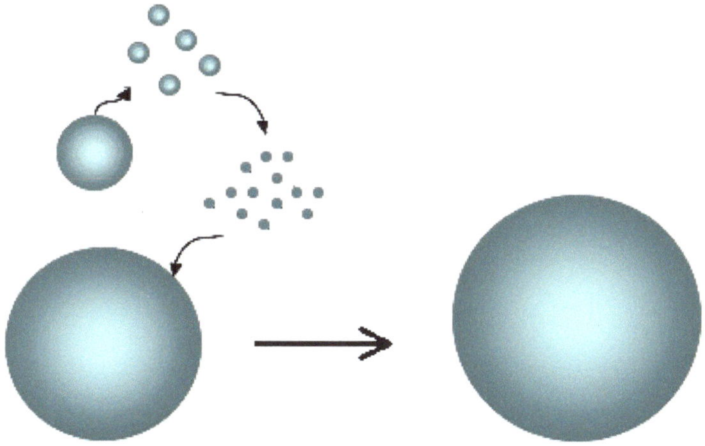

Figure 7. Picture of the Ostwald ripening mechanism: the small particles dissolve in the constituent elements which re-aggregate on the larger particles, determining their unbounded growth.

In general, the viscosity of dispersions is governed by the Einstein equation

$$\eta(\phi) = \eta_0(1 + \frac{5}{2} \cdot \phi)$$

where η_0 is the viscosity of the continuous phase, in which the aggregates are dispersed, and ϕ is the volume fraction of the dispersed phase.

The volume fraction of the aggregates is given by

$$\phi = \frac{V_B}{V}$$

where V_B is the volume of the dispersed phase and V is the total volume of the dispersion. Therefore, the *volume fraction* is proportional to the *concentration* of the dispersed phase and, assuming the unit density, coincide:

$$\phi = \frac{V_B}{V} = \frac{\rho M_B}{V} = \rho \cdot B = B$$

The BRG model consists of three steps depending on the degree of the coarsening progress. For still-small aggregates, the unbounded growth aggregation mechanism (Ostwald's ripening) prevails (1); when the aggregates have become sufficiently large, the negative feedback is triggered the breakup of the clusters due to applied shear rate (2), and the elementary particles adsorbed by the growing clusters are released. Then, the loose particles aggregate again, and so on. Finally, a steady state is reached in which the processes of formation (the feedforward of the surface tension) and destruction (the negative feedback of the shear rate) reach equilibrium (3). The result, as we will see, is an asymptotic plateau trend of the cluster concentration in agreement with the observed sigmoidal viscosimetric curves.

In the initial ripening step, we represent the gelation process by an autocatalytic process, in which the elementary particle A "reacts" with the cluster B_n to give the cluster larger by one unit B_{n+1} in the coarsening process:

$$A + B_n \rightarrow B_{n+1}$$

Figure 8 schematizes the autocatalytic process in which we assume the concentration of the species A is constant.

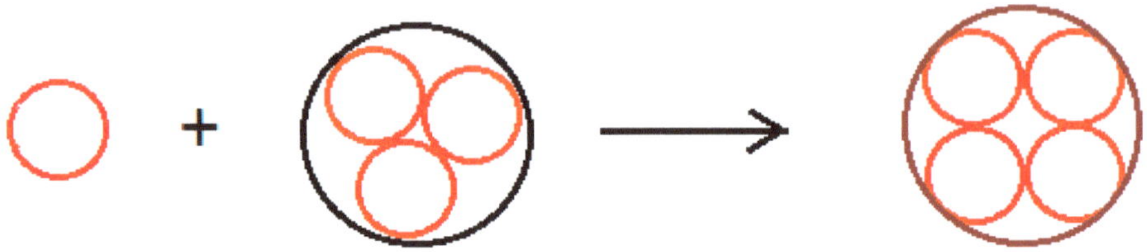

Figure 8. Picture of the autocatalytic process $A + B_n \rightarrow B_{n+1}$.

This results in the first order kinetic equation are written as

$$\frac{dB}{dt} = k_1 \cdot B$$

The solution of which is the exponential growth of the concentration of the species B over time:

$$B(t) = B_0 \cdot \exp(k_1 \cdot t)$$

According to Einstein's equation, the viscosity of the dispersion also varies exponentially:

$$\eta(t) = \eta_0(1 + k_E \cdot B(t))$$

4.2. Instability of the Clusters

During the viscometric experiment, the shear stress τ on the fluid is proportional to the shear rate ν of the fluid according to Newton's law:

$$\tau = \eta \cdot \frac{du}{dt} = \eta \cdot \nu$$

where u is the linear flow rate.

Due to the shear rate, the dispersed aggregates experience a mechanical moment that keeps the particles rotating around the axis, passing through the center of gravity and perpendicular to the flow direction (vorticity axis); the instability of liquid rotating particles is the basis of the breakup mechanism of dispersed clusters that are too large.

The dynamics of an isolated rotating particle in the flow field was first addressed by Einstein [18] for the case of a newtonian medium. Under steady low shear, the sphere translates in the flow direction, while rotating around the vorticity axis. Thus, in a frame translating with the sphere center, the sphere just rotates in time with a constant angular velocity ω [19].

Einstein, and subsequently Jeffery [20], demonstrated that under no-slip boundary conditions at the particle surface, the angular velocity is independent of particle size $\omega = \frac{\nu}{2}$. Furthermore, the rotating spherical particle of radius R experiences a centrifugal force (gyrostatic pressure) with a magnitude at the surface dependent on the size and angular velocity $F_c = m\omega^2 R$.

Plateau [21] found that as the angular velocity increased, a liquid sphere suspended in a liquid medium progressed through a sequence of shapes which evolve to ellipsoidal and lobed shapes and, finally, breakup. These experimental works have been repeated with basically the same outcome [22,23].

The equilibrium shapes of a rotating drop held together by surface tension are governed by the Brown and Scriven nonlinear differential equation [24]:

$$2\gamma \cdot \nabla^2 R(r, \vartheta, \phi) = \Delta p + \frac{1}{2}\omega^2 r^2 \cos^2 \vartheta \cdot \Delta\rho$$

$R(r, \vartheta, \phi)$ is the surface of the particle represented by the surface vector $\vec{R}$ in spherical coordinates; γ is the surface tension; $\Delta\rho$ is the density difference between the liquid of the drop and the surrounding fluid; ω is angular velocity of the drop; $r\cos(\vartheta)$ is the perpendicular distance from a point on its surface to the axis of rotation; and Δp is the Laplace pressure across the drop surface.

As the angular velocity increases, the particle surface vector $R(r, \vartheta, \phi)$ progresses through a sequence of shapes, ellipsoidal axisymmetric at first, then no-axisymmetric and lobed shape. The no-axisymmetric shapes are stable at low rotational rates but lose stability at the bifurcation to lobed drops. Then, we have two lobed shapes: the symmetrical Darwin's dumbbell shape [25] or the asimmetrical Poincarè pear shape [26]. In any case, they undergo fission into two ovoid particles of the same or different size [27].

What happens as the size of the rotating particles increases while keeping the angular velocity constant? This is what concerns the ultimate fate of the particles in our dispersion. The aggregates all rotate with the same angular velocity; however, the angular momentum is greater for larger particles. This means that the instability of the larger aggregates is favored for the same angular rotation. By means of the rotation of the dispersed aggregates and by the low surface tension of the aggregates, they undergo beakup at a critical dimension, thus, establishing a negative feedbeak loop to the formation of larger aggregates. On the other hand, the particles that are too small are unstable at Laplace pressure and dissolve into the constituent particles. The free elementary particles reaggregate according to the Ostwald mechanism and fuel the equilibrium of the *Bounded Ripening Growth* (Figure 9).

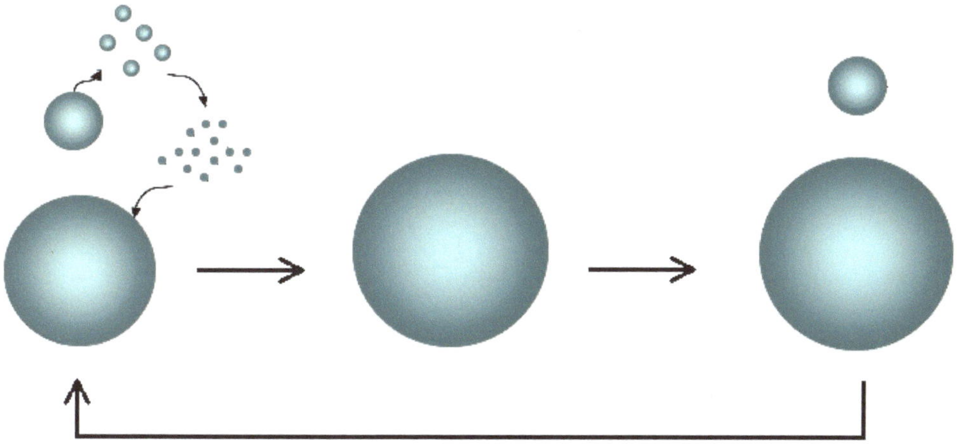

Figure 9. Picture of the autocatalytic mechanism of *Bounded Ripening Growth* in which the unbounded growth of Ostwald ripening is bounded by the fission of larger aggregates.

4.3. *Kinetic Equation of the Bounded Ripening Growth*

When the aggregates break down, a reverse process with negative feedback overlaps with the direct formation process with the feedforward effect. In this way, the exponential growth is replaced by bounded growth kinetics of the logistic type, according to the equilibrium equation (Figure 10)

$$A + B_n \leftrightarrow B_{n+1}$$

The kinetic constant becomes dependent on the concentration of the clusters B, on the forward k_1 and reverse k_- kinetic constants:

$$k(t) = k_1 - k_- \cdot B(t)$$

This gives rise to the logistic kinetic equation with the constants controlled by surface tension $k_1(\gamma)$ and shear rate $k_-(\nu)$:

$$\frac{dB}{dt} = (k_1 - k_- \cdot B) \cdot B$$

$$\frac{dB}{dt} = k_1(\gamma) \cdot B - k_-(\nu) \cdot B^2$$

The logistic non-linear differential equation admits the sigmoid function (or sigmoidal curve) $B(t)$ as the analytical solution:

$$B(t) = \frac{B_\infty}{1 + \frac{B_\infty - B_0}{B_0} \cdot \exp(-k_1 \cdot t)}$$

where k_1 incorporates the concentration of the species A, considered constant, and B_∞ is the concentration at equilibrium:

$$B_\infty = \frac{k_1}{k_-} = \frac{k_+ \cdot A_0}{k_-}$$

The solution depends on the initial conditions. For $B_0 < B_\infty$, we have a sigmoidal trend of $B(t)$ and, consequently, of $\eta(t)$; however, for $B_0 > B_\infty$ we have an exponential decay to the equilibrium value in excellent agreement with the observed viscosity curves (Figure 11).

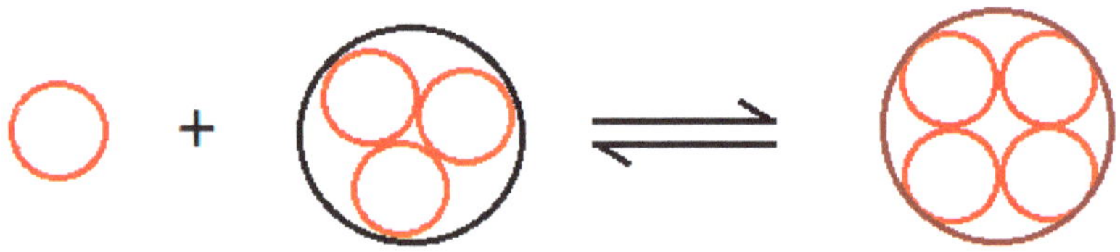

Figure 10. Picture of the bounded autocatalytic process $A + B_n \leftrightarrow B_{n+1}$.

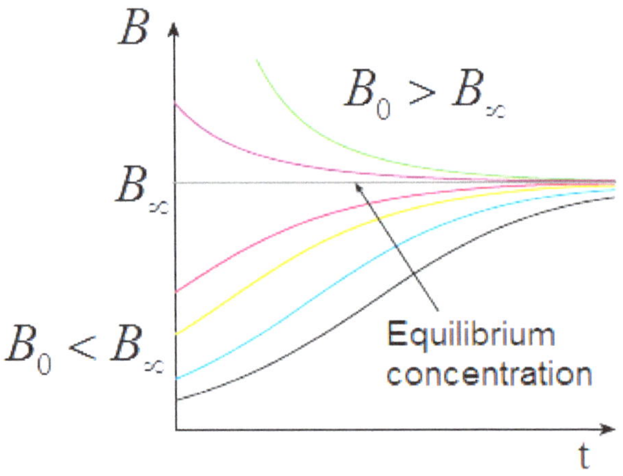

Figure 11. Solutions of the logistic equation: sigmoidal trend for $B_0 < B_\infty$ or exponential decay for $B_0 > B_\infty$.

The viscosity curve of the sample homogenized at 45 °C presents the typical relaxation of a supersaturated solution in agreement with the proposed logistic model. However, the kinetics converge to increasingly higher equilibrium concentrations by iterating the homogenization treatment.

Homogenizing the material at 50 °C, we observe the characteristic viscosity curves of an undersaturated solution, with a progressive increase in the equilibrium concentration by iterating the treatment.

Therefore, the cluster disaggregation modifies the final equilibrium B_∞ by varying the initial concentration A_0 of the free species by increasing its concentration at 45 °C or decreasing it at 50 °C.

4.4. Dimensionless Sol-Gel Equilibrium Equation

At hydrostatic equilibrium, the Laplace pressure and the shear stress in the Newtonian flow give the constitutive equation:

$$\eta\nu - \frac{2\gamma}{R} = 0$$

Then,

$$We = \frac{R \cdot \eta\nu}{2\gamma} = 1$$

where the *Weber number We* is defined by the ratio of shear stress to surface tension [28]. At steady state, the creation–destruction processes balance and the Weber number is unity:

$$We - 1 = 0$$

On the contrary, far from hydrostatic equilibrium, in conditions in which surface tension and, therefore, the creation process prevails (at low shear rates or for small particles), we have

$$We < 0$$

At enough high shear rates or particle sizes, the destruction process prevails, and we have

$$We > 0$$

If J is the flow of particles then J_+ and J_- are the transport of matter into the cluster or out of the cluster, respectively, where the positive flow is representative of aggregation; negative flow is the disaggregation of the clusters; and zero is the steady state. For $We > 1$, dispersed particles undergo breakup with the release of small particles.

The set of constitutive equations and inequations of the Weber number

$$We - 1 = 0 \qquad We - 1 < 0 \qquad We - 1 > 0$$

are reduced to a single dimensionless equation based on the difference between the Weber number and the number Wi:

$$We - Wi = 0$$

where Wi is given by

$$Wi = \frac{J_-}{J_+} = \frac{k_-}{k_+} = \frac{1}{K} = \frac{A_0}{B_\infty}$$

where K is the equilibrium constant of reaction.

5. Discussion Section: Experiments vs. Theory

Consistent with the viscosity curve of Figure 1, the *Bounded Ripening Growth* predicts a sigmoidal trend in the concentration of the dispersed phase during the gelation. Consistent with the solutions of the logistic equation of Figure 11, the sigmoidal trend depends significantly on the initial concentration of the dispersed particles.

The negative feedback due to the shear rate as predicted by the model is consistent with the viscosity curves of Figure 2; as the shear rate increases, the viscosity is reduced and the final steady state is favored.

The solutions of the logistic equation account for the observed rheological histories. They depend on the initial conditions for $B_0 < B_\infty$ (undersaturated dispersion), where we have a sigmoidal trend of predicted $B(t)$ and observed $\eta(t)$; for $B_0 > B_\infty$ (supersaturated dispersion), we have an exponential decay to the equilibrium value. A supersaturated state occurs in the flow–pause–flow experiment of Figure 3; during the pause, the concentration of the dispersed phase increases in an unbounded way, and the expected exponential decay is observed in the final flow curve. Furthermore, the expected trends are observed in the flow curves of Figures 4 and 5, which run from the undersaturated state at 45 °C or from the supersaturated state at 50 °C after homogenization of the clusters. Furthermore, the kinetics converge to increasingly higher equilibrium concentrations in both cases in agreement with the proposed model: the disaggregation of the hydrogel modifies the final equilibrium B_∞ values depending on the concentration of the free species A_0, which is increased in both cases due to the homogenization process.

The gelation of the two-component agarose-hyaluronic chains of Figure 6 is consistent with the gelation logistic kinetics. The deep compatibility of these systems of increasing complexity is of technological interest.

The microscopic mechanism of *Bounded Ripening Growth* is the basis of macroscopic logistic kinetics, and the low surface tension of the particles of growing hydrogels accounts for the instability of the large particles at the applied shear rates.

The determination of the kinetic constants of the logistic equation that governs the gelation kinetics and the extension of the theory to further and more complex experimental cases are the subject of ongoing work.

The study of viscosity flow curves allows determining the onset of the sol-gel transition in a simple way through the appearance of the characteristic viscous steady state: this may have useful real-life applications. The behavior is viscous, as it is related to the formation of a fluid dispersion in which the particles are isolated and do not form a connected network. At temperatures lower than the onset value, the formation of an extended network finally prevails and the transition from the viscous dispersion to the viscoelastic gel state occurs, whose behavior is being studied using viscoelastic characterization according to loss and storage moduli.

6. Conclusions

The complexity of the gelation kinetics of aqueous agarose-based solutions was addressed from a viscometric and theoretical point of view. The sigmoidal trend of the viscosity curves as a function of time and temperature, the dependence of the trend of the curves on the applied shear rate and rheological histories were highlighted. The kinetics of the transition were described using an autocatalytic process with negative feedback. A logistic equation was obtained as a function of the concentration of the dispersed phase, in which the forward constant is governed by the surface tension of the dispersed particles, and the inverse constant is governed by the applied shear rate:

$$\frac{\partial B}{\partial t} = k_1(\gamma) \cdot B - k_-(\nu) \cdot B^2$$

The solutions of the logistic equation account for the trend in the sigmoidal or exponential decay viscosity curves.

The gelation process, at equilibrium and far from equilibrium, is controlled by the dimensionless equation

$$We - Wi = 0$$

in which the hydrostatic balance is given by the difference between the Weber number We and the dimensionless ratio of the inverse kinetic constant Wi.

The driving force of the aggregation process is due to the minimization of the surface tension of the dispersed phase according to the Ostwald ripening. However, an antagonistic factor is due to the instability of enough large aggregates that deform and eventually breakup, releasing small aggregates that are unstable from the point of view of the surface tension. Thus, unstable large aggregates to the shear rate represent the bounding growth factor, and unstable small aggregates to the surface tension is the aggregate growth factor. In this way, a viscous steady state is due to small particle ripening and disaggregation due to the size instability of the clusters that are too large.

In general, Ostwald ripening is the microscopic process underlying the autocatalytic process with indefinitely growing matter transport, described by a first-order kinetic equation. However, as in our case, negative feedback is present, a bounded autocatalytic process results, and given by the microscopic process of bounded ripening growth, the observed logistic kinetics corresponds to this microscopic process.

The complete description of the *Bounded Ripening Growth* at the microscopic scale requires a system of differential equations of Ostwald ripening and the Laplace equation of rotating particles. To take into account the deformation of the spherical particles and the diffusion-controlled growth process, it is necessary to consider equations in which the particle surface vector is time dependent $R(r, \vartheta, \phi, t)$. Therefore, we must write

$$2\gamma \cdot \nabla^2 R(r, \vartheta, \phi, t) = \Delta p + \frac{1}{2}\omega^2 r^2 \cos^2\vartheta \cdot \Delta\rho$$

$$\frac{\partial R(r, \vartheta, \phi, t)}{\partial t} = \frac{\nu}{4\pi R^2} D \oint_S \nabla c \cdot dS$$

We have a complex system of partial differential equations whose analytical and numerical solutions are the subject of a work in progress.

Funding: This research received no external funding.

Informed Consent Statement: Informed consent was obtained from all subjects involved in the study.

Data Availability Statement: Data are contained within the article.

Conflicts of Interest: The authors declare no conflict of interest.

References

1. Ahmed, E.M. Hydrogel Preparation, Characterization, and Applications: A Review. *J. Adv. Res.* **2015**, *6*, 105. [CrossRef]
2. Nath, P.C.; Debnath, S.; Sharma, M.; Sridhar, K.; Nayak, P.K.; Inbaraj, B.S. Recent advances in cellulose-based hydrogels: Food applications. *Foods* **2023**, *12*, 350. [CrossRef]
3. Nath, P.C.; Debnath, S.; Shrindkar, K.; Inbaraj, B.S.; Nayak, P.K.; Sharma, M. A comprehensive review of food hydrogels: Principles, formation mechanisms, microstructure and its applications. *Gels* **2023**, *9*, 1. [CrossRef]
4. Wang, H.; Wang, X.; Lai, K.; Yan, J. Stimulus-responsive DNA biosensors for food safety detection. *Biosensors* **2023**, *13*, 320. [CrossRef]
5. Gyles, D.A. A review of the designs and prominent biomedical advances of natural and synthetic hydrogel formulations. *Eur. Polym. J.* **2017**, *88*, 373. [CrossRef]
6. Villani, V. *Lezioni di Chimica e Tecnologia dei Polimeri*; Aracne Editrice: Rome, Italy, 2021.
7. Baxter, R.J. Percus–Yevick Equation for Hard Spheres with Surface Adhesion. *J. Chem. Phys.* **1968**, *49*, 2770. [CrossRef]
8. Dickinson, E. Hydrocolloids at interfaces and the influence on the properties of dispersed systems. *Food Hydrocoll.* **2003**, *17*, 25. [CrossRef]
9. Liu, Y.; Dai, C.; Wang, K.; Zhao, M.; Zhao, G.; Yang, S.; You, Q. New insights into the hydroquinone–hexamethylenetetramine gel system for water shut-off treatment in high temperature reservoirs. *J. Ind. Eng. Chem.* **2016**, *35*, 20. [CrossRef]
10. Beenakker, C.W.J.; Ross, J. Theory of Ostwald ripening for open Systems. *J. Chem. Phys.* **1985**, *83*, 4710. [CrossRef]
11. Voorhees, P.W. The theory of Ostwald ripening. *J. Stat. Phys.* **1985**, *38*, 231. [CrossRef]
12. Lifshitz, M.; Slyozov, V.V. The Kinetics of Precipitation from Supersaturated *Solid* Solutions. *J. Phys. Chem. Solids* **1961**, *19*, 35. [CrossRef]

13. Alexandrov, D.V.; Alexandrova, I.V. From nucleation and coarsening to coalescence in metastable liquids. *Phil. Trans. R. Soc. A* **2020**, *378*, 20190247. [CrossRef] [PubMed]
14. Blaser, S. Forces on the surface of small ellipsoidal particles immersed in a linear flow field. *Chem. Eng. Sci.* **2002**, *57*, 515. [CrossRef]
15. Higashitani, K.; Inada, N.; Ochi, T. Floc breakup along centerline of contractile flow to orifice. *Colloids Surf.* **1991**, *56*, 13. [CrossRef]
16. Sonntag, R.C.; Russel, W.B. Structure and breakup of flocs subjected to fluid stresses: II. *Theory. J. Colloid Interface Sci.* **1987**, *115*, 378. [CrossRef]
17. Dai, B.; Matsukawa, S. NMR studies of the gelation mechanism and molecular dynamics in agar solutions. *Food Hydrocoll.* **2012**, *26*, 181. [CrossRef]
18. Einstein, A. Eine neue Bestimmung der Moleküldimensionen. *Ann. Phys.* **1906**, *19*, 289. [CrossRef]
19. D'Avino, G.; Hulsen, M.A.; Snijkers, F.; Vermant, J.; Greco, F.; Maffettone, P.L. Rotation of a sphere in a viscoelastic liquid subjected to shear flow. Part I: Simulation results. *J. Rheol.* **2008**, *52*, 1331.
20. Jeffery, G.B. The motion of ellipsoidal particles immersed in a viscous fluid. *Proc. Roy. Soc. Lond. A* **1922**, *102*, 161.
21. Plateau, J. *Statique Experimentale et Theorique des Liquides Soumis aux Seules Forces Moleculaires*; Gauthier-Villars: Paris, France, 1873.
22. Lee, C.P.; Anilkumar, A.V.; Hmelo, A.B.; Wang, T.G. Equilibrium of liquid drops under the effects of rotation and acoustic flattening. *J. Fluid Mech.* **1998**, *354*, 43. [CrossRef]
23. Aussillous, P.; Quéré, D. Liquid marbles. *Nature* **2001**, *411*, 925. [CrossRef] [PubMed]
24. Brown, R.A.; Scriven, L.E. The shape and stability of rotating liquid drops. *Proc. Roy. Soc. A* **1980**, *371*, 1746.
25. Darwin, G.C. On Jacobi's figure of equilibrium for a rotating mass of fluid. *Proc. Roy. Soc. Lond.* **1886**, *41*, 319.
26. Poincare, H. Sur l'equilibre d'une masse fluide animee d'un mouvement de rotation. *Acta Math.* **1885**, *7*, 259.
27. Chandrasekhar, S. *Ellipsoidal Figures of Equilibrium*; Yale University Press: New Haven, CT, USA, 1969.
28. Walstra, P. Principles of emulsion formation 77–92. In Proceedings of the Conference The Preparation of Dispersions Veldhoven, The Netherlands, 14–16 October 1991. IACIS conference; Laven, J., Stein, H.N., Eds.

MDPI AG
Grosspeteranlage 5
4052 Basel
Switzerland
Tel.: +41 61 683 77 34

Molecules Editorial Office
E-mail: molecules@mdpi.com
www.mdpi.com/journal/molecules

www.ingramcontent.com/pod-product-compliance
Lightning Source LLC
LaVergne TN
LVHW072322090526
838202LV00019B/2336